Becoming a THIRD EDITION Personal Support Worker

Becoming a THIRD EDITION Personal Support Worker

LYNELLE A. HAMILTON

Contributors

SHEILA RITCEY

ARLENE WOLKOWYCKI

PEARSON

Prentice Hall

Toronto

Library and Archives Canada Cataloguing in Publication

Hamilton, Lynelle A. (Lynelle Anne), 1956–
    Becoming a personal support worker / Lynelle A. Hamilton. — 3rd ed.

Includes index.
ISBN 978-0-13-205070-8

1. Home care services—Textbooks. 2. Home health aides—Textbooks. I. Title.
RA645.3.H35 2009   362.14   C2007-906989-4

ISBN-13: 978-0-13-205070-8
ISBN-10: 0-13-205070-6

Vice President, Editorial Director: Gary Bennett
Acquisitions Editor: Michelle Sartor
Marketing Manager: Colleen Gauthier
Senior Developmental Editor: Madhu Ranadive
Production Editor: Imee Salumbides
Copy Editor: Audrey Dorsch
Proofreader: Valerie Adams
Production Coordinator: Patricia Ciardullo
Composition: Jansom
Photo and Permissions Research: Sandy Cooke
Art Director: Julia Hall
Cover and Interior Design: Anthony Leung
Cover Image: Veer Inc.

4 5 6 7 8 9   14 13 12 11

Printed and bound in Canada.

To my mother, Velma Hamilton Williams, and my grandmother,
Nellie Hamilton, whose guidance was abundant and beneficial.

To my uncle, Robert Hamilton, and aunt, May Denton, from
whom I have learned much and continue to learn.

To Alexandra and Steven, who give me faith in the future.

To Maddie, who gives me hope.

Brief Contents

Table of Contents

PART 5 Assisting in Special Situations   *466*

List of Procedures

Preface

A CANADIAN TEXT

We have always needed a Canadian text for support workers. I am immensely pleased to have been asked to write this text. Finally, we now have a Canadian book that covers the unique ways in which we across the country provide support services in our multicultural society.

This third edition is significantly expanded and—at last—in full colour. Like its predecessors, it includes material requested by teachers, employers, and students. The result is a text that provides significantly more information in a format that is easy to read and use.

CONTENT

Support services are by nature diverse. Services vary from province to province, and support workers help people of all ages, people who have a wide range of conditions and needs, and people who live and work in a variety of settings.

To address this diversity, *Becoming a Personal Support Worker* incorporates the following important characteristics:

- It covers the entire spectrum of support work, from community to facility services. Students no longer need two texts to address the range of settings in which they may work.
- It reflects the current view that support work includes social and emotional support as well as physical assistance.
- It emphasizes multicultural issues that the worker should consider.
- It reflects the current range of client needs. The book prepares support workers to work with people of all ages who need support. It also demonstrates how to meet the needs of adults with impairments who direct their own care.
- It includes information relevant to the diverse role of the support worker across Canada. The text includes an expanded chapter on cognitive impairment, as well as chapters devoted to mental health, medications, abuse, and childcare.
- It includes information on employability and guidance on obtaining employment in the field.
- This third edition adds a chapter on human growth and development, additional information on cognitive impairment, and more in-depth discussions on providing support in a diverse society.

ORGANIZATION

Becoming a Personal Support Worker is organized into 28 chapters, grouped into six main parts. Part One (The Role of the Support Worker) consists of six chapters that examine the roles and functions of personal support workers and the various settings in which they can work. Chapter 3, on ethics, encourages students to consider how they provide support. Part Two (The Client) consists of two chapters that focus on the client setting and the client-worker relationship.

Parts Three, Four, and Five provide the information and skills that support workers require to perform their duties competently. Part Three (Fundamental Skills) consists of five chapters that address important aspects of communication, safety, time management, problem solving, and care planning. Part Four (Assisting with Routine Activities) consists of eight chapters that focus on the skills commonly used in support work. Part Five (Assisting in Special Situations) consists of five chapters that focus on the skills used to support clients with complex needs.

Part Six (Gaining Employment) consists of two chapters that provide the student with information and skills necessary to gain employment.

FEATURES

An effort has been made to incorporate special features in the book to facilitate the learning and application of the material:

- An introductory section entitled **How to Use This Text** provides valuable guidance to the student.
- The entire book is written in an informal style that is easy to read.
- Each chapter opens with a set of **Learning Objectives**, a **Chapter at a Glance** section, and a list of **Terms You'll Use** with their definitions.
- Key terms are defined at the beginning of each chapter, boldfaced in the body of the text, and collated with their definitions in a **Glossary** at the back of the book.
- Procedures are highlighted throughout the book. For convenience, a **List of Procedures** is presented following the **Table of Contents** at the front of the book.
- **Stop and Reflect** boxes throughout the book pose questions that encourage students to relate the material being discussed to their own personal experiences.
- **Case Example** boxes throughout the book present realistic situations that students are likely to face when they begin working in the field. The third edition includes questions for some case examples.
- **Spotlights** examine specific issues relevant to the chapter in which they are placed.
- Multicultural issues are addressed wherever appropriate throughout the book. For convenience, the Canadian Charter of Rights and Freedoms is reproduced in **Appendix A** at the back of the book.
- **Questions for Review** at the end of each chapter test the student's factual recall of information and concepts.
- **Questions for Discussion** at the end of each chapter require students to apply their learning to realistic scenarios.
- An annotated list of National and Provincial Long-term Care Associations, support worker associations, and other agencies that may be of interest is provided in **Appendix B** at the back of the book.

SUPPLEMENT

An *Instructor's Manual* is available to facilitate teaching. This guide includes teaching suggestions, notes on the Stop and Reflect boxes, answers to the review questions, answers to the discussion questions, and suggested class activities.

ACKNOWLEDGMENTS

This text would not be as comprehensive as it is without the contributions of others. I am indebted to the following people who, in addition to sharing their health care expertise, also drew upon their experience as teachers to make contributions that strengthened the text:

- Arlene Wolkowycki, for her time and contribution to the chapters on Human Development and Growth and Understanding Elements of the Body.
- Susan Barton-Blay, R.N., B.A.S., who contributed many care procedures and significantly revised the chapter discussing the body systems.
- Sheila Ritcey, B.Sc. P.T., M.A., Ph.D, who significantly revised the chapter on mobility.
- Karen Mayer, R.N., B.Ed., who offered many useful suggestions used in the text.

My thanks also go to the teachers of the Personal Support Worker Programmes of the York Region District School Board for their comments, suggestions, and support as this book evolved.

I am also grateful to the following instructors who provided formal reviews of part or all of the manuscript:

Sharon Dixon, Camosun College, Lansdowne Campus
Julia Liska, Humber College Institute of Technology & Advanced Learning
Sally R. Malicki, Confederation College
Karen Mayer, Loyola Community Learning Centre
Judy MacInnis Risebrough, Nova Scotia Community College
Joanne Roberts, St. Lawrence College, Cornwall Campus
Ann Robinson, ARC Advantage
Karen VanNiejenhuis, Norquest College
Debra Walker, Confederation College
Arlene Wolkowycki, Norquest College

I owe an additional thanks to Susan D. Wilson of the West Coast College of Health Care for checking the entire edited manuscript.

I'd also like to express my appreciation to the many people who provided photos or gave of their time to pose in photographs. Specifically, I'd like to thank Preferred Health Care, Leisureworld Preferred Institute, Leisureworld Incorporated, Community Home Assistance to Seniors (CHATS), the CHATS' Day Program, Maple Health Centre, and Forget's Aurora IGA, and the following people: Marya Grad, Tim Valyear, Milan, Arisa, and Kiara Valyear, Marlene Parsons, Jacqueline Carabott, Robert Harmon, Cynthia Brodeur, Alexandra Brown, Faye Gardner, A. Kuminthini Ponniah, Esme Cyrus, Marylou B. Marqueses, Hyacinth Daley, Suzanne A. England, Isaac Armstrong, Avril Murdock, Shirene Maillet, Phyllis Fuller, Lui Fung Ming, Gloria Yeung, Christine Watson, Sophia Spence, Manuel Soriano, Jeena Sajan, Mary Robinson, Giti Ramezan, Consuelo Maxion, Jong Gap Kym, Lorna Rhea G. Harrison, Navour Douglas, Lurline Brown, Grace Brown, Denise Boulgrave, Hing Tse Chan, as well as clients of CHATS and CHATS' Day Program.

Finally, I would like to express my appreciation to those Personal Support Worker students who gave me feedback and suggestions. Student input helped me keep the text focused on what really matters.

SCOPE OF THIS TEXT

This text is intended to provide a reference for you as you develop skills in providing personal support. It is not intended to replace a course or program, nor will it provide all of the information you'll need as you work in the field. It is a companion to the classroom sessions in which you'll participate. At the conclusion of the course or program, it can serve as a reference for many years. We also hope that it will encourage you to go on and read more about topics that interest you.

You may find that you may not be able to use all of the information and/or skills described in this text. Your employer may not allow you to do certain tasks, or you simply may not have clients who require you to use all your skills. Your practice should always be within the bounds set by your employer, your training, and your client's needs.

Using the Information

Keep in mind that knowledge and skill often become stale if not used for a period of time. Before you use any skill, ask yourself the following questions:

Am I competent? Can I perform the skill properly?
Am I current? Have I used this skill recently?
Am I comfortable performing the skill?

Only proceed if the answer to all three questions is yes. If you need to review the procedure or information, do so. Ask a teacher, supervisor, or a skilled colleague to go over the information with you. If you need to practise, ask a colleague to assist you. Review and practise until you feel comfortable.

How the Text Is Organized

In each chapter, you'll find:
- Objectives: the things you'll learn by reading the chapter
- Key terms introduced in the chapter
- Information and/or procedures
- Case studies, examples, biographies, spotlights
- Questions for review
- Questions for discussion

Suggestions for Using This Text

As an adult learner, you probably want to learn information and skills that are useful to you. Keeping this in mind, try the following to get the most out of the textbook.

Read the chapter before you discuss the topic in class. Reading the chapter beforehand prepares you to take full advantage of the teacher's presentation, take part in the class discussions, as well as get answers to your questions about the topic. The text is broken down into chapters that will relate to one or more classes. If you're not sure which chapter you should read, ask your teacher.

Review the chapter first, making note of the question boxes, headings, and key terms. Relate your answers, the headings, and key terms to your work and your learning needs. Does the chapter contain information that helps you to better understand or meet a client's need? Is there information that you already know and use? This process helps you to connect the information in the text with your own work.

Identify the questions you have with regard to the chapter. You may want to make a written list of the questions as you go along.

Read the chapter. Have you ever heard the advice, "Spread the butter thickest where it will do the most good"? In this context, it means to spend more time on the information that is new to you, or that answers questions you have. Spend less time on the information with which you are already familiar.

As you read, relate the information to the clients with whom you work and to the settings in which you work. Many times, the information in the text will remind you of a client or a situation. Thinking of the information in connection with your client will help you to retain the information. The question boxes will help you to connect the information to your work. The case studies in each chapter also give you an opportunity to see the information applied in a "real" setting.

Make notes or highlight information you want to remember. Many students find that making written notes best helps them to remember information, particularly if they put the information into their own words as they make the notes. Some students prefer to underline or highlight information in the text. Experiment to see which method works best for you.

Complete the review questions at the end of the chapter. This review makes you connect the information to your own experiences and helps you to retain the information. Once you are finished, compare your answers to those in the text. Review material you found difficult.

Discuss the chapter with classmates or colleagues. This activity has many benefits. You can share information with each other, thus helping each other to understand difficult parts. Also, as you put the information into your own words, you, once again, are connecting the information to your own experience.

Apply the reading to class discussions. Use the information to participate in class discussions, case studies, and other activities.

Ask questions in class. Sometimes, it's hard to "get" a concept or to understand information. This happens to everyone. We all have topics that are harder for us to understand as well as topics that come more easily to us. Don't be afraid to ask questions. Chances are that you are not the only person who has that question.

Apply the information you learn. Make a point to apply the information and concepts you learn to your work. Remember, you retain, on average:

10% of what you read
20% of what you hear
30% of what you see
50% of what you see and hear
70% of what you say
90% of what you say and do

Notices

NOTICE ON CARE PROCEDURES

The material in this book contains the most current information available at the time of publication. However, national, provincial and local guidelines concerning clinical practices, including, without limitations, those governing the scope of the support workers' role, infection control and universal precautions, change rapidly. The reader should note, therefore, that new regulations may require changes in some procedures.

It is the responsibility of the reader to familiarize themselves with the policies and procedures set by national, provincial, and local agencies as well as the institution or agency where they are employed. The authors and publisher have taken care to make certain that these procedures reflect currently accepted clinical practice; however, they cannot be considered absolute recommendations. The authors and the publisher of this book disclaim any liability, loss, or risk resulting directly or indirectly from the suggested procedures and theory, from any undetected errors, or from the reader's misunderstanding of the text. It is the reader's responsibility to stay informed of any new changes or recommendations made by any national, provincial, or local agency as well as by their employing institution or agency.

NOTICE ON DRUGS AND DRUG DOSAGES

Every effort has been made to ensure that the information concerning the administration and usage of drugs and/or dosages presented in this book are in accordance with nationally accepted standards. It is the responsibility of the reader to be familiar with regulations in their province that concern the support worker's administration of medication and to practise accordingly.

A Great Way to Learn and Instruct Online

The Pearson Education Canada Companion Website is easy to navigate and is organized to correspond to the chapters in this textbook. Whether you are a student in the classroom or a distance learner you will discover helpful resources for in-depth study and research that empower you in your quest for greater knowledge and maximize your potential for success in the course.

Companion
Website

[www.pearsoned.ca/hamilton]

PEARSON
Prentice
Hall

Jump to... http://www.pearsoned.ca/hamilton ⬍ Home | Search | Help | Profile

Companion
Website

Home >

Companion Website

Becoming a Personal Support Worker, Third Edition
by Hamilton

Student Resources

The modules in this section provide students with tools for learning course material. These modules include:

- Review of Learning Objectives
- Critical Thinking Questions
- Practice Quizzes, including multiple-choice, true and false, and short-answer questions
- Case Studies
- Glossary Flashcards

In the quiz modules students can send answers to the grader and receive instant feedback on their progress through the Results Reporter. Coaching comments and references to the textbook may be available to ensure that students take advantage of all available resources to enhance their learning experience.

Instructor Resources

The modules in this section provide instructors with additional teaching tools. Downloadable PowerPoint Presentations, Test Bank, and an Instructor's Manual are just some of the materials that may be available in this section. Where appropriate, this section will be password protected. To get a password, simply contact your Pearson Education Canada Representative or call Faculty Sales and Services at 1-800-850-5813.

Chapter 1

What Is Personal Support?

Learning Objectives

Through reading this chapter, you'll be able to

1. Describe the five main types of activities that personal support includes.
2. Distinguish between short-term and long-term support.
3. Outline how personal support has developed as a distinct career in Canada.
4. Describe some of the factors that may affect support work in the future.
5. Distinguish between a training title and a job title.
6. Describe the three main types of clients who use personal support.

Chapter at a Glance

- The Purpose of Personal Support
- Personal Support as a Career
- Regulation and Personal Support
- Who Uses Support Services?
- Settings

Terms You'll Use

Acute Care Facility A setting in which a person receives treatment for a specific medical condition on a short-term basis. This is another term for a hospital.

Assisted Living A setting in which clients live in their own apartments or townhouses but receive services from an agency in the building. Assisted living is also called supportive housing or assisted housing.

Attendant A person who assists a client with physical disabilities, who directs his or her own care.

Caregiver A person who assists the client. Caregivers can include people who are not paid (e.g., family, friends, neighbours, and volunteers) as well as those who are paid (e.g., support workers or companions).

Client A person who uses community support services. However, for clarity, throughout this text, we will use the term client to refer to clients, residents, and consumers.

Community A setting in which a person lives in her or his own home (house or apartment) without support services located in the same building.

Consumer In this book, we use the term to describe a person with temporary or permanent physical disability who uses support services.

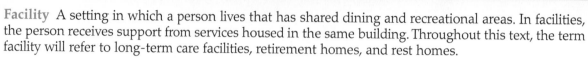

Facility A setting in which a person lives that has shared dining and recreational areas. In facilities, the person receives support from services housed in the same building. Throughout this text, the term facility will refer to long-term care facilities, retirement homes, and rest homes.

Long-Term Care Facility A setting in which a person lives and receives assistance with routine activities of living as well as some nursing care.

Patient A person who is in an acute care facility (hospital).

Resident A person who lives in a long-term care facility, or retirement or rest home.

Retirement Homes or Rest Homes Settings in which older adults live where some laundry and homemaking services are provided.

Support Worker A worker who provides personal support. Support Worker may or may not be the title of the program you are taking. Different provinces have different titles to describe the worker who provides personal support.

STOP AND REFLECT

How would you define personal support?

_____

What types of activities do you think personal support includes?

_____

_____

If you had to describe the typical person who would need personal support, what would you say? How old would the person be? Would the person be male or female? What other characteristics would the typical person have?

_____

_____

Compare your answers with those of your colleagues or other students.

Did you find that your answers were different than those other people had? You likely identified some things that were the same and some that were different. That's because the need for personal support activities can vary a great deal from person to person.

THE PURPOSE OF PERSONAL SUPPORT

When I assist a person, I have to work really hard at learning what the person needs me to do and how the person needs me to do it. I have to know when—for that person—I can go ahead and do something without waiting to be asked and when I should wait for the person's direction.

Melanie, an attendant

The purpose of support work is to assist clients to accomplish the tasks of everyday living so that they can get on with their lives. This is much easier said than done, as you might have guessed from the quote at the beginning of this section. Providing personal support is both tremendously challenging and extremely rewarding.

As you saw earlier, support means different things to different people. Consider the following examples.

CASE EXAMPLE 1-1

Sara Ramkissoon is 42. Since her stroke at age 29, she uses personal support services to help her get up, wash, dress, and eat before she goes to work. She uses a wheelchair to get about, as her right leg is weak. She advises her attendant as to how she wants things done.

How do you think you might work with the person described in this Case Example?

CASE EXAMPLE 1-2

Gary Fulton is 88. He has Alzheimer Disease and lives in a long-term care facility. He is able to get dressed by himself if his support worker hands him his clothes in the order he needs to put them on. He often forgets where he is and becomes frightened. Staff members *spend a great deal of time comforting and reassuring him, as well as making sure that he is safe.*

How do you think you might work with the person described in this Case Example?

CASE EXAMPLE 1-3

Sue and Gene Angelotti recently had triplets. They also have a five-year-old daughter. Sue had a Caesarean section and is still quite weak. Sue and Gene prefer to provide most care to the newborns and prefer that the support worker assist Sue with bathing and dressing, help in the care of their older daughter, help with laundry, *and perform household chores so that Sue and Gene can spend as much time as possible with their children.*

How do you think you might work with the people described in this Case Example?

With which person, from any of the Case Examples, would you most like to work? Why?

As you can see from the examples, support means many things to many people. Furthermore, even though the same kind of support might be provided (for example, assistance with dressing), how it is provided may be very different, depending upon the person's needs and preferences. For example, both Sara Ramkissoon and Gary Fulton require assistance to get dressed. However, the way in which the support worker assists them is very different. Sara Ramkissoon guides her support worker in doing what she needs done, while Gary Fulton relies on his support worker to guide him.

Some Basic Definitions

There are many different terms used to describe people who use support services and people who provide those services. It can be confusing! In this section, well discuss some of the more common terms used.

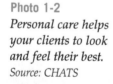

Photo 1-1
Household tasks, such as meal preparation, are an essential component of personal support.

The term **clients** is often used to describe people who use community support services. People who live in long-term care facilities are often called **residents**. People who direct their own care are often called **consumers**. **Patients** are people who are being cared for in acute care facilities. Some agencies use terms such as *care recipient, guest* or *patron* to describe the people who use their services. In this text, we'll use the term client to describe all people who use support services.

Some terms used to describe people who provide support evolve from the nature of the work or the type of work relationship. The general term **caregiver** includes people who assist the client but are not paid (volunteer, family, friend, and neighbour) and those who are paid (support workers). The term **attendant** is used to describe people who are employed to assist people with physical disabilities who direct their own care. In this text, we'll use the term **support worker** to describe workers who provide personal support to clients.

Despite the differences in how support is carried out and the different terms used to describe people, personal support can be divided into five general categories: home management, personal care, assisting with family responsibilities, assisting with a client at work, and assisting a client to take part in social and recreational activities.

Home Management

Home management refers to the many tasks that are involved in the running of a household, such as shopping, house cleaning, and meal preparation (Photo 1-1). It is a significant part of personal support.

The specific tasks vary according to where the person lives and what other services and assistance he or she has. For example, some workers prepare a noon meal for a client whose family is able to do the shopping and housekeeping, but who can't be at home when the client eats lunch. Other workers may shop for a client as well as prepare meals. Sometimes, the help that the worker provides seems unusual. Some workers in northern areas must melt snow in the winter to get drinking water for their clients! Other workers assist clients who have no running water in their homes or who heat their homes by means of a wood-burning stove.

Photo 1-2
Personal care helps your clients to look and feel their best.
Source: CHATS

Personal Care

Personal care refers to help with dressing, bathing, toileting, grooming, mobility, and other routine activities of living. Many clients will require some assistance with personal care (Photo 1-2). Some will require a great deal of help; others will require very little. Because personal care is so intimate, it can be the most challenging type of care to provide.

Supporting a Person at Work or School

Many clients work or attend school—or do both. Support workers may be asked to assist the person with many tasks. These tasks can be very distinct; for example, a support worker might assist a person by taking notes in class, by providing personal care, by carrying a lunch tray, or by assisting the person to travel to and from work or school.

Family Responsibilities

Family responsibilities refer to things that the client is responsible to do as a husband or wife, a parent, or even as an adult child. Support workers may be asked to care for children, to prepare meals for the family, or to do the family's laundry (Photo 1-3). In keeping with the purpose of helping clients to do what they need to do, support workers are often asked to assist with or complete some things that are not directly related to the client's care.

Social and Recreational Activities

Social and recreational activities refer to activities for enjoyment and interaction with others, such as accompanying clients on outings or helping the client to do things with others or take part in activities. Support workers in assisted living settings or long-term care facilities might help clients plan a tea party or encourage residents to visit one another. Some support workers have been hired by clients to accompany them on a vacation.

Photo 1-3
Caring for a client's children may be a part of the support you are asked to provide. It should be seen as part of the support your client needs, not as an "extra" duty.
Source: Preferred Health Care

STOP AND REFLECT 1-2

If you work in the field . . .

What kinds of support service do you provide?

_____

_____

Do your colleagues provide other types of support?

_____

_____

If not, which ones are provided?

_____

_____

If you are new to the field or do not work in the field . . .

Find out who provides support services in your community. What services do these agencies provide?

_____

_____

Do all agencies provide the same types of services?

_____

_____

Do any agencies specialize in providing one type of service (for example, homemaking) or serve only one type of client (for example, older adults)?

_____

Short-Term and Long-Term Support

Not all support work is provided on a long-term basis. Some services are provided for a short period of time. Examples of situations in which you might be asked to provide short-term support include:

- Assisting a person who is recovering from an illness, an operation, or an accident
- Assisting a new mother
- Assisting a person while his or her primary caregiver (spouse or family member) is away
- Assisting a person who has moved from a long-term care facility to a more independent living arrangement

STOP AND REFLECT ((1-3))

Have you ever had help on a short-term basis? Perhaps someone came to help when you or your spouse had a child. Maybe you had help if you had an operation and were recovering. Perhaps you were ill and had someone help you out for a bit.

How did you feel about needing help?

_____

_____

How did you feel about having that person who was helping you in your home?

_____

_____

How did you feel when the person no longer came to help you?

_____

_____

Would you have felt differently if you had to have help for a long period of time? If so, how?

_____

_____

Did you have mixed feelings about the support you had? Perhaps you appreciated the help, but at the same time you were uncomfortable with having someone else in your home. Perhaps the person was very nice but did not do things the way you would do them.

When the person left, you might have been a bit sad and a bit glad. Compare this to how you might have felt if you needed the help for a much longer period of time. Chances are, you'd feel differently about longer-term support.

Needing support for a short time is different than needing it for a long period of time. Short-term support is often seen as meaning that the person will recover and be able to go back to a previous lifestyle after a while, or that the person will be able to move on to a new, more exciting phase in life.

Assisting a client on a short-term basis requires you to quickly learn your client's preferences and the basic information you need to assist. You'll also have to adapt to changes in routine as your client's condition improves. When the client no longer needs you, you may find yourself feeling a little sad that you didn't get to know him or her better. This is perfectly normal.

Photo 1-4
Provide assistance in a way that respects your clients' needs and preferences.
Source: CHATS

Needing long-term support can make a person feel dependent, frustrated, and very sad. It may take time for the person to adjust to the change in lifestyle and to begin to see the support needed as something that helps them to get on with life.

As a support worker, you always want to assist your client in a way that makes the person feel valued and that respects their needs and preferences (Photo 1-4). Working with a client who has just begun to use long-term support will require you to be particularly sensitive to the effect that needing your help has on the client. You'll also have to be particularly flexible as you learn about your client's ways of doing things. You'll have to adapt your approach to support each individual client.

SPOTLIGHT 1-1 WHAT'S IN A NAME?

As you'll learn in this chapter and those that follow, support workers are known by many names. In addition, the programs that train support workers have many different titles. A *training title* describes the name of a particular training program. Training titles vary by province. A *job title* describes an occupational title. It may or may not be the same as the name of a training program. It's also important to remember that a person who has a specific job title that is the same as a training title does not necessarily hold the certificate. For example, a person may work as a health care aide, but not have a health care aide certificate—or any certificate at all.

PERSONAL SUPPORT AS A CAREER

Although this type of work has been done for decades, personal support work is a relatively new career in Canada. Support work has its roots in the health care aide and homemaker training programs developed in the late 1970s and early 1980s. In many areas, support workers now require a provincially recognized certificate to work in most settings. However, support workers who assist adults with physical disabilities, where the client directs her or his own care, are often trained by their employers and may not be required to take a provincial training program.

Personal support training programs differ from province to province. Some provinces have one program that prepares workers to work in both community and facility settings. Others have separate training programs for facility and community support workers. Table 1-1 illustrates selected training programs of some provinces and territories in 2007. It's important to note that there may be more than one training program available in your province. As well, specific employers may prefer a particular training program or provide their own.

Although training programs across the country have much in common, the programs do vary from province to province. A certificate valid in one province may not be seen as equal to another province's certificate. However, many schools have experience in reviewing out-of-province certificates for equivalency.

REGULATION AND PERSONAL SUPPORT

You may hear colleagues speak of regulation of support workers. In health care, regulation is one way that a province determines which professions may perform certain activities that are considered to pose too great a risk for most people to perform.

Many health professionals are regulated. Each province determines which professions must be regulated. Regulation usually involves at least these three things: identifying what education is required for the profession and how that education is assessed, establishing what activities may be done by the profession, and establishing a disciplinary procedure to handle complaints about members of the profession. Usually, a regulated profession establishes a college or professional association to carry out these duties. In order to work in the profession, a person must be a member of the appropriate college or association.

Support workers are unregulated. Though a support worker may choose to belong to a provincial association, there is no requirement that he or she do so. Most importantly, you, as a support worker, are responsible to make certain that your work is always within the bounds set by your training, your employer, and any legislation that applies to your work, whether or not you belong to a provincial association and even if you are not regulated.

TABLE 1-1	Selected Training Programs across Canada	
Province	**Community Support Work**	**Facility Support Work**
Alberta	Personal Care Attendant	
British Columbia	Home Support/Resident Care Attendant	
Manitoba	Home Care Attendant	Health Care Aide
Nova Scotia	Continuing Care Assistant	
Ontario	Personal Support Worker	
Prince Edward Island	Primary Health Care Worker	
Quebec	Santé, assistance et soins infirmiers (Health Care Aide) Auxiliaire familiale et sociale (Home Support Worker)	
Saskatchewan	Home Care/Special Care Aide	
Northwest Territories	Homemaker/ Personal Care Attendant	Long-Term Care Aide
New Brunswick	Health Care Aide	
Newfoundland	Personal Care Worker	

SPOTLIGHT 1-2 THE FUTURE OF SUPPORT WORK

What are the trends in support work? To answer this question, we have to examine a few factors: population distribution, life expectancy, the impact of chronic conditions, and policy trends.

Canada is culturally and ethnically diverse and is becoming more so. In 2001, 18.4 percent of Canada's population was born outside Canada—the largest percentage in 70 years. As well, more than 50 percent of Canada's population is not of British or French ancestry.

A 2003 Statistics Canada survey found that approximately 5 percent of the population over 18 received some form of government-funded home care in the 12 months preceding the survey. This percentage is likely to rise as our population ages. (Statistics Canada, Canadian Community Health Survey, 2003)

Life expectancy has increased steadily since the 1900s. In 1900, a person could expect to live until age 50. A woman who is 65 today can expect to live another 20.8 years; a 65-year-old man can expect to live another 17.4 years. (Deaths 2003, Statistics Canada, 2005)

Another factor is how long people may live without requiring significant support. In 2002, the most recent year for which figures are available, a person could expect to reach age 78 without requiring significant support. Many factors influence this: how physically fit a person is, whether the person has a healthy lifestyle, as well as availability of health care.

The incidence of disability rises with age. (Statistics Canada, Profile of Disability, 2001) Conditions that often cause disability—obesity, arthritis, and high blood pressure rates—have risen among seniors.

Facilities continue to provide support for a significant number of Canadians. According to the 2001 Canadian census (the most recent for which figures are available), approximately 7 percent of persons over 65 live in a long-term care facility. This percentage is essentially the same as reported in the 1991 census. However, people over 75 were actually *less* likely to live in a long-term care facility than they were in 1991.

Despite all this, Statistics Canada found significant differences among provinces. There are also differences among communities. Government policies, population mix, geography, population density, and community-specific factors such as availability of services/workers all affect an individual setting.

So, what does all this mean? Though no one can predict with absolute certainty, it's likely that adult clients in the future will be older, represent many communities, and hold a wide variety of traditions. They will more likely live at home and have more complex support needs for a longer period of time. These general factors, as well as those affecting your specific area, will determine what it means for you in your community.

What factors do affect your local community? What are the trends where you live and work?

WHO USES SUPPORT SERVICES?

As you might guess from the beginning of this chapter, clients come from all age groups. While it is true that most clients are older adults, a significant number are younger adults and children. A Statistics Canada study found that one-third of the clients of the provincial home care programs were children or adults under the age of 65. (Statistics Canada Health Reports, vol. 10, no. 1, Summer 1998)

We can distinguish three main categories of clients. It's important to remember that a client may belong to more than one of these general categories described below. It's also important to remember that each client is an individual with specific needs and preferences. The support service you provide to a specific client depends as much upon who they are as it does upon their chronological age.

Photo 1-5
Many—but not all—clients are older adults.
Source: *Preferred Health Care*

Older Adults

Older adults account for nearly two-thirds of the community services and most of the facility support services used (Photo 1-5). Although many older adults use support services for a long period of time, some older adults use services on a short-term basis to recover from an injury or illness. Most older adults receive support services in their homes—only approximately 7 percent live in a long-term care facility.

Adults with Physical Disabilities

Adults with disabilities make up approximately 10 percent of the population over age 18. Most adults with physical disabilities use services on a long-term basis (Photo 1-6). Like an older adult, the adult with physical disabilities may require a different type of service on a short-term basis (for example, help while the person recovers from surgery or an illness). The vast majority of adults with disabilities live and receive services in their own home.

Services provided to adults with disabilities may be provided in a way that differs from those provided to older or younger clients. Adults with disabilities who work may require assistance getting ready for work, or they may require assistance at work. They may also require assistance to travel for work or pleasure.

Photo 1-6
Most younger adults with a disability will use support services for many years.

Children

Most children who receive support services directly receive them because of the effects of a physical or developmental condition. Many children also receive rehabilitation services (services aimed at helping them to recover ability), and support workers may be asked to assist in certain activities related to rehabilitation under the direction of the health professional who is working with the particular child. Some children receive support services at school. A support worker may also accompany children on the way to and from school (Photo 1-7).

Children can also receive services indirectly because of a caregiving parent's illness or disability or because the family has had a new child or children.

Photo 1-7
Children with disabilities may receive a variety of support services, both at home and at school.
Source: CHATS

SETTINGS

People who use support services have the right to participate fully in life. Support service is provided wherever the client is located—at home, at work, on the way to and from locations such as a mall or the movies, or in facilities. A **community** setting is one in which a person lives in his or her own home without support services in the same building. **Assisted living** is a setting where clients live in their own apartments or townhouses but receive services from an agency in the building. This is also called supportive housing or assisted housing. **Facilities** are settings in which people share dining and recreational areas and receive support from services housed in the same building. In this text, the term facilities will be used to refer to retirement homes, long-term care facilities, rest homes, and acute care facilities. **Retirement homes** are settings in which older adults live where some laundry and homemaking services are provided. Personal care may or may not be available, and residents are usually able to perform most routine activities of independent living. In general, care is not regulated to the same extent that it is in long-term care facilities.

Long-term care facilities are those in which a person lives and receives assistance with routine activities and some nursing care. Each province has different names for these facilities, including nursing homes, board and care homes, special care homes, and homes for the aged. **Acute care facilities** are settings where people receive treatment for specific medical conditions on a short-term basis. Hospitals are examples of acute care facilities. Each setting is different, and how you carry out your duties will vary by the setting in which you work. In the next chapter, we will discuss the major types of settings in more detail.

Questions for Review

Answer each of the following. Then check your answers with the text.

1. What are the five major categories of personal support work?

2. How is short-term support different from long-term support?

3. Do you need a provincially recognized certificate to work as a support worker in most provinces?

4. What is the difference between a job title and a training title?

5. When might you be trained by your client?

6. How are patients and residents different?

7. What are the three main categories of clients?

8. What are the trends in support work? What community-specific factors affect these trends?

Questions for Discussion

1. Talk to a person who uses support services. How does the person describe the services he or she receives? Does this person's definition match yours? In what ways is it similar? In what ways is it different?

2. Talk to a person who has been providing personal support for five years or more. According to that person, how has the career changed over that time?

3. Imagine that you have broken your leg and must wear a cast from toes to groin for six weeks. You can't walk even a short distance without crutches, and even then, getting around is difficult. You must use a wheelchair if you want to go out of your home. What help would you need? How do you think you would feel about needing this help? How would you feel about asking another person to provide it? Would your feelings be different if the person helping you was a family member, friend, or a personal support worker?

Chapter 2

Work Settings

Learning Objectives

Through reading this chapter, you'll be able to

1. List five requirements of the *Canada Health Act* that ensure everyone has access to necessary health care.
2. List nine types of settings in which you may work as a personal support worker.
3. Discuss the common characteristics of the nine settings.
4. Describe how to select the type of setting that is best for you.

Chapter at a Glance

- The Canadian Health Care System
- The Variety of Settings
- The Variety of Job Titles
- Direct Employment by a Client
- Community Outreach, Including Respite Care
- Day, Social, and Recreational Programs
- School or Work Support
- Assisted Living, Cluster Care, and Supportive Housing
- Retirement Homes
- Group Homes
- Long-Term Care Facilities
- Other Centres
- Which Setting Is Best for You?

Terms You'll Use

Acute Care The type of care provided in hospitals. Clients in an acute care setting are usually called patients.

Chronic Care The type of care provided to people whose condition is stable, but who need more professional care than residents of long-term care facilities. Some provinces have separate buildings for chronic care facilities; others provide chronic care services in acute care centres.

Continuing Care The type of care provided on a long-term basis. Continuing care can refer to long-term services provided in facilities or for people who live in their own homes.

Day Program Programs that provide clients an opportunity to take part in activities and be with others in a secure setting. Some day programs offer rehabilitation services to help clients recover from illness or injury. Other programs are geared toward clients with specific conditions, such as clients who have dementia or who have had a stroke.

Group Home A home in which a small number of people live—in most cases, no more than eight people. The group home has round-the-clock staff members, and it is usually located in a residential neighbourhood.

Home Care Services provided to clients in their own homes through a provincially funded program. Different provinces include different services, although most include personal support as well as nursing, physiotherapy, and occupational therapy services.

Mental Health Facility A facility designed to provide service to people with mental health concerns. Many such facilities provide both short-term and long-term services. Some mental health facilities are located in acute care settings, whereas others are completely separate. Increasingly, mental health services are provided to clients who live in their own homes.

Multidisciplinary Teams A support team made up of members from different professions or backgrounds.

Outreach Services Services that are provided to clients in their own homes, not in facilities, assisted living, or supportive housing.

Rehabilitation Centre A facility that provides rehabilitation services to patients to help the patient recover from surgery, illness, or injury. Patients usually stay in rehabilitation centres for only a short period of time.

Respite Care A type of service provided to a client and the client's caregiver, so that the caregiver can be relieved from the responsibilities of caring for the client and has the opportunity to take a break. Respite care is provided in the client's home and in many long-term care facilities. Respite care is also called caregiver relief.

THE CANADIAN HEALTH CARE SYSTEM

Canada has a nationwide system of health care. This system is governed by federal legislation, specifically the *Canada Health Act*. It requires each province and territory to ensure that its residents have access to necessary health care, according to five criteria:

1. Universality. All residents of the province/territory are entitled to public health insurance coverage.
2. Accessibility. No fees or other barriers prevent residents from receiving medically necessary services.
3. Comprehensiveness. All medically necessary services are covered by provincial/ territorial health insurance.
4. Portability. People have coverage if they move from one province or territory to another within Canada.
5. Public Administration. The health insurance plan is administered by a not-for-profit, public organization.

Many people think of Canada's health care system as socialized medicine. It is not. It is a system of provincial insurance programs that cover the costs of necessary services. Hospital care, most physician services, and some rehabilitation services, as well as long-term (or continuing) care services, are covered under these provincial plans. However, provincial plans do vary according to exactly what is covered.

Extended Health Care

The *Canada Health Act* includes many extended health care services—the type of ongoing care that many personal support workers help provide. This care includes services provided to clients who live in their own homes, as well as residents of approved long-term care facilities. There are three types of care discussed in this book: acute care, chronic care, and continuing care. **Acute care** is the type of care provided in hospitals, while **chronic care** is provided to people whose conditions are stable but who need more care than people in long-term care facilities. **Continuing care** is provided on a long-term basis in facilities or in a client's home. Health Canada estimates that continuing care is the third-largest program funded under the *Canada Health Act*, and that it is the fastest growing of all types of health care covered by the Act. (Health Canada, Reports of the Continuing Care Symposium, 1995)

Most provinces have a **home care** program whose purpose is to provide services to clients who live in their own homes. Clients who receive service from this program are assessed to identify their needs and to determine the services that the program will provide. Some provinces provide extended health care services at no charge to the client. Other provinces charge a co-payment for all extended health care services. The rest of the provinces charge a co-payment for some services and provide some services at no charge to the client.

Each province has established specific types of long-term care facilities that may receive extended health care funds. In such facilities, the insurance program covers medically necessary services. However, residents in long-term care facilities may be required to pay part of the portion of the cost of their room and board. This payment by residents is often called a co-payment.

THE VARIETY OF SETTINGS

Support workers can work in a wide variety of settings and under many different employment arrangements. Some support workers work in more than one setting, while others work in only one. In this chapter, we will examine some of the more common settings in which you might work. We can identify the following nine types of work settings:

- Direct Employment by a Client
- Community Outreach, including Respite Care
- Day, Social, and Recreational Programs
- School or Work Support
- Assisted Living, Cluster Care, and Supportive Housing
- Retirement Homes
- Group Homes
- Long-Term Care Facilities
- Other Centres (including Chronic Care Centres, Mental Health Facilities, Rehabilitation Centres, and Acute Care Centres)

In what kinds of settings do support workers in your community work? Aside from being in different locations, how do these settings differ?

_____

_____

If you work in the field, do you work in more than one type of setting? If so, is what you do—or how you do it—different in the different settings? In what ways?

_____

_____

_____

_____

Each setting has different rules, regulations, and expectations of support workers. Furthermore, each facility or agency has its own policies and procedures. You will have to adapt your work habits to meet the expectations of your employer. If you work in more than one setting, you'll have to learn to adapt to the different procedures each uses. However, it's important to remember that no matter where you work, you must always perform your duties to the best of your ability. You owe your clients and yourself nothing less than your best.

THE VARIETY OF JOB TITLES

As you read this chapter, you'll come across many different job titles. In Chapter 1, we discussed the difference between training titles and job titles. Each employer determines the title they will use for workers providing personal support. Moreover, your job title may not exactly match the title of the training program you are taking. For example, you may receive a certificate in personal support, yet work as a home-maker or care aide.

DIRECT EMPLOYMENT BY A CLIENT

Some clients prefer to employ support workers directly. There are a number of reasons why a client might hire a support worker. In some provinces, persons with disabilities may receive funding to employ support workers directly, rather than receiving services through an outreach agency. Some clients need to have support services at times when local agencies do not offer services. The client's needs may change, or the times at which they need assistance may change from week to week. Others simply prefer to select, orient, and supervise the support worker themselves.

Sometimes, a client or family will hire a support worker to assist a client who lives in a retirement home or long-term care facility. This arrangement is often called private-duty work.

When you work directly for a client, the client is your supervisor. Like any other employer, the client determines what his or her needs are, the tasks you'll perform, and, often, when you'll need to perform them. The client may provide you with additional training or ask that you take additional training in order to provide the right support.

CASE EXAMPLE 2-1

Olivia has worked for her client for many years. Over time, her duties have changed. At first, she assisted her client with household tasks, usually for a few hours one day each week. When her client was recovering from a fractured ankle, Olivia was asked to increase her time to include shopping once a week and visiting three mornings a week to assist in exercises and other follow-up care.

Recently, Olivia's client has had an illness and is recuperating at home. Olivia now spends several nights with her client. She also drives the client to medical appointments three times each week. Olivia has arranged with

her client to have time off during the day to visit her other clients.

Olivia is an employee of her client. Therefore, the client handles deductions and premium payments. As the client's needs have changed, she and Olivia have worked out a schedule that has allowed Olivia to meet her obligations to her other clients while still meeting this client's needs.

What are some of the benefits of working directly for a client? What are some of the challenges?

Terms of Employment

Working directly for a client can be very rewarding. However, you need to make sure that both you and the client agree on the terms of your employment: in particular, your wages, your hours of work, whether the hours will change from day to day, and how you will handle any problems that come up.

It's especially important to know if you or the client is responsible for submitting taxes and other benefit payments from your salary. Some clients act as employers, meaning that they deduct from your salary any taxes, Canada Pension Plan premiums, and Employment Insurance premiums required. When the clients do this, they are responsible for sending the monies deducted to Canada Revenue Agency.

Some clients prefer to hire you as a contractor. In most cases, this means that you are responsible for paying taxes and other premiums on your income. If you are considering taking a contract position, you should contact an accountant for advice.

Challenges

Working on Your Own

Some support workers who work directly for clients can feel alone. Because of the nature of the work arrangement, the support worker may have no one with whom to discuss problems or stresses that may arise related to the work. Be certain that you are comfortable working without the support of co-workers before you accept this type of position.

Resolving Problems

Because there is no agency to help you resolve any problems, it's important to work out with your client a way to resolve differences of opinion or disputes. You must make sure that you and your client are comfortable discussing issues or concerns, so that neither of you becomes frustrated with the arrangement.

Keeping Busy and Balancing Commitments

When a client employs you directly, you and your client will determine the amount of time that you will work. If you need additional work, it will be your responsibility to find it. You may choose to work for another client directly or to seek part-time employment through an agency. Whichever you choose, you will be responsible to make sure that you have enough work.

You will also be responsible to make sure that you can meet all the commitments you make (Photo 2-1). You must not lower your standard of service to a client because you have taken on too many obligations. Before you take on a new position, you should carefully consider its requirements to ensure that you can meet them along with your other obligations.

Be sure to discuss the time and location requirements with a new client so that you are well aware of the scope of the assignment before you take it on. For example, will you be required to stay with the client overnight? Travel with the client? Provide service at different times on different days? The answers to these questions will help you to determine whether you can fulfill the assignment if you accept it.

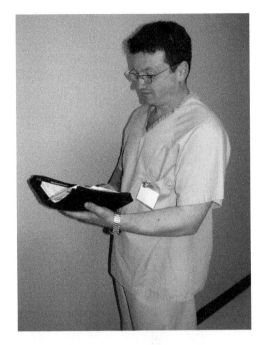

Photo 2-1
Support workers must be well organized to be able to meet schedule commitments.

Responsibility for Your Actions

When you work directly for a client, you must make certain that you are trained and legally permitted to perform the activities your client requests. You are responsible for the activities you perform, even if you do so at your client's request. If you perform an activity incorrectly or perform a task you are not legally permitted to do, you may be held legally responsible for your actions.

COMMUNITY OUTREACH, INCLUDING RESPITE CARE

Many support workers work for agencies that provide outreach services or services to clients in their own homes, not in facilities, assisted living, or supportive housing (Photo 2-2). The agencies may be not-for-profit or for-profit. Some agencies may provide service to individual clients who call them directly. Others may take referrals from a third party, such as a home care program or an insurance company. Some agencies do both.

Support workers who work for agencies providing outreach may perform a wide variety of tasks. Some agencies offer many types of outreach, such as basic personal care, homemaking, new mother and childcare, convalescent care, as well as assistance to the person who is dying. **Respite care** is another type of outreach in which the support worker relieves the client's caregiver in the client's home or in a long-term care facility. This allows the caregiver to take a break from his or her responsibilities while making sure that the client is cared for. Support workers may be hired to provide service in one or more of the programs the agency offers.

Working for an agency that provides outreach can be very rewarding in many ways. On one hand, the opportunity to work with a single client at a time is attractive to many support workers. They enjoy having the opportunity to personalize their service, as well as not having to juggle the needs of many clients at the same time. On the other hand, working with a number of different clients provides variety and the opportunity to get to know many people.

Photo 2-2
Many support workers work through an agency. They receive assignments from the agency, not directly from clients.
Source: CHATS

Terms of Employment

In most cases, support workers hired by agencies are hired as employees. The worker's time is scheduled by the agency. The agency also determines which worker is assigned to a particular client. This does not mean that the worker is not consulted about when he or she is available, or about the type of work he or she performs. In fact, the worker is consulted. However, the agency usually retains the right to make assignments. Many agencies will attempt to accommodate a worker's schedule when possible. Some agencies offer support workers full-time work. Other agencies offer only part-time or casual (occasional) assignments.

Most outreach agencies require support workers to have provincially recognized training. In addition, most agencies provide an orientation program to help new workers become familiar with the agency's philosophy, policies, and procedures. New workers may accompany an experienced worker for a visit or two to see how things are done. Agencies often provide additional training (often called inservice training) to help workers meet clients' needs.

In most cases, the support worker reports to a coordinator or supervisor. The worker may also take assignments from another person called a scheduler. In some agencies, the supervisor or coordinator also assigns the visits.

Following Agency Policies and Procedures

When you are hired by an agency, you'll be asked to follow the agency's policies and procedures for support work. These policies and procedures may change according to the type of service you are providing.

As well, an agency may provide a particular type of service to a particular type of client, but not provide that service to other clients. For example, an agency may allow support workers in respite care to set a client's hair with rollers, even if this is not done for clients receiving service through another program. Sometimes, the agency that refers the client sets out what can and cannot be done for that client.

It is up to you to be aware of your agency's policies and procedures and how they affect the type of service you are providing.

CASE EXAMPLE 2-2

Claire has been an employee of a small homemaking agency for more than 10 years. She takes pride in doing her job well. Claire has four clients she sees each week. The local home care program refers two clients, and a third client receives service directly from the agency. Her fourth client receives respite care that helps the client's spouse to get some needed rest and relaxation.

Claire's duties vary with each client's needs and the requirements of the specific program. For example, each home care client's service plan specifies the exact tasks that Claire is to perform during her visits.

However, Claire has been asked to work out with her other two clients the tasks each client would like done, within the bounds of her training and agency policy.

Claire enjoys her work and the different people she meets. If she has a problem she cannot work out with the client, she discusses it with her supervisor. She relies upon her supervisor to assign her to clients whose needs match her abilities.

What are some of the benefits of working for an agency? What are some challenges?

Challenges

Isolation

The support worker providing outreach does not have day-to-day contact with other support workers. The worker does, however, have the opportunity to speak with his or her supervisor to discuss concerns. Many agencies will arrange for a regular time for support workers to meet and share concerns. As well, most agencies set aside time for support workers who share the care of a client to meet to discuss issues related to that client.

Travel

Support workers in outreach must travel from one client's home to another throughout the day. Agencies try to schedule visits to keep travel to a minimum. Nonetheless, travel can be considerable, particularly in rural areas. It also can be hazardous in severe winter weather. Some agencies require support staff to have a driver's licence and reliable transportation. Agencies located in cities often expect workers to use public transit to get from client to client. It is your responsibility to be sure that you can travel to each client you are assigned.

Working with Personnel from Other Agencies

Many clients receiving outreach services also receive visits from other health professionals or agencies.

It is important to make sure that you know your responsibility with regard to the other members of the support team. You may, from time to time, be asked to take direction from a nurse or therapist also visiting the client, even though that person is not an employee of your agency. Sometimes, another member of the support team may assume that you can perform activities your agency actually forbids you to do. Always clarify your role with your supervisor prior to taking on any new tasks or responsibilities assigned by other members of the support team. In Chapter 5, we will discuss support teams in more detail.

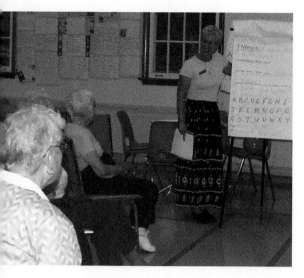

DAY, SOCIAL, AND RECREATIONAL PROGRAMS

One relatively new area of employment is in day, social, and recreational programs. Support workers assisting clients in these settings often assist clients with recreational activities such as baking, crafts, and games, as well as assisting the clients with any personal care they may need (Photo 2-3). In some provinces, you will need additional training to work in this setting.

Day programs provide support workers the opportunity to expand their skills in small group work and recreation. They offer the worker the opportunity to get to know clients (and, sometimes, the clients' families) over a period of time.

Photo 2-3
Support workers employed by day programs often conduct activities or other social events.
Source: CHATS

Terms of Employment

Support workers are generally considered to be employees of the day program. The program supervisor will schedule the support worker's time. The program supervisor is the person to whom the worker would go to resolve any work-related problems.

Working Closely with a Team

Support workers in day programs work closely with a team. This team usually consists of a program supervisor and other support workers. It may also include nurses, social workers, and therapists. Working in a team is a challenge but also a benefit, as the team can easily work together to resolve concerns and assist each other.

Following Agency Policies and Procedures

Day programs, like outreach programs, have policies and procedures that the support worker must know and follow.

Challenges

Balancing Multiple Demands

There may be a number of clients taking part in the day program. Support workers have to be able to balance multiple demands upon their time. The worker must also be able to easily shift attention from one client to another as each client's needs require. The worker has to be able to set priorities, manage time well, and quickly solve problems.

SCHOOL OR WORK SUPPORT

Some support workers find employment in schools or work sites. Generally, support workers in these settings provide personal care and other support to one or more clients in the setting. The specific personal support duties will vary with the employing agency, and may be affected by provincial legislation. The worker may or may not function as a member of a team.

Terms of Employment

The worker is usually employed by the organization (such as the school board or the agency for whom the client works), not the individual clients she or he assists.

Challenges

Following Agency Policies and Procedures

School or work support programs have policies and procedures that the support worker must know and follow.

Balancing Conflicting Demands

Sometimes the client's needs or preferences may conflict with the employer's policies. Support workers must develop skill in working through these problems.

ASSISTED LIVING, CLUSTER CARE, AND SUPPORTIVE HOUSING

Support workers working in assisted living settings provide service to clients who live in an apartment block or condominium development. The terms cluster care and supportive housing are also used to describe these settings. Each client has his or her own apartment or condominium unit. Support workers provide service to a number of clients each day. Clients who live in assisted living do not necessarily receive the same amount of service each day. Because all clients are located in the same area, it is easier than in other settings for the support worker to provide service when the client needs it.

Terms of Employment

Generally, support workers in assisted living settings are hired and scheduled by an agency. The agency schedules the worker's shifts. However, the individual workers in supportive housing often talk with the clients to identify the actual tasks they will do each day.

The support worker usually reports to a coordinator who is responsible for the services provided. The coordinator may be responsible for more than one supportive housing site. The coordinator may have an office at the site or may make regular visits to the site.

Like outreach programs, many assisted living programs require workers to have provincially recognized training. Many provide an orientation program and regular inservice training to their staff members.

Photo 2-4
Planning helps support workers work together to make certain that all clients receive service when they need it.
Source: Leisureworld Preferred Institute

Working as Part of a Team

Support workers in assisted living settings often work in teams to help a group of clients (Photo 2-4). This arrangement allows workers to share responsibilities. The support workers also work closely with the coordinator.

Sometimes, a supportive housing client receives nursing, therapy, or other services. When this happens, the support workers involved with the client must work with the client and the coordinator to identify any changes in the worker's routine.

Following Agency Policies and Procedures

Assisted living programs, like outreach programs, have policies and procedures that the support worker must know and follow.

Challenges

Balancing Multiple Demands

Because the support worker has to meet the needs of several clients each day, the worker has to be able to prioritize needs with clients, to solve problems, and to be flexible. For example, a support worker may make breakfast for one client. While the client eats, the worker may assist another client to dress. Once the second client is dressed, the worker may return to the first client to assist with a bath. If two clients have needs that they want met at the same time, the worker must work out a suitable arrangement with them.

Photo 2-5
Residents of retirement homes usually have their own rooms yet share common living areas, such as the sitting room in this photo.

RETIREMENT HOMES

Some support workers work in retirement homes. Retirement homes provide housekeeping, laundry, and meals to clients (often called residents) who live in the facility. Residents usually have their own bedrooms, but they share the living and dining facilities with other residents (Photo 2-5). In some provinces, retirement homes are regulated.

It is important to remember that retirement homes are not long-term care facilities. The residents living in retirement homes are generally able to perform most routine activities of living on their own.

Terms of Employment

Support workers are most often employed by the retirement home itself. However, some retirement home residents employ support workers to provide assistance. As we mentioned earlier in the chapter, this is often called private-duty work.

When employed by the retirement home, support workers may report to a director of client service, a guest services coordinator, or to the administrator of the home. When employed by a resident, the support worker would report directly to the resident.

Working as Part of a Team

Support workers in retirement homes work as a part of a team that may include a supervisor, an activity director, and other support workers, as well as dietary, house-keeping, and laundry staff. Nurses or therapists may also form part of the team if a resident receives their services.

Following Agency Policies and Procedures

Retirement homes have policies and procedures that the support worker must know and follow. Some of these policies and procedures may be in place to meet provincial regulations. As in all other settings, it is important for you to know and follow the policies and procedures that apply to your work.

Challenges

Balancing Multiple Demands

Support workers in retirement homes are often responsible for assisting a number of residents. As in assisted living and day programs, here the support worker must be able to set priorities, solve problems, and be flexible in order to meet each resident's needs.

GROUP HOMES

Group homes are small facilities, often located in residential neighbourhoods (Photo 2-6). In many cases, no more than eight people live in the home. Residents of a group home usually have their own bedrooms, but share living, dining, and other facilities. They often require supervision as well as assistance with routine activities of living. Staff members provide service twenty-four hours a day.

People of any age may live in a group home. However, most residents of group homes are younger adults or children who have physical or developmental disabilities or both.

Photo 2-6
Group homes are designed to blend in with the neighbourhood. It's often impossible to tell a group home from any other home in the area.

Terms of Employment

Support workers employed in group homes are usually employed by the organization operating the home. Terms of employment are very much like those for supportive housing. Support workers usually report to a supervisor or coordinator. The supervisor or coordinator may have an office in the group home, or may make regular visits to the home.

Challenges

The challenges of working in a group home are very much like those identified for assisted living—namely, the challenge of balancing multiple demands and the challenge of working as a team member.

CASE EXAMPLE 2-3

Inderjit works in a group home for adults with cerebral palsy. Six people live in the bungalow located in a new housing development. The home looks like any other on the street. Two of the residents work part-time, one goes to community college, and three residents attend day programs.

Inderjit works the 11 p.m. to 7 a.m. shift. She is usually the only person on duty. Her tasks include assisting two residents to bed just after 11 p.m. She is also responsible for assisting a resident to get up at 6 a.m. to get ready for school. Overnight, she assists residents as they require it. She may assist someone to use the commode, change an incontinent brief, or reposition a resident who cannot do so herself. In slow periods, she does laundry and some cleaning, and makes up grocery lists

for the day staff. Sometimes, the evening worker has told her about other tasks scheduled for the night. If so, Inderjit fits them into her schedule.

Inderjit has gotten to know the residents and looks forward to spending some time talking with those who happen to be up late when she's working. On some Friday nights, she is responsible for ordering the pizza that residents usually get at midnight.

Inderjit spends a few minutes at the end of her shift filling in the day staff about any significant events that occurred overnight.

Can you identify some of the challenges Inderjit faces?

LONG-TERM CARE FACILITIES

As we discussed in Chapter 1, residents of long-term care homes receive assistance with routine activities of living as well as nursing care. Long-term care homes are regulated by the province in which they are located. Provincial regulations vary, as do the names by which these homes are known. Some of the more common names are nursing homes, special care homes, board and care homes, or homes for the aged.

Terms of Employment

Support workers in long-term care homes may be called by various titles, such as personal care aides or health care aides. They are normally hired by the facility.

Support workers in long-term care homes are usually members of the Nursing Department and report to a charge nurse. The charge nurse, in turn, reports to a Director of Care or Director of Nursing. Some support workers work in Activity Departments and report to the Activity Director.

Most long-term care homes require support workers to be available to work shifts. As a support worker, you may be required to be available to work day, evening, and night shifts.

Long-term care homes usually require support workers to have provincially recognized training. In addition, they may require or provide additional training to help support workers meet specific resident needs. Most facilities provide orientation and inservice training to their staff.

Working as Part of a Team

Support workers in long-term care homes work as a part of the team, which includes their supervisor, the facility's pharmacist, the resident's doctor, nurses, the activity director, activity aides, dietary aides, housekeeping aides, and laundry aides, as well as clergy, families, and volunteers (Photo 2-7). Therapists may form part of the team if the resident receives therapy. Teams in long-term care homes are often called **multidisciplinary teams**, as they bring together staff members from various disciplines to assist in the care of the resident.

Photo 2-7
The team is key to good support.
Source: Leisureworld Preferred Institute

The high level of support that long-term care home residents require means that the team must work very closely to provide good service. The team must share information and tasks, and must problem-solve together daily.

Challenges

Needs of Residents

More and more, residents in long-term care facilities have complex care needs. Many residents may have dementia. Most residents move to long-term care facilities when they can no longer remain at home. Many residents must cope with the effects of their condition and the losses that they experienced when they had to leave their homes.

Making a Homelike Setting

A long-term care home is a place where people live. However, most of us would not say that it's like our homes. You may hear people speak of long-term care facilities as though they are places where no one would want to live. Though it's likely true that most of us would prefer to live in our own homes until we die, it's also true that long-term care homes provide an opportunity for a sense of belonging and community, as Jaber Gubrium wrote in his book *Living and Dying at Murray Manor*, a portrait of a long-term care home.

> *. . . Life at Murray Manor is filled with intimate social ties, the celebration of small accomplishments, agonizing losses, boredom, conspiracies, anger, pride, humiliation, trust, love, hope, despair—in short, all the complexities that occur when a groups of people spend their daily lives together.*
> Jaber Gubrium, *Living and Dying at Murray Manor*

Making the long-term care home as much like a person's own home as possible is one of the most important challenges that support workers are expected to meet.

SPOTLIGHT 2-1 THE IMPORTANCE OF INTERACTION

As you might have guessed from the description of life at Murray Manor, a long-term care home is a community. In a very real sense, your actions create the world for the residents.

As a support worker in that community, what you do and how you do it will affect the lives of the residents. Perhaps you've heard someone say, "It wasn't *what* she did, it was *how* she did it that upset me." The manner in which something is done often has as much of an effect as the activity itself. This is especially true in a long-term care home, as a great deal of the residents' day is made up of communicating and interacting with staff.

As a support worker, your words and actions must always tell the resident that you value her or him as a person. This is easier said than done, particularly when you are rushed or a resident does not wish to do what you have asked. Review Case Example 2-4. How does Kevin show residents that he cares for them as individuals?

Balancing Multiple Demands

Support workers in long-term care homes are responsible for assisting a number of residents with many tasks. The level of resident need means that demands are greater than in other homes. The worker must work as efficiently as possible, yet be caring, kind, and gentle. Support workers must be able to set priorities, solve problems, and be flexible in order to meet each resident's needs.

CASE EXAMPLE 2-4

Kevin Morris works in a long-term care home in which 110 residents live. He works the day shift. Kevin shares with another support worker the responsibility of caring for 22 residents in a unit of the home. He and his co-worker help the residents get up, washed, dressed, and to breakfast each morning.

When he arrives, Kevin attends the unit's morning report. He learns of any new residents and any changes in each resident's condition. He also goes over the shift duty roster to confirm his schedule. If he has any questions, he discusses them with the charge nurse. He then gets on with the duties of the day.

Many of Kevin's residents have some type of dementia. Some do not always remember where they are, and

they become very frightened when first awakened. Although he is very busy, Kevin has to make sure that he approaches people calmly and gently so that he does not make them more frightened.

In order to make the best use of his time, Kevin has learned who can get dressed alone and who needs help. He also knows who just needs a bit of time to adjust to the new day before getting out of bed. He plans his morning rounds to spend the time with the residents who need him most. He also works with his co-worker to assist residents who need the help of more than one person.

What are some of the challenges associated with working in a long-term care home? What are some of the benefits?

OTHER CENTRES

Other centres have begun to hire support workers. They include:

- Chronic Care Centres
- Rehabilitation Centres
- Acute Care Centres
- Mental Health Facilities

People using these centres are often called patients. Patients do not usually stay in acute care centres or rehabilitation centres for a long period of time. Mental health facilities provide both long- and short-term services to patients with mental health concerns. However, patients in chronic care centres may live there for many months or years, much like residents of long-term care facilities. Rehabilitation centres are facilities that provide services to help patients recover from surgery, illness, or injury. Patients in these centres have conditions that may change, or they may require professional services on a regular basis.

Some hospitals offer all three types of service in separate wings. A hospital may have a rehabilitation unit, a chronic care unit, and a mental health unit, as well as acute care and emergency units.

Some chronic care centres, rehabilitation centres, mental health facilities, and acute care centres have employed support workers for many years. Others have only recently hired support workers. Some of these centres do not hire support workers at all.

Terms of Employment

Support workers in chronic care centres, rehabilitation centres, and acute care centres may be called health care aides or patient care attendants. The centre usually hires them. The organization in which they work is often much like that of a long-term care facility, although it is usually larger and has more specialized services. For example, a hospital may employ support workers to assist patients in its medical unit or new mothers on the maternity ward. Patients have medical or rehabilitation needs as well as needs for assistance with routine activities.

The role that the support worker fulfills may be much different than it would be in the long-term care facility. In chronic care centres, rehabilitation centres, and acute care centres, support workers assist patients with routine activities of living while the patient is receiving other types of care. Support workers must be careful not to exceed the bounds of their training or legislation when assisting patients in these centres.

Most support workers are members of the Nursing Department and report to a Charge Nurse. The Charge Nurse reports to a Unit Director, the Director of Care, or Director of Nursing. In some centres, support workers may be hired to work in rehabilitation or other departments. In these situations, the worker reports to the department supervisor.

These centres usually require support workers to have provincially recognized training. Because not all provincial training programs include a great deal of training in this area, many centres require or provide additional training to help support workers meet the centre's needs. In addition, most centres provide orientation and inservice training to their staff.

Working as Part of a Team

Support workers work as a part of a team that includes physicians, pharmacists, other nursing staff, rehabilitation staff, dietary staff, and housekeeping staff, as well as clergy, families, and volunteers. Because most patients' conditions are changing, this team has to work very closely to make sure that appropriate care is given and that the appropriate person provides the needed care. The team must share information and tasks and problem-solve together daily.

Challenges

Patient Need

Patients have complex care needs that may change rapidly. Usually, the patient is coping with an illness or condition that has changed his or her life, if only for a little while. Furthermore, the patient is in unfamiliar surroundings. All these things can make it difficult for the patient to cope. The patient may become frustrated or irritated at things. You must be able to appreciate the patient's perspective. You must be able to put yourself in the patient's shoes, so to speak, and provide care as you would like it to be provided to you.

Balancing Multiple Demands

Support workers in centres are responsible for assisting many patients with many tasks. Patients' conditions may change rapidly. Their need for support may change from day to day. Emergencies may disrupt the normal workflow of the unit or cause other members of the team to be called away. Support workers must be able to set priorities, solve problems, and be flexible in order to meet each patient's needs.

Respecting the Scope of Your Role

Many patients will have needs that the support worker is not trained or permitted to meet. Sometimes, the worker is very familiar with what needs to be done. However, the worker should never exceed the bounds of his or her role, no matter how seemingly simple or familiar the task. Support workers must report to their supervisor as soon as possible about any needs for care that lie beyond the scope of their training or their role.

WHICH SETTING IS BEST FOR YOU?

No one setting is the best setting. Each has its benefits and challenges. The one that's right for you depends upon what you want to do. Many factors should be considered when you seek employment (Figure 2-1).

FIGURE 2-1
Many factors determine which setting is best for you.

- Does the type of work interest me? Am I excited by the job?
- Can I perform the tasks required? Do I have all the training I'll need?
- Do I like working with people in that kind of work setting?
- Can I get to the work site? Can I travel from client to client if the job requires it? Do I like the amount of travel required?
- Am I comfortable with the agency or client who is hiring me? Will I be proud to work for them?
- Are the wages and benefits (if any) competitive?
- Is there an opportunity to learn additional skills and take on different responsibilities if I would like to?

Employers may differ in the type of working arrangements, wages, policies, and procedures. One employer may offer things another does not. It is up to you to find out what each employer offers in order to determine which setting and which employer is best for you.

Questions for Review

1. What are the five requirements set out by the *Canada Health Act* to ensure that everyone has access to necessary health care?

2. List the nine major types of settings in which support workers may work.

3. What are two of the challenges in working directly for a client?

4. In which settings might you need additional training?

5. In which settings do you work as part of a team?

6. How might working in an acute care centre be different than working in a long-term care facility?

7. What must you have in order to work in most settings?
   a) A reliable car
   b) The ability to be flexible and to problem-solve
   c) A uniform
   d) Thorough knowledge of the agency's history

Questions for Discussion

1. In which setting do you prefer to work? Why? Compare your preferences with those of your colleagues or classmates.

2. What agencies in your community offer the types of support discussed in this chapter? With three other classmates or colleagues, draw up a list of the agencies. Compare your answers to those of other groups.

3. You have recently been offered employment by a community agency offering respite care and outreach services to a rural community near where you live. What factors should you consider in deciding whether or not to take the position offered by the agency? What characteristics would be positive factors for you? What characteristics would be difficult for you to accept?

Chapter 3

Ethics and Personal Support

Learning Objectives

Through reading this chapter, you'll be able to

1. Define the term *ethics*.
2. Describe the personal ethics you use in everyday life.
3. List and discuss six important principles of the ethics that apply to providing personal support.

Chapter at a Glance

- What Are Ethics?
- The Ethics of Personal Support

Terms You'll Use

Autonomy Each person's right to have his or her decisions respected.

Beneficence The obligation to prevent or remove what is bad and to promote what is good.

Confidentiality The obligation to keep the client's personal information private.

Ethics The principles that guide how people behave.

Nonmalificence The obligation to do no harm to another person.

Privacy The right we all have to choose to share or not share personal information, or to restrict the distribution of information we have shared.

Security The obligation to keep others' information safe and away from those who are not authorized to see it.

WHAT ARE ETHICS?

STOP AND REFLECT 3-1

Imagine that you are going to a friend's house. On the sidewalk, just steps away from her home, you find a $20 bill. You put it in your pocket.

When you get to your friend's house, her neighbour is there. This neighbour has not been nice to you in the past. Today, she is upset and barely notices that you have arrived. Your friend tells you that this neighbour has lost $20—money she needed to help pay her telephone bill.

What do you do?

_____

_____

Why?

_____

_____

Did you find yourself thinking of the "right" thing to do? If so, you've relied upon your **ethics**—the principles that guide behaviour. We all have them, although we may not all have exactly the same ones. Sometimes, ethics are called morals or precepts.

Personal Ethics

> *What you do not want done to yourself, do not do unto others.*
>
> Confucius

Each of us has personal ethics—the principles that guide how we behave in everyday life. The principle expressed by Confucius is one of the most common—treat others as you'd like to be treated. There are many others.

We can become so used to these principles that we use them without thinking. Sometimes, when we feel bad about something we did, we realize that we have gone against a principle in which we believe.

STOP AND REFLECT 3-2

What principles do you try to live by?

_____

_____

Are you always aware of these principles?

_____

_____

Have you ever done something that went against your principles? Did you know it at the time? How? What did you do about it?

_____

_____

Compare your answers with those of your colleagues. In what ways are your answers similar? Different? Did you find that you and a colleagues called a principle by different names, but you both meant the same thing?

Sometimes, we share a principle but differ in the way that the principle should be shown. For example, some people feel that a person shows respect by making eye contact with the person to whom he or she is talking. Others feel that this eye contact is tremendously disrespectful.

This is one of the problems with Confucius' principle. When we treat someone as we would want to be treated, we may be ignoring how that person would want to be treated. This may cause the person to feel that his or her needs are not valued or as important as ours.

Many of these differences are rooted in our personal culture—how we have been taught to demonstrate ethical principles. We'll discuss personal culture in Chapter 7.

Common Personal Ethics

Many of us might say that we live by the Golden Rule—to treat others as we'd like to be treated. What, though, does that mean? The following principles might be included:

- **Honesty:** To not lie or mislead. Honesty also means not misleading by leaving something out—in other words, to tell the "whole truth."
- **Integrity:** To mean what we say, say what we mean, and do what we say we will do.
- **Caring:** To have concern for other people, their feelings, and their needs.
- **Fairness:** To do what we feel is right and just in a situation.
- **Consistency:** To apply the same standard to all; to not have a double standard, nor to change how we apply a standard.
- **Acceptance:** To respect each person as an individual, despite differences in appearance, background, situation, or behaviour.

While the principles might appear clear, the way in which we use each of them is sometimes a bit complicated. For instance, imagine that your best friend has just had her hair cut (Figure 3-1). Your friend asks you how you like it. From how your friend

FIGURE 3-1 *Balancing the principles of personal ethics. Imagine your best friend has just had her hair cut in a style you don't think is right for her, and she asks what you think. How would you answer her?*

looks at you, you know that she wants you to approve. You think that the style is all wrong for her. What do you say? Complete honesty may hurt your friend. Yet, you may not want to lie just to make her feel good. How do you balance these principles?

THE ETHICS OF PERSONAL SUPPORT

Health care and human service workers have codes of ethics that relate to the performance of their duties. These ethics are in many ways similar to the ones we have for ourselves. Most are extensions of personal ethics, applied to common work situations. Most codes of ethics reflect the personal ethics described above. The ethics of personal support include six important principles that are described in the following sections.

1. Privacy and Confidentiality

Privacy and confidentiality are two of the most fundamental concepts of personal support ethics. Although they are closely related, privacy and confidentiality are not the same. In this section, we'll discuss both concepts.

Privacy

STOP AND REFLECT **3-3**

Imagine that you were using a support service and had someone assisting you. How much would that person learn about you?

_____

_____

How might you feel about your support worker knowing this information?

_____

_____

_____

How would you feel if the worker shared the information with others, or told a story to her co-workers about you?

_____

_____

Privacy refers to the right that we all have to share or to refuse to share information. We often think of privacy as *physical* privacy. For example, we often remind others to close the door when a person is dressing—to maintain the person's privacy. It actually means much more, including information about the person, the person's situation, and his or her activities.

When you provide support to a person, you often learn a great deal about the person. This often includes information that is not necessary for the support that you provide. You'll also learn information that is necessary for the support you provide, but is not appropriate to share with other people who provide other types of support.

Confidentiality and Security

Confidentiality refers to your obligation to keep the client's personal information private. Security describes how you do this—by not discussing or leaving client information where others may overhear or see it.

Support workers often spend a great deal of time with clients. They get to know the client and, often, the client's family and friends. As a result, the support worker usually learns a great deal of personal information that the client wouldn't share with most other people.

Federal and Provincial Privacy Legislation

It's extremely important to respect the person's privacy and to refrain from sharing information when it is not appropriate to do so. It's also the law. As of January 1, 2004, a person's information privacy is protected by federal and/or provincial legislation. On January 1, 2004, federal legislation—the *Personal Information Protection and Electronic Documents Act* (PIPEDA) was extended to apply to commercial activity federally and provincially, unless a province put substantially similar legislation in place. Thus, a person's privacy is protected, but exactly how it is protected varies from province to province. Nonetheless, the basic principles of the legislation are the same.

Not all provinces have privacy legislation. Those provinces that don't must follow the federal legislation. Some provinces have privacy legislation that covers certain types of information. For example, Ontario has the *Health Information Protection Act* (HIPA), which deals with the privacy of health information. Personal information that is not health information (or used in the context of health care) is governed by PIPEDA.

PIPEDA and most provincial privacy laws are based upon 10 privacy principles, as set out in Figure 3-2. The most important guidelines for support workers include the following:

- Know what kind of client information is necessary and which isn't. Don't collect or document unnecessary information.
- Never reveal to an unauthorized person any information that could breach the client's privacy. Know the persons with whom you can share information, and always make certain you cannot be overheard when you are sharing necessary information.
- Document clearly, accurately, and carefully so as to give an accurate picture to the reader. Do not pass on information as true unless you know for certain that it is true. As well, don't use language that might mislead. For example, if your client was crying because of happiness, you might give another person the wrong impression if you said your client was upset.
- Keep secure any client information in your possession. Use a separate appointment book for client information, and keep your personal information in another book. When you're using client information, make certain that unauthorized people can't see it. Have you ever been on a bus and been able to look over someone's shoulder and see what the person was reading? You must be careful to not allow client information to be seen in that way.
- Keep information in a secure binder or satchel when you're not using it. Don't leave client information where unauthorized people may see it.

FIGURE 3-2 *Privacy principles underlying PIPEDA and provincial privacy legislation*
Source: PIPEDA

The 10 Privacy Principles

(Accountability, Challenging Compliance, Individual Access, Openness, Safeguards, Accuracy, Limiting Use Disclosure & Retention, Limiting Collection, Consent, Identifying Purposes)

STOP AND REFLECT ((3-4))

Sometimes, it's difficult to maintain someone's privacy. For example, what do you do if you must accompany your client to an appointment? It's important that you complete the task, but it's also important to not breach the client's privacy. The client may not want everyone to know that you are a support worker.

How could you do your best to maintain your client's privacy? Here are a few ideas.

- When escorting a client, put your nametag in your pocket or purse. This way, you're not identifying yourself as a support worker—and your client as a client.
- Don't talk about your client as a client when others can overhear you. For example, saying "Mrs. Rampersand, I can talk to my supervisor to see if we can get more hours for you," tells everyone who can hear you that Mrs. Rampersand is a client.
- Respect that the client can share information about his or her status because it is the client's information. If the client chooses to introduce you as "my support worker," it is her or his right—it is the client's information to share. It is not acceptable for you to do this without the client's permission or for you to share information with a person just because the client has identified you as a support worker to that person.

Can you think of other ways you can maintain the client's privacy in this situation?

_____

_____

_____

_____

STOP AND REFLECT ((3-5))

What privacy legislation applies in your province?

_____

_____

_____

What is the name of the legislation?

_____

_____

What government agency enforces it?

_____

_____

When You Must Share Information

As a support worker, you have an obligation not to share this information with others. There is one exception to this rule: you must share with your supervisor any information that is essential to the client's health or well-being.

STOP AND REFLECT ((3-6))

You are a support worker assigned to Mrs. Cabriole. Mrs. Cabriole does not speak a great deal of English. You have been assigned extra hours, as her family is on vacation for the next four weeks and cannot visit her as they normally would.

While you are tidying her kitchen, you accidentally drop her mail on the floor. As you pick it up, you notice a disconnection notice for Mrs. Cabriole's telephone. It says that if the bill is not paid this week, the service will be disconnected. You know that Mrs. Cabriole needs to have her phone in case of an emergency. You also know that her family pays her bills.

What do you do?

_____

_____

In this case, you should contact your supervisor to advise her or him of the situation. It would not be appropriate to share this information with a co-worker or anyone else.

At times, you may share the care of a client with another support worker. Then, you may have a legitimate need to discuss client care with the co-worker, particularly if the client has complex needs. Even so, you must not do so in a way that allows the information to be overheard by unauthorized persons. It is never appropriate to discuss client concerns in public areas such as a lunchroom or a store.

It is best to use your agency's staff conference room or other private room to meet. If you work in the community, ask your supervisor to arrange for a meeting with you and your co-worker so that the information may be shared in private.

Confidentiality also applies to any written information you may have about a client, such as a referral form, a duty roster, or any other item that includes personal information about clients or their needs. You must be extremely careful not to allow unauthorized people to see this information. In most cases, your agency will have guidelines about what written information you may have and how it must be kept. Be sure to follow those guidelines.

Maintaining confidentiality is more difficult when you have known the client before he or she became a client—perhaps because the client is a relative of a friend or was a neighbour of yours. In these situations, you must be particularly cautious of what you say to others, so as not to share information you have gained through your work. Responding to the simplest questions can be difficult. Consider what you would say in the following situation.

STOP AND REFLECT

You have just finished your shift at the long-term care home and are at the post office. One of your neighbours sees you and inquires about a resident who used to live across the street from you both. She asks whether the resident is happy living in the home and if she and her roommate are now getting along.

What do you say?

_____

_____

_____

_____

_____

There are two issues here. First, you are in a public place where you could be overheard. Second, some of the information your neighbour is asking for is information you have gained through your professional relationship with the client. In order to avoid a breach of confidentiality, you might ask your neighbour to wait until you are both outside and away from others, and then you might suggest that your neighbour visit the resident.

2. Respect for a Person's Right to Make Decisions and Take Risks

Respecting a person's right to make decisions and take risks is also called respecting the person's **autonomy**. We all have the right to make decisions that affect our lives. Most of us, at one time or another, have made a decision with which our close friends or family did not agree. Sometimes, we ourselves have disagreed with a decision a friend or family member has made. When these differences of opinion happen, the person making the decision can feel as though she or he does not have the right to make the decision after all. The person can become angry. Consider the following situation.

STOP AND REFLECT ((3-8))

After thinking about it for a while, you have made the decision to return to school to become a personal support worker. Your closest friend thinks that this is not a good idea. She says that you have too much to do already and that your family will be neglected. She also tells you that you are doing fine as you are now, so you shouldn't change anything. She points out that you will not earn any more money and may have to work night shifts.

How do you feel about your friend's comments?

_____

_____

What would you say to her?

_____

_____

_____

Would you rethink your decision?

_____

_____

Like you, clients have the right to make decisions about things that affect their lives. It is your responsibility not to attempt to influence your client's decisions simply because you don't think that the client's choice is a good one.

In some situations, it's pretty easy to apply this principle. For example, your client may prefer a particular brand of canned corn. It may happen to be one you don't feel is as good as another. However, it's likely that you'll respect the client's right to select the brand that he or she prefers. You would probably not even say anything to the client about it.

It becomes more difficult when the client's choice seems to be risky. For example, how would you feel if your client asked you to purchase something you know he or she is not allowed to eat? Would you react differently than you might to the choice of canned corn?

Respecting a person's right to make decisions becomes much more difficult when the client has a condition (such as a dementia) that affects his or her ability to make decisions. In these cases, you will have to work closely with the support team to identify what decisions the client can safely make and what decisions the client cannot.

3. The Obligation to Do No Harm

The obligation to do no harm is called **nonmalificence**. As a support worker, you must not do things that would cause your client harm. This seems pretty clear and, in most cases, it is. However, this principle also includes not doing harm unintentionally if you should have known that the activity would cause harm. For example, running a client's bath without checking the temperature of the water could cause harm if the water was too hot. As a support worker, you should know to check the water temperature before the client gets into the tub.

The obligation to do no harm requires that you know the correct procedure for doing the tasks you are assigned to do. You must also be aware of how to safely use different types of household equipment in order to avoid damaging the client's property.

4. The Obligation to Prevent or Remove What Is Bad and to Promote What Is Good

The obligation to prevent or remove what is bad and to promote what is good is called beneficence. As a support worker, you are obliged to do your best to promote the client's well-being. However, you must balance this principle with the need to respect the client's right to make decisions and take risks. Sometimes, clients make decisions that are based on priorities that others around them do not share. The client weighs the risk with the benefit and makes a decision.

Sometimes a decision or situation may seem to you to be too risky. Before you say anything, you must always ask yourself if excessive harm will be caused by not acting, or whether you will simply be uncomfortable with the situation. You may want to talk over the situation with your supervisor. Consider the following situation.

STOP AND REFLECT **3-9**

Your client lives alone in a two-storey house. He has had several falls, all related to a balance problem. The last time, he could not get up and lay on the floor for 14 hours before someone found him. He wants very much to stay in his own home, yet he will not allow more help. He also won't let his family rearrange his furnishings so that all he needs would be on the ground floor. Today, you arrived to find him at the foot of the stairs, bruised and unable to get up. He was taken to hospital, checked over, and released.

How do you feel about the risks your client is taking?

_____

_____

Would you feel better if he moved or rearranged the furnishings in his home?

_____

_____

What, if anything, would you say to him about this situation?

_____

_____

Compare your answers with those of your colleagues.

Did you find that you wanted the client to be safe? Perhaps you wanted to protect him from the harm that might come from living the way he does. Yet, you must balance your feelings with respect for his right to make choices and take risks. As with other ethical problems, you might want to discuss your thoughts and feelings with your supervisor.

5. The Obligation Not to Take Advantage of a Person

We take advantage of a person when we use our power over them to make the person do something we want. Your client may see you as being more powerful, simply because you are coming to help. Like the obligation to do no harm, the obligation not to take advantage of a person seems pretty clear. Most of us would not intentionally use our position to make someone do something. Sometimes, though, we may use this power unintentionally. Consider the following situation.

STOP AND REFLECT ((3-10))

You have been assigned to a new client, Mrs. Lai. She is quite capable, alert, and oriented. A recently fractured hip has meant that she needs some help with her homemaking and getting around.

As you're helping Mrs. Lai dry off after her bath, she asks you to get her body lotion. As you hand her the Avon lotion, she remarks that the bottle is almost empty and that she has to remember to order more. "Some neighbour sells it," she tells you. "I don't really know her, but she lives a few houses down." She also says she buys some stocking stuffers (cologne and other things) from the catalogue because it's "easier than going to the store."

You sell Avon. While you don't make a lot of money at it, it helps pay for the incidentals.

Do you tell Mrs. Lai that you sell Avon?

_____

Why or why not?

_____

_____

Would you take an order for Avon from her?

_____

Compare your answers with those of your colleagues.

Would you be taking advantage of Mrs. Lai by telling her you sell Avon? By taking an order from her? Deciding whether or not you should tell her probably wasn't as easy as you thought.

Sometimes you can figure out if something is not a good idea by looking at it from the client's point of view. For example, would Mrs. Lai possibly feel obligated to buy Avon from you? Would she feel that your relationship with her would be different if she chose not to buy Avon from you? If the answer to these questions is yes, you should not tell her you sell the products. In such situations, you should also make sure that you are familiar with your agency's policy on selling items to clients.

Accepting tips and gifts may make the client feel obligated to give them in the future. This may also be seen as taking advantage. Again, you must obey your agency's policy on accepting gifts and tips. Even if they are permitted, you must be particularly careful not to take advantage of a client.

You don't have to be selling something or accepting something to take advantage of a client. It can happen whenever your client feels obligated to do something you suggest. For example, suppose you visit a particular client each Thursday. This Thursday, your sister is coming to visit for two days on her way to Mexico. You haven't seen her in two years and want to spend the day with her. However, you don't want to lose the work. You tell your client about your sister's visit. You also say how much it would mean for you to be able to spend the day with your sister, but that you can't afford to lose the work. You let the client know that you hope the client will agree to have you come on Wednesday this week, even though you know that Wednesday is not a good day for the client. In this instance, the client may feel obligated to change the day.

6. The Obligation to Use Best Efforts

Support workers must always use their best efforts to assist the client. This principle means many things: doing your best at all times, using your skills to the best of your ability, and learning any skills you need to learn (within the bounds of your role) to assist your client.

Keeping your skills and knowledge up to date is one important way of meeting this obligation. Taking a personal support training program will prepare you to work in the field. You will also find that you will want to take additional training to enhance your skills and knowledge. If you work for an agency, make sure to take part in the inservice training your agency provides. Find out what training is offered by other organizations. For example, you may learn a great deal about assisting a person who is dying by taking a course offered by your local palliative care or hospice service.

Once skills are learned, you must then keep them up to date. Wherever possible, you must use the skills you've learned. If you cannot, you must make sure that you can perform the skills properly. You can do this by taking a refresher course or workshop, or by having your supervisor review your skills and observe you performing them.

Your supervisor can be of great help in identifying and meeting your learning needs. In addition, skilled and experienced co-workers, as well as other team members, can also be tremendous resources.

Questions for Review

1. What do we mean by the term *ethics*?

2. Name four personal ethics. For each, give one example of how it would apply to everyday life.

3. Name and describe six important ethical principles that apply to support work.

4. How could the obligation to do no harm be applied to assisting a client to bathe and dress?

5. What do we mean by the term *privacy*? How is it different from *confidentiality*? Why is it important to maintain both?

6. What legislation protects the privacy of health information in your province? What privacy rights do clients in your province have?

7. Why should you keep your skills and knowledge up to date?

Questions for Discussion

1. Discuss what you would do in the following situation:

   Suppose that you are visiting Mrs. Schmidt, a client who has had severe diabetes for many years. You have been cautioned not to add sugar to anything you cook for her.

   Today, when you're going shopping, you notice that chocolate bars are on the shopping list. When you ask Mrs. Schmidt what kind, she looks embarrassed and says, "Any kind will do. They're for my grandchildren, you see."

   You get a sense that this is not the case. For one thing, Mrs. Schmidt's grandchildren live out of town and are not coming to visit for at least three weeks.

   What would you do in this situation? What principles would guide you?

2. Speak with an experienced support worker who has faced an ethical problem. How did the support worker solve it?

Chapter 4

You, the Support Worker

Terms You'll Use

Accountability Being personally responsible for your actions.

Code of Conduct A statement that is intended to guide support worker practice. It is often made up of ethical principles, support worker qualities, and skills. It is sometimes called a code of ethics.

Distress Stress that prevents us from functioning in the way we would like.

Stress A psychological and physiological condition that arises when we respond to stimulation or adjust to changes and demands.

Stressor A particular source of stress.

Wellness A process of becoming aware of and practising healthy choices to attain a sense of balance and well being.

THE VALUE OF SUPPORT WORK

STOP AND REFLECT ((4-1))

Imagine that you have been asked to speak to a community group about what you do. The group would like you to focus on the benefits that support work provides to clients.

What would you say?

_____

_____

In what way do you think clients benefit from support services?

_____

_____

_____

In what way do you benefit from providing support?

_____

_____

_____

Support work is more than housekeeping and physical care. It involves a relationship between you and the client. That relationship provides support and comfort to the client. It usually benefits both the client and the worker.

The value you place on providing support will directly affect the benefit you get from providing it. If you do not see the role as rewarding, you will not put much effort into performing your duties and will probably not get much benefit from them.

How you provide support is also affected by other beliefs you may have. For example, if you feel very strongly that families should care for a person who needs support, you may find it difficult to work for a client whose family cannot, or chooses not to, provide that support. Similarly, if you feel very strongly that a person is responsible for what happens to her or him, you might find it difficult to provide support to a person who feels that her or his situation is beyond her or his own control.

This does not mean that holding such beliefs is a reason not to become a support worker. It is important to know what beliefs you hold so that you can guard against letting them affect your work. You may find that your beliefs change over time as you work.

PERSONAL QUALITIES AND ATTITUDES

Many personal qualities and attitudes are essential in providing effective personal support. If you are working in the field, you likely are familiar with some of these. We'll identify fifteen qualities here.

1. Interest in People

Photo 4-1
Support work requires you to work with many people. Here members of the team gather to discuss a client concern.
Source: Leisureworld
Preferred Institute

It is very difficult to work in such a people-oriented career unless you have a genuine interest in people. All of your working time will be spent in direct contact with others, including your client, co-workers, other members of the team, the client's family and friends, and your supervisor (Photo 4-1). Your day will be very long indeed if you do not have an interest in people.

2. Positive Outlook

Photo 4-2
Is the glass half full or half empty?

Look at Photo 4-2. Is the glass half empty or half full? Having a positive outlook will help you see the best in situations. You will have hope, and you will be better able to provide encouragement. Bear in mind that a positive outlook must also be genuine; you should not be falsely optimistic or unrealistically positive, as this can mislead or offend the client.

STOP AND REFLECT ((4-2))

A client has just learned that a very close friend has had a serious stroke and is in the intensive care unit at hospital. She is unconscious. The client is very frightened and sad. Her support worker says to her, "Don't worry. I'm sure she'll be just fine."

How do you think that the client might feel?

_____

_____

Why might the worker have said this?

_____

_____

_____

What might the support worker have said instead?

_____

_____

_____

3. Sensitivity

The nature of many support tasks and the closeness of your relationship with clients require you to be sensitive to your client and your client's needs. This includes becoming sensitive to each client's nonverbal communication and preferred ways of doing things. Sensitivity includes being alert for subtle communication and the importance of the client's routine and ways of problem solving.

As we'll discuss in Chapter 7, sensitivity is particularly important when your client's preferences, practices, and methods differ from your own.

CASE EXAMPLE 4-1

Kadhyia provides support to a client who uses a special rug when she prays. Kadhyia knows how sacred the prayer rug is and treats it with the care that her client prefers. When her supervisor came to visit, Kadhyia advised her of the rug's purpose and the importance of not stepping on it.

Have you ever been in a situation where you upset someone without meaning to? What did you learn from that situation? Has it made you more aware of what you need to know before you act?

---

4. Caring

Have you ever been cautious about how you said something to avoid hurting another person's feelings? That's an example of caring. Caring is a special quality that is related to many of the others in this list. Having a caring nature means many things: that you do not want to harm people in any way; that you think about how your actions affect others; that the effect you have on other people matters to you.

5. Sense of Personal Responsibility

Many people will rely upon you to do your job and to do it well. You must take responsibility for your own actions. Personal responsibility is also called accountability. You must also honour your commitments. Unless there is an emergency that prevents you from fulfilling your duties, you must complete any assignment you accept, arrive at work on time, and do the tasks assigned to the best of your ability.

If you have made a commitment to an employer or agency, you must make sure that you are able and available to fulfill it. If you tell your employer that you are available for certain shifts, you must accept them when asked. When you accept a shift, you must arrive on time, and you must work the entire shift.

Personal responsibility also means making sure that you are mentally and physically prepared to complete any assignment you have accepted.

You must complete all tasks assigned to you if possible. If you cannot complete all the tasks assigned, you must advise your supervisor of those tasks that remain and the reason you could not complete them.

Personal responsibility also includes handling mistakes properly. You should admit any mistake you make. You should also take action to correct the mistake and use your best efforts not to repeat it.

CASE EXAMPLE 4-2

Sarah Green works part-time for a home support agency. Every other weekend, she also works for a long-term care facility. Sarah knows that her employers, clients, and co-workers depend on her. She is accountable to them to do her part and therefore makes certain that she is on time, works effectively, and completes her shift.

In addition to those mentioned, in what other ways might you be accountable to a client? To an employer?

How are you accountable to your colleagues? To your teacher?

6. Maturity

The ability to see the other person's perspective, make thoughtful decisions, and take responsibility are part of maturity. Mature people constantly grow and develop. They know that no one is perfect. They have the ability to accept constructive criticism, listen to the wisdom of others, and learn from their mistakes.

7. Patience

You may have heard the phrase "Patience is a virtue." In support work, patience is essential. Patience is the ability to slow your pace, repeat instructions, and respond to repetitive questions without frustration. Many people with disabilities and many older adults take longer to do things. So do people adjusting to a new condition who must adapt old techniques or learn new ways of doing things. Support workers must constantly demonstrate patience.

8. Skill

To be skilled means to be competent, current, and comfortable. These are called the Three Cs. You must know the right technique (be competent). You must practise the technique so as to keep your skills up to date (be current). You must feel confident performing the technique (be comfortable). Only if you meet the Three Cs will you perform your tasks safely, efficiently, and properly.

9. Accuracy

Have you ever tried to follow a recipe without measuring the ingredients? Chances are that your food didn't turn out properly. Your work must be accurate and complete. This includes the tasks done for the client as well as any reporting or documenting that you do.

10. Attention to Detail

It's the little things that mean a lot. Paying attention to details is essential, whether that means completing all the elements of a task or paying close attention to how you do the task. The extra step it may take to put a client's water glass just where he likes it, fold the towels the way she likes them, or make sure that the dishes are fully dry before you put them into the cupboard will please your client and make you feel good about what you do.

11. Personal Cleanliness and Appearance

As a support worker, you will be in close physical contact with clients. Personal cleanliness is a must (Photo 4-3). You should shower or bathe daily and use an effective unscented deodorant or antiperspirant. You should not wear strong colognes or fragrances at any time. Bear in mind that, because of their condition, some clients may not be able to tolerate any scents at all. Keep your fingernails short and smooth.

Employer dress codes vary. Over the past few years, many agencies have relaxed their dress codes. Some employers may allow you to select a uniform from several options. Other employers may no longer require uniforms at all.

What you wear may also vary because of the setting in which you will be working. You would probably not wear a uniform if you were assisting a client who is attending a business meeting. You may dress professionally but casually if your duties require you to assist residents on an outing.

Whether or not your employer has a dress code, you must dress appropriately for the work you are to do and the setting in which you are to do it. Your clothing should always be clean, neat, and in good repair. Do not wear stained clothing, even if it is freshly washed.

Keep your jewellery to a minimum. Rings with sharp edges or raised stones can catch and tear the client's skin or clothing. Do not wear them. Refrain from wearing long, dangling necklaces or bracelets, as they can catch, scrape, or tear. Hoop earrings can easily be caught on many things and may tear your earlobe. Wear small studs or post-style earrings if you must wear any at all.

Photo 4-3
A well-groomed and well-dressed support worker conveys a professional appearance.
Source: Leisureworld
Preferred Institute

12. Flexibility

You will work with many clients with different personalities and ways of doing things. Flexibility is essential. You must be able to adapt your style to how the client does things or would like them done. This is harder than it sounds. We all have preferred ways of doing things. We often resist changing our ways because we are comfortable, not because an alternative is wrong or unsafe.

CASE EXAMPLE 4-3

Susan works for Mrs. Georgeopolous. Each week, Susan does the laundry. She notices that Mrs. Georgeopolous does not seem to be really pleased with how she does this task. Susan asks Mrs. Georgeopolous if there is something she should do differently. After a bit of hesitation, Mrs. Georgeopolous explains that she would like her towels folded in a different way and that she would prefer her blouses to be hung on hangers to dry. She shows Susan how to fold the towels and tells her where the plastic hangers can be found. Mrs. Georgeopolous is happy that her laundry is done the way she prefers.

Susan feels appreciated and pleased that she has met her client's needs.

What are some feelings that you experience when you learn that you are doing something in a way that displeases someone else?

Imagine that your teenaged son has promised to clean the kitchen after making a pizza with his friends. He does not clean the kitchen the way you like it and many things are left undone. How do you feel? What would you say to your son? How might you resolve the situation?

Sometimes, illness, pain, or stress will affect a client's interest or participation in the tasks planned for a particular visit. You will have to be flexible. For example, a client who usually helps you perform certain tasks may not feel like doing so if he or she has a cold. A client who is having a particularly good day may want to do tasks she or he doesn't usually do. You must be able to reorganize your visit to adapt to these changes.

13. Creativity

Creativity is the ability to look at things in different ways. Support workers must be creative. They help clients decide priorities for support. They adapt their approach to their clients and figure out how best to help each client do what the client needs to do.

14. Organizational Skills

Support workers must be extremely well organized. You often will have a great number of tasks to do for a client within a short period of time. You must be able to plan your tasks so as to accomplish priorities and get as much done as possible in the time available. If you work for more than one employer, you must also carefully organize your schedule to avoid conflicts and to make sure that you don't miss appointments.

15. Respect

Although it's mentioned last in this section, respect for people really is a part of all of the qualities we've discussed. Respect means taking someone's feelings, thoughts, needs, and desires into account when you do something. It can be shown both in words and in actions, but we tend to place more weight on the actions that convey respect for a person.

When you show genuine interest in a person as a person, and not as a representative of a group (for example, as a "child" or an "old person" or "Pakistani") you are conveying respect.

CODES OF CONDUCT

Many agencies combine ethical principles, support worker qualities, and skills into a *Code of Conduct* or a *Code of Ethics*. A **Code of Conduct** is intended to guide support worker practice in the agency. An example is given in Exhibit 4-1.

How many of the personal qualities described in this chapter did you find in this code? Can you see where the ethics we discussed in Chapter 3 are included?

Note that this code is signed by the support worker. When you are first hired, many agencies require you to read their code and agree to work in accordance with the code.

BALANCING YOUR COMMITMENTS

In the previous section, we discussed the need for organization. As a support worker, you will have many different demands placed on your time. You will have to identify priorities, organize your time, and manage the positive and negative stress that you will experience.

You likely found that you have a number of commitments. You may have family obligations such as making sure that you are there when your children or spouse need

**Preferred Health Care
Code of Ethical Practice**

It is the responsibility of all staff members to practise in a manner based on respect for the client, his or her caregivers, and others involved in providing care.

All staff members are expected to:

1. Work in a manner which supports client well-being.
2. Respect and support client choice.
3. Respect client privacy and the right to confidentiality of their information.
4. Respect the client's views on the sanctity of life, within the bounds of legislation and professional standards of practice.
5. Respect the role of the substitute decision maker (if any) with regard to client support and care.
6. Maintain commitments to clients:
   a. Assume responsibility for their own actions, admit mistakes, take corrective action, and take steps to prevent repetition of a mistake.
   b. Be reliable and consistent, arrive at work on time at the right location, and complete the full assignment.
   c. Dress appropriately for the assignment.
   d. Remain available to the client at all times during the assignment.
   e. Give reasonable notice if changes need to be made in the work schedule.
   f. Comply with the policies (if any) of the setting in which they are working.
   g. Treat the client with respect at all times.
   h. Treat the belongings of the client with respect and care.
   i. Refrain from requesting tips, loans, or other gifts. Seek guidance from supervisor before accepting tips or gifts.
   j. Ensure that personal activities and needs do not interfere with judgment and performance of the job.
   k. Refrain from involving the client in their personal problems.
   l. Refrain from acting as a witness to the signing of any legal document.
7. Maintain commitment to their designated profession:
   a. To practise in accordance with the standards established by their training.
   b. Maintain commitment to Interface Personnel.
   c. To accept the job requested by Interface Personnel and to advise Interface Personnel if unable for any reason to complete the assignment.
8. To raise issues with regard to employment and client service and to actively participate in the resolving of those issues.
   a. Actively take part in furthering the quality of Interface Personnel's client service.
   b. Ensure that personal activities and needs do not interfere with judgment and performance of the job.
9. Maintain commitment to personal professional development:
   a. Identify areas for professional development and to actively seek opportunities to meet those needs.
   b. Practise in an honest, equitable, and fair manner.

I have reviewed this Code and commit to practise in accordance with its tenets.

Date   Signature

EXHIBIT 4-1

A sample Code of Conduct

Source: Preferred Health Care

STOP AND REFLECT ((4-3))

What are your current commitments?

To your family:

_____

_____

To your job:

_____

_____

To yourself:

_____

_____

you, doing household chores, getting your children to school, and making sure that lunches are made.

If you are currently working, you will have a number of work commitments such as arriving at work on time and doing your job properly. We often say that a full-time job is a 40-hour week. In reality, you probably spend closer to 55 hours per week if we count getting ready for, going to, and coming from a full-time job.

You should also be sure you fulfill your commitments to yourself. Training for a new career, getting enough rest, or taking time to relax for a bit are common examples. You need to do these things in order to feel good about yourself and to have the energy to meet your other commitments. In Chapter 11, we will discuss time management in detail.

WELLNESS

You may have heard the term wellness. **Wellness** is a process of becoming aware of and practising healthy choices to attain a sense of balance and well being. It includes getting enough rest, eating a healthy diet, exercising, balancing your commitments, and managing stress. Wellness requires that you take active control of the things that affect your life and that you get the information you need to make sound decisions on diet, lifestyle, and health care.

A wellness plan is your personal plan to maintaining a good quality of life. Use Stop and Reflect 4-4 as a guide for your wellness plan.

STOP AND REFLECT 4-4

The activities in the left-hand column of the table are some of the more common wellness-oriented activities. For each, identify how often you practise the activity and what you might do to improve the activity.

Activity	How often I do this	How I might improve this activity
I get enough sleep.		
I minimize and/or avoid the use of nicotine, alcohol, caffeine, or illegal drugs.		
I eat a balanced diet.		
I exercise three to five times a week.		
I express my feelings openly.		
I take time out for meditation or "quiet time."		
I treat myself as well as I would treat my best friend.		
I enjoy my schooling.		
I enjoy my job.		
I listen to and consider ideas that are different from my own.		
I read about and/or listen to the news of the world.		
I spend time with a really close friend.		
I take time out to laugh, relax, and play.		
I take the time to enjoy my children.		
I put things in perspective and don't let minor things take on too much importance.		

BOUNDARIES

Karen is a support worker in assisted living. She works with clients who are on a fixed income. Because three of her clients have physical problems, Karen does grocery shopping for them.

Over time, Karen has gotten to know her clients' favourite foods. Occasionally, she has even picked up a favourite item using her own money. This has stretched Karen's budget at times.

Her clients are always grateful for these "treats." Although they have never indicated that they expect these things, Karen has begun to feel that she should make these purchases. She has begun to see it as a way of showing how much she cares.

Karen realizes that she must rethink the value she puts on caring when she finds herself putting back a treat for her own child so that she can afford to buy a treat for a client.

Chances are, you had some concerns about what Karen was doing. You might have thought that Karen "crossed a line" or "got too close." In other words, Karen may have crossed a boundary.

Have you ever had to set limits on the caring you do for others? How did you do this? Was your decision easy? Why or why not?

Both you and your client have boundaries—a limit that defines you as separate from others. We have many types of boundaries: professional, physical, emotional, interpersonal, social, and sexual. In a very real sense, boundaries help to define who we are and define our role responsibilities. As such, they provide a source of protection and predictability.

We tend to think of boundaries as rigid. They are not. They are flexible and constantly shifting to accommodate specific situations. They must also accommodate unavoidable situations and take into account cultural impacts upon boundaries. As you get to know someone, your boundaries will likely change. For example, you may have greater comfort sharing personal information as you get to know the person.

When you work closely with a person, it is easy for boundaries to become blurred. Though we often think of crossing a boundary as a clear-cut "crossing of a line," the reality in most cases is not so clear-cut. Boundary crossings can happen in stages, and at times seem to occur without notice. Boundary issues often result from intent. For example, is having a coffee at a Tim Hortons a boundary issue? It might—or might not be. It depends upon what the expectations of the activity are for both the attendant and the consumer. If the intent by either party is to move into a romantic relationship, then a boundary has been crossed. If the intent is to have a refreshment at the end of an outing, the activity may not cross a boundary at all.

What would you do in the following situation?

You assist a client. As you get to know the client, you discuss music and find you both like the Tragically Hip. Today, your client tells you that the Hip are doing a concert in town, with the proceeds going to a local shelter. He asks if the two of you want to go together. The concert is on your night off and you have no other plans. What do you do? What factors would you consider?

Many boundary issues result from situations in which you and the client have dual roles, where you have other relationships outside of the therapeutic. Some may be quite fine: for example, you both may take the same general interest course at a local college. Others may spark an extension of your work relationship or evolve into another type of relationship and run the risk of harm. You likely thought of these things as you decided what to do in the situation presented above.

Warning Signs

Frederic Reamer, a researcher and writer on professional ethics, identifies five common types of boundary issues:

- Intimate relationships (explicit or subtle)
- Relationships that meet an attendant's emotional needs (to be needed or address personal issues)
- Relationships that personally benefit the attendant (gifts, bartering, or special deals)
- Altruism—caring too much, being too available
- Unavoidable/unanticipated—when personal/professional crossover cannot be avoided

Most of us have experienced one of these during our work life. It's important to be sensitive to warning signs so that you can respond to a potential problem before it gets out of hand. It's also important to set clear boundaries so as to help prevent boundary issues.

Boundaries That Work

As a support worker, we have greater responsibility to prevent boundary issues. You have the responsibility to protect the client/worker relationship. This will require you to examine not only what you do, but why you do it.

As a result, you should set clear boundaries and monitor them. This doesn't mean that you make artificial boundaries, but that you are clear and kind when describing your limits.

Qualities of Effective Boundaries

There are five qualities of effective boundaries:

1. Clear and specific: easily understood by others
2. Respectful of yourself and not intentionally hurtful to others
3. Proactive: developed before the need arises
4. Positive: framed in gentleness, consideration for how the message is delivered
5. Consistent

Boundary issues can be difficult. Sometimes, it's helpful to get the perspective of a trusted other (peer or supervisor) who can help you work through the situation and provide another perspective.

STRESS

When we hear the word stress, we often think of negative things. This is a misconception: everything we do causes stress. Stress is a psychological and physical condition that arises when we respond to stimulation or when we adjust to changes and demands.

Stress can be both good and bad. In fact, we all need some stress to live. However, each of us functions best at a different level of stress. You might be able to handle more demands and changes than a friend. In turn, another friend may be able to handle more changes and demands than you can and still do quite well.

All of us experience distress. We can define **distress** as stress that prevents us from functioning in the way we would like. We'll discuss how to cope with distress later in this chapter.

Where Does Stress Come From?

Anything can cause stress. A particular source of stress is known as a **stressor**. In support work, it's helpful to think of stress as coming from four main sources: the changing expectations of support work, our expectations of ourselves, the meaning we give to the demands we feel are made of us, and the value we place on caring for or supporting others. Let's examine each of these sources.

Changing Expectations of Support Work Like many health and human services, support work is changing. Client needs are becoming more complex, and client expectations are increasing. Support workers, like all other workers, are expected to do more and to do it more efficiently. In this type of environment, the support worker must be especially careful to monitor and cope with stress.

Our Expectations of Ourselves On one hand, setting realistic goals or expectations can be very motivating. Attaining a realistic goal can give us a sense of accomplishment. On the other hand, setting unrealistic goals or expectations for ourselves can create distress. These goals may be related to what we feel others expect of us, but, in fact, we are the ones setting these expectations.

The Meaning We Give to the Demands We Feel Are Made of Us It's fine to attach importance to others' needs. You wouldn't be very caring if you didn't. However, you must keep others' demands in perspective.

The Value We Place on Caring for or Supporting Others You always must balance caring for others with caring for yourself. If you do not, you run the risk of expending all of your energy caring for others without taking the time to restore your own resources. In extreme cases, you can become bitter or burned out.

WHEN IS STRESS DISTRESS?

As we mentioned earlier in this chapter, stress becomes distress when it prevents us from functioning in the way we would like. The same demand or change may not create distress in every person. Much depends upon the following six factors:

1. You
2. Where the stress is coming from (who or what is causing it)
3. How you see the stress and what meaning you attach to it
4. How much control you have over the stress
5. Your coping mechanisms
6. What other changes and demands you must deal with at the same time

Consider the following situation.

STOP AND REFLECT 4-5

Imagine that you are a support worker in a long-term care facility. You are a new employee and want to do everything perfectly. Tonight, several residents are coming down with the flu and the staff are very busy trying to keep up. Because you are new, you are slower than the other support workers. Just as you are getting towels to wash a resident who vomited, one of the most experienced support workers says to you: "You're going to have to be a lot more organized if you're going to keep working here."

How do you feel? Are you experiencing distress? Look at the stress you are feeling in this situation in light of the six factors listed above. Would your level of stress have changed if:

- You had been more experienced?
- You had worked at that facility before?
- The residents weren't coming down with the flu and needing more care than usual?
- So many things hadn't happened at the same time?

We can change the meaning of the stress we experience by looking at stress in a different way and changing what it means to us.

RESPONDING TO YOUR OWN DISTRESS SIGNALS

There are many distress signals. These signals are your body's way of telling you it is having trouble coping with the level of stress you are having. The signs may vary from person to person. Some physical and emotional signs are given in Table 4-1.

TABLE 4-1	Some Common Signs of Distress
Physical Symptoms	**Feeling or Thinking Symptoms**
shallow breathing	panicky
headache	uncertain
backache	agitated
diarrhea	irritable
pounding pulse	sad
red face	unfocused
breathlessness	forgetful

It's important to be aware of the stressors that cause these symptoms. When you notice these symptoms, try to identify the cause.

BURNOUT

Burnout occurs when stress becomes so great that the person is unable to cope. Burnout can be emotionally, physically, and mentally draining.

Some of the common signs and symptoms of burnout are listed in Table 4-2.

TABLE 4-2	Some Common Signs of Burnout

Feeling irritable

Distrusting others' intentions

Lacking creativity

Lacking physical or emotional energy

Attempting to feel good about yourself by focusing on how much you do

Feeling overly emotional or not emotional at all

Feeling pessimistic

Sweating at night

Grinding your teeth when asleep

Burnout is a serious condition. Some health studies link burnout to illness. If you start to experience some of the signs listed in Table 4-2, you should seek help. You may want to talk with your supervisor, your doctor, or another trusted and knowledgeable person about how to manage the distress you are experiencing.

MANAGING STRESS

Don't sweat the small stuff.

You should learn to manage stress before it becomes distress and leads to burnout. You will find it easier to manage stress if you first separate the stresses you can change from those you cannot. Take a good look at each stressor and ask yourself three questions:

1. Is the stressor really a threat to me? In other words, will I be harmed if I just ignore it?
2. If the stressor is a real threat, is it worth the stress I'm feeling?
3. If the stressor is a threat and is worth the stress I'm feeling, could I change the stressor if I wanted to?

If the answer to any of these questions is no, it's either not important or out of your control. Either way, you will be better off changing the meaning you have given to this stressor. View it differently and reduce its effect upon you. If necessary, accept that you cannot change the stressor.

If you've answered yes to any of the questions, you can change the effect the stressor has on you. You can do this by using the following techniques:

- Change your routine so that the stressor no longer affects you.
- Change how you react to the stressor.
- Strengthen your stress-management skills so that you can better respond to the stressor.

Sometimes it's easy to change your routine so that the stressor no longer affects you. For example, if driving to work through heavy city traffic is stressful, you might try taking public transit.

At other times, it's not easy, or even possible, to change your routine to eliminate the stressor. Then, you'll need to focus on how you react to the stressor. Have you ever said to yourself, "I'm not going to let this get to me?" Were you able to change how you responded? If so, you've changed how you react to a stressor. Changing your response may be all you need to do to reduce the stress to a manageable level. Sometimes, changing your response is difficult. You may have to work on a particular response for a while, each time getting closer to how you want to respond.

Finally, you may want to strengthen your stress-management skills so as to be better able to handle stress. Many stress-management skills also help you to balance your need for work, rest, and recreation. Stress-management skills include relaxation techniques, exercise, recreation, and creative hobbies.

Some people attempt to manage stress through things that are harmful, such as drinking, taking drugs, and smoking. These activities, which do you harm, provide only temporary relief from your stress. Focus on stress-management techniques that give you good value—those that do not harm you or take more energy to use than they give back.

STOP AND REFLECT ((4-6))

What are the major stressors in your life?

_____

_____

What do you do to manage them?

_____

_____

What stress-management techniques give you good value?

_____

_____

Which stress-management techniques do not give you good value?

_____

_____

What new stress-management technique do you think you would like to try?

_____

_____

Questions for Review

1. How can your beliefs about the value of support work affect how you provide support? Using your own beliefs, give two examples.

2. Describe fifteen personal qualities and attitudes that are important in providing effective personal support.

3. What are the Three Cs? Why is each important?

4. What is a Code of Conduct? Why is it useful to you as a support worker?

5. What is a boundary? Why is it important?

6. How might you be able to tell that you may have crossed a boundary?

7. What is stress? Where does it come from? Is it always bad?

8. What are some common signs of distress?

9. What are some common signs of burnout?

10. What three questions should you ask about any stressor?

11. Describe three effective ways of managing stress.

12. What is wellness? What are three wellness-oriented activities?

Questions for Discussion

1. With five other colleagues, develop a Code of Conduct for personal support workers.

2. Share with your classmates the stress-management techniques that work for you. Do you use some of the same techniques as others in your group? Do you use techniques that others don't? Did you learn about any new techniques?

3. If you felt that you were experiencing some of the signs of distress or burnout, with whom would you talk?

4. Imagine that you are a support worker working for two community agencies. Although you were hired on a part-time basis, you often are scheduled for 30 hours per week or more by each agency. You also work for a local facility on a casual basis (they call you when they are short of staff for a shift). You want to work as much as possible so that you can earn enough money to provide well for your family.

   Over the last two months, you have averaged 66 hours of work each week. This week, you have agreed to work 70 hours for the community agencies. You will be working six days this week. You are not scheduled to work Friday and are really looking forward to having this one day off, as you are tired and want to spend some time with your children. In fact, you have planned to take your two children to a movie Friday night.

   On the Thursday, you receive a call from the facility, asking you to work the Friday evening shift. The rate of pay the facility offers is very good and you really enjoy working with the facility's residents.

   You are tempted to work this shift, as you will earn much-needed money. However, it would mean giving up your only day off and cancelling your plans with your children. You find yourself feeling resentful that the agency called you. You are also beginning to feel that none of your employers appreciate you.

   What stressors can you identify? What signs of distress or burnout can you identify? What actions would you take to respond to the stressors and reduce the distress you are experiencing?

5. Is it ever okay to become friends with your client? How might becoming friends affect you? Your client? Your ability to work with the client?

6. You have gotten too close to a client. What might you do to re-establish a positive working relationship?

Chapter 5

The Support Team and Its Members

Learning Objectives

Through reading this chapter, you'll be able to

1. Tell what a team is and give examples of the kinds of teams to which you belong.
2. List the five major benefits of teams.
3. Name the two major types of support teams.
4. Identify the purpose common to all support teams.
5. Distinguish between support teams organized for community services and support teams organized in facilities.
6. Describe the role of the support worker as a member of the team.
7. Identify the eleven most common members of the support team and describe each member's key responsibilities.

Chapter at a Glance

- What Is a Team?
- The Benefit of Teams
- Purpose of the Support Team
- Types of Support Teams
- Contributing to the Support Team
- Members of the Support Team

Terms You'll Use

Care Plan A written document that outlines the support a client is to receive. This document often describes client needs and support goals, and includes names and contact information for family members and other services involved in the client's support. There are many forms of care plans. These plans are also called support plans or service plans.

Service Agreement A document that spells out the services to be provided, but does not usually include goals or client needs. Service agreements may be called service contracts.

Team The term used to describe the group of people who work together (and depend upon one another) to provide support to a client.

Therapists Professionals who help the client regain ability or adjust to changes.

WHAT IS A TEAM?

A **team** is a group of people who work together toward a common interest or a common goal. In a team, members rely upon one another to get tasks done (Photo 5-1). This is called interdependence.

All of us are members of teams. In a sense, we and our families form a team. We might even say that a group of friends is a team. We don't often think of these groups as teams, but they are. Each is a group of people who share common interests or goals and who rely upon one another to do tasks related to those interests or goals. Let's take a look at the life of Robert, a support worker.

Photo 5-1
The team works together to meet the client's needs. Here, the client and her daughter discuss an issue.
Source: CHATS

CASE EXAMPLE 5-1

Robert is a support worker. He is also a husband and father of two young girls. He lives in Vancouver, near his brother, sister, and parents. He is a member of many "teams."

As a member of his family team, Robert is responsible for sharing the care of his children with his wife. He is also responsible for contributing to the family's income and for helping keep the family's home clean and in good repair. In turn, Robert relies upon the other members of the team (his wife and daughters) to perform certain tasks. For example, his wife also contributes to the family's income and shares in household duties. Robert's children have been assigned chores that help contribute to a clean, safe, and comfortable home. All members are affected if one member does not do his or her part. If Robert is ill, his wife must take on some of his responsibilities. Likewise, if Robert's wife is away, Robert must take on some of the tasks she would usually do.

Along with his brother, sister, and parents, Robert is also a member of another family "team" focused on caring for Robert's grandparents. Robert's grandfather is 88 and has some problems getting around after his stroke. As Robert is a support worker, he helps his grandfather with some personal care. His sister assists their grandmother with shopping. Robert's brother and his father help out with the upkeep of the grandparents' home. In this team, each person contributes what she or he can do best. They rely upon each other to do their respective parts.

Robert is a support worker for a home support agency. He also works in a local facility. Each of Robert's clients has a support team, and Robert is a member of each. Robert has specific responsibilities as a member of each team, as we'll see later.

As you can see, Robert's two family teams are essential to the health and well-being of each of the teams' members. Members share goals and interests and work together to get tasks done.

STOP AND REFLECT ((5-1))

To what teams do you belong?

_____

_____

Who else is a member of each team?

_____

_____

_____

What are your responsibilities as a member of each team?

_____

_____

_____

Have you ever been unable to fulfill your responsibilities to the team? If so, what happened? Did other members take on some of your responsibilities? Did some tasks remain undone?

_____

_____

_____

_____

How did the other members feel about this?

_____

_____

_____

How did you feel when you were unable to complete your responsibilities?

_____

_____

THE BENEFIT OF TEAMS

Have you heard the expression, "Two heads are better than one"? There are five major ways that teams make working together easier and more effective. Teams provide their members with the opportunity to see situations in many different ways, to solve problems, to share information, and to share responsibilities. Teams can also bring together people with different strengths and abilities. Each of these benefits is described below.

Different Views Each team member brings a unique perspective to the team. The team provides the opportunity to see a situation from many different points of view.

This can help all team members understand a client's situation or better understand an issue. Have you ever shared an issue with other people and found that they saw the issue differently than you saw it? It's likely that looking at the issue in a different way made it easier to understand.

Varied Strengths and Abilities The team brings together people who have different training, experience, and skills. This variety means that the team can apply a great deal of expertise to resolving issues and problems.

Information Sharing Through team meetings and established ways of communicating, members of the team can easily share information. This means that information is less likely to be lost.

Problem Solving By sharing information with each other, the team can examine a problem in many different ways and identify many approaches to solving it.

Responsibility Sharing As you saw in Case Example 5-1, members of the team share the responsibility for any tasks. Because the team brings together people with different strengths and abilities, it's often easy to find the right person to perform a task.

PURPOSE OF THE SUPPORT TEAM

Client Focused

The general purpose of a support team is to provide the best support possible to the client. Each team will have specific goals that relate to the needs of the client for whom the team is formed. The team develops a plan to help address the needs of the client. A **service agreement** is a document that spells out the services to be provided. It does not always include goals or client needs. It may also be called a service contract. **Care plans** are written documents that outline the support a client is to receive and often describe client needs and support goals. The contact information for family members is included, and other services involved in the client's support are listed. Care plans come in many forms and are also called support plans or service plans.

Regardless of the level of participation the client has in the team's activities, the client is the focus of the team's activities. The client should always feel a part of the team and feel free to speak openly to members of the team.

TYPES OF SUPPORT TEAMS

We'll define two general types of teams: those common to community settings and those common to facility settings. We'll discuss each team's characteristics in terms of membership, leadership, and communication.

Remember that each support team is unique. A specific client's team will be made up of the people involved in that client's care.

Community Support Teams

Membership and Leadership

The community team usually includes the client, involved family members, support workers, a support worker supervisor, the client's case manager, therapists (if involved in the client's care), as well as other caregivers. **Therapists** are professionals who help the client regain ability or adjust to changes. A specific client's team may include many other people, such as a pharmacist, clergy member, friends, neighbours, or volunteers.

The case manager is often the person responsible for organizing and leading the activities of the community support team. A family member or other team members may perform this role. A client may also take on the leadership of a support team.

Communication

Community teams usually communicate *indirectly*; that is, they do not necessarily meet on a regular basis. In fact, the team may meet only when there is an issue that requires all the members to be present. Day-to-day communication is often done through telephone calls among members of the support team, progress notes, or entries in communication logs. Most agencies have specific policies and procedures and forms for communication. You are responsible for using the method approved by your agency.

CASE EXAMPLE 5-2

As we mentioned earlier, Robert's position as a home support worker requires him to take part in a different support team for each of his clients. For example, when Robert provides respite care to his client Mr. Ross, Robert is a member of a support team that includes Mr. Ross, Mr. Ross's wife and daughter, as well as the nurse who visits, and Robert's supervisor.

Robert doesn't often see all the other members of the team. In fact, Robert's visits are scheduled so that he is not at the Ross home when the nurse is there. As well, Robert's visits enable Mrs. Ross to get out to do some shopping and to relax. She usually doesn't stay in the home when Robert is there.

Robert does communicate regularly with members of the team. Robert usually speaks briefly with Mrs. Ross when he arrives, to get an update on Mr. Ross's status. In turn, Robert reviews his visit with Mrs. Ross when he is getting ready to leave.

Robert keeps in regular contact with his supervisor. He immediately reports any significant change in Mr. Ross's status, any needs beyond the scope of his role, or any problems that cannot be resolved. In addition, he submits to his agency monthly support worker reports that provide an overview of Mr. Ross's situation and support.

Occasionally, Robert is asked to attend a meeting of Mr. Ross's support team. These meetings are scheduled to discuss significant changes in Mr. Ross's care or to deal with specific problems that have arisen.

How do you communicate with members of your family or work teams?

Is communication with the other members of your teams easy? What problems have you encountered with this type of communication?

Facility Support Teams

Membership and Leadership

The facility support team members may include many people: registered nurses and support workers, the client's physician, therapists (if the client receives therapy), as well as the facility's pharmacist, activity director, and other staff members. The team may include the client and the client's family, as well as professionals from other agencies involved in the client's care.

Often, a registered nurse is responsible for organizing and leading the team. Sometimes other members may take on this role. It is less common (although not impossible) for a client to lead the facility team. This is because many clients living in facilities have conditions that make support team leadership difficult for them.

CASE EXAMPLE 5-3

Robert's work as a care aide in a local facility requires that he be a member of a different type of support team. The facility support team differs from the community support team in two ways. First, almost all members of the support team work in the same location. As a result, it is easier for Robert to meet with members of this support team. Second, the same support team assists all of Robert's residents. (Only the client and family members are different.) This means that the team has many opportunities to work together.

Because it is easy for facility support team members to speak with one another, information sharing is often verbal. Each team member must be particularly careful to make sure that necessary information is communicated to all team members who need it and, where appropriate, that the information is written on the appropriate form.

When Robert arrives, he checks in with the charge nurse to receive his schedule and up-to-date information about his clients. At 11 a.m., Robert advises the activity director that a client, Mrs. Reager, asked about attending a

program. This is the first time that Mrs. Reager has expressed any interest in activities, and Robert wants to make sure the activity director knows about her interest.

Just after lunch, another client asks Robert for help changing clothes, as the client is going out with her daughter. Robert checks with the charge nurse to make sure that the appropriate arrangements have been made. While at the nursing station, Robert makes a note in Mrs. Reager's chart about her interest in activity programs and his discussion with the activity director.

At 2:30 p.m., Robert attends a team meeting to discuss Mrs. Chang, one of Robert's clients. The team meets monthly to discuss each client. At this meeting, Mrs. Chang's support plan will be reviewed and updated.

Consider the teams of which you are a member. In which do you take a leadership role? In which are you under another's leadership?

Is leadership shared in some teams? If so, how does this happen?

CONTRIBUTING TO THE SUPPORT TEAM

As you've learned so far, communication is essential to the work of the support team (Photo 5-2). If members do not share information and work together, the team will not attain its purpose of providing the best support possible to the client.

Each member has the responsibility to share information with the other members of the support team. Because each team member has a different role with the client, each member sees the client in a different way. If members do not freely share their views and observations, the support team will not have a complete picture of the client, and the support provided to the client may suffer as a result. It's a bit like putting together a puzzle when you don't have all the pieces. The picture will be incomplete, and you will likely end up a bit frustrated.

Each support team member's information is equally important. You should never feel that your information is less important than that of another member. In fact, you may be the team member

Photo 5-2
Support workers discussing the support provided to a facility resident.
Source: © Directphoto.org/ Alamy

who spends the greatest amount of time with the client and thus you may have a great deal of useful information to share.

When you share your observations with the team, it is important to gather your thoughts and present them clearly. What information do other team members need to hear? What is most important? Sometimes, other team members may not recognize the value of your observations. In this instance, you will have to clearly show why the information is important. It is equally important to listen carefully to the reports of other team members.

In Chapter 10, we will discuss team communication.

MEMBERS OF THE SUPPORT TEAM

As we discussed earlier in this chapter, some types of professionals and other caregivers are more likely to be members of a support team. Table 5-1 identifies the most common members of the support team. Be aware that the descriptions provided here include the general tasks of the profession. Provincial and agency regulations will determine each professional's scope of practice in a specific setting. Also, remember that the client, the client's family, as well as volunteers are members of the team. Finally, an individual client's support team is made up of the people who work together to assist that client and may well include people not listed.

TABLE 5-1	Common Members of the Support Team			
Profession	Regulated by	Training	Common Duties	Common Relationship to Support Worker
Activity Director	No mandatory regulation	Provincial requirements vary. Common preparation includes gerontology programs, social service rehabilitation diplomas and/or degrees. Some provinces have developed specific training programs.	Coordinates social programs and conducts groups in long-term care facilities Some Activity Directors work in day programs, day hospitals, and seniors' centres.	Support Workers may assist with programs, transport residents to programs, and coordinate assistance to residents so that they can attend programs.
Adjuvant Activity Aide	No mandatory regulation	Provincial requirements vary. Common preparation includes health care aide training, personal support training, rehabilitation aide training, as well as gerontology.	Usually works in facility settings Assists Activity Director with small groups, therapy follow-up, etc.	Support Workers may assist with programs, transport residents to programs, and coordinate assistance to residents so that they can attend programs.

▶▶|

TABLE 5-1	Common Members of the Support Team *(continued)*			
Profession	Regulated by	Training	Common Duties	Common Relationship to Support Worker
Clergy	Determined by religious organization	Determined by religious organization	Religious/spiritual guidance, counselling	Support Workers may be asked to assist with specific practices (for example, assist a person to kneel to pray) or to observe specific food preparation guidelines.
Dietitian	Professional College	University degree	Assess nutritional needs; devise special diets; provide public education	Support Workers may implement a diet prescribed by a dietitian.
Doctor (M.D.)	Provincial Professional College	University and medical school degrees	Diagnosis, treatment, able to perform all 13 controlled acts defined by the RHPA	Support Workers may receive direction from M.D.
Homemaker Supervisor	No one	No specific program. Training may include nursing, social services, or other health/ human service training. Some supervisors are former Support Workers.	Supervise, guide (and sometimes schedule) Support Workers	Supervisory
Occupational Therapist	Provincial Professional College	University degree	Assistance with meaningful movement (e.g., regaining of life skills, etc.) and vocational rehabilitation.	May treat the client the Support Worker sees; may give some guidance to Support Worker as per specific needs of clients (for tasks within Support Worker's role).
Physical Therapist	Provincial Professional College	University degree	Assistance with adaptation and/or regaining movement, including range of motion, walking, positioning, as well as breathing assistance (postural drainage, chest clapping, etc.)	May treat the client the Support Worker sees; may give some guidance to Support Worker as per specific needs of clients (for tasks within Support Worker's role).

⏭

TABLE 5-1	Common Members of the Support Team *(continued)*			
Profession	**Regulated by**	**Training**	**Common Duties**	**Common Relationship to Support Worker**
Registered Nurse	Provincial Professional College	Diploma program from provincial college, or university program. A Registered Nurse may hold either a degree or a diploma—the title refers only to membership in the provincial professional college.	Assists the client to solve actual or potential health problems. The scope of practice is controlled by the regulating college.	May treat the client the Personal Support Worker (PSW) sees; may give some guidance to PSW as per specific needs of clients (for tasks within PSW's role).
Registered Practical Nurse/Licensed Practical Nurse	Provincial Professional College	College diploma	Subset of Registered Nursing duties Actual scope of practice varies among provinces.	May care for the client the PSW sees; may give some guidance to PSW as per specific needs of clients (for tasks within PSW's role). In a long-term home, a LPN or RPN may supervise support workers. Some LPNs/RPNs have specific training (for example, in foot care) and may provide specialized services to the client.
Nurse Practitioner	Provincial Professional College	University degree	Extended class of a registered nurse	May provide ongoing medical care to the client the PSW sees.
Respiratory Therapist	Provincial Professional College	University degree	Assist clients who have respiratory problems, implement respiratory therapy and treatment	May treat the client the PSW sees; may give some guidance to PSW as per specific needs of clients (for tasks within PSW's role).
Speech Language Pathologist	Provincial Professional College	University degree	Assisting clients to regain speech/language; assist clients with swallowing disorders	May treat the client the PSW sees; may prescribe adaptations to client diet; may provide guidance to PSW regarding specific needs (for tasks within PSW's role).

▶▶

| TABLE 5-1 | Common Members of the Support Team *(continued)* | | | |
Profession	Regulated by	Training	Common Duties	Common Relationship to Support Worker
Social Worker	Varies from province to province	University degree	Counselling, group work related to psychosocial and emotional issues	May treat the client the PSW sees; may give some guidance to PSW as per specific needs of clients (for tasks within PSW's role).

Questions for Review

1. What is a team? To what kinds of teams do you belong?

2. What are the five major benefits of teams? Using one of the teams you listed in your answer to Question 1, give an example of each benefit.

3. What are the two major types of support teams? What is one major difference between these two types?

4. What is the one purpose common to all support teams?

5. Are support teams organized for community services and for facilities different? If so, how?

6. What is the support worker's role as a team member?

7. Name eleven possible members of the support team. What are each member's key responsibilities?

Questions for Discussion

1. How do you resolve disagreements in the team?

2. Is there ever a time when a team approach is not the best way to assist a client? If so, under what circumstances is another approach better?

3. Are support workers always equal members of the client's support team? What specific contributions do support workers make to the team? Do other team members always listen to the support worker's views? What can you, as a support worker, do to make sure your contributions to the team are heard by the other members of the team?

Chapter 6

Human Growth and Development Across the Life Span

Learning Objectives

Through reading this chapter, you'll be able to

1. Explain why it is important for you to know about human growth and development.
2. Discuss the seven principles of growth and development.
3. Describe the commonly used theories of growth and development.
4. Discuss life span perspective and relate it to personal and client situations.
5. Discuss major influences/factors affecting a client's growth and development.
6. Describe activities associated with infancy, childhood, adolescence, young adulthood, middle age, young-old age, middle-old age and old-old age.
7. Identify ways you can apply knowledge of growth and development to the support you provide.

Chapter at a Glance

- The Challenge
- Describing Growth and Development
- Principles of Growth and Development
- Theories of Human Development

Terms You'll Use

Adolescence The period from 12–19 years of age.

Development The progression from simple to more complex communication, language, thinking, movements, and behaviours.

Developmental Achievements The expected physical, emotional, or psychological and social skills at a particular age, stage, or situation.

Developmental Delays When physical skills and behaviours expected at a particular point in an individual's life are not present.

Fine Motor Skills The delicate movements of the human body that require small muscles and coordination.

Gross Motor Skills The movements of the body that primarily involve the body's large muscles.

Growth A measurable increase.

Heredity The traits and attributes a person inherits from his or her parents.

Life Span Perspective The development of a person that occurs from birth to death.

Maturation The sequence of growth and development.

Milestone The time at which particular events, skills, or behaviours are generally expected to occur.

Motor Skills The coordinated movements of the human body that require either large or small muscles.

Personality The psychological traits that each person has.

Psychomotor Development The ability to sequence movements in purposeful groups.

Stage A period of time in the human life span.

THE CHALLENGE

> *We believe that each older person is unique. Each person has values, goals, strengths, limitations, rights and responsibilities. Each person develops within a society and influences and is influenced by societal attitudes, culture, spiritual beliefs and the environment.*
>
> Canadian Gerontological Nursing Association

As the quote above indicates, our growth and development is a result of many things. Some of the things are biological or environmental. Others are social or are rooted in our family, culture, or society. Scientists have long debated just what influence each of these elements has, but most agree that all have some impact on the person.

We are often concerned about growth and development. For example, we may imagine what our children will look like when they grow up, if they will have particular talents or skills, and what their personalities will be like. We may worry about our parents or grandparents. We may eagerly look forward to our first (or next) grandchild.

We also think about what makes each of us a unique person. Have you ever looked at two siblings and wondered how they could be so different? Born to the same parents, raised in similar ways, yet they are *so* different. If you've had this experience, you understand the challenge that researchers face: just what causes this to happen? Different genes? Changes in parenting? What could it be?

In this chapter, we'll describe human growth and development and how you can apply this knowledge to the support you provide. As you read this chapter, you'll likely also learn information that will help you understand your own development and that of your family.

DESCRIBING GROWTH AND DEVELOPMENT

Philosophers and researchers have examined growth and development for centuries. However, it wasn't until the late 1800s that this examination became a scientific discipline.

Sometimes the terms growth and development are used together or interchangeably, but they have somewhat different meanings. Growth relates to an increase in physical size and includes changes in appearance and body functions. Growth is considered objective data, as it can be measured. For example, a newborn baby's weight and height can easily be measured.

Development is a process of gradual changes that take place. These changes range from the simple to the more complex. They are acquired from learning and growth. Development occurs in many different spheres: psychological, emotional, social, spiritual, as well as physical. Developmental changes are gradual and may be affected by many factors, so they are often more difficult to measure objectively.

We use the term developmental delays to describe when physical skills and behaviours expected at a particular point in an individual's life are not present.

We use the term maturation to describe the sequence of growth and development. You've probably heard someone use the word *mature* to refer to someone who is able to handle the challenges expected of him or her. However, maturity also refers to the ability of the nervous system to handle developmental tasks. For example, certain activity milestones require a particular level of brain and spinal cord development.

PRINCIPLES OF GROWTH AND DEVELOPMENT

There are seven commonly accepted principles of growth and development:

- Growth and development are continuous.
- Many factors affect a person's development: biology, lifestyle, access to nutrition, education, access to social and family supports, among others.
- People experience three types of changes: universal, group specific, and individual.
- Growth and development move from simple activities to complex activities.
- Physical growth and development occur in specific directions.
- Developmental milestones refer to an age range, rather than a specific age.
- Expectations of a person at a particular age or stage must be based upon factual information and not stereotypes.

We'll discuss these seven principles in this section.

Human Growth and Development Are Continuous They continue throughout the life span until death. One skill builds upon another and in turn makes further development possible. For example, a child learns to grasp a chubby pencil and then develops the skill to hold a regular pencil. Similarly, first the child scribbles, then prints, then writes.

Cognitive/emotional skills develop in the same manner. For example, the child learns to recognize another person's view. As the child develops, she becomes able to understand that a different point of view is not necessarily wrong. She also learns to identify similarities between her view and the view of another person. Using this as a base, she develops skill in problem solving when these differences must be resolved.

Your own learning bears this out. For example, you had to (or will have to) develop skill in assisting a person to transfer from a bed to a chair or into or out of a wheelchair, or help a person with limited use of his arm to dress. Chances are, you'll be much better at these tasks as you understand the procedure, as you practise the procedure, and as you gain confidence. The term life span perspective is used to describe this process.

Many Factors Affect a Person's Development Biology, nutrition, and education, among others. We can't measure growth and development by physical development alone. In fact, most physical growth is actually complete by the late teens. For example, you might notice that a parent and child act very much alike. You might attribute this to heredity (the traits and attributes inherited from parents). However, it's quite possible that the child *learned* the behaviour from the parent or someone else, and it is not caused by heredity at all.

An individual's personality (the psychological traits that each person has), life experiences, resources, coping mechanisms, and attitudes are major influences on the potential for human development.

A number of other factors influence a person's growth and development. The World Health Organization has identified factors that can affect a person's health. As Spotlight 6-1 on page 72 describes, these factors include things you might not think of as helping to determine a person's health.

STOP AND REFLECT 6-1

How do you think a person's development might be affected if:

- His family did not have enough money to feed him properly?
- He lived in an area where the air and water were heavily polluted?
- His parents were unable to care for him and he had to live with another family?
- His home was in an unsafe neighbourhood?
- He was physically abused?
- He was bullied by other children at school?
- He had to leave school at 16 to help support his family?
- He lost almost all his vision at 18 because of an inherited condition?

You might have found it difficult to respond to these statements without saying that the answer would depend upon a number of things. If so, you would be right. No single factor will determine a person's development. Development is the product of *many* factors.

CASE EXAMPLE 6-1

René Sylvester is 29. He has been legally blind for 10 years, and for the past two years has had no sight at all. This is due to an inherited condition. René knew at age 11 that he would eventually lose his sight. He began to prepare for the loss by developing skills that would let him use his memory, hearing, and other senses to make up for what his eyes could not provide. As a result, René has developed skills that most other people haven't and has gained confidence in his ability to function. He works full-time and lives with his wife and three small children.

In what ways do you think he has developed differently than he might have if he'd remained sighted?

Do you think you might have responded the same way, if you were in René's situation? How might you be different? How might your life?

SPOTLIGHT 6-1 HEALTH AND DEVELOPMENT— THE WORLD HEALTH ORGANIZATION'S VIEW

In Chapter 14, we discuss the World Health Organization's definition of health as "a state of complete physical, social, and mental well-being, not merely the absence of disease or infirmity." In this context, there is a clear link between what determines health and what determines "normal" growth and development. The World Health Organization identifies the following as determining a person's health. (WHO, *Health Impact Assessments, Determinants of Health, 2007*)

- Income and social status—Higher income and social status are linked to better health. The greater the gap between the richest and poorest people, the greater the differences in health.
- Education—Low education levels are linked with poor health, more stress and lower self-confidence.
- Physical Environment—Safe water and clean air; healthy workplaces; and safe houses, communities, and roads all contribute to good health.

- Employment and Working Conditions—People in employment are healthier, particularly those who have more control over their working conditions.
- Social Support Networks—Greater support from families, friends, and communities is linked to better health.
- Culture—Customs and traditions, and the beliefs of the family and community all affect health.
- Genetics—Inheritance plays a part in determining life span, healthiness, and the likelihood of developing certain illnesses.
- Personal Behaviour and Coping Skills—Balanced eating, keeping active, smoking, drinking, and how we deal with life's stresses and challenges all affect health.
- Health Services—Access and use of services that prevent and treat disease influences health.
- Gender—Men and women suffer from different types of diseases at different ages.

Let's apply this to a client situation.

CASE EXAMPLE 6-2

Mabel Sawyer is 74. She lives alone in a small one-bedroom apartment with a tiny refrigerator and a two-burner stove. She has osteoporosis, arthritis, and has recently been diagnosed with diet-controllable diabetes. A widow, she did not work at a job that provided a pension. Her husband's pension ended when he passed away five years ago. She lives on government pensions. She does not have a car and cannot usually afford taxis. She walks or takes the bus when she needs to go somewhere. She is saving money to have several teeth repaired, but will not have saved enough to have this done for another year or so.

Mrs. Sawyer is referred to a dietitian to help her plan meals that will help her control her diabetes. As they plan, they face the following challenges:

Income—Mrs. Sawyer has a very limited income. This affects several things: the amount and type of food she can purchase, her housing (with its limited food storage), how quickly she may have her teeth repaired, and her inability to take taxis. All these factors combine to make it harder for her to eat properly.

Physical Environment—Mrs. Sawyer lives on the second storey of a building that has no elevator. She must

carry her groceries to the bus and then up to her apartment. Her arthritis makes this especially painful and difficult. As a result, she often avoids foods that would be nutritious but are heavy to carry.

Social Supports—Mrs. Sawyer has no children and no close friends in the area. She has not used any support services. To this point, she has relied only on herself to meet her needs.

Health Services—Mrs. Sawyer says she was never one "to run to the doctor for every little thing." She remembers the time before medicare, when you paid for each doctor's visit. She also avoids medications, partly because she was "raised not to take pills" and partly because of their cost. As a result, she has often gone without treatment for her osteoporosis and arthritis, likely making it harder for her to do what she needs to do.

All these challenges make treating her health conditions difficult.

If you were a support worker assigned to assist Mrs. Sawyer, how might you be able to help her overcome these challenges?

People Experience Three General Types of Changes: Universal, Group Specific, and Individual. An individual's development is a function of all three.

Universal changes happen to everyone at a certain age or age range, but group-specific and individual changes may or may not happen at a specific time in a person's life. In fact, they may not happen at all.

Universal changes come from our biological makeup. For example, we know that all human beings eventually die—there is a finite *life span.* We also know that middle-aged adults experience sensory changes. Our ability to hear high frequencies diminishes, and we have trouble seeing well in low light.

It's important to note that though these changes do happen to everyone, they don't happen to everyone at the exact same age. In some cases, the range is narrow: we expect babies to learn to walk within a four-month range around age twelve months. In other cases, the range is wider: age-related changes in vision might occur over a five- to ten-year range.

Group-specific changes happen to people in specific groups in a particular setting or area, or subject to a specific historical event. For example, war brides (those marrying Canadian military men who were stationed in Europe during World War II) experienced a specific set of changes that other groups did not. They usually had no family or support system in Canada and had to adapt to a new country and new ways without that support. As a result, the members of this group—the war brides—developed somewhat differently than did women of the same age who were not members. The experience of First Nations people who were sent to residential schools is another example. Taken from their homes and ways of living when they were children, these individuals were placed in unfamiliar surroundings without any family support. The effect this experience had on them has lasted their entire lives.

We are all members of various groups. For example, we may belong to a political party or an ethnic or religious group. We will likely have different experiences as the result of our membership in that group. We may also experience changes because we belong to a group of people who share a particular characteristic, such as being a single parent or being a person who has a child with special needs or who has come to Canada from another country.

What types of group-specific changes do you think the individuals in the following case examples have experienced?

CASE EXAMPLE 6-3

Mrs. Dodor is 84. She lives in rural Saskatchewan. She was born and raised in England. In 1943, Mrs. Dodor met a Canadian serviceman stationed in England. After a two-week courtship, they married. She remained in England, living with her parents until 1944, when the Canadian government arranged for her to travel by ship to Canada. When Mrs. Dodor arrived, she travelled by train to Saskatchewan, where she lived with her husband's parents until he was discharged from the military. She had no friends or family in Canada. She tells you that it was hard to be alone, but she and her husband learned to love each other and to make a good life.

CASE EXAMPLE 6-4

Sheryl is the mother of triplet girls, born one month premature. She has found it hard to cope with so many babies at once. A group for parents of multiple births has helped her deal with some of the issues common to this group. Though she has much in common with the other parents, she feels a bit out of place, as she was 38 when her daughters were born, and seems to be almost 10 years older than the other moms in the group.

CASE EXAMPLE 6-5

Mr. Singh is 72 years old. His daughter was a financial analyst who died in the World Trade Center attack. He tells you that his life "stopped" on that day and hasn't been the same since. He has formed relationships with other families of victims and tells you that he finds comfort in these relationships. "We have all lost," he says. "Other people don't really understand fully."

Individual changes occur in specific situations and are generally unexpected. For example, a young child does not expect to experience the death of a parent. Similarly, a parent does not generally expect to outlive her children. An adolescent who receives a scholarship that enables him attend university—something he did not think was possible—will have different experiences and develop differently as a result.

Not all people will react the same way to a similar change. For example, different parents of triplets will respond to the pressures of a multiple birth in different ways and have different experiences. This is one of the reasons that development is so complex. How a person responds to these changes is a function of who she is, her personality, her resources, and previous experiences. Many, many factors make us who we are.

STOP AND REFLECT ((6-2))

What experiences have influenced who you are?

_____

_____

What universal changes have you experienced?

_____

_____

What group-specific changes have you experienced?

_____

_____

What individual changes?

_____

_____

How do you think that this has influenced who you are?

_____

_____

What other factors have played an important role?

_____

_____

Growth and Development Move from Simple Activities to Complex Activities

Have you ever heard the term "baby steps"? Perhaps you've heard someone say, "You have to learn to walk before you can run." These are both examples of this principle. Growth begins with the simple and moves to the more complex.

For example, a baby learns to hold his head up before he can attempt to sit unassisted. A child learns simple arithmetic before she proceeds to fractions and more complex mathematics.

As adults develop, they become more able to handle complex psychological tasks. The Harvard *Longitudinal Study on Aging* identified the following skills that are generally done best by older adults:

- Identity: a sense of one's own self and personal values; respect for where personal values end and social values begin
- Intimacy: the ability to form strong, nurturing relationships
- Generativity: the ability to share of oneself and to guide younger persons
- Integrity: acceptance of one's personal life cycle as having a beginning and an end. (*Longitudinal Study on Aging*, 2006)

Photo 6-1
An older adult works on a task with a teen.
Source: U.S. Department of Health & Human Services, Administration on Aging.

This progressive attainment of skills and abilities is often called making **developmental achievements** or attaining developmental tasks. We often use the term **psychomotor development** to describe the person's ability to sequence movements into purposeful groups.

Physical Growth and Development Occur in Specific Directions Growth and development proceed from the head to the toe and from the inner part of the body outward. One example of this is illustrated by the development of **motor skills** (the coordinated movements of the human body). For example, an infant's arms begin to develop before the fingers; **gross motor skill** (the movements of the body that primarily involve the body's large muscles) develops before **fine motor skill** (the delicate movements that involve fine muscles—such as those in the hand—and coordination).

Photo 6-2
Until the child's fine motor skill develops, he will find it easier to handle larger blocks. As he develops, he'll be able to manipulate smaller ones.
Source: Shutterstock

You might have noticed that a child's ability to use fingers for fine, detailed tasks (such as picking up small toy parts) develops later than the ability to grasp objects. This is an example of directional growth. A young child plays with large blocks, and then gradually develops the ability to manage smaller ones, as Photo 6-2 illustrates.

Developmental Milestones Refer to an Age Range, Rather than a Specific Age **Milestones** are described as the point at which particular events or behaviours are generally expected to occur. When we think of milestones, we often think of a specific point in time. However, the age range for some milestones may be measured in months or in years. Aging, growth, and development are all ongoing processes—nothing in this process happens to everyone at the same single point in time. For example, most babies will walk at around 12 months. However, some babies walk at ten months; others may not do so until 14 months or later.

You'll often hear descriptions of **stages**. Stages are periods of time in the human life span. For example, you might hear someone talk about infancy (the period between birth and 2 years of age) or of **adolescence** (the period from 12 to 19 years of age). Some stages are less age-specific. For example, "middle-age" may describe a person who is anywhere from 30 to 60 years of age, depending upon the perspective of the person.

STOP AND REFLECT ((6-3))

Your seven-month-old son requires a large pillow behind his back to sit up on the carpet. Your friend has a five-and-a-half-month-old baby boy who is already sitting independently and starting to crawl.

How does this make you feel?

_____

_____

What might you do?

_____

_____

> *Never trust anyone over 30.*
>
> Jerry Rubin

Expectations of a Person at a Particular Age or Stage Must Be Based Upon Factual Information and Not Stereotypes Perhaps you remember hearing the quotation above. At the time, Jerry Rubin was in his 20s. His comment was based upon a stereotype of people over 30 as controlling, conservative people who hated younger people—something that many researchers have disproved. Figure 6-1 describes some common stereotypes.

In Chapter 7, we discuss stereotypes. People hold stereotypes about many groups: women, men, children, members of ethnic communities, people who belong to a specific religion, economic group, or age group. Stereotypes about growth and development can dramatically affect how we treat a person and may well be harmful. For example, suppose a person said to a parent of a 12-month old, "There must be something wrong if she's not walking by now." This could affect how the person treats the infant, and possibly could affect how the parents interpret what the infant is able (or not able) to do.

Stereotypes may also affect the person him- or herself. The person who is constantly told that he is unable, or is treated in a way that reinforces that he is unable, may begin to believe that he actually is unable. Spotlight 6-2 illustrates the experience of a "new senior"—in her own words.

SPOTLIGHT 6-2 THE AT OUR AGE NOW CLUB

This is a portion of an essay submitted to the Ontario Advisory Council on Senior Citizens. The author is a woman in her 60s.

I have found that the glow of the Golden Age can be tarnished rather quickly. I emerged, flushed and expectant, into the after-sixty world. I was ready for all those things I always wanted to do and never had the time. I was unprepared for the push . . . into the Senior Citizen class. The deflation came not only from the attitude of younger, but middle-aged and older people as well. On the job, I drove the daily rush hour traffic and the weekend highway stream for thirty years. Now if I plan to go over twenty-five miles or if a few snowflakes appear, I hear concerned remarks, "Surely you're not going to drive. Why not take a bus or taxi?" Not the least among the discouragers were some of my contemporaries. I dubbed them the A.O.A.N. Club—At Our Age Now Club. Just when I had planned to master the Art of Living or felt inspired to live creatively, charged by the examples of Grandma Moses, Picasso, and Bernard Shaw, I ran into a member of this group. "What can we expect at our age now?" she lamented. One sparkling winter day that set me wondering if I could pick up cross-country skiing, since I was formerly a weekend skier of sorts, I met another one. "Well, don't you think, at our age now, we have to curtail our activities?"

THEORIES OF HUMAN DEVELOPMENT

Many theorists have attempted to describe human development. These theories can be grouped into general categories:

- Psychoanalytic theories
- Cognitive theories
- Multi-faceted theories

Each theory has its strengths and weaknesses. No one theory explains all aspects of human development. You'll likely find that one theory may help you to understand certain aspects of a person's development, while another theory helps you to understand other aspects.

Within each of the three general categories are two types of approaches: those that see development as a series of stages that must be completed in a set order, and those that see development as the result of tasks that a person may or may not have in a specific order at a specific time.

In this section, we'll discuss some of the better-known theories in each category.

"You can't teach an old dog new tricks"

"She's still wet behind the ears"

"He's old and set in his ways"

"Ahh...the enthusiasm of youth"

"Too young to understand"

Figure 6-1
Common stereotypes about various ages

Psychoanalytic Theories

Psychoanalytical theorists focused on the person's internal drive and emotion as the driving force behind a person's development. Sigmund Freud, Erik Erikson, and Abraham Maslow are among the best-known theorists in this group.

Sigmund Freud

Sigmund Freud was a behavioural scientist who explored how personality develops, how the human mind works, and how sexuality develops in humans. He is perhaps best known for his work describing the conscious and unconscious processes of the personality. Freud felt that a person's drive for pleasure was present at birth and is what motivates the person to develop. He identified phases of development that he called *psychosexual stages.* Under Freud's theory, childhood development determined whether or not the person would function in adulthood. Good development meant that a person became a well-functioning adult; poor childhood development led to problems as the person grew up.

Freud stated that personality has three aspects: the *id* (part of the brain that makes up a person's basic sexual and aggressive responses), the *ego* (the "thinking" element of personality), and the *superego* (the part responsible for moral development). Freud saw each aspect as playing a specific role in determining a person's behaviour.

Erik Erikson

Erik Erikson is known for his psychosocial theory that revolves around eight stages of the human lifespan: from infancy to old age. He felt that the person develops as the result of the interaction of internal drives and external demands. Each of his eight stages is represented by a "crisis" that the person must resolve. He strongly believed that "success" at each life stage included increasing independence and self-esteem for individuals and others. Erikson's stage theory is one of those often used today in health education.

Abraham Maslow

Abraham Maslow is probably the best known among the humanist theorists. Humanist theorists hold that a person's drive to achieve is the strongest motivator. Maslow saw development in terms of a person's drive to meet needs. He is best known for his *Hierarchy of Needs* (see Chapter 7, page 98), one of the best-known concepts in health care. Maslow felt that a person has needs that must be fulfilled before the person can meet other needs. He also felt that a person may move up and down the hierarchy, depending upon his or her circumstances at the time. Maslow's work has also been applied to management and organizational theory. We'll discuss Maslow in greater detail in Chapter 7.

Cognitive Theories

Jean Piaget

Most current researchers view cognitive theories as useful to explain some, but not all, aspects of human development. However, the work of one cognitive theorist, Jean Piaget, has been seen as useful in explaining how thinking may develop.

Piaget studied cognitive development. He was most concerned with how an individual develops his intelligence and thought processes. He believed that children increased their intelligence as they adapted to their environments. Thus, Piaget saw development less as internally driven and more as a result of interaction. Infants begin with identification of objects in their environments and then progress to mastering language skills. At about age six, the child begins to use logic and apply rules. When an individual is fully mature, he or she is able to think and reason in abstract terms and is able to predict specific outcomes.

Subsequent research has shown that the ages at which these changes occur are probably different than Piaget stated, and that the way in which the abilities develop is less global than he felt. Nonetheless, his theories provide a unique way of looking at how thinking develops.

STOP AND REFLECT 6-4

Think of a child you know well and have known since she or he was a toddler. Can you apply the concepts Piaget identified to the child (discussed in the section above)? Did some things happen earlier or later than Piaget described?

_____

_____

_____ ∎

Multi-Faceted Theories

Lev Vygotsky

Some of the more recent theorists have looked at the influence of interaction on human development. Canadian researchers have begun to look at the socio-cultural theory developed by Lev Vygotsky. While Vygotsky's work shares the interactive approach

Piaget used, he felt that a child's development was to be led by a guide: a more knowledgeable person, such as a parent, older sibling, or teacher. The guide would use an approach Piaget called *scaffolding*. In scaffolding, the guide is responsible to do three things: get the child's attention, demonstrate the skill to be learned, and structure the interaction to meet the child's needs so that the child can learn. For example, an adult might use this approach when helping a child learn to tie his shoelaces.

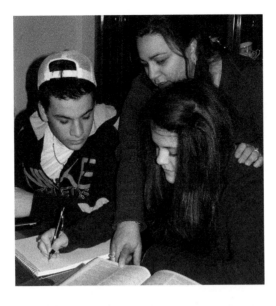

Photo 6-3
A parent guides her child's learning.

CASE EXAMPLE 6-6

Ndidi works with Jeremy, a seven-year-old with some developmental issues. As a part of her role, Ndidi is helping Jeremy learn to read simple books. She is careful to select a book of the appropriate reading level that interests Jeremy, so that she can get and keep his attention. Ndidi reads from the book (demonstrating), and then helps Jeremy sound out the sentences (structuring the interaction). With Ndidi's guidance, Jeremy learns to read the book.

STOP AND REFLECT 6-5

Recall a time you had to teach a person something or had to help him or her learn something. For example, you might have had to help your child learn a concept taught at school or help a friend learn to bake or sew; or you might have helped a client learn a skill. Recall that experience. Did you use the scaffolding approach Vygotsky described when you were teaching? If so, how did you:

Get the person's attention?

_____

_____

_____

Demonstrate the skill?

_____

_____

_____

Structure the interaction to help the person learn?

_____

_____

_____

Bronfenbrenner

Have you ever heard the phrase "It takes a village to raise a child"? In some ways, this phrase describes Bronfenbrenner's approach. Bronfenbrenner's Ecological Theory (Figure 6-2) focuses on development as a product of interactions between many factors: the person, his or her family, neighbourhood, community, society, beliefs and values, the environment, as well as the person him- or herself.

FIGURE 6-2
Bronfenbrenner's
Ecological Theory
Source: Copyright
Nicole A. Sage

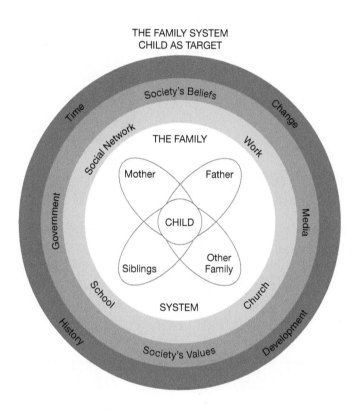

THE FAMILY SYSTEM
CHILD AS TARGET

Bronfenbrenner felt that an individual develops within a *context* or what he called an *ecology*. This ecology has three levels: the *microsystem*, the *mesosystem* and the *macrosystem*.

The earliest and most significant level is the microsystem. Within this system, there are many influences: those of the family and its culture, the local neighbourhood or community institutions such as school, religious institutions and peers.

The mesosystem describes work, social, and community influences upon the person. This includes the work "culture" and its expectations, the influence that school has upon a person, the influence of the broader community/society in which the person lives.

The third level is the macrosystem. It includes influence from the most distant sources: global issues, government, media, and general societal values.

While the macro level is the most intimate, all three levels may exert influences on the person—and that influence may be intense. For example, a person may be significantly influenced by a social issue such as poverty or discrimination, without having had personal experience with either.

Table 6-1   Developmental Tasks Commonly Associated with Age

Bear in mind that this table provides information about general milestones and patterns. Like any generalization, it is only a guide and will not accurately describe any one person. People grow and develop in response to many factors, not simply chronological age. For instance, a person's ability to eat properly, attend school, and have a sense of security will affect communication, psychosocial, and cognitive development to a far greater degree than will chronological age. Personality, access to resources, as well as any illness, impairment, or injury will all affect a person's development.

Stage	Major Tasks/ Milestones	Physical Changes	Motor Skills	Communication/ Language	Psychosocial Skills	Cognitive Development
Infancy (birth to one year) Chapter 21 covers this period in greater depth	Increasing gross and fine motor skills, which culminate in walking Feeding self and tolerating solid foods Communicating needs and wants with a few words or actions Sleeping and resting patterns become more stable Playing becomes a large part of infant's environment	Weight at six months double that at birth; weight at 12 months triple birth weight Length usually increases to at least 150 per cent of length at birth A newborn's head is large compared to the rest of the body	Rapid progression in gross and fine motor skills Holding head up by about four to six weeks of age Learns to roll over and sit	Initially communicates exclusively by crying By end of period, can communicate simple wants, approval or disapproval of specific things	Recognizes mother's face within the first few weeks Initially cannot recognize that a person is present, if not seen (e.g., behind the infant) By about seven or eight months of age, becomes distressed if primary caregiver leaves. Older infants smile and laugh frequently, particularly when they interact with others	Identifies impact of crying as signalling needs Explores environment by feeling, sucking on, and manipulating objects Usually likes to play simple games like "peek-a-boo" and "pat-a-cake"
Toddlerhood (1 to 3 years of age)	Communicating with short sentences and phrases	Extremities grow much faster than the trunk	Further development of gross and fine motor skills	Uses words and gestures to communicate needs	Can clearly indicate preferences, make simple decisions	Able to state her or his name and identify toys and body parts

Table 6-1 Developmental Tasks Commonly Associated with Age (continued)

Stage	Major Tasks/Milestones	Physical Changes	Motor Skills	Communication/Language	Psychosocial Skills	Cognitive Development
	Developing control of bowel and bladder functions Increasing independence of activities of daily living (toileting, feeding, dressing) Becoming less dependent on his primary caregiver	Toddler takes on a more proportioned appearance than in infancy Rate of head growth slows down compared to infancy	Able to climb stairs, kick a ball, and run A three-year-old can usually hop, stand on one foot, and walk several steps on tiptoe Feeding, dressing, and playing all illustrate fine motor skill development	Will point at things he or she wants Can say a few simple sentences or sing a simple song		Begins to learn the relationships between persons and things May be toilet trained or nearly toilet trained
Preschool (4 to 6 years)	Increasing use of language and communication skills Increasing independence in routine activities of living (toileting, feeding, dressing, bathing) Developing gross and fine motor skills Learning right from wrong	Extremities grow faster than the trunk Head size more proportionate to the body Muscles grow and strengthen, leading to more erect posture and less clumsiness. Require sleep/rest of 10 to 12 hours per night	Capable of running, skipping, catching a ball, and balancing on one leg Show interest in sports, dance, or other coordinated movement	Communicates first and last names, addresses, and telephone number Able to tell simple stories	Likes to try different roles and use active imagination Engages in many different structured and unstructured play activities Able to take turns, share, and follow rules or directions Becomes aware of sexual identity and is curious about the differences between female and male bodies	Learns by imitating others in her or his environment Active imagination may cause him or her to embellish or enhance stories Reasoning skills remain limited May overestimate physical skills

Table 6-1	Developmental Tasks Commonly Associated with Age (continued)					
Stage	Major Tasks/ Milestones	Physical Changes	Motor Skills	Communication/ Language	Psychosocial Skills	Cognitive Development
	Expanding social relationships by forming family ties and playing with others Learning more about his or her environment Play is an extremely important part of a preschooler's day					
School Age (6 to 12 years)	Growth remains stable and steady until puberty Muscular strength, coordination, and balance develop Moves from family relationships toward peer relationships Becomes less self-centred and more achievement-directed	Slow and steady physical growth; much more rapid at start of puberty Sex organ and secondary sex characteristics begin to develop	Significant improvement in gross and fine motor skills over previous stages Marked increase in muscle mass and strength Great deal of energy	Communicates effectively Generally able to solve conflicts by using words as opposed to crying and gestures	Able to act independently, but is still emotionally close to caregiver Able to gain satisfaction from accomplishments Responds best to positive reinforcement Privacy becomes important Begins to develop a sense of responsibility	Learns quickly about objects and her or his relationships to other objects and self Able to classify things in an orderly sequence and understand concepts of numbers, matter, length, area, width, volume and height In the later period, develops abstract thinking

Table 6-1	Developmental Tasks Commonly Associated with Age *(continued)*					
Stage	Major Tasks/ Milestones	Physical Changes	Motor Skills	Communication/ Language	Psychosocial Skills	Cognitive Development
	Learns basic skills such as reading, writing, and mathematics Develops a conscience and knows right from wrong Develops self-esteem				Develops concern for other living things	
Adolescence and Puberty (12 to 19 years)	Developing independence Dealing with changes in body and physical appearance and coming to term with their self-image Entering into appropriate male and female relationships Accepting increased responsibility at work, home, and school	Rapid physical growth, increase in height and weight, development of sex characteristics Girls usually begin their growth spurts earlier than boys Girls: ■ breast size increases ■ menstruation begins ■ pubic and axillary hair develop ■ fatty deposits contribute to the rounding of the hips	Gross motor capabilities improve and are comparable to that of adults Fine motor coordination also improves Some adolescents experience awkwardness or clumsiness as they learn to deal with increases in size and rapid growth	Vocabulary increases, language skills very close to that of an adult	In early phase, a time of deep emotions and reactions that vary from minimal to intense, and may change rapidly In later phase of stage, intense emotions usually subside Often a preoccupation with body image and attractiveness	Able to understand abstract concepts such as illness, death, and the future Can imagine a sequence of events and consequences Increasingly able to use reasoning and logic in forming opinions and decision-making, although not yet at adult level

Table 6-1   Developmental Tasks Commonly Associated with Age (*continued*)

Stage	Major Tasks/Milestones	Physical Changes	Motor Skills	Communication/Language	Psychosocial Skills	Cognitive Development
	Using appropriate behaviours to deal with issues related to family and members of the opposite sex Developing and testing values, beliefs, and attitudes	Boys: ■ voice deepens ■ facial, axillary(armpit), and pubic hair develop ■ muscle strength increases ■ shoulders and upper body develop Both sexes see an increase in sweat gland and oil gland activity				
Young Adulthood (20 to 40 years)	Starting careers or attending educational institutions Developing friendships and expanding social networks Finding a live-in partner or marrying Dealing with pregnancy and starting a family and home Finding ways for satisfactory intimacy or sexual expression	Physical growth is completed; body systems and organs are fully developed and are usually in peak functioning order	Good endurance, flexibility, and stamina Fine motor skills and coordination are at peak	Fully developed	Usually has established identity and lifestyle Learns to live and share with others in a domestic setting	Fully developed Able to accept other points of view Expresses opinions freely Uses information and learns to deal with conflicts

Table 6-1	Developmental Tasks Commonly Associated with Age *(continued)*					
Stage	**Major Tasks/ Milestones**	**Physical Changes**	**Motor Skills**	**Communication/ Language**	**Psychosocial Skills**	**Cognitive Development**
Middle Adulthood (40 to 65 years)	Adapting to varied energy levels and physical changes Maintaining healthy lifestyles and well-being Adjusting to new family roles with grown children, grandchildren, and elderly parents Making time for leisure activities Planning for second career or retirement options	Some loss of height Body fat tends to accumulate around the trunk of the body Skin becomes less elastic and wrinkles become more pronounced Muscle tone and strength decreases Bones become more porous Heart and lungs lose some capacity Hearing and visual acuity decline Increased likelihood of onset of a chronic condition	Energy levels and endurance decrease somewhat	Able to communicate appropriately with persons from different age groups Some verbal skills improve	Confidence with knowledge and experience Some review their lives to this point and make changes or take on different activities Adjusting to new family as children leave home or have families of their own is common Some will adapt to the demands of caring for their parents	Peak memory and mental abilities Most middle-aged adults are able to use past knowledge and experience to make appropriate decisions and may assist others in doing so
Young-old (65 to 75 years)	Adjusting to reduced physical strength and any chronic illness Adjusting to retirement or a second career Establishing new activities/sources of meaning	Progression of changes seen in middle adulthood	Gross and fine motor skills may diminish somewhat	Language skills remain intact	Adaptation to retirement, career changes May provide assistance to own parents, children, and grandchildren	Remains cognitively intact Benign forgetfulness occurs with all adults

Table 6-1	Developmental Tasks Commonly Associated with Age (*continued*)					
Stage	Major Tasks/ Milestones	Physical Changes	Motor Skills	Communication/ Language	Psychosocial Skills	Cognitive Development
Middle- to Old-Old (75 to 85 and beyond)	Identifying new ways of meeting needs and attaining life satisfaction when previous activities are no longer available	A continuation of the changes identified in middle adulthood	Stable unless affected by impairment or by effects of medications or treatment	Stable	Stable	Stable
	Adjusting to death of spouse/partner, siblings, or friends	Chronic conditions more often present				
	Conveying knowledge to others					
	Undertaking interdependent relationships					
	Developing a sense of generativity					
	Developing a sense of balance					
	Developing a perspective on one's own life and life cycle					

Developing Well

Humans are complex creatures and, as we've seen from this chapter, no one theory of development completely describes the processes by which we become who we are. As well, there is no one theory that tells us how to develop well—to become the best we can possibly be. Development is far more complex than any single set of "rules."

Development is also ongoing. We live—and develop—until we die. You are not exactly the same person you were five years ago; nor are you exactly the same as you will be five years from now.

Consider your own situation. Chances are, you learn every day. Perhaps you're reading this text because you're in school. If so, the course you are taking is providing you with new experiences, new information, and new ways of applying the information you already know. If you're reading this text for interest, you are also growing. This too, is development.

Though there is no one theory that tells us how to develop well, there are notions of what makes up a "good age." Spotlight 6.3 describes one researcher's criteria for aging well.

SPOTLIGHT 6-3 AGING WELL

Aging Well—Some Advice from the Harvard University *Study of Adult Development* (George E. Vaillant, M.D.)

- It is not the bad things that happen to us that doom us; it is the good people who happen to us at any age that facilitate enjoyable old age.

- Healing relationships are facilitated by a capacity for gratitude, for forgiveness, and for taking people inside. (By this metaphor I mean becoming eternally enriched by loving a particular person.)

- A good marriage at age 50 predicted positive aging at 80. But surprisingly, low cholesterol levels at age 50 did not.

- Alcohol abuse—unrelated to unhappy childhood—consistently predicted unsuccessful aging, in part because alcoholism damaged future social supports.

- Learning to play and create after retirement and learning to gain younger friends as we lose older ones add more to life's enjoyment than retirement income.

- Objective good physical health was less important to successful aging than subjective good health. By this I mean that it is all right to be ill as long as you do not feel sick.

Interesting, isn't it? These results clearly show the effect that many factors have on development. Our relationships with others and our ability to cope with changes have a significant effect on our ability to age well.

STOP AND REFLECT ((6-6))

Do you agree with Dr. Vaillant's advice?

_____

_____

_____

_____ ■

Share your ideas with your classmates.

Questions for Review

1. Why is it important for support workers to have an understanding of the factors that influence human growth and development?

2. How do physical changes involve growth?

3. Describe what development is and give an example.

4. Describe factors that may influence growth and development.

5. State the seven general principles of growth and development and give an example of each.

6. Identify developmental tasks that an adult will likely complete.

7. What are some milestones and events of infancy?

8. What are the major developmental milestones of toddlers?

9. According to the Harvard _Longitudinal Study of Aging_, what developmental tasks do older adults do well?

10. According to the Harvard University _Study of Adult Development_ (Spotlight 6-3), how can a person "age well"?

Questions for Discussion

1. What factors have influenced your own development? How have these factors shaped who you are today? What factors do you think will affect who you are as you age? Share your thoughts with your classmates. Where are your thoughts similar to your classmates? Where are they different?

2. Read over the six principles for aging well identified by the Harvard study. Relate them to your own life. Relate them to one of your older relatives or to a client. Do your experiences prove or disprove the six characteristics? Do the experiences of your older relative or your client prove or disprove them?

3. You are assisting the Smith family with household management and childcare while the mother is recovering from surgery. While their mother is resting, Emily, the two-year-old, grabs a favourite stuffed toy from her four-year-old brother, Adam. Adam begins crying and attempts to hit Emily, who now has the toy. Emily screams and runs with the toy.

   How do you respond to the two children? How does your knowledge of growth and development help you in dealing with this situation?

Chapter 7

The Client

Learning Objectives

Through reading this chapter, you'll be able to

1. Describe individuality.
2. Describe holistic as it applies to a person.
3. List the five major aspects that make each person's life unique.
4. Discuss the five needs most people have and, for each, describe common ways that people might meet these needs.
5. Describe the relationship between common roles people have and life satisfaction.
6. Tell what personal culture is and apply the concept to your life.
7. Identify support systems and the components of a support system.
8. Describe the usual responsibility a support worker has in helping to meet a client's needs.

Chapter at a Glance

- Individuality
- Holistic Approach
- Needs of the Individual
- Social Roles
- Culture
- Family and Other Members of the Client's Support System
- Applying What You've Learned About Yourself to Your Work with Clients

Terms You'll Use

Ethnicity A person's ethnic origin.

Holistic Approach A way of seeing all aspects of a person instead of just one.

Life Satisfaction Being content with our lives.

Need Something we must meet in order to survive or feel satisfied with our lives.

Personal Culture The mix of many factors, including ethnicity, religion, race, and experience, that make a person unique.

Personality The psychological traits that each person has.

Personhood The characteristics, attributes, and strengths of an individual.

Sexuality Our sense of ourselves as sexual beings.

Social Role Activities that are grouped together because of the expectations of a group or society.

INDIVIDUALITY

In order to be irreplaceable, one must always be different.

Coco Chanel

STOP AND REFLECT ((7-1))

Who are you?

_____

_____

How would you describe yourself as a person?

_____

_____

How would a friend describe you?

_____

_____

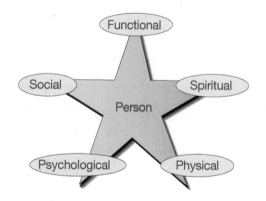

FIGURE 7-1
The personhood star

In Chapter 6, we discussed the various ways we develop. In this chapter, we'll look at how those factors combine to make us each a unique individual.

This chapter will examine what makes us individuals. We'll talk about what shapes our sense of **personhood**—the characteristics, attributes, and strengths that make us a unique individual (*Personhood: A Teaching Package*, Educational Centre for Aging and Health, McMaster University, 1993). Personhood includes five aspects of a person: the physical, psychological, spiritual, social, and functional (Figure 7-1).

The Physical Aspect

Take a look at your answers to Stop and Reflect 7-1. Did you first describe yourself in terms of being male or female, your age, your health or fitness, the colour of your hair, or other physical characteristics? Our physical characteristics play a significant role in how we define ourselves (Photo 7-1). Changes in health and body image can affect our sense of personhood. Some people's sense of personhood is affected by age.

The Psychological Aspect

The psychological aspect includes many things, including our personality, our patterns of behaviour, and our sexuality. You probably described some of these things when you described yourself on the previous page. We'll discuss each below.

STOP AND REFLECT ((7-2))

Have you ever experienced a change in your body image? Perhaps you broke a leg or arm and had to wear a cast, or had to wear an obvious bandage because of an injury or surgery.

_____

_____

Did you feel that this change affected how you saw yourself? Did this change affect how others saw you?

_____

_____

_____

Were there differences in these views? If there were differences, what were they?

_____

_____

_____

Sexuality

Sexuality refers to our sense of ourselves as sexual beings. It is an important part of our sense of personhood. We'll discuss sexuality in greater detail later in this chapter.

Personality

Personality refers to the psychological traits we have. For example, you might describe yourself as shy and quiet or outgoing and bubbly. You might say that another person is sweet or pleasant. These terms describe the traits that help to make us unique.

Like the other factors, personality is determined by our biology and how we have developed in relation to other people.

For example, you may know someone who lived through the Great Depression in the 1930s. Chances are that person's experience (what happened to the person and

how they coped with it) has had an effect on who that person is today. Similarly, a person who was raised in a strict, conservative manner is shaped by that experience. Bear in mind that the result is unique—it is not necessarily true that the same experience will have the same effect upon the person.

Photo 7-1
Our physical images form a part of our sense of personhood.
Source: Leisureworld Preferred Institute

STOP AND REFLECT)) 7-3))

Recall the discussion of life span development in Chapter 6. Consider your own life in light of the three types of events described by the life span development model—universal, group specific, and individual. In what way has each type of event affected you? For each type, identify the event and how it has helped shape who you are.

Age-Related Events (such as marrying at an older or younger age than was expected of you)

_____

_____

Historical Events (such as having a family member in Bosnia, or having lived through a flood or forest fire)

_____

_____

Unexpected Events (such as an accident or untimely death of a family member or close friend)

_____

_____

If you like, compare your answers with those of your colleagues.   ■

We do not see the whole person if we separate the person from her or his past. Consider the following essay in Exhibit 7-1.

Patterns of Behaviour

Have you ever travelled with another person? If so, did you find that the other person had very different ways of doing things? Perhaps you were a morning person and your travelling companion was a night owl. Perhaps you liked to plan events in advance and your companion preferred doing things on the spur of the moment. Our patterns of behaviour are how we go about doing things. These patterns are influenced by our personality. Because they are behaviours and are more readily seen by others, it's often easier to describe them than it is to describe personality traits. Think back to how you described yourself. You likely included some of your patterns of behaviour.

The Spiritual Aspect

The spiritual aspect (*spirituality*) includes the need for meaning or a purpose in life—hope. It can be defined as a part of oneself that is separate from the material world (Denton, 1999). Spirituality often includes, but is not limited to, religious beliefs. Keep in mind that holding religious beliefs or belonging to a particular religion is not essential to having a sense of spirituality. A person can be spiritual without being religious.

The Social Aspect

The social aspect is concerned with the way we are shaped by our relationships with others, such as family, colleagues, or other members of our community. The social aspect includes the roles we have (as a parent or a sibling, for example), as well as the concept of culture. These concepts will be discussed later in this chapter.

EXHIBIT 7-1
*Life span development
in the first person*

*Source: Are You
Listening?: Essays by
Ontario senior citizens on
what it means to be a senior.* © Queen's Printer for
Ontario 1989. Reproduced
with permission.

This essay is taken from Are You Listening? *It was written by Gladys C. Atkins,
an older adult.*

I am a senior citizen, but, as well, I am a person—the product of heredity, environment and of all the events of my life. The happiness, sorrows, achievements and
disappointments have given me the ability to see life with a clarity of perception
and appreciation not possible 50 years ago.

The beauty of a sunset, the flash of a hummingbird poised over a flower or the
smile of a child can move me to tears. But, on the other hand, the slights or hurts,
real or imagined, can wound more deeply than ever. I resent being ignored or
merely tolerated, left out of a conversation or disregarded by a waitress. It doesn't
happen often.

I love this beautiful world and have compassion (not pity) for its under-privileged,
perhaps because I remember the years of Depression. The social benefits which
seniors now enjoy compensate somewhat for the hard years and we should be
grateful. We are able to live in a dignified manner with a sense of independence.

I am, though widowed, fortunate to be in my own home, to drive my car and be able
to travel. My life might be compared to a river flowing along smoothly but with
undercurrents below the surface. Under the serenity of small-town life, family and
volunteer work, lies concern for personal, social, political and international
problems. The media keep me informed. I avoid self-pity and I do not worry for "to
worry is to pay interest on a loan before it is due." I strive "to have the serenity to
accept the things I cannot change, the courage to change the things I can, and the
wisdom to know the difference."

The future, in my view, holds great promise. Everywhere I see goodness and
kindness, especially in time of need. This far outweighs the adverse aspects of
crime, greed and so on. Our young people are enterprising, imaginative and innova-
tive far beyond my generation. Of course, their education and opportunities exceed
ours in the same proportion. Or so we like to think.

As the eddies surface on the river, so, in the silence of the night or in the darkest
hours before the dawn, a thought emerges in my mind. "I love this world but I must
leave it—perhaps soon." But I have lived and loved. I have children and grandchildren of whom I am very proud. Somewhere along the way I must have done some
good or left a pleasant memory. If so, I have not lived in vain. The future holds no fear.

The Functional Aspect

The functional aspect includes *how* we do the things we need to do. Our sense of self
is affected by our ability to perform as we prefer. If you have ever had to change your
activities because of an injury, you might have felt frustrated that your normal activities were impaired.

This aspect includes the ability to do things as a result of physical ability, cognitive
ability, psychological readiness, or opportunity. A person's function may be affected
just as significantly by anxiety or fear (psychological preparedness) as it might by a
physical barrier. Similarly, a person may be affected by a loss of opportunity that does
not allow the person to do what he or she wants. For example, an older person may
be able to and be interested in having a romantic relationship with another person but
not have the opportunity because of a lack of suitable persons, or because the person
is told that a romantic relationship is "inappropriate" at the person's age.

The functional aspect may be very significant to your clients. Your clients will likely
have experienced losses and changes that affect how they function. The emotions that
arise from not being able to do what the clients want to do can be very frustrating. Your

role as a support worker will require you to work with clients to help them cope with challenges to their functional aspect.

HOLISTIC APPROACH

A **holistic approach** requires us to see all aspects of a person, not just one or two. You are practising a holistic approach when you take the time to learn about your client as a whole person—a unique individual who is not just a diagnosis, an old person, or a disabled person. The poem in Exhibit 7-2 illustrates this concept.

EXHIBIT 7-2

The Crabbit Old Woman, author unknown

The Crabbit Old Woman

The Crabbit Old Woman
What do you see?
What are you thinking when you are looking at me?
A crabbit old woman not very wise
Uncertain of habit with far away eyes
Who dribbles her food and makes no reply,
When you say in a loud voice 'I do wish you'd try'
Who seems not to notice the things that you do
And forever is losing a stocking or shoe
Who, unresisting or not, lets you do as you will
With bathing and feeding the long day to fill
Is that what you're thinking? Is that what you see?
Then open your eyes nurse,
You're not looking at me.

I'll tell you who I am as I sit here so still
As I use at your bidding, as I eat at your will.
I'm a small child of ten with a father and mother
Brothers and sisters who love one another,
A young girl of sixteen with wings on her feet,
Dreaming that soon now a lover she'll meet:
A bride soon at twenty my heart gives a leap
Remembering the vows that I promised to keep:

At twenty-five now I have young of my own
Who need me to build a secure and happy home.
A young woman of thirty my young now grow fast
Bound to each other with ties that should last:
At forty my young ones now grown will soon be gone
But my man stays beside me to see I don't mourn
At fifty once more babies play round my knee,
Again we know children my loved one and me,

Dark days are upon me, my husband is dead
I look at the future I shudder with dread
For my young ones are all busy rearing young of their own,
And I think of the years and the love I have known
I'm an old woman now and nature is cruel
'Tis her jest to make me age like a fool
The body it crumbles, grace and vigour depart,
There now is a stone where I once had a heart:
But inside this old carcass a young girl still dwells,
And now and again my battered heart swells,
I remember the joys, I remember the pain,
And I'm loving and living my life over again
I think of the years all too few — gone too fast,
And accept the stark fact that nothing can last

So open your eyes, open and see,
Not a crabbit old woman
look closer—see ME.

NEEDS OF THE INDIVIDUAL

A **need** is something we must meet in order to survive or to feel satisfied with life. We all have the same range of needs, but the priority (that is, how important a particular need is) may vary over time and from situation to situation.

Abraham Maslow is a well-recognized researcher on needs. His *Hierarchy of Needs* provides a useful way of examining common needs. It categorizes needs into five groups: physical needs, safety and security needs, social needs, esteem needs, and self-fulfillment needs (see Figure 7-2). Here, we have adapted Maslow's hierarchy to include some examples of the needs in each of his categories.

Physical Needs

Physical needs are those needs essential to our survival. Air, food, and water are clearly linked to our survival. At first glance, the link between touch and reproduction and survival may seem less clear. Let's examine these needs more closely.

The need for *touch* has been well documented in research. In fact, studies have shown that infant primates (high-functioning mammals who share many characteristics with humans) who are not touched often die before they reach the age of one year.

How, where, and by whom a person prefers to be touched is highly individual (Photo 7-2). You should not assume that all clients prefer to be touched in the same way, or that they appreciate touch from you. Preferences for touch differ from one person to another and are heavily influenced by our *personal culture.*

Biologists have identified that the need to *reproduce* is essential to ensure that the species does not become extinct. This does not mean that every person is equally driven to reproduce. Rather, the intensity of this need, like that of touch, differs from person to person. It is, however, essential if the human race is to survive.

Photo 7-2
Touch is an important need. Still, you must be careful to respect a person's wishes for how he or she prefers to be touched.
Source: CHATS

Security and Safety Needs

Security and safety may seem to mean the same things. They do not. Safety refers to the need to *be* safe. Security refers to the need to *feel* safe. For example, if you are riding on a roller coaster, you might not feel secure, even though you are safe.

Included in this group are needs that contribute to feeling secure: stability, territoriality, and privacy. Stability refers to the need for things to be predictable and known. Territoriality refers to the need to have one's own space. The need for privacy refers to the need to keep personal business private.

Social Needs

Social needs are those needs that are met through communicating with, and being accepted by, others. Meeting social needs makes us feel less alone and more a part of a community. The need to be recognized by others as a sexual being is a part of the need to be accepted. The need for intimacy refers to a particular kind of closeness that requires acceptance, communication, and a sense of belonging. The concept of interdependence—the reliance we all have upon others for some things—is a social need.

FIGURE 7-2
Human needs

Maslow's Hierarchy of Needs (Adapted)

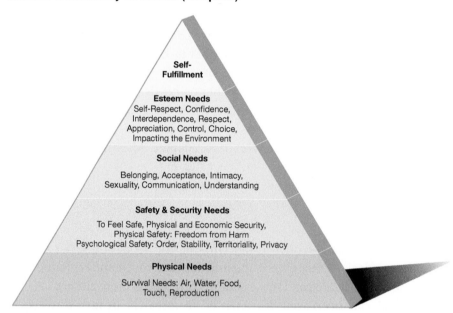

Esteem Needs

Esteem needs are needs that are met through one's activities with others. These needs are met in two ways: through the response of others to how we perform activities, and through the personal satisfaction we get from doing them. One example of this is the need to make choices in one's life. We can meet esteem needs when we have the opportunity to make choices and have the satisfaction of making choices in a way that satisfies us (e.g., making the "right" choice).

Self-Fulfillment

Self-fulfillment means attaining a goal one sets for oneself. Unlike social and esteem needs, self-fulfillment is met primarily through the person's own measure of his or her own activities. For example, only you know whether you have tried your best at a task.

Attaining one's potential is very much a personal thing. Only you can set your personal goals and know when you have put your best efforts toward achieving them.

STOP AND REFLECT

Imagine that you are on holidays with friends. Look at Figure 7-2 above. What needs would be most important to you?

Now, imagine that you have been robbed while on this holiday. Though you are physically unhurt, your car has been broken into and all of your possessions have been ransacked. Some items of sentimental as well as monetary value have been taken. Look again at Figure 7-2. What needs are most important to you now? Are these needs the same as those you identified above?

_____

_____

_____

_____

_____

In the first instance, you probably identified needs like belonging, acceptance, or perhaps self-fulfillment. In the second instance, you might have identified safety or security.

SOCIAL ROLES

Social roles are activities that are grouped together because of the expectations of a group or of society. For example, the role of mother includes the things that society expects of mothers, such as caring for their children, providing guidance, and providing a stable home environment. In turn, these expectations help us to know what we need to do in order to fulfill the role—to be "moms."

We hold many roles throughout life (Photo 7-3). Recall your answers to Stop and Reflect 7-1 on page 92. You likely included such roles as parent, worker, friend, or spouse. Table 7-1 describes some of the roles we may have over our lifetime.

As we age, we discard some roles and take on others. Sometimes, the activities associated with a role change as we grow older. For example, your role as a child changes as you grow up. You might discard a role because you can no longer do it. For example, your role of child will end when your parents die. Similarly, you may take on new roles, such as that of grandparent or of your family's breadwinner.

Some roles change because society changes its expectations of the role. For example, the role of mother is different today than it was 50 years ago.

Photo 7-3
We all have many roles: worker, consumer, family member.

TABLE 7-1	Common Social Roles	
Worker	Handy Person	Comic/Jokester
Grandparent	Attractive Dresser	Leader
Consumer/Buyer	Cook	Organizer
Religious Person	Student	Decision Maker
Friend	Gourmet	Singer
Sister/Brother	Gift Giver	Sports Fan/Spectator
Citizen	Boss	Musician
Lover	Supporter	Breadwinner
Voter	Helper	Hunter
Spouse	Traveller	Head of Household
Homemaker	Advice Giver	Child
Significant Other	Athlete	Stimulator/Idea Generator
Mother/Father	Expert	Problem Solver
Attractive Person	Game Player	Master of My Own Destiny
Hostess/Host	Reader	
Dancer	Group Member	

Roles and Life Satisfaction

Roles provide us a way of meeting our needs. Fulfilling roles can cause us to be accepted and respected by others and to have a sense of self-fulfillment through accomplishing a personal goal. Through this process, we can attain life satisfaction, or being content with our lives.

STOP AND REFLECT ((**7-5**))

Look over the roles listed in Table 7-1. What roles do you have now?

_____

_____

_____

Which roles are most important to you?

_____

_____

_____

Sexuality

As we discussed earlier in this chapter, sexuality is the term we use to describe ourselves as sexual beings. Often, people assume that sexuality means sexual activity. This is only partly true. You likely noticed that Maslow's *Hierarchy of Needs* included sexuality and that Table 7-1 included "attractive person" in the list of roles. Though sexuality includes sexual activity, it also includes how we see ourselves as male or female, the qualities we desire in ourselves as a man or woman and how much we feel that we possess those qualities.

Part of our sexuality is rooted in biology—we are born with it. Other aspects of our sexuality are learned from others. From the time we are born, people treat us as boys or girls. As a society, we still often identify roles or activities as masculine or feminine. For example, you may still hear people refer to a nurse who is a man as a "male nurse." Sex roles can and do change over time, as society changes its concept of what is inherently "male" or "female."

Social concepts also influence what people see as desirable. Research suggests that people who are part of a culture that respects people's right to express themselves as sexual beings throughout the life span tend to view themselves as sexual beings throughout life. Members of cultures that emphasize the desirability of a particular age group are more likely to reflect the culture's view. For example, North American culture is seen as emphasizing the desirability of youth: young people, specific body types, smooth, unwrinkled skin. A person who is older, or has wrinkles or sees him- or herself as having a less than ideal body type may feel less attractive or desirable.

Others' stereotypes about age and impairment can also affect one's sexuality. For example, some people may assume that a person using a wheelchair is not attractive or even that the person does not have sexual feelings. Similarly, an older person may be seen as sexless. Neither of these assumptions is valid.

Some people may view older adults' sexuality in a way that is very similar to thinking about their parents' sexual activity. They may be uncomfortable seeing older adults as sexual beings because they have difficulty seeing their parents in this way. It may cause the person to treat an older person differently or even to indicate disapproval of the elder's actions.

STOP AND REFLECT ((7-6))

How might you define your own sexuality? What does it mean to you? How do you express it? Are there times when others seem not to respect your sexual identity? When? How does this make you feel?

_____

_____

_____

_____

_____

Supporting the Person's Sexuality

Others' opinions or comments about sexuality may affect how a person sees himself or herself as a sexual being. Consider the following case example.

CASE EXAMPLE 7-1

Nimmi's client is Mrs. Guiterrez, an 88-year-old woman. Today, Nimmi and her client are shopping for a dress for the client to wear to her granddaughter's wedding. Mrs. Guiterrez has tried on several dresses, but none so far seem to suit her. You are just bringing another dress to the dressing room when a sales clerk says to you. "She's old. Who cares what she looks like? She should just wear something comfortable." You know that Mrs. Guiterrez overheard the sales clerk's comment.

How do you think Mrs. Guiterrez might feel?

Do you think it would affect her interest in finding a dress?

How do you feel about the sales clerk's comments?

Do you think that the sales clerk intended any harm by her comment?

Would you say or do anything in response? Why or why not?

As a support worker, your approach and responses may have significant effect upon your client's sense of sexuality. As Chapter 8 discusses, the nature of your relationship may cause the client to give more weight to your comments. The following seven guidelines will help you to demonstrate respect for the client's sense of sexuality:

1. **Show the client that you know that attractiveness includes a person's physical being as well as his or her psychological being.** What makes a person interesting and attractive is not limited to the person's physical condition or how he or she dresses.

2. **Respect the client's boundaries with regard to what you say and how you say it.** Some clients may not appreciate a comment about their appearance or attractiveness. Others may ask your opinion. Make certain to learn and respect the client's boundaries.

3. **Respect the client's relationships with other people.** Avoid trivializing or teasing the client about a relationship. You may have heard someone "tease" a client about

having a "boyfriend" or "girlfriend" in a way that makes the client feel uncomfortable. These comments often have a way of making the client feel as though any relationship (romantic or not) is inappropriate. They also invade the client's privacy. As with people of all ages, relationships between persons may be intimate or platonic. The people involved have a right to relationships without having to endure comments by others.

4. **Assist the client to dress or groom in the way he or she prefers.** A client may want to dress in a certain way or to wear makeup or jewellery. Assist your client to do so.

5. **Encourage a client who needs support to feel attractive.** A client may feel that it's no longer "worth it," that "no one cares how I look." Support your client's sense of self-worth and attractiveness. Be certain that any comment you make is both genuine and sensitive to the person's needs.

6. **Respect a client's right to privacy in relationships, whether intimate or not.** In most cases, you will not need to be involved in a client's relationships, beyond knowledge that the relationships exist. Respect your client's boundaries with regard to discussing personal relationships.

> *We see what is behind our eyes.*
>
> Chinese proverb

7. **Speak up if others make inappropriate comments about a client's sexuality.** It's important to let others know that you don't agree that it's acceptable to make these types of comments. Do so respectfully, however.

CULTURE

What Is Culture?

Culture refers to the patterns of learned behaviours that are shared among members of a group. Anthropologists Kevin Avruch and Peter Black explain the influence of culture this way: "One's own culture provides the 'lens' through which we view the world; the 'logic'... by which we order it; the 'grammar'... by which it makes sense." (Avruch and Black, 1993)

In a very real way, our personal culture shapes how we see the world and how we interpret others, their words, and their actions.

You may hear people speak of the "Italian culture" or the "Chinese culture." These are usually references to ethnic practices or influences. Many people assume that culture is the same as ethnicity. It is not. Culture is a very complex issue. Culture includes many things: ethnicity, language, religion/spiritual beliefs, race, gender, age, sexual orientation, geographic origin, education, upbringing, life experiences, and rites of passage. **Ethnicity** refers to a person's nation of origin. Figure 7-3 illustrates a number of aspects that may make up a particular individual's culture.

Personal culture refers to the way in which culture affects the individual, given the individual's personality. Personal culture is the result of the way in which the individual relates to and balances the demands of his or her culture (Figure 7-3). For example, second-generation Canadians may have to balance the demands of their ancestral cultures with their current cultures.

Significant Relationships • Age • Values and Beliefs
Geographic Origin   Rites of Passage
Life Experiences   Language
Education   Gender
Religion   Family
Ethnicity   Race

FIGURE 7-3 *Many aspects can make up one's personal culture.*

STOP AND REFLECT ((7-7))

What is your personal culture? Examine the aspects of personal culture identified in this section.

Which of these have most influenced you?

_____

_____

In what way did these aspects influence you?

_____

_____

Have you had any "cross-cultural" interactions—for example, marrying into another religious or ethnic group, or working with people who have different backgrounds? If so, how did you learn about the other culture? How did you share your culture with the others?

_____

_____

_____

The Dangers of Stereotyping

A *stereotype* is a fixed set of ideas or assumptions about a group of people. For example, many people have stereotypes about older adults, or about people from an ethnic group, religion, or race. We often stereotype by sex, calling certain jobs "women's work" or "men's work." Stereotypes are dangerous because they can cause a person to forget that everyone is a product of her or his own personal culture.

Stereotypes can often make it harder to get to know an individual. They can lead to misunderstandings that may make both parties uncomfortable. As a support worker, you must be careful to examine the beliefs you have about people to make sure that you do not hold stereotypes. When working with clients, you must always focus on the client's personal culture.

STOP AND REFLECT ((7-8))

What stereotypes have you encountered? Has anyone made assumptions about you because you were a man or a woman, or because of your age, or how you looked?

_____

_____

_____

If so, how did you feel?

_____

_____

Share your answers with your colleagues. In what ways were your experiences and feelings similar?

_____

_____

_____

Working with People from Different Cultures

We are all different from other people because each of us has a unique personal culture. In some cases, these differences do not significantly affect how we work together with other people. In other cases, the differences are significant and make working together a challenge. This can be because there are a number of differences or because a single aspect (for example, language) is very different.

You might have expected this passage on culture to include a list of characteristics considered to be common to particular groups. There's a good reason why you won't find lists like those here: they might be as misleading as they could be helpful, as they can promote stereotypes or simply make it harder to get to know the person as a person. We can make some general statements about the types of things people may see differently as the result of the culture in which they live.

Communication Styles Patterns of verbal and nonverbal communication, how decisions are made, and ways of problem solving are often specific to a particular culture.

Significance of Life Events and the Life Course Some cultures may see a life event as a response to something done earlier in life. For example, an illness may be seen as the result of the way a person lived earlier in life, even if there is no biological link.

Significance of Time and Activity In some cultures, tasks are the first priority and are expected to be done quickly. Other cultures value the relationships involved in doing a task more than the task, and have less emphasis on a rapid pace.

Different Attitudes Toward Disclosing Some cultures are very open about personal issues. Others are very closed and may even see the sharing of a personal issue as bringing shame upon the person or family. These differences can also affect a person's use of health care or support services.

As a support worker, you must work with clients to make sure that you develop the best working relationship possible. In order to do this, you must have the knowledge, skills, and attitudes necessary to address cultural differences. We'll examine each in this section.

SPOTLIGHT 7-1 FUNDAMENTAL QUALITIES

Awareness of your own values, cultural biases, and stereotypes and how they might affect the way you work with the client

Acceptance that there are many different ways of communicating or doing things

Openness and willingness to learn about a client's practices and beliefs as they relate to the support provided

Sensitivity to different methods of communicating, problem solving, and handling conflict

Respect for client boundaries and for what is taboo or inappropriate

Attitudes

In order to work effectively with people whose culture differs from yours, you will need to be aware of your own values, cultural biases, and stereotypes and how these may affect your work with clients. For example, if you were raised to believe that family members should care for an older adult, you may find it difficult to work with a client whose family does not share in the client's support. If you are not aware of the effect your belief might have on the support you provide, you might unknowingly behave in a manner that indicates you disapprove of the family's decision.

Several other attitudes are useful. As you saw above, you must be *open* to examining (and possibly changing) your own views. You must be *sensitive* to any differences and *respect* your client's preferences and practices, no matter how different they may be. Finally, you must be *flexible* so that you may adapt your approach to best support the client.

Knowledge

You'll need to learn about your client's significant cultural practices and beliefs. If your client speaks a different language, you should learn words and phrases in the client's language. (If you have ever been in a country where no one spoke your language, you'll have a sense of how wonderful it is when you hear words in your own language.)

As you learn about your client's practices, remember that he or she has a personal culture. Your client's practices may not be the same as other members of his or her religion or ethnic group. Learn from your client and your client's family.

Some specific techniques you might use include the following:

1. Showing interest in the client's foods, dress, and other habits. For example, you might ask the client for favourite recipes and then prepare them.
2. Respecting the client's values, beliefs, attitudes, traditions, and rituals.
3. Encouraging the client to tell you about his or her culture. You may share information about your culture if it helps clients to tell you about theirs.
4. Asking family members for information, if appropriate.

It is sometimes helpful to read about the client's culture. If you do, keep in mind that the person may not hold all the beliefs or values or take part in all the rituals and traditions that are considered to be a part of the overall culture. Always verify this information with your client.

Personal culture is just that—personal. Your client's personal culture will reflect a wide range of influences. The following questions should help you support the client more effectively. You'll need to balance your need to understand the client's personal culture with the client's right to privacy.

What language does the client speak? If it is not one you also speak, can you learn some basic phrases or find another way of reliably communicating?

How does the client feel about needing support? Does the client feel that it is an embarrassment or the result of a previous activity?

How does the client indicate approval, discomfort, or disapproval? You might learn these things only through observation as you work with the client.

Does the client have specific practices or ways of doing things?

FAMILY AND OTHER MEMBERS OF THE CLIENT'S SUPPORT SYSTEM

What Is a Support System?

A support system is the network of people upon whom we rely to help us meet our needs. Have you ever heard the saying "No man is an island"? We all have support systems to help us. Most of us are part of one or more support systems that help others.

STOP AND REFLECT 7-9

Various types of support are listed below. Read over each type, thinking carefully about the sources you have for each. Sources can include your family, friends, or people you know through your work or your participation in organizations, community services, or agencies.

Type of Support	Source(s)

Admiration

Who praises me, gives attention to me, or shows an interest in me?

Satisfaction

Who expresses pleasure at what I give to or do for them?

Love

Who cares for me, gives me affection?

Physical intimacy

With whom are you able to be physically intimate?

Type of Support	Source(s)
Companionship With whom do I share activities or have a sense of belonging or togetherness?	
Encouragement Who gives me emotional support and reinforcement, and expresses confidence in me?	
Acceptance Who gives me respect, has empathy for me, trusts me, understands me, and is a good listener for me?	
Comfort Who reassures me, is someone I can rely upon?	
Example Who is my role model or mentor?	
Guidance Who gives me advice, direction, or spiritual help?	
Help Who gives me material assistance, does things for me?	
Knowledge Who shares expertise with me, gives me information, or teaches me things?	
Honesty Upon whom can I rely for honest feedback, to be a sounding board for my thoughts?	

Take a look at your answers. Who does your support system include? Does one person provide more support to you than the others? You likely listed family and friends in your support system. You may have listed some people many times and other people only once. If you compare your answers to those of your colleagues, you will probably find that their support systems are different from yours.

Each of your clients has a unique support system. Like yours, it may be made up of a combination of family members, friends, and others. Who provides each type of support may differ, as may the total number of people involved in the system.

We often think of the client's family as the client's support system. Though family members commonly make up an individual client's support system, there may be other people to whom the client is close and who provide support. Some clients have no living family or no family who live nearby. Their support systems may be made up of friends or neighbours. You must remember that one client may be just as close to a friend or neighbour as another client may be to a spouse or child.

CASE EXAMPLE 7-2

Mrs. Antonov is an 80-year-old widow and retired farmer. Since 1960, she has lived on a farm outside Regina. She has two daughters, both of whom live in Ontario. Mrs. Antonov has four very close friends who live in her community.

Mrs. Antonov's support system is made up of her family, her friends, and other people from her community. For example, she relies upon her friends for social support and emotional support. However, when Mrs. Antonov was approached to sell her farm, she sought the advice of her daughters.

Mrs. Antonov provides support to her friends and family. She provided advice when her grandson was thinking of buying a farm. Now that her broken arm has mended, she volunteers to bring meals to members of her church who cannot cook for themselves.

When Mrs. Antonov broke her arm last year, her friends brought meals and helped with her housekeeping. A member of Mrs. Antonov's church cut her lawn. Her daughters were not able to visit but kept in contact in order to provide emotional support.

> Who makes up Mrs. Antonov's support system? What kinds of help does each member provide? Did you notice that Mrs. Antonov is part of other support systems?

STOP AND REFLECT 7-10

Whom do you support? Pick three people (other than clients) to whom you provide some kind of support. Then, complete the table below.

My relationship to the person	Person # 1	Person #2	Person #3
I provide this kind of support to the person			
How emotionally close to this person am I?			
How geographically close to this person am I?			

What did you learn about the support you provide? Do you always have to live near the person to be emotionally close to them? Are you related to all three people you listed? Are you closer to some friends than to some relatives? Do you provide support to people who also provide support to you?

Working with a Client's Support System

The support team we discussed in Chapter 5 usually becomes part of the client's overall support system. It's important to remember that the support team does not replace the client's support system. It simply makes the system a bit larger and adds more resources to assist the client. Consider the following situation.

CASE EXAMPLE 7-3

Mr. Rampersaud came to Canada in 1994, after his wife died. His six children all live in Canada and all had asked Mr. Rampersaud to move in with them, as it is considered a blessing in their culture to provide one's children the opportunity to learn from an elder. Mr. Rampersaud asked his children to decide with whom he would live, as he did not want to cause hard feelings.

The children met and decided that Mr. Rampersaud would live with his youngest son and daughter-in-law. The family also decided that the daughter-in-law would take a leave of absence from work to help Mr. Rampersaud move and become settled. His daughter-in-law has helped Mr. Rampersaud find a doctor and

receive health care. Mr. Rampersaud takes part in family activities and helps around the house. When a problem arises in the family, Mr. Rampersaud asks his eldest son to help resolve it.

Mr. Rampersaud is looking forward to spending the summer with his eldest daughter, her husband, and family, who live in Vancouver. He regularly talks with his other children by phone and often visits his eldest son, who lives nearby.

What kinds of support do Mr. Rampersaud's children provide? What kinds of support do you think a support worker might provide to Mr. Rampersaud?

Each client's support system has a unique way of working. This pattern is usually established over a number of years. It may be handed down from generation to generation. For example, some support systems are traditionally led by the eldest male of the family. The eldest female leads others. The members of one system may discuss things openly. The members of another support system may not.

Remember, your client's support system may not work the way your own support system works. You must always respect the way the client's system works, even if it is not the way you would like it. Because the client's support system becomes part of the overall support team, it is important to find a way of working together that allows everyone to provide the best support possible to the client.

CASE EXAMPLE 7-4

Mrs. Jukas uses home support services. Susan is her support worker. Susan comes from a family where members openly stated their opinions and ideas.

Susan's client is very different. Mrs. Jukas has always been uncomfortable stating her own opinions and ideas. She has always relied upon her eldest daughter to speak for her.

When she was first assigned to Mrs. Jukas, Susan found it difficult to adapt to Mrs. Jukas's way of communicating her preferences. She felt a bit hurt that Mrs. Jukas was not comfortable enough with her to speak openly.

Susan mentioned her concern to Mrs. Jukas's daughter. The daughter explained to Susan that Mrs. Jukas has always communicated in this way. She told Susan that her mother had always deferred to her husband when he was alive. "Once Dad died, Mom simply started relying upon me to do what Dad did," the daughter said. Susan then recognized that she must adapt to Mrs. Jukas's communication style, even though it is not the way Susan would communicate.

Consider your support system. Do some members communicate differently than others?

APPLYING WHAT YOU'VE LEARNED ABOUT YOURSELF TO YOUR WORK WITH CLIENTS

In many ways, the same types of things that affect you affect your client. Each person will respond differently to the same situation. Take a moment to complete Stop and Reflect 7-11.

STOP AND REFLECT ((7-11))

Talk to a person whom you know well, who is at least 20 years older than you are.

Are there events (such as wars, deaths, successful careers) in the person's life that have shaped him or her? If so, how?

_____

_____

_____

Were there events in the person's personal life that were unusual (such as the loss of a parent at an early age, an early or late marriage, or the loss of a child)? How did these shape the person?

_____

_____

_____

What sorts of roles has the person had over time? What roles have been most satisfying to the person? What meaning did the person attach to changes in roles? What roles does the person see himself or herself as having now?

_____

_____

_____

How does the person describe himself or herself?

_____

_____

_____

What sorts of things make up the person's personal culture? How has that culture shaped the person?

_____

_____

_____

If the person had the opportunity, would she or he choose to be 18 years old again? Why or why not?

_____

_____

_____

Pay attention to your responses to the person's comments. How do the person's comments change your perception of him or her?

_____

_____

_____

Questions for Review

1. How would you describe yourself in terms of the five aspects of a person that were discussed in the chapter?

2. Review the Hierarchy of Needs. What needs are most important to you? How do you meet these needs?

3. Speak with a colleague. What roles give him or her satisfaction in life? What makes these roles so satisfying?

4. What is a holistic approach? How does it relate to the aspects of a person that were discussed in this chapter?

5. What is sexuality? What seven things can you do to support a client's sense of sexuality?

6. What is culture? What are four fundamental qualities for learning about a client's culture?

Questions for Discussion

1. How would you define yourself in terms of your culture? Compare your responses with those of your colleagues. Look for similarities and differences in your responses. Are you and your colleagues more or less alike than you thought?

2. Most families have traditions around major life events. What are the traditions that your family has when a family member gets married? Compare your traditions with those of your colleagues. In what ways are your traditions similar? In what ways are they different?

3. Read over the following case study. Respond to the questions at the end.

Jessica Wieldon is a new client. She is 39 years of age. Three months ago she was seriously injured in a car accident that killed her husband and injured her two children. Mrs. Wieldon has just returned home from a rehabilitation hospital. Her leg is in a cast and has several pins holding it secure. She can move around the house in a wheelchair but cannot get up and down the stairs. As a result, her bedroom has been moved to the first floor. Mrs. Wieldon's children are being cared for by her husband's parents. The children have largely recovered from their injuries, but are still dealing with the loss of their father.

Mrs. Wieldon is currently on leave from her job as a bank manager. You are aware that she was well respected in her job and that she took pride in getting things done for her customers. She is a detail-oriented person, always the one who makes sure that loose ends are tied up and that everything required is done perfectly. She has been active in her children's school and on a local recreation committee. You are also aware that she has had to stop all activities in order to recover.

Mrs. Wieldon has a devoted family (one sister and one brother) in addition to her husband's parents. She also has a small circle of close friends, many of whom have offered help. You, along with four other support workers, have been assigned to provide 24-hour support for Mrs. Wieldon. You know that she wants to recover as quickly as possible so that her children may return home. She has also stated that she is anxious to get back to work. Additionally, she is grieving the loss of her husband and adjusting to life without him.

What do you think Mrs. Wieldon's needs are at this time? Upon whom might she rely to help her meet these needs? What needs might she rely upon you to meet?

Chapter 8

The Client–Worker Relationship

Learning Objectives

Through reading this chapter, you'll be able to

1. Explain the importance of the client–worker relationship.
2. List five fundamental abilities that characterize a positive personal relationship.
3. Portray interdependence as it applies to you and to your work with clients.
4. Identify the three stages of a client–worker relationship.
5. Outline the rights that clients enjoy.
6. Outline the rights that support workers enjoy.

Chapter at a Glance

- The Client–Worker Relationship
- Fundamentals of Positive Relationships
- The Power Balance
- Interdependence and the Client–Worker Relationship
- The Three Stages of the Client–Worker Relationship
- Client and Worker Rights

Terms You'll Use

Communication The ability to share your ideas, explore others' ideas, and resolve conflicts. The aim of communication is to understand and to be understood.

Empathy The ability to sense what others are feeling while respecting that you will never fully understand their emotions.

Flexibility The ability to adapt to changes in a relationship, setting, or situation.

Independence The ability to do things for oneself.

Interdependence The reliance we all have on others to help us do things.

Mutuality The ability to see how both people in a relationship benefit from it.

Respect The ability to recognize and accommodate others' thoughts, opinions, behaviours, needs, preferences, and decisions.

Right Something we have the authority to do.

THE CLIENT–WORKER RELATIONSHIP

> *The quality of our human existence is grounded in our relationships.*
> John Powell, *The Secret of Staying in Love*

A relationship can be described as the feelings that exist between two people. It is made up of a series of expectations, ways of doing things (behaviours), and psychological and emotional distance. Your personality and the other person's personality will also help determine the quality of the relationship you have with each other.

Relationships—even brand-new ones—give meaning to our lives. Consider the following situation.

STOP AND REFLECT 8-1

You are shopping with your best friend. You enter a store that boasts about its wonderful selection, reasonable prices, and good service. The store is clean, well organized, and attractive.

After some time, you select an outfit and take it to the sales counter. As the clerk starts to ring up your purchase, you ask her if the store carries luggage. The clerk looks at you, rolls her eyes, and says to you, "What do I look like, the answer lady?"

How do you feel about the store? What has influenced your feelings?

_____

_____

_____ ■

It's likely that your feelings about the store were most influenced by the exchange you had with the clerk, not how clean or attractive the store appeared, or even the attractive prices. Our need to communicate and to make connections with other people leads us to place importance on human interactions.

Each Relationship Is Unique

Each relationship is the product of the two people who are involved in it. As a result, each relationship is unique. Relationships can be close or distant, good or bad, healthy or unhealthy. It is even possible for each person in the same relationship to have a somewhat different view of it.

A relationship requires some commitment from both people involved. Sometimes, this commitment is voluntary, such as when you want to make friends with someone. The relationship exists as long as the two parties want it to or as long as they are brought together by circumstances, whether or not the people are in daily contact.

Relationships can be personal or professional. Occasionally, some relationships start out as one type and become another. This can pose problems for both people involved, as the personal relationship may make it harder to do what you need to do in the professional relationship. The nature of the work you do will often cause you to work with clients over a long period of time. You and your client will likely get to know each other well, making this personal–professional distinction hard to define. Consider the following client viewpoint.

CASE EXAMPLE 8-1

When asked, a consumer of attendant services defined the relationship she has with her support staff (attendants) in this way.

The relationship between my attendants and me is almost impossible to define. It isn't a parent–child relationship, as we need each other. I need services, and my attendants need work meaningful to them. It's more of an adult–adult relationship. The relationship is sometimes that of employer and employee, but, at other times perhaps surprisingly, the relationship is one of friendship. I don't want someone who adopts a paternal stance toward me or assumes I am "sick" rather than a well person with a disabling condition. My attendants and I must be able to "get along" on a personal level for the overall relationship to work.

How would you define your role as a support worker assisting this consumer?

CASE EXAMPLE 8-2

A support worker was asked to describe how he saw the relationship between the client and himself. He said:

"It's not just that I have to get to know my client and what he needs me to do, I have to know how he wants me to do these things, and not just the method he prefers. I need to learn when I'm expected to wait for his instruction or request and when I'm to simply go ahead and do whatever needs to be done. It takes time, effort and patience on both our parts to get it right. And, it's that way for every client I support."

Compare the support worker's answer with your own. How is your response similar? How is it different?

FUNDAMENTALS OF POSITIVE RELATIONSHIPS

STOP AND REFLECT ((8-2))

Think about a really positive working relationship you have with another person. Perhaps this relationship is between you and a co-worker. It might be between you and a supervisor or between you and a client.

What makes the relationship such a positive one for you?

_____

_____

_____

Would the other person involved see this as a positive relationship? If so, what makes it that way?

_____

_____

What makes your relationship so positive? It's likely that you listed such things as: we like the same things, we see things the same way, I can really talk to her, or I can count on him.

Five abilities are fundamental to your ability to form and maintain a positive relationship with another person: communication, respect, mutuality, flexibility, and empathy. We'll discuss each in this section. These abilities are necessary for *any* positive relationship, not just one you would have with your client.

Communication is essential to sharing your ideas and exploring the other person's ideas, as well as to resolving any conflicts that might arise. In Chapter 9, we will discuss communication skills further.

Respect means several things. It means recognizing and accommodating a person's opinions, patterns of behaviour, and preferences. It includes respecting the other person's needs and behaving in a way that does not intentionally hurt the other person. Respect also means that you respect the person's *boundaries*, the limits we all set on the information we share and the things we will do. Boundaries change with each relationship. For example, your client might not wish you to know very much about his or her relationship with a family member, even though the client may freely share this information with another person.

Mutuality is the ability to see how you both benefit from the relationship. Despite the fact that your client benefits from the support you provide, it's quite likely that you also benefit from the relationship. Give some thought to the following questions.

STOP AND REFLECT 8-3

Think of a situation where you have provided support or assisted another person. This can be a work situation, a volunteer situation, or any other where the reason for the relationship was your helping the other person.

How did you benefit from this relationship? For example, did you learn from the other person or attain a sense of satisfaction?

_____

_____

_____

Flexibility includes the ability to adapt to changes in a relationship. Most of us have good days and bad days. We may be tired one day and energetic the next. Clients are no different. As you'll learn in the next section, relationships change over time. You must be flexible in your approach so that you can respond appropriately to your client.

Empathy is the ability to sense what the other person is feeling, while respecting that you will never fully *understand* the person's emotions. Empathy includes respect for the person's boundaries as to what they will share with you. It also includes the person's right to have feelings to which you cannot relate or with which you do not agree.

THE POWER BALANCE

In every relationship, there is a sense of equity (an equal balance of power) or a sense of imbalance in the power one person has relative to another. Consider the following situation.

STOP AND REFLECT 8-4

Recall a time that you needed help from another person for help with everyday activities (for example, when you were recovering from surgery, or recovering from a broken leg or arm). If you cannot recall such a time, try to imagine yourself in one of these situations.

How did you feel when you had to rely upon this person?

_____

_____

_____

Did you find that your feelings affected how you related to this person?

_____

_____

Did you feel as though you were dependent upon the person? Even if you had a good relationship with the person who helped you, you may have felt that you were not quite equals.

The balance of power is affected by the degree of *interdependence* between the parties involved.

INTERDEPENDENCE AND THE CLIENT–WORKER RELATIONSHIP

Interdependence can be defined as the reliance we all have on other people for some things. You will often hear colleagues talk about independence (the ability to do things for oneself). Remember that no one is completely independent. The ability to do certain things for oneself is a goal for many clients. However, many clients have a preferred mix of activities they would prefer to do independently and activities with which they would prefer help. Consider the following situation.

CASE EXAMPLE 8-3

Erin Young is 35 years old and a senior manager in an insurance company. Five years ago, Erin was diagnosed with multiple sclerosis and has lost strength in her arms. As a result, she finds that her ability to do certain tasks (such as those that require her to open and close jars or to grip items firmly) is diminished. Additionally, her energy level has diminished to the extent that performing many routine activities, such as making a meal, leaves her exhausted.

For the past eight months, Erin has received frozen Meals on Wheels. Seven meals are dropped off at Erin's home each Monday night. Erin takes one to work with her each day, heating it in the staffroom of her office.

Erin's use of the frozen meals means that she is able to save her energy for more important things in her life. If she had to make meals each day, she would not have the energy to bathe, dress, and get herself to work. If she were to use "fast foods," she would not be able to eat the balanced diet she needs.

Ironically, by being more physically independent by making her own meals at home, Erin might, in fact, become financially dependent through the loss of her ability to work because of the resultant exhaustion.

What things do you rely upon others to do, even though you could do them yourself? How does this affect your sense of independence?

Can you understand why Erin has made the choices she has? Like all of us, she has made decisions as to when she will rely upon others and when she will do things for herself. This is much the same as a decision you might make to hire someone to paint a room for you or to mow your lawn. It is not to say that you cannot do those tasks; you may be perfectly able to do them. You simply have chosen to do other things.

Some caregivers find it difficult to accept a client's decisions as to what tasks he or she prefers to rely upon others to do, particularly when the caregiver feels that the client *could* do the task. Did you find yourself thinking about Erin—*She could make herself meals if she wanted to?* If so, you can understand the caregiver's view. Many of us are raised to believe that a person must be as independent as possible. This can make it difficult for us to understand a person's decision not to do something of which he or she is capable. We all make these choices, and you must respect your client's right to do so (Photo 8-1).

Photo 8-1
Mutual respect is essential to good client–worker relationships.
Source: CHATS

THE THREE STAGES OF THE CLIENT–WORKER RELATIONSHIP

Your relationship with the client can be described in three phases: the introductory phase, the productive phase, and the parting phase. Each phase is described in this section.

The Introductory Phase   This is the phase during which you and your client get to know each other. Your tasks in this phase include identifying your client's preferences as to what needs to be done and how it will be done; learning your client's ways of communicating; problem solving; and learning what the nature of the client–worker relationship will be. It is natural for both you and your client to be a bit anxious during this phase.

The Productive Phase   This is the phase during which you and your client should feel comfortable. You appreciate each other's preferences and habits, and you have worked out ways to resolve any conflicts that arise. Your working relationship is a good one, and there is enough consistency in the routine that it is predictable without becoming tiresome. Your tasks in this phase include making sure that you remain responsive to your client's preferences and needs, even if the routine does not change for a long period of time.

The Parting Phase   This is the phase in which you wind down your relationship, usually because you will no longer be visiting the client. The task here is to acknowledge the change and to recognize that you both have benefited from the relationship. It is not unusual for both you and your client to feel a sense of loss when you are leaving a relationship.

CLIENT AND WORKER RIGHTS

We can define a **right** as something that we have the authority to do. People speak about rights in many ways, such as legal rights, moral rights, and human rights.

Sometimes, a person has certain rights because he or she is in a particular situation. For example, a person has certain rights as a worker, as a client of an agency, or as the purchaser of some property. (Table 8-3 describes some common rights affecting workers.)

Legislated Rights

Many rights are legislated or regulated; that is, they are written into law or into the regulations that governments establish to implement the law. Sometimes, the rights are combined together into a *bill of rights*. Other times, the rights are simply stated in the law. These rights do not usually change quickly.

Rights Established by Associations and Agencies

Some rights are established by voluntary associations, such as long-term care associations. These rights do not have the force of law, but the association that establishes them usually requires its members to agree to respect them as a requirement of membership.

Some rights, like those accorded to someone who uses the services of a particular agency, are determined by the agency and may be changed whenever the agency decides to do so, provided that they do not conflict with any rights also guaranteed by legislation or other means.

Client Rights

Most provinces have several types of legislation that provide for client rights: a human rights code, long-term care services acts, and acts that protect the confidentiality of client records. Some provinces provide for client rights in landlord and tenant legislation (if the client lives in a retirement home). Each province has different titles for these pieces of legislation. Table 8-1 highlights the rights that each type of legislation typically includes. Table 8-2 describes the *Bill of Rights* for Ontario's long-term care facility residents.

TABLE 8-1	Typical Client Rights
Legislation Type	**Rights**
Human Rights Code	Prohibits discrimination on the basis of: race, ancestry, place of origin, colour, ethnic origin, citizenship, creed, sex, sexual orientation, disability, age, marital status, family status, record of offences.
Long-Term Care Act	Provides a *Bill of Rights* for persons receiving long-term care services in the community and in a facility. Some provinces use separate legislation to guarantee rights in each setting.
Health Records or Privacy Act	Usually protects patient health information. Provides guidelines as to how it can be accessed by clients as well as shared among providers.
Guardianship, Power of Attorney Act	Usually allows you to appoint someone to look after your affairs. Different provinces may have very different provisions with regard to people's rights under this legislation.

TABLE 8-2	*Bill of Rights* for Ontario's Long-Term Care Facility Residents

Residents' Bill of Rights

Every licensee shall ensure that the following rights of residents are fully respected and promoted:

1.   Every resident has the right to be treated with courtesy and respect and in a way that fully recognizes the resident's dignity and individuality and to be free from mental and physical abuse.

2.   Every resident has the right to be properly sheltered, fed, clothed, groomed, and cared for in a manner consistent with his or her needs.

3.   Every resident has the right to be told who is responsible for and who is providing the resident's direct care.

4.   Every resident has the right to be afforded privacy in treatment and in caring for his or her personal needs.

5.   Every resident has the right to keep in his or her room and display personal possessions, pictures, and furnishings in keeping with safety requirements and other residents' rights.

6.   Every resident has the right,
     i.   to be informed of his or her medical condition, treatment, and proposed course of treatment,
     ii. to give or refuse consent to treatment, including medication, in accordance with the law and to be informed of the consequences of giving or refusing consent,
     iii. to have the opportunity to participate fully in making any decision and obtaining an independent medical opinion concerning any aspect of his or her care, including any decision concerning his or her admission, discharge, or transfer to or from a nursing home, and
     iv. to have his or her medical records kept confidential in accordance with the law.

7.   Every resident has the right to receive reactivation and assistance towards independence consistent with his or her requirements.

8.   Every resident who is being considered for restraints has the right to be fully informed about the procedures and the consequences of receiving or refusing them.

9.   Every resident has the right to communicate in confidence, to receive visitors of his or her choice, and to consult in private with any person without interference.

10. Every resident whose death is likely to be imminent has the right to have members of the resident's family present twenty-four hours per day.

11. Every resident has the right to designate a person to receive information concerning any transfer or emergency hospitalization of the resident and where a person is so designated to have that person so informed forthwith.

12. Every resident has the right to exercise the rights of a citizen and to raise concerns or recommend changes in policies and services on behalf of himself or herself or others to the residents' council, nursing home staff, government officials, or any other person inside or outside the nursing home, without fear of restraint, interference, coercion, discrimination, or reprisal.

TABLE 8-2	*Bill of Rights* for Ontario's Long-Term Care Facility Residents *(continued)*

13. Every resident has the right to form friendships, to enjoy relationships, and to participate in the residents' council.

14. Every resident has the right to meet privately with his or her spouse in a room that assures privacy and, where both spouses are residents in the same nursing home, they have a right to share a room according to their wishes, if an appropriate room is available.

15. Every resident has a right to pursue social, cultural, religious, and other interests, to develop his or her potential, and to be given reasonable provisions by the nursing home to accommodate these pursuits.

16. Every resident has the right to be informed in writing of any law, rule, or policy affecting the operation of the nursing home and of the procedures for initiating complaints.

17. Every resident has the right to manage his or her own financial affairs where the resident is able to do so and, where the resident's financial affairs are managed by the nursing home, to receive a quarterly accounting of any transactions undertaken on his or her behalf, and to be assured that the resident's property is managed solely on the resident's behalf.

18. Every resident has the right to live in a safe and clean environment.

19. Every resident has the right to be given access to protected areas outside the nursing home in order to enjoy outdoor activity, unless the physical setting makes this impossible. R.S.O. 1990, c. N.7, s. 2 (2); 1999 c. 6, s. 46 (3); 2004, c. 3. Sched. A, s. 92 (1); 2005, c. 5, s. 49 (4).

TABLE 8-3	Common Rights and Obligations
Legislation	**Usually Includes**
Employment Standards Act	Basic rules about worker entitlement (minimum wage, vacation pay, public holidays, hours of work, etc.)
Labour Relations Act	Right to form and/or join a union, take part in lawful union activities, allow your union to negotiate wages and other working conditions with your employer on your behalf, to strike (and the employer's right to lockout), and identify the criteria for unfair labour practices
Workplace Safety Act	Issues of workplace injury and compensation, worker and employer rights when an injury occurs
Human Rights Code	Prohibits discrimination on the basis of: race, ancestry, place of origin, colour, ethnic origin, citizenship, creed, sex, sexual orientation, disability, age, marital status, family status, record of offences There are limitations to the extent of prohibition in many cases.

TABLE 8-3	Common Rights and Obligations *(continued)*
Community Long-Term Care Act	What services are covered, a definition of personal support services, how services are to be provided, what records to be kept Sometimes includes criteria for providers
Long-Term Care Facilities Act	Sets out requirements for the operation of long-term care facilities Includes regulations specifying records to be kept, documentation, the level of training required to administer medications, etc.
Health Records or Privacy Act	Rights and rules about access, disclosure, and retention of client health records (including community support agency records)

Questions for Review

1. Why is the client–worker relationship important?

2. Select a positive personal relationship you have now or have had. How did that relationship reflect the five fundamental abilities discussed in this chapter?

3. What legislation protects clients in your province? What branch of the government administers this legislation?

4. What legislation protects workers in your province? What branch of the government administers this legislation?

Questions for Discussion

1. Select a *professional* relationship you currently have. This could be a relationship between you and a client, or a relationship between you and another person. How does the concept of interdependence apply to this relationship? How many examples of interdependence can you define?

2. Read the following case study and then discuss the questions that follow.

   You work with Mrs. Brown, a 55-year-old client who has lung cancer. She has been receiving chemotherapy that has eased her symptoms. She is aware that the treatment will not cure the cancer but that it will reduce the effects of the disease and prolong her life. Mrs. Brown is a lifelong smoker. She has continued to smoke, despite the link between cigarette smoking and lung cancer. You have grown fond of Mrs. Brown and worry that her continued smoking will offset the benefits of the chemotherapy.

   How do you feel about this situation? What are Mrs. Brown's rights in this situation? How might you demonstrate respect for Mrs. Brown's rights?

3. Assume that you and three or four of your colleagues are in the following situation. Discuss the questions at the end of the situation.

   You and your colleagues are residents of a long-term care facility. You have been asked to develop a residents' bill of rights. Instead of using the bill of rights presented earlier in this chapter, you want to write your own.

   What rights do you think you—and the other residents—should have? List at least ten rights.

Chapter 9

Basic Communication Skills

Learning Objectives

Through reading this chapter, you'll be able to

1. Describe how we communicate.
2. Tell why good communication skills are important in support work.
3. Explain what good communication is.
4. Express the three principles of communication.
5. List the two common types of communication.
6. Tell what the process of communication is.
7. Describe how culture affects and shapes communication.
8. Discuss ten ways that you can make cross-cultural communication more effective.
9. Outline common barriers to communication with clients and, for each, list one thing a support worker can do to try to overcome the barrier.
10. Use the ten principles of client teaching to assist a client to learn and practise a new skill or relearn an old one.

Chapter at a Glance

- What Is Communication?
- Communication and Support Work
- What Is Good Communication?
- The Process of Communication
- Filters and Barriers
- Culture and Communication
- Understanding and Being Understood
- Client Teaching

Terms You'll Use

Barriers Things that prevent the message from getting across when communicating, such as language or hearing impairment.

Body Language Communication through posture, facial expressions, and movements. This is often called nonverbal communication.

Client Teaching The instruction given to a client by a support worker.

Content Information communicated through words.

Feelings Emotions communicated through words and body language.
Filters Things that affect how we communicate, including body language, mood, and stress.
Learning Changes in behaviour that result from new information.

WHAT IS COMMUNICATION?

Communication is depositing part of yourself in another person.
Anonymous

Communication is essential to our everyday life. Researchers have linked communication to physical well-being, to our ability to define who we are, and to our ability to form relationships. We also must communicate in order to make our needs known.

Despite the time we spend doing it, we generally spend very little time thinking about communication and how we communicate. We often take it for granted—until something goes wrong!

STOP AND REFLECT ((9-1))

Try this test. When you are with a group of friends or family, try not to communicate for five minutes. Pay particular attention to what happens when you do this.

How easy was it to not communicate? Did you find that you were tempted to talk? Did you try to use gestures and facial expressions to communicate your needs?

_____

_____

_____

_____

How did the people you were with react to you? Did they attempt to communicate with you? If they did, how did they try to communicate?

_____

_____

_____

Did the other people think you were communicating? If so, what message did they think you were sending?

_____

_____

_____

You probably found it very difficult to do this exercise. Even if you did try not to communicate, chances are that you did. You likely received communication from the others (perhaps through their reactions and their comments). It's also likely that the other people felt that you sent a message. In this exercise, you have proved several principles. This section discusses three principles of communication.

You cannot not communicate. Your "body language," your posture, facial expressions, and movements all send messages, even if you don't say a word. Recall the way the other people reacted to your attempt to not communicate. They likely thought you were communicating some message.

You communicate, whether or not you mean to communicate. When you tried the exercise above, did you find that the other people around you thought you were sending a message, even though you were attempting not to communicate? We often communicate without meaning to, through how we look. Some of us are better at filtering our body language. For example, you may know someone who is said to have a "poker face" because it's hard to read emotions from his or her body language. Nonetheless, everyone communicates.

You cannot undo communication. You've probably watched a television show in which a jury was listening to testimony. A witness says something to which the defendant's lawyer objects. The judge tells the jury to "disregard the witness's statement." Do you think that the jury really could act as though they never heard the statement? Probably not.

COMMUNICATION AND SUPPORT WORK

As a support worker, you will constantly communicate with clients. How you communicate can make the difference between a positive experience for you both or one that you both dread. Many clients will have difficulty communicating, and you will have to adapt your methods to make the communication as positive as possible.

WHAT IS GOOD COMMUNICATION?

STOP AND REFLECT ((9-2))

If you had to tell someone what "good" communication is, what would you say?

_____

_____

_____ ■

Good communication can be described as "understanding and being understood." If your definition is close to this, you have the right idea.

You may have described communication as involving listening and asking questions. If you did, you've included some of what we can call the process of communication. These are the techniques that help us to understand and be understood. The more we know about the process and the techniques, the better able we are to make sure that good communication takes place—or to figure out what went wrong when it doesn't.

THE PROCESS OF COMMUNICATION

The process of communication is presented in Figure 9-1. It involves a sender and a receiver. In most communication, each person is alternately a sender and a receiver, depending upon whether or not the person is giving or getting a message.

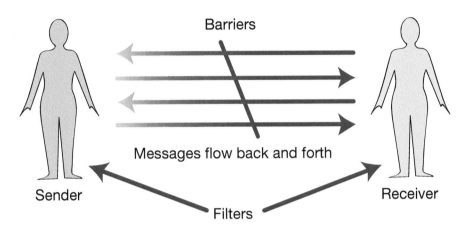

FIGURE 9-1 *The process of communication*

Getting the Message

Messages generally come in two parts: feelings and content. **Feelings** are emotions communicated through words. **Content** is factual information communicated through words. Not all messages have both; some messages have content only. For example, giving someone directions to the mall might not involve much feeling, but the message contains a lot of content. Table 9-1 describes some characteristics of feelings and content.

TABLE 9-1	Characteristics of Feelings and Content	
Feelings	**Content**	
▪ Expressed in both words and body language	▪ Usually expressed in words	
▪ Are neither good nor bad	▪ Often are based in facts, describing events, desires, issues, acts, etc.	
▪ Can conflict with one another (e.g., be happy and sad at the same time)	▪ Can conflict with other parts of the message	
▪ Always make sense to the person	▪ Always make sense to the person	
▪ Denial will not make them go away	▪ Denial will not make them go away	

FILTERS AND BARRIERS

If all we had to do is speak and hear in order to have good communication, it would be easy. Alas, there are many things that can affect the transmission of the message.

Filters

Filters affect how we say or hear things. They may even make us not say or hear things. Filters include the following:

Body Language
Past Experiences with the Person or Situation
Whether or Not the Person Is in a Position of Authority
Attitudes and Stereotypes
Mood, Personality
Words, Tone of the Other Person
Stress, Physical Health

Nonverbal Behaviour (Body Language)

It's important to remember that we get a great deal of information from another's nonverbal behaviour (body language). Some studies suggest that most of the message we get comes from the nonverbal communication. Likewise, *our* body language tells others a great deal about us. Many of the filters listed above will show up in your body language. Some people naturally show more body language than others.

Body language includes a number of things: facial expression, how we sit or stand, the gestures we use, how we move about, whether we sigh or yawn, as well as the tone and pace of any words we use.

STOP AND REFLECT ((9-3))

Try this exercise with a friend or colleague. Ask the other person to pretend that she or he is mad at you for some reason. Look at the person's nonverbal behaviour and answer the following questions.

How does the person's face (eyes, mouth, brow) look?

_____

How does the person stand or sit?

_____

Where does the person put his or her hands?

_____

Does the person cross her or his arms?

_____

Does the person clench his or her fists?

_____

If the person spoke to you, how did she or he sound?

_____

Did the person speak rapidly or slowly?

_____

It's sometimes difficult to describe these things. You might have been tempted to say that the person "looks angry." That's what you asked for! But, what is it about how the other person looks that makes you say the person looks angry? The physical appearance is what conveys the feeling.

STOP AND REFLECT   9-4

Take a look at the following situations. Describe how you would show your feelings in each situation. Be sure to describe how you would look. For example, what would your face look like? What would your posture be?

Situation	How you'd **show** it
You're taking a walk with someone. You're walking in an area in which you feel uncomfortable. You're becoming frightened.	
You've planned an evening out with a friend who is visiting your city. Your husband was supposed to look after your three children. He comes home three hours late, saying that he forgot. You are angry that you have had to cancel your plans.	
You've just started visiting a new client. She is a bit forgetful, and although you've been taught how to respond, you haven't practised very much. You really don't feel too sure of yourself or your skills.	
You are going out with a good friend. She wants to do something that you really don't want to do. You don't want to hurt her feelings, but you really don't want to do what she wants.	

Share your responses with your colleagues. Would you all show the same feelings in the same way? Were there feelings you showed differently? Which ones?

It's just as important to learn to read the other person's body language (Photo 9-1). Along with tone of voice, body language can tell you much about the other person's message and possibly about how your message might be filtered. Keep in mind that

Photo 9-1
Who would you rather see?
Source: Leisureworld Preferred Institute

this is a two-way street—your body language and tone of voice will tell the other person about you. If your body language does not match your words, you'll likely confuse the other person.

How we see the person can also affect not only what we say and how we say it, but also how we interpret the message that person sends to us. Our attitude toward another person, and whether or not we've had any past experiences with the person, can affect the current communication. For example, we often speak and listen differently to children than we do adults, or to a co-worker differently than a supervisor. Likewise, if we've shared good experiences when we last spoke with that person, we are more likely to see the current communication as positive.

Appearance also affects how we interpret the other person's message. Looking too old or too young, too dressed up or too casually dressed, or unclean or unshaven can greatly affect the way communication happens. In Chapter 4, we discussed the need for a professional appearance. Dressing appropriately and professionally will affect how others see you and your role.

Culture directly affects how we interpret other people's messages. For example, people of British descent place great value on making eye contact when communicating. You might ask someone to look you in the eye when they are speaking to you, or you may refer to "seeing eye to eye" with another person. People from other cultures may see direct eye contact as offensive or disrespectful. You must always make sure to appreciate how other people's culture affects their interpretation of messages.

Finally, our mood and whether we're stressed or feeling unwell can affect how we give a message and how we interpret what we hear. If you've spoken sharply to someone because you weren't feeling well, you know what this can be like.

Because filters can dramatically alter the message you send and receive, pay particular attention to them. You should examine your responses to filters to make sure that you are not making communication more difficult.

Barriers

Barriers are things that actually prevent the message from getting to the other person. Many barriers have to do with the environment, but some have to do with the receiver.

STOP AND REFLECT ((9-5))

What things do you think might be barriers to communication? List your ideas below.

_____

_____

_____

_____

_____

_____

A number of things can become barriers, including the following:

- Sensory loss
- Environmental causes
- Background noise
- Distractions
- Environment too hot or cold
- Offensive smells
- Furniture or décor
- Lack of a common language
- Nonverbal communication that is misinterpreted or not understood
- Jargon
- Poorly worded or disorganized messages
- Interruptions
- Lack of attention
- Not listening

Sensory Loss

Losses in vision, hearing, and touch affect a person's ability to communicate. Communication is diminished if the words and gestures can't be heard, seen, or felt. Additionally, because so much of communication is nonverbal, vision problems can directly affect the message a person gets. In Chapter 10, we will discuss some of the ways you can adapt your communication to meet the needs of the person with changes in vision, hearing, or touch sensation.

Listening Skills

> *When you talk, you repeat what you already know.*
>
> *When you listen, you often learn something.*
>
> Jaren Sparks

Good listening skills are essential to understanding the other person's message. They are a learned behaviour. If you don't practise good listening skills, you'll lose them. Try these tips to increase your listening skills:

- Judge the speaker's content, not delivery.
- Listen for ideas. What is the speaker trying to tell you?
- Work at listening. Pay attention to what the speaker says.
- Make certain that your body language says that you're listening. Lean forward, make eye contact if appropriate, and stop doing other tasks.
- Avoid distractions.
- Avoid getting upset over emotionally charged words or phrases. Focus on the content.
- Get into the habit of listening first, *then* deciding what you will say. Avoid thinking up a response before the person has finished speaking.

CULTURE AND COMMUNICATION

You are standing outside an apartment complex built for Greek seniors. You are talking with the complex's coordinator. She is fluent in Greek and often speaks Greek to the tenants.

While you are there, a tenant who has been out shopping comes to the door. She has difficulty unlocking he door and getting her bundle buggy inside. When the coordinator asks her—in Greek—if she needs a bit of help, the tenant straightens up, glances at you, and says—in English—"No, I am fine."

What factors do you think might have affected this communication?

You might have identified things such as the woman not knowing whether you spoke Greek and not wanting to be impolite, not wanting to appear to need help, wanting to be clear. Any of these things could well have influenced the woman's response.

In Chapter 7, we discussed personal culture. Awareness of another's personal culture is fundamental to communication. Culture affects communication in many ways. Some are obvious: people from different cultures may not use the same words to describe things. Gestures and other nonverbal communication may mean different things to people of different cultures. Common sayings may not have the same meaning—or any meaning at all to a person from a different culture. Sometimes, the differences are funny. Have you ever heard a person from England talk about being "knocked up"? In England, this means to be awakened, while in Canada, it means to become pregnant.

Some of the other ways culture affects communication are not nearly as obvious. They have much more to do with how well we think we are communicating or how comfortable we feel with the person. Because these are not easily traced to different words, gestures, or language, they are harder to identify.

You've probably had the experience of talking to a person you didn't know well. You might have found that communication was a bit harder. Perhaps you weren't certain that you were being understood or weren't even certain that the person was listening to you. You might have sensed that the other person was having difficulty too, even if she or he didn't say anything. You may not have been at all certain that you and the other person would ever get along well. These differences in communication can lead to a lack of trust between the sender and the receiver.

However, after you got to know the person, it's likely that communication felt easier and more comfortable. Why did the communication become easier? Chances are that you developed a sense of familiarity and comfort with the other person's *way* of communicating—and the other person became more comfortable with yours. In a sense, you adapted and became more comfortable with each other's *personal culture*.

Sometimes, even the more obvious things are hard to define. We may see nonverbal behaviour but not realize at first that it is the nonverbal behaviour to which we're reacting.

As discussed earlier in this chapter, many people of British descent want a person to look at them when the person is speaking. However, many Canadians from other

FIGURE 9-2
*Cultural differences can
have a significant effect
on communication.*

cultures feel that making eye contact with another person in this way is a sign of disrespect. Figure 9-2 illustrates what may happen when a person needs to make eye contact when communicating and the other person cannot. Understanding and developing a sense of comfort with one another becomes very difficult. It may also be difficult for each party to identify exactly why communication is difficult; we often respond to another's nonverbal behaviours without thinking about it. Thus we react to the eye contact (or lack of eye contact) but may not realize that we're reacting to it.

Some people have difficulty understanding why it is important to take another's personal culture into account. For example, you may have heard someone say, "If she's living here, she'd better learn to get along as we do." This view does not take into account how difficult it would be for anyone to change something as fundamental as communication. Recall a time when you were asked to behave in a way that is not "like you." How easy was it to do? Did you feel that your communication was "natural" or "easy"? Probably not.

CASE EXAMPLE 9-2

Jacob is 15 years old. He is Cree. He lives with his parents in Winnipeg. Jacob and his parents have adopted some Western styles of communicating. For example, Jacob and his parents often engage in lively discussions about issues, with each person asserting his or her perspective.

When Jacob visits his grandfather in Western Ontario, he has to adopt a different style of communication. He

learns to listen, then to ask questions. It often takes Jacob a day or two to relearn this pattern each time he visits. His grandfather is patient as Jacob makes this adjustment.

What factors influence these different styles? Is one style "better" than another? Is one style more productive? Do you feel that Jacob's grandfather should adapt to Jacob's style? Why or why not?

Communicating Across Cultures

Communicating well always requires interest, sensitivity, and patience. Communicating well when we don't share common "culture" requires more of you. Practising the following will help you to better understand—and be understood:

Seek first to get to know the person as a person, not as a representative of a particular culture or group. None of us are "cultural" representatives."

Recognize that you too have a personal culture, even if you don't notice it much. The story is told of a support worker who was asked to describe herself in terms of her culture. She thought for a moment and said, "I'm Scottish. We don't have a culture!" Often the dominant culture—the one that is most prevalent in a society—becomes almost invisible to its members. It is not invisible to people who are not a part of the dominant culture, however. The person with whom you're communicating is as aware of your personal culture as you are of his or hers.

Don't assume that communication styles that differ from your own are wrong. There are many ways to get a message across. The right way is the one that works for all people involved.

Try to see the communication from the other person's perspective. The better you understand how the other person sees things, the easier and more effective the communication will be.

Respect the other's preferences for style and pace in communicating. Don't demand that communication be done your way. Can you find a method that respects both your needs?

Respect the other's boundaries for what, when, and how much is shared. Some things may be very uncomfortable or even impossible for a person to discuss. As well, recognize that some things that are easy for the other person to discuss may be difficult for you.

Listen actively and with flexibility. Don't jump to conclusions or react too quickly to words without ensuring that your interpretation is correct. Explore, don't explode!

Problems in communication must be solved by all parties. It isn't helpful to blame a person for something he or she did "wrong." Focus instead on how to solve the problem and avoid it in the future.

Use generalizations about other groups carefully. Knowing how a particular community has often responded may give you a place to start when trying to communicate with a person. It will not likely tell you exactly what to do, and to assume so stereotypes the person.

Work at communicating. Don't let a bad experience cause you to avoid or limit future communication. Learn from what has happened, and use that information to improve future communication.

UNDERSTANDING AND BEING UNDERSTOOD

In many situations, good communication is reasonably automatic. We send and receive messages with little difficulty. Table 9-2 lists some desirable qualities of messages. Yet,

TABLE 9-2	Desirable Qualities of a Message

	Is Your Message...
✔	Clear?
✔	Culturally Responsive?
✔	Complete?
✔	Congruent?
✔	Sent in the Right Climate?
✔	Caring?

there are times when even the best communicator has problems understanding and being understood.

If any of the following are present, you need to be particularly careful to make sure that your message gets across.

- Barriers
- Different communication styles
- First-time communication
- Filters that will hamper communication (yours or the other person's)
- A complex or difficult message
- An emotionally charged message

Asking yourself the following six questions will help make you more easily understood by others:

- **Is your message clear?** Are you saying what you want to say? Have you put your message in simple language? Are you using words that you know the other person will understand? Are you taking into account the other person's style?
- **Is your message culturally responsive?** Have you taken the other's personal culture into account? Have you made certain that your message is sent in a manner that will make it easier for the other to understand?
- **Is your message complete?** Have you left any gaps? Will the person have to "fill in any blanks"?
- **Is your message congruent?** In this instance, congruent means that your body language matches your words. For example, if you're concerned, do you look concerned? If you're happy, do you look happy?
- **Is your message sent in the right climate?** Have you picked the right setting to say what you have to say?
- **Is your message caring?** Have you picked words that will not needlessly hurt the person? Even when you are upset with something that a person has done, you can let the person know without being mean to the person. Table 9-3 gives some examples of caring and uncaring communication.

TABLE 9-3		Which Would You Rather Hear?
"You're so lazy."	**or**	"I'm angry because you didn't do the chores I asked you to do."
"Why can't you do anything right?"	**or**	"I'm upset about the mess that you left in the kitchen."
"Can't you see that I'm busy?"	**or**	"Could we talk about this later, after I finish this phone call?"

CLIENT TEACHING

What Is Learning?

Learning is a change in behaviour that results from new information. This information can be in the form of knowledge, such as knowing the signs of shock. It can also be in the form of skill, such as the ability to safely assist a client to transfer from a bed to a chair. Finally, it can be in the form of information that causes you to re-examine your attitudes, such as information that causes you to examine a stereotype.

We often think of learning as a formal process that occurs in school. In fact, we learn every day of our lives. Many things that we learn, we learn informally from other people, from things that we read, even from television.

Adult Learning

Have you ever heard the statement: "I'm just too old to learn"? It's not true! We can and do learn well into our 80s and 90s. As Photo 9-2 illustrates, *how* we learn does change, though. As adults, we learn differently than we did when we were children. There are several major differences, as we'll see in this section.

Purpose in Learning Adults generally want their learning to meet a need or to have a direct link to some benefit. There are three types of purpose: achievement, self-fulfillment, or social. Sometimes, this purpose is achievement—to learn a task (such as to operate a new appliance). At other times, the purpose is self-fulfillment—meeting a challenge one sets for oneself or overcoming a barrier (such as learning a new way of getting dressed) so that the client is no longer dependent on others. Sometimes, the need is social, such as when a client learns ways of communicating that allow him or her to connect with other people.

Learning Style Adults are usually practical learners. We tend to learn best by doing the task being taught or by applying information to "real world" case studies. We also tend to be social learners, learning best when we can discuss things and ask questions, as well as when we have the support of others.

Learning Ability In general, adults take longer to learn new things. Adults are also more susceptible to interference—things

Photo 9-2
Learning is a lifelong activity. Here, two day centre participants discuss the centre's "Thought for the Day."
Source: CHATS

that distract us or make it harder for us to concentrate. For example, fatigue, anxiety, and illness can all make learning more difficult. Trying to take in too much information at one time can be overwhelming and make it harder for the client to learn.

We all have the opportunity to be teachers. Most of us have shown someone how to put together a child's toy. We often tell someone how to cook something. Many of us have taught a child how to tie a shoelace. When you teach someone, you probably find out that there are certain ways to teach things that make it easier for the person to learn.

STOP AND REFLECT ((9-6))

Recall a few people who have taught you something. They could have been formal teachers, or simply someone from whom you learned something.

What did they do that made it easier for you to learn?

_____

_____

_____

_____

How did they help you to learn?

_____

_____

_____

_____

Was your "teacher" supportive? Did he or she give you time to practise? Did the person find a way to make the information interesting and easy to learn? These approaches make the information easier to learn. They are often called *teaching strategies* or teaching techniques.

Strategies Useful in Client Teaching

The teaching that you do as a support worker is similar to the teaching you have done all your life. Some strategies are the same, such as providing support and encouragement. Others are different. In this section, we'll discuss the ten strategies useful in client teaching, or the instruction that you give to clients.

1. **Find out what the client is interested in learning.** The client may be more interested in learning one task than another. Adults are more motivated to learn when the task interests them.
2. **Break the task into smaller activities.** Even a simple task, such as making a cup of tea, actually has several steps. Take a moment to identify the activities that make up the task. Teach one activity at a time.
3. **Organize the information.** Group information to make it easier for the client to remember. Use verbal clues, or help the client develop a mental image of the task. For example, you might remind a client that his or her water glasses (something that

holds water) are in the cupboard nearest the sink (where the client would get water). Similarly, you might help a client who is relearning to grocery shop to organize the list by food type.

4. **Put the client at ease.** Reassure the client. Try to have some fun.

5. **Let the client set his or her own pace.** People learn at different rates. Some tasks will naturally be easier for the client to learn. Illness and fatigue will also affect the pace. Give the client time to rest when he or she needs to. Realize when it is best to leave the task for the day.

6. **Start at the easiest.** How did you learn to ride a bicycle? You likely started with a tricycle and then moved to a two-wheeler bike with training wheels before attempting a 10-speed. Use the same approach with the client. Start with the easy steps. The client will more easily master the task. The satisfaction of completing the easy task builds a sense of accomplishment, making it psychologically easier to attempt the next more difficult task.

7. **Practise the "tell-show-do-review" model.** (1) Tell the client the steps of the task. (2) Show the client the steps. (3) Let the client attempt the task. (4) Review the client's success.

8. **Appreciate "almost right."** Don't be unrealistic in your expectations. Encourage your client to be realistic in his or her expectations. Few of us perform a task perfectly the first time. Be sure to recognize the parts of the task done well, even when other parts need more work.

9. **Provide support and encouragement to the client.** Learning takes time and effort.

10. **Let the client practise what he or she learns.** Give the client ample opportunity to practise. This helps the client retain the information and gives you an opportunity to offer praise and encouragement.

Questions for Review

1. Recall a recent conversation in which you felt that communication really went well. What made the communication so good?

2. Recall a time that communication went wrong. What happened? Looking back, what could you do to correct the process?

3. How would you attempt to communicate with a new client?

4. What are five desirable qualities of a message?

5. How can culture affect communication? What can you do to help make cross-cultural communication more effective? Identify five ways.

6. Recall a communication situation in which you felt that the other person was not saying what she or he really felt because the person's body language did not match the words used. Describe the body language and define why you felt that it did not match the words.

7. Look at each of these drawings. What does the person's body language tell you?

Questions for Discussion

1. What techniques can you use (or have you used) to improve communication with a client whose cultural background is not the same as yours? Share your ideas with your colleagues.

2. You are assigned to a new client. You know that this client had a worker she really liked, but that worker has moved and can no longer visit. You also know that this client takes a long time to "warm up" to anyone. She is Ukrainian and has spoken Russian most of her life. She learned English in her 60s and still has some difficulty finding the words she wants to use. She is also a bit hard of hearing. When you first meet her, she says, "You look awfully young." What things filter your communication with her? What things do you think filter the client's communication? Are there any potential barriers you can identify? What are they?

3. Read the situation below. Then discuss the questions with your colleagues.

   You have been assigned to assist Mr. Singh. He is recovering from a stroke, and you have been assigned to assist him as he relearns how to cook and do laundry. These are tasks that Mr. Singh only started to do six years ago when his wife died.

   What factors would you consider when you work with Mr. *Singh*? How might you help him to learn more easily?

Chapter 10

Adaptive and Augmentative Communication

Learning Objectives

Through reading this chapter, you'll be able to

1. Describe adaptive communication.
2. Define augmentative communication and list common communication aids.
3. Explain aphasia and fifteen techniques you can use to assist the person with aphasia to communicate.
4. Define apraxia and dysarthria and identify two techniques you can use to assist a person with either condition to communicate.
5. Describe the communication barriers posed by sensory loss. For each type of sensory loss, identify three techniques you can use to help overcome the barrier.

Chapter at a Glance

- What Is Adaptive Communication?
- Augmentative Communication
- Common Conditions Requiring Adaptive or Augmentative Techniques
- Aphasia
- Tips for Communicating with the Person with Aphasia
- Dysarthria and Apraxia of Speech
- Tips for Communicating with the Person with Dysarthria or Apraxia of Speech
- Communication Aids for Language or Speech Production Conditions
- Sensory Loss
- Assisting the Person with Sensory Loss
- Communication Aids to Compensate for Sensory Loss

Terms You'll Use

Adaptive Communication A form of communicating in which a group of techniques is used to adapt communication to the specific needs of the sender or receiver.

Aphasia The complete or partial loss of language skills because of an injury to the brain.

Apraxia A condition that results from an injury to the brain, making voluntary, physical control of purposeful movement difficult.

Augmentative Communication A form of communicating in which physical aids are used in communication.

Dysarthria A condition that results from a weakness or lack of coordination in some of the muscles involved in speaking.

Presbyopia An inability to focus on close objects due to age-related changes in the lens of the eye.

Sensory Loss Changes in the senses that result in a loss of hearing, smell, touch, taste, and sight.

WHAT IS ADAPTIVE COMMUNICATION?

Adaptive communication refers to the group of techniques used to adapt communication to the specific needs of the sender or receiver. Most often, adaptive techniques are used to help people overcome a language problem (such as aphasia) or a sensory loss (such as hearing loss).

CASE EXAMPLE 10-1

Maggie James has hearing loss that resulted from an infection she had as a 50-year-old. Her type of hearing loss cannot be helped by a hearing aid. As a result, Maggie has learned to lip-read and has become quite good at picking up conversation. In fact, many people do not know she has a hearing problem and don't realize that she needs to see the person speak in order to "hear." Maggie then has to remind the person to face her directly.

As you can see in Case Example 10-1, the client's condition makes the adaptation necessary. As a result, the adaptations are often put in place by the person speaking to the client (such as facing the client when speaking). Some clients use various techniques themselves. For example, a visually impaired client may write memos to himself in large block letters on a white board (Photo 10-1).

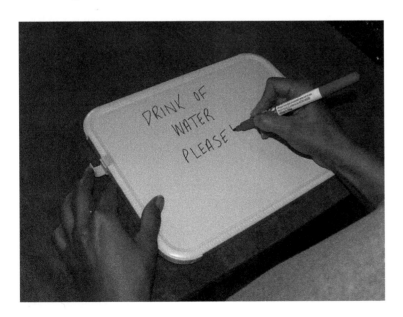

Photo 10-1
A whiteboard can be a useful communication aid.

CASE EXAMPLE 10-2

Mrs. Fried has macular degeneration. She cannot easily discriminate among dark colours, such as navy, black, dark green, or brown. As a result, Mrs. Fried has worn clothing that does not match. Occasionally, she has worn dirty clothing, as she cannot easily see the soil. This has embarrassed Mrs. Fried.

As a result, Mrs. Fried has devised a system that helps her to wear matching and clean clothes. After each wash, she asks her daughter to colour-code her outfits.

Mrs. Fried's daughter puts a fluorescent paper sticky dot on the label of each item. Each navy item receives a fluorescent green dot, each dark green item receives a fluorescent pink dot, and each brown item receives a fluorescent yellow dot.

Mrs. Fried can easily distinguish the fluorescent colours and thus knows what articles of clothing match. She removes the dot as she puts on each item. This way she knows that the item was worn and may be soiled.

Adaptive approaches are *techniques*, such as using large type, changing the pace of the communication, or using short sentences. These approaches often require little "technology." Most techniques have been developed through trial and error.

It's quite likely that you will encounter clients who use adaptive techniques. Remember that each person who uses adaptive approaches has usually tried a number of techniques before selecting those that best fit his or her needs. Remember also that necessity is the mother of invention. Many clients will have developed very creative techniques that work for them. Always take the time to learn the specific techniques your client prefers. If a client has a technique you've never seen before, take the time to find out how it works.

If you have learned of a technique that seems particularly useful, you may choose to tell other clients about it. This is fine, as long as you do not force the idea upon the client or breach confidentiality in describing the technique (by divulging the first client's name or other identifying information).

AUGMENTATIVE COMMUNICATION

Augmentative communication techniques include all approaches that use some form of communication aid. For example, the person who cannot speak but communicates by pointing to various words on a page is using an *augmentative* device—the paper with the words written on it. A hearing aid is another augmentative device, as are the FM devices provided by some theatres to their hearing-impaired patrons.

A computer that synthesizes voice (such as the one used by theoretical physicist Stephen Hawking) is a high-tech augmentative device. However, many devices are much less technologically sophisticated (Photo 10-2). Strictly speaking, eyeglasses are augmentative devices!

Most people with communication problems use a communication aid. Low-tech aids are more common, in part because of their affordability and simplicity. Some clients, particularly younger ones, may use more technologically advanced aids.

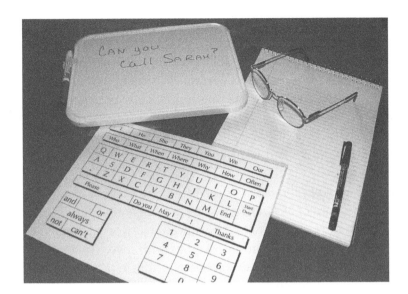

Photo 10-2
Augmentative devices need not be expensive or complex.

COMMON CONDITIONS REQUIRING ADAPTIVE OR AUGMENTATIVE TECHNIQUES

Many conditions can create the need for some change in communication techniques. Some conditions are the result of aging; others result from disease or injury. In this section, we will discuss four common types of conditions: *aphasia*, *dysarthria* or *apraxia*, *sensory loss*, and *cognitive loss*. There are many other conditions that may affect communication. As well, a particular condition will probably affect different people differently. The need to determine what works best for your client is essential.

It is extremely important to remember that a person who has problems communicating does not necessarily have a dementia (a condition discussed in Chapter 22). The person may be able to problem-solve, understand, and remember very well. She or he simply has a problem communicating.

Overcoming a communication problem takes time, patience, and creativity. It also can take a great deal of energy. The ongoing difficulty in getting one's message across can be extremely frustrating. Recall how difficult it was for you when you were not able to communicate.

APHASIA

CASE EXAMPLE 10-3

Mrs. Retman had a stroke two years ago. As a result, she lost most of her ability to use language. Through speech therapy, Mrs. Retman has regained some of this ability. She can now use approximately one hundred words easily.

She has also learned to alter the way in which she says key words so that she can make the best use of the

vocabulary she has. Support workers assisting Mrs. Retman have learned what the variations of these words mean, making it easier for Mrs. Retman to have her wishes understood. Support workers also assist Mrs. Retman to practise tasks assigned by her speech-language pathologist.

Aphasia is the complete or partial loss of language because of some disease or injury to the brain. Aphasia can affect all forms of language, for example, using words to speak, understanding others, writing, reading and gesturing. Aphasia is not the same as apraxia or other problems in language production. According to the Aphasia Institute, 100 000 Canadians are living with aphasia. This number is expected to rise as Canada's population ages.

There are four general causes: physical assault to the brain (such as a stroke), dementia, primary progressive aphasia, and transient aphasia. Each is described in this section.

One of the most common causes of aphasia is a stroke (cerebral vascular accident). The Aphasia Institute states that one-third of all stroke survivors are diagnosed with aphasia (Aphasia Institute, 2007). Aphasia can also be caused by a head injury or brain tumour. Aphasia that results from these causes often improves over time with speech therapy.

One type of aphasia, called primary progressive aphasia, results in the progressive loss of language *without* any loss of other cognitive functions. Usually, people with primary progressive aphasia gradually lose the ability to speak. They often retain their ability to understand.

Transient aphasia is a temporary aphasia. It may be caused by an infection, a transient ischemic attack (TIA), or other illness. It might last only a few hours or days. Most people with transient aphasia recover fully.

Dementia and Language Loss

Some dementias, such as Alzheimer Disease, Pick's Disease, or Creutzfeldt-Jakob Disease, can cause language loss. Language loss resulting from dementia is one of many symptoms of cognitive loss. This type of language loss becomes worse over time. Some researchers call this type of language loss aphasia. Others feel that this language loss is not aphasia. Chapter 22 discusses dementia and its effects on communication in greater detail.

The Extent of Aphasia

The extent of aphasia is determined by the area of the brain that is affected and its size. Aphasia can range from minor word-find problems to the total inability to understand what is said or to create meaningful sentences. Sometimes, only one aspect of language is lost (such as the ability to spell). Usually, more than one aspect of language is impaired. Bear in mind that a person's lifestyle may be significantly affected, even if the extent of aphasia is limited.

Types of Aphasia

There are five major types of aphasia: global, Broca's, mixed non-fluent, Wernicke's, and anomic. Although most people with aphasia have one of these five types, some people may have other, less common forms, such as *alexia* (a disorder of reading). Each type of aphasia has specific characteristics, as we'll discuss in this section.

It's important to have some idea of the various types of aphasia that exist so that you can understand that there are many ways this condition can impair a person's ability to communicate. A particular client may have symptoms of more than one type. You must always use communication techniques that work for your client, according to the type of aphasia he or she has.

Global Aphasia This is the most severe form of aphasia. People with global aphasia cannot read or write; nor can they understand language or produce meaningful language. Global aphasia may occur right after a trauma or stroke. It may improve very quickly after the incident.

Broca's Aphasia Broca's aphasia usually affects the person's ability to express language. The person may speak only in short phrases and may have great difficulty speaking them. Usually, people with Broca's aphasia have difficulty writing, although the person may be able to read and to understand written and verbal communication.

Mixed Non-fluent Aphasia Mixed non-fluent aphasia is similar to Broca's aphasia, except that the person's ability to understand language and to read are also impaired.

Wernicke's Aphasia Wernicke's aphasia is often called fluent aphasia, because the person's ability to string words together is not impaired. However, the words the person says often have no meaning or don't make sense in the sentence. Sometimes, the words are not words at all—the person makes them up. People with Wernicke's aphasia usually have difficulty understanding spoken language, as well as difficulty reading and writing.

Anomic Aphasia Anomic aphasia is the inability of a person to find and use significant words (usually nouns or verbs). The person's spoken language may be very difficult to follow, as it often lacks many of the key words.

TIPS FOR COMMUNICATING WITH THE PERSON WITH APHASIA

1. **Do not exclude the person from social contact.** Remember, the person may well be able to understand you even if he or she cannot speak. The opportunity to interact is important. Even if the person's ability to understand is impaired, she or he will benefit from the sense of being included.
2. **Speak to the person naturally.** If the person appreciates being cued to respond, you can ask questions. If the person becomes frustrated in attempts to respond and prefers not to be asked questions, then form your communication in statements or use questions that can be answered by a yes or no (by a nod or shake of the head).
3. **Speak to the person as an adult.** Loss of language does not mean that the person is confused. Speak with the person as you would like someone to speak to you.
4. **Minimize background noise and other distractions.** Doing so makes it easier for you both to concentrate on the communication.
5. **Make sure your nonverbal communication shows that you are listening.** Make eye contact, do not do other tasks when the person is speaking to you, and listen actively (Photo 10-3).
6. **Be sensitive to the person's nonverbal communication.** Learn what the facial expressions and gestures mean.
7. **Find out what communication is reliable and use it.** For example, the person may be able to reliably tell you yes by a nod of the head. You can then phrase your communication to the person in a way that allows him or her to respond with the gesture.

Photo 10-3
Facing a person when speaking to him or her makes communication easier.
Source: CHATS

8. **Encourage social communication.** The language associated with greetings and other frequently used social behaviours may be more easily picked up by the person.

9. **Use short sentences that highlight the key words.** This allows the person to focus on a few words at a time.

10. **Speak slowly and pause between sentences.** Experiment to find the right pace for each person.

11. **Give the person time to respond to statements.** Resist the temptation to answer on his or her behalf. Respond for the person only if he or she signals to you that the inability to respond is quite distressing and the person prefers that you respond on her or his behalf.

12. **If the person has difficulty understanding, rephrase your sentences or use other words that mean the same thing.** Some words are more easily understood than others.

13. **Be creative in your attempts to understand the person's language.** Look for clues. Does the person use words that describe the use of an item, even though he or she cannot name it? Does she or he use gestures or point to something? Does a particular phrase usually mean a particular thing? Try to look at all the ways you might be able to make sense of the person's statements. Be sure to test out your assumption by asking the person to show you (by whatever means is reliable for the person) that you have the right idea.

14. **If you cannot figure out what the person means, try changing the subject for a bit.** The person's ability to use language may vary from hour to hour. Come back to the issue at a later time.

15. **Don't show concern about the person's speech.** The person is doing the best that he or she can.

16. **Do not force the person to speak in front of others.** This can be embarrassing to the person and actually make speaking more difficult.

17. **Support the person's efforts to speak.** If, after repeated tries, the person says something that is still not clear, rephrase the person's statement and ask for confirmation. Remember that the person needs to practise his or her language skills.

The Aphasia Institute offers the following tips to help a person with aphasia to communicate (Aphasia Institute, Canada, 2007):

- Encourage the person with aphasia to write down a word or draw if they can.
- Encourage the person with aphasia to point to something.
- Attempt to identify the general topic first and then move onto understanding the details. For example, –"Are you talking about your family?"–"Are you talking about your daughter?"–"Are you wondering if she is coming to visit today?"
- Ask yes/no questions.
- Use a written yes/no if needed.
- If you do not have the time to communicate, explain this and give a time when you will return to finish your conversation. Make sure you do return.
- Encourage the person with aphasia to use some of the words you have written down to communicate. For example, "I have heard you are a big fan of music What kind of music do you like?"
  – OPERA
  – CLASSICAL
  – BLUES
  – OTHER

DYSARTHRIA AND APRAXIA OF SPEECH

Dysarthria and *apraxia* of speech are conditions that arise from the brain's inability to properly and consistently control the physical aspect of speaking. Although these conditions seem to result in the same type of impairment, dysarthria and apraxia of speech are different. Dysarthria is the result of some weakness or lack of coordination in some of the muscles involved in speaking. Apraxia results from an injury to the brain that makes the voluntary control of speaking difficult.

People with either condition can have difficulty forming words, pacing their speech, and breathing at the right point in communication or rhythm. As a result, their words may be poorly formed. They may rush through a sentence or take a long time to say a few words. People with apraxia may also have inconsistent sound substitutions. For example, a person with apraxia may say the word "fence" as "pence," "tense," "shentz," or "fesce."

These conditions are often confused with aphasia. People with dysarthria or apraxia of speech do not necessarily have aphasia, although many people with apraxia of speech have some level of aphasia. A person with severe apraxia of speech may only have a mild form of aphasia.

Dysarthria and Apraxia of Speech Are Not Dementia

The speech of a person with either dysarthria or apraxia of speech may sound very different. It may be very difficult to understand. However, this has nothing to do with the person's ability to understand or to think. The person with dysarthria or apraxia of speech simply has a problem performing the mechanics of speech.

CASE EXAMPLE 10-4

Ramiro is a 26-year-old man with cerebral palsy. His ability to produce speech has been impaired by his condition. As a result, Ramiro's speech is slower than that of most other people and some words sound different than when others say them.

Because of this, Ramiro has found it difficult to use a telephone. People often hang up on Ramiro because they assume that the call is a prank because of his

speech. He also finds that people often assume that he has difficulty understanding and thinking as a result of his speech.

Ramiro has taken the time to work with the people around him so that they can more easily understand his speech. He is well able to communicate with his staff to fulfill the responsibilities of his job, and with his support workers to ensure that his requests are understood.

TIPS FOR COMMUNICATING WITH THE PERSON WITH DYSARTHRIA OR APRAXIA OF SPEECH

Many people with apraxia also have aphasia. If this is true for your client, you may want to try the tips listed earlier in this chapter. Some of the tips listed below are similar to those we listed for working with people with aphasia. However, you must remember that the person with dysarthria or apraxia of speech can likely use language.

1. **Do not exclude the person from social contact.** Remember, the person understands you even if he or she cannot speak well. The opportunity to interact is important.

2. **Speak to the person naturally.** If the person appreciates being cued to respond, you can ask questions. If the person becomes frustrated in attempts to respond and prefers not to be asked questions, then form your communication in statements or use questions that can be answered by a no or yes (by a nod or shake of the head).

3. **Speak to the person as an adult.** Speak with the person as you would like someone to speak to you.

4. **Minimize background noise and other distractions.** Doing so makes it easier for you both to concentrate on the communication.

5. **Make sure your nonverbal communication shows that you are listening.** Make eye contact, do not do other tasks when the person is speaking to you, and listen actively.

6. **Learn the person's way of saying common words and phrases.** A person with dysarthria may be consistent in how he or she says something, even if the word or phrase does not sound the same as when you say it.

7. **Ask the person to speak more slowly.** This may make it easier for you to determine breaks between words.

8. **Ask the person to rephrase the sentence.** Sometimes using different words makes the communication more clear.

9. **Ask the person to repeat the statement if you cannot understand.** The repeated phrase may be clearer. If you got part of the message, repeat it and ask the person to start from there.

10. **Have patience.** The person may speak slowly, or may have to repeat words or phrases a number of times before you can understand. Time spent learning a pattern (if the person's speech is consistent) will make future communication much easier.

11. **Pay particular attention to the person's gestures and nonverbal communication.** These signals may provide valuable clues as to the message the person wants to convey.

12. **Consider writing or the use of a letter or word board when verbal communication does not work.** Some people with dysarthria may be able to write down the message for you to read. Other people may benefit from a word list, as described in the section on communication aids.

Photo 10-4
Some people find word lists helpful. Pointing to words on a list helps the person to more easily communicate.

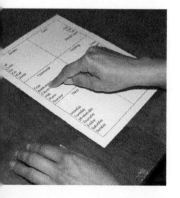

COMMUNICATION AIDS FOR LANGUAGE OR SPEECH PRODUCTION CONDITIONS

Augmentative devices range from the simple (paper and pen) to the complex. This section focuses on items that are common or easy to create. Always be observant of the techniques your client uses. Another client may also find them useful as well.

1. **Word boards and word lists.** If the person has some language, he or she can point to words to communicate. Some boards have many items printed on them. Others are made up of one list, usually containing words that are similar in use (Photo 10-4). Lists can be purchased or made up at home. Some people place word list cards in a photo book or binder. The person flips to the page containing the words he or she wants to use.

2. **Letter cards or letter lists.** Letter cards or lists are similar to the word lists described above. In this instance, the alphabet is printed out. The person points to the letters he or she wants, composing words (Photo 10-5).

3. **Photo or picture albums.** These aids can assist the person who cannot use word lists. Photos or drawings illustrating things the person usually wishes to communicate are put into an album. The person can then point to the appropriate photo or drawing to convey a message. The books may also include information the person likes to share, such as photos of memorable family or social events or photos of favourite places. It can include items the person needs or wants (such as a photo of a hairbrush) or desired activities (such as a photo of a few compact discs to indicate a desire to listen to music).

4. **Yes/no or smile/frown cards.** These cards can be used when the person can reliably indicate yes or no by pointing to the correct word or to the appropriate face (smile means yes, frown means no).

5. **Cards with pictures of commonly used items or tasks.** The person simply selects the appropriate card. Some people use flash cards for this, but care must be taken to make sure the drawings are simple but not childish.

6. **An object basket.** Some people relate best to the actual item in need. A basket, box, or plastic carryall is filled with items that the person might use. For example, the basket might contain a cup, toothbrush, hairbrush, empty shampoo bottle, and a razor (with blade removed). The person simply selects the specific item to indicate what he or she wants or wants to do.

Photo 10-5
A person uses a letter/word board to communicate.

SENSORY LOSS

Sensory losses refer to changes in hearing, vision, touch, taste, and smell. It's important to remember that sensory loss can't easily be seen. Though you may be able to notice that a person has a vision or hearing problem by how he or she does certain tasks, you'd likely have to watch the person for a while. You wouldn't be able to tell by just looking at her or him (Figure 10-1).

FIGURE 10-1 *Can you tell whether this woman has impaired hearing?*

Many of the communication problems you will encounter are the result of age-related sensory changes that happen to everyone if they live long enough. Age-related changes usually develop gradually over a long period of time. The change is so gradual that we often don't realize that changes are taking place. For example, most of us don't even notice that our vision is changing until we can't easily read the print in the telephone directory.

Age-related changes usually add to the sensory problems a person may have had all his or her life. Many of us have worn eyeglasses since we were children; some of us have used hearing aids. The conditions that made the glasses or the aid necessary don't get better as we age, and sometimes the age-related changes make them harder to cope with.

Changes in Vision

Vision makes communication easier. We use our sight to recognize body language, to know when someone is speaking to us, as well as to communicate nonverbally with others. Changes in vision can certainly hamper communication.

Vision changes can happen to people at any age. In fact, some babies are *born* with vision problems such as blindness, cataracts, or the inability to focus. It's not unusual for children to have vision problems that require them to wear glasses.

There are many age-related changes in vision. The lens of the eye, the liquid that fills the eye, and the pupil all change with age, as do the *rods* and *cones* (parts of the inner eye that translate images to impulses that can be understood by the brain). The most common problems are described below:

Photo 10-6

Rapid changes in levels of light may make it difficult for an older person to see.
Source: *Leisureworld Inc.*

- **Changes in colour perception.** The lens of the eye yellows, making it difficult to distinguish between greens and blues or pink and melon colours.
- **A need for more light to see well.** This is due to a decrease in the size of the pupil as well as changes in the rods' ability to react. It is estimated that the average 80-year-old needs three times the amount of light a 20-year-old needs to see well.
  - **A slowing of the pupil's ability to react to changes in levels of light.** This slowing can make it difficult for a person to see well indoors after coming in from outside on a sunny day (Photo 10-6).
  - **Difficulty focusing on things close up.** Reading a prescription label may become very difficult or even impossible. This condition is called **presbyopia**.
  - **Problems with glare or the inability to see things near a source of bright light.** For example, written material printed on high-contrast paper (such as black print on fluorescent pink paper) is very difficult for older people to read. It's also very difficult for many older people to see the facial expression of a person who is standing in front of a source of bright light (such as standing in front of a window on a very bright day). This is similar to a photograph of people taken when the photographer was facing the sun. You probably cannot see any detail in the subjects' faces.

Some vision diseases are more common in older people. These are not age-related changes, though, and do not affect everyone who is older. Some researchers estimate that 40 percent of residents living in nursing homes have significant vision loss. Some of these conditions are macular degeneration, cataracts, glaucoma, diabetic retinopathy, and detached retina.

Changes in Hearing

It is estimated that more than 50 percent of the population over age 60 has some level of hearing loss, and that the percentage of those experiencing hearing loss increases with age. Yet, many people do not want to admit to hearing loss and tend to be uncomfortable about wearing a hearing aid.

Age-related hearing loss starts at age 20 and develops gradually. It is largely the result of changes in the middle ear and usually affects a person's ability to hear high-pitched sounds first, such as the sounds made by many consonants. (Consonants are the letters of the alphabet other than a, e, i, o, u.) In particular, s, c, sh, ch, th, st, and words starting with g, b, or d can be difficult. The person's ability to hear low- and mid-pitched sounds is usually not affected. Often, this can cause other people to assume that the person chooses not to hear things when, in fact, the person cannot.

Most of us experience some hearing loss over our lifetimes (Table 10-1). Much of this loss likely results from everyday "injuries" to our ears, such as those that result from exposure to loud noise. Infections and injuries to the ear can also diminish hearing. This type of hearing loss can make all sounds more difficult to hear.

TABLE 10-1	Do You Have Hearing Loss?

Check off the number of statements that apply to you.

1. People tell me I raise the volume of the radio or television too high.
2. I frequently have to ask people to repeat their message because they mumble.
3. I cannot tolerate loud sounds or voices.
4. I sometimes don't hear the telephone or the doorbell.
5. I have more trouble hearing female voices than hearing male voices.
6. I find it difficult to understand others' speech when there is background noise, such as difficulty in carrying on a conversation while the television is on, or difficulty following conversation in group situations.
7. I find it hard to tell the direction from which sound is coming.
8. I find myself turning one ear or tilting my head toward the person who is speaking.
9. I have ringing or buzzing in one or both of my ears.
10. When I use the telephone, I find it hard to hear the other person.

More than three checkmarks may mean that you have difficulty hearing. Hearing loss should be thoroughly investigated by the appropriate health care professional.

Changes in Sensitivity to Touch

Touch is considered a basic human need. Physical contact with other people and objects is considered to be a necessary part of life satisfaction. The decrease in sensitivity to the sensation of touch is of great importance because it makes it more difficult for us to meet our need to touch and to communicate.

Sensitivity to touch actually refers to four things: texture, temperature, pressure, and pain. Not all researchers agree that a person's sensitivity to touch changes with age. However, illness, injury, and some medications can change a person's sensitivity to touch.

Your use of touch with a client must always be guided by the client's preferences for touch. The client may have preferences for where, when, and by whom he or she is touched. Always ask if the client appreciates a hug or gentle squeeze of the shoulder before you do these things.

ASSISTING THE PERSON WITH SENSORY LOSS

Be aware that the person with sensory loss has a great deal of experience coping with the loss. Always take the time to find out how the person copes with the loss and what techniques the person finds successful.

Photo 10-7
What do you see?
Source: CHATS

Compensating for Vision Changes

1. **Don't stand in front of a bright source of light when speaking to a person.** The person will find it very difficult to see your face (Photo 10-7).
2. **Stand so that the person can see you.** Experiment with the distance and position that works best for your client.
3. **Tell the person where you are and what you are doing.** If you are walking or riding with a person, describe the surroundings.
4. **Be specific in your communication.** Saying to the person, "It's over there" is of little help. Say something like, "The chair is about two steps away, on your right."
5. **Let the person know if you leave the room.**
6. **Use large type (or write in large letters) when writing information.**
7. **Avoid decorative fonts, all capital letters, or underlining information.** In fact, all of these things make printed information *harder* to read.

Compensating for Hearing Changes

1. **If the person uses a hearing aid, make sure that it is in place and working properly.**
2. **Make sure the person is wearing his or her glasses, if needed.** This is particularly important if the person reads lips.
3. **Use notes or sign language.**
4. **Avoid shouting.** It can be painful and make understanding more difficult.
5. **Speak using your face, your hands, and your eyes.** Use gestures, and point to objects that will help you get your message across.
6. **Stand or sit where your face can be easily seen.** Make sure that the person is able to read your lips.
7. **Be sure that you have the listener's attention.** Does he or she know you are talking to him or her? Always try to communicate at eye level and establish eye contact.

8. **When you speak, don't chew gum, smoke, or put your hand over your mouth.** These things distort normal lip movement and make lip reading impossible.

9. **Move away from background noise** (such as an air conditioner, television, or a crowded room).

10. **If you are not understood, rephrase your statement using different words.** For example, substituting a phrase like "false teeth" for the word "dentures" may make it easier for the person to understand.

11. **Be positive. Have patience.**

12. **Bear in mind that an ill or tired person will not hear as well as he or she might when rested or well.**

13. **Lower the pitch of your voice, but keep the volume up.** Experiment with different volumes and different tones.

14. **Vary your position relative to the person.** Some people hear better when the sound comes from a particular direction.

15. **Decrease your rate of speech.** We all speak much faster than we think we do!

16. **Avoid words with double consonants if you can.** Double consonants like ss, ch, st, and ch are particularly difficult to hear. If possible, substitute a word without these combinations.

17. **Learn and use sign language.**

Compensating for Changes in Touch Sensitivity

1. **Make use of opportunities for touch.** A handshake, hug, walking arm in arm, and gentle rubbing of arms or shoulders are ways of communicating by touch. Be careful, though, not to force touch on a person who does not want it. We all vary in the amount of touch that we need.

2. **Use touch to get the person's attention.** A brief touch on the arm will let the person know where you are.

3. **Let your touch linger for a moment.** A quick, gentle pat on the hand may be fine for a teen, but an older person may not realize you have even touched him or her.

COMMUNICATION AIDS TO COMPENSATE FOR SENSORY LOSS

Many of the following items can be purchased at variety stores or made by you.

Aids to Compensate for Vision Loss

1. A magnifying glass can enable a visually impaired person to read directions or other small print (Photo 10-8). Magnifying bars and sheets are also available (Photo 10-9).

Photo 10-8
A magnifying glass can enable a visually impaired person to read directions or other small print.

Photo 10-9
Magnifying sheets are also available.

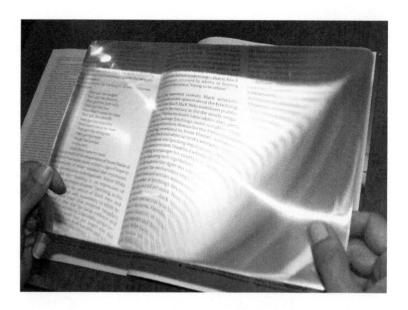

2. A clamp-on lamp with a magnifying lens in its centre provides illumination as well as magnification (Photo 10-10).
3. Increasing the lighting in frequently used rooms (without creating glare) can make it easier for a person to see faces and gestures.

Photo 10-10
A clamp-on lamp with a magnifying lens in its centre provides illumination as well as magnification.

Aids to Compensate for Hearing Loss

1. **Flashing lights for doorbells and telephones.** These items flash when the doorbell or phone rings.
2. **Pen and paper.** Some people find it easier to lip-read if the topic of the conversation is written down. Others prefer to jot notes to communicate.
3. **A hearing aid.** Encourage the person to contact the appropriate health professional if the person feels the aid is broken or not suitable. Many problems can be eliminated through adjustments to the aid or to its settings.

4. **Systems to assist a hearing-impaired person with the phone.** One kind uses typewriter-style machines to allow the person to type messages that are sent to tele-type terminals. Another, more sophisticated kind, is a computer-based system which allows the person to select predetermined phrases that are then converted to speech and subsequently transmitted to another person.

Questions for Review

1. Describe the difference between adaptive and augmentative communication.

2. Identify at least six approaches you can use to assist a client with aphasia to communicate.

3. What are three techniques you might use to assist a person with aphasia to get his or her message across?

4. Describe two augmentative communication aids.

5. You are working with a client with hearing loss. What are three things you can do to make communication easier with your client?

6. What guideline should you follow when learning about the level of touch your client prefers?

7. List two ways of helping a client meet his or her needs for touch.

8. How might you better communicate with a person who has apraxia of speech? List at least five methods.

Questions for Discussion

1. Imagine that you could not express yourself verbally. How would you feel? How would you make your needs and wants known?

2. Review Case Example 10-4 on page 145. How would you feel if you were Ramiro? Share your answers with those of your colleagues.

3. Develop your own personal word list (as described in the section on communication aids). What words would be important to include? Compare your list with those of your colleagues. How do their lists differ from yours? Does this reflect the differences in your hobbies and other activities?

Chapter 11

Setting Priorities and Working Effectively

Learning Objectives

Through reading this chapter, you'll be able to

1. Describe the three elements of effective time management.
2. Discuss the importance of setting goals.
3. Generate SMART goals.
4. Describe balance in time management.
5. Depict overlapping tasks and apply the technique to manage multiple tasks.
6. Define assertiveness and describe behaviours that indicate assertiveness.
7. List the four skills involved in problem solving.
8. Discuss how your personal culture might affect how you resolve problems.
9. Apply the problem-solving process to address a problem.
10. Identify situations where you must decline a task and apply the five principles when you must decline a task.

Chapter at a Glance

- The Elements of Time Management
- Time Management in Support Work
- Assertiveness
- What Is Assertiveness Training?
- Problem Solving

Terms You'll Use

Assertiveness A technique that helps you respect others' views, concerns, and needs while not compromising your own.

Clarifying Describing things clearly so that others understand or asking questions so that you understand.

Negotiating The give-and-take used in problem solving.

Overlapping Tasks Tasks that are started and allowed to continue while another task is finished or begun.

Priorities Goals that you want to attain before others.
SMART Goals Criteria for describing the effectiveness of goals.
Time Management Making the most of the time you have, in light of your priorities.

THE ELEMENTS OF TIME MANAGEMENT

The secret of life is enjoying the passage of time.

James Taylor

Do you have enough time? You probably said no. The truth is, you have all the time there is to have. **Time management** means making the best of the time you have. This means developing skills in three things: knowing what your goals are, disciplining yourself to stay focused on those goals, and using techniques that make the best use of your time.

In this chapter, we'll make a distinction between managing your personal goals and time, and managing work goals and working efficiently. Each is different, but still essential to effective personal support work.

What's Important? Setting Personal Goals

Personal goals are the things you as a person want to attain. At least some of them are probably linked to your decision to become a support worker. Knowing what your goals are helps you to attain them (Figure 11-1). In fact, some research suggests that a person becomes more effective at managing time *simply* by defining his or her goals.

FIGURE 11-1
Spheres of goals

"To learn how to best work with clients with dementia"

"To read a book for pleasure each month"

"To lose 5 kg"

"To spend one night each month on a 'date' with my spouse – without children"

"To improve my communication skills"

"To exercise at least twice a week"

We have many types of personal goals. We have goals related to our work and goals related to our own personal life. Remember, the work goals we talk about here are *your* goals for *your* professional development. These are different from the work goals you set with an individual client in order to work effectively.

STOP AND REFLECT ((11-1))

What is most important to you? For each heading below, write three goals you want to attain.

Personal Goals

_____

_____

_____

_____

Work Goals

_____

_____

_____

SMART Goals

To be effective, goals must also be SMART:

   Specific
   Measurable
   Attainable
   Require resources that are available
   Timely

Have you ever started a fitness plan? If so, chances are you had a goal in mind, such as to be able to do 50 sit-ups at a time or to be able to run two kilometres. These goals are specific and measurable. Whether they are attainable depends upon your overall health status. Similarly, the amount of time you could devote to the goal is an indication of whether you have the resources.

A timely goal is one that is measured in a reasonable time period. There is no set definition of a reasonable time period; it depends upon the other factors. For example, allowing enough time to attain the goal is a function of how much work you must do to be able to complete the 50 sit-ups or run the two kilometres and how many resources you can devote to it. For example, if you have never even walked two kilometres, it would likely be unrealistic to expect that you could learn to run two kilometres in, say, two weeks.

You always must be realistic when you set time frames. Setting your goals too high—expecting to attain too much—can discourage you. Similarly, setting your goals too low often results in little satisfaction because the goal was too easy.

You should plan in blocks of three months. If you have ultimate goals, such as to complete a course or to have children within the next five years, give some thought to what you have to do in the shorter run to make the ultimate goal attainable. These short-run goals are the ones to focus on now.

STOP AND REFLECT ((11-2))

Take another look at the goals you set for yourself in the previous Stop and Reflect box. Rate each goal against the SMART criteria, using a time period of not more than three months. For example, if you had listed the goal "eat better," you might rewrite it as "by the end of three months, I will eat balanced meals at least four days per week." Rewrite your goals here.

Personal Goals

_____

_____

_____

Work Goals

_____

_____

_____

It's important to keep your goals in mind. You might want to write them on a card that you keep in your wallet. You might find that writing them in your appointment book helps you to keep your goals in mind.

Setting personal goals can help you attain wellness, as was discussed in Chapter 4. Setting SMART goals can help you regularly practise the activities associated with wellness.

Getting There

Knowing your goals is important. However, you'll still need a plan to get there. There are often many steps involved in attaining the goal. Consider the following situation.

CASE EXAMPLE 11-1

Fatima is a support worker at a seniors' day program. For some time now, she has wanted to lose 10 kilograms and to become more fit. However, she has not been able to do so.

Fatima mentions her frustration to a friend. As they discuss the issue, Fatima identifies two actions she could take to attain her goal. First, Fatima can start walking to and from work. This will require her to leave for work 15 minutes earlier than she currently does, and she will *get home 15 minutes later. Second, Fatima can replace the convenience foods she currently brings for lunch with healthier choices.*

Through these two actions, Fatima is able to lose 10 kilograms in 14 weeks. She feels better and has the satisfaction of having attained a much-desired goal.

How can Fatima's plan to lose 10 kilograms be expressed as a SMART goal?

Managing Your Time

Setting SMART goals and identifying approaches to attain those goals are necessary components of time management. As singer Willie Nelson said, "If you don't know where you're going, you're liable to end up somewhere else." The third step requires you to evaluate what you do against your *priorities*, making changes so that most of your time is spent attaining your goals. Priorities are those things that you want to do first. Consider the following case example.

CASE EXAMPLE 11-2

Yuri is a support worker. He is also taking a course to upgrade his skills. He plans to attain his certificate in the spring. With a certificate, Yuri will receive a raise that will allow him to better provide for his family.

He attends class one night each week. This week, a classmate asks Yuri to join him for a coffee after class. Even though Yuri has to work the next morning at 7 a.m., he agrees.

The classmate tells Yuri about a personal problem. He is very upset over a break-up with a girlfriend. By the time Yuri leaves his classmate, it is 3 a.m. Yuri heads home.

Yuri's wife wakes him at 6:30 a.m. He rushes to get ready, but knows that he will be late for work. As he is leaving, the building custodian stops him. "I need your door keys," the custodian tells Yuri. "We're changing the locks, and I may as well give you your new keys now." Although Yuri's wife will be home to let him in when he returns from work, Yuri follows the custodian. Fifteen minutes later, he has his new keys.

By the time Yuri gets to work, he is 45 minutes late. He apologizes to his co-worker (who has had to work extra hard because Yuri was not there) and does his best to catch up. He also has to explain his lateness to his supervisor.

What do you think Yuri's goals are?

Which of his activities did not support his goals?

What would you have done differently?

Making sure that your activities support your goals doesn't mean that you are selfish. It is still important to help others. You must learn to balance your needs with those of others. For example, you may well have done what Yuri did—helped a classmate. You might not have stayed out until 3 a.m. with that friend, though.

TIME MANAGEMENT IN SUPPORT WORK

Managing your time at work is a bit different than managing your personal time. At work, your priority is to provide the best service possible to your client. In a very real sense, your goal is to help your client attain his or her goals.

In Case Example 11-3, Karen illustrates three principles of time management with clients: she knows her clients' preferences and goals; she has planned her work with the clients; and she makes the best use of her time by *overlapping* tasks. We'll discuss each of these principles in this section.

Learning Your Client's Goals and Priorities

One of your first tasks when assigned a new client should be to talk with the client to find out his or her goals and priorities as they relate to your work with him or her. This includes two things: what the client wants to attain, and how the client would like you to assist.

If you work in the community, prior to your first visit you may receive a referral form for each client that describes the client's general goals and tasks you are to do. If you work in a facility, you will likely learn this information through a care conference

CASE EXAMPLE 11-3

It's 7:05 a.m. Karen has just started her shift. She is responsible for 12 residents, all of whom need some help getting up and dressed before breakfast at 8:10 a.m.

Three residents take a great deal of time to get started in the morning. Four need assistance with toileting as well as complete help with dressing. Three need someone to lay out their clothes in order. Two need reminders to dress and someone to do up shoelaces, buttons, and zippers.

Karen knows her residents well. She knows who likes to rise early and who wants to stay in bed until the last minute. She knows who needs 30 minutes to adjust to waking up and who does not. In the first room on her assigned unit, Karen begins with the residents who like to rise early and need time to adjust. She wakes Mrs. Baker, leaving her to rouse as she wakes and assists Mrs. Morse into the washroom. When Karen returns to the room, she lays out Mrs. Baker's clothes in the order Mrs. Baker will put them on. (Mrs. Baker prefers to dress herself, even though her arthritis makes this very difficult.) Karen then helps Mrs. Morse dress. The room's third resident, Mrs. Veenstra, likes to sleep in, so Karen leaves her and proceeds to the next assigned resident room. She'll return to wake Mrs. Veenstra after all her other residents are cared for.

In what ways does Karen manage her time well? How does she manage time and give good support to her residents?

or from the charge nurse when you report for work. The information you get before you meet the client can help you plan your work. Still, you should talk with your client to determine her or his priorities for your visit and *how* the client would like you to do what you are assigned to do.

Keep in mind that priorities may change from day to day. A client whose family member is coming to visit may prefer that you spend more time helping him or her get washed and dressed. A client who normally has a bath during your Wednesday visit may ask that you assist her on another day.

A client's goals may also change over time, just as your goals do. Sometimes, a goal is attained and replaced by a new one. For example, a client who is recovering from a stroke may have set a goal of being able to get dressed without help. You may have helped the client practise techniques that made it easier to accomplish this goal. However, once the goal was attained, the client may have set another. You would then assist the client with attaining that new goal.

Planning Tasks Together

If at all possible, plan your tasks with the client. This gives you three benefits. First, you let the client know that her or his priorities are important to you. Second, you learn from the client what is important to her or him. You can ask questions so that you actually understand the client's needs. Third, you learn how the client would like you to assist, including the parts of any assigned tasks that the client would like to do.

Organizing Overlapping Tasks

Like Karen's job, most of your work will require you to perform a number of tasks in a short period of time. You must develop skill in scheduling **overlapping tasks**—those you start and then can leave for a bit while you do something else.

Most of us have some experience in organizing overlapping tasks. For example, you likely do other things while your laundry is in the wash. Chances are, you start the washer and then do other things while the cycle runs. You come back to the washer when the cycle is finished. If you take your laundry to the laundromat, you bring along something to do while your clothes are in the machines.

STOP AND REFLECT ((11-3))

How do you make best use of your time by organizing overlapping tasks? List at least five tasks you do while waiting for something else to finish.

_____

_____

_____

_____

Share your answers with your colleagues. Do they use different techniques? Are there any techniques they use that you might try?

_____

_____

_____

ASSERTIVENESS

STOP AND REFLECT ((11-4))

Imagine the following situation.

You are the health care aide assigned to Mrs. Fasikas. Today, just as you're about to leave Mrs. Fasikas's room, she begins to tell you about her sister's visit. While you would like to hear about the visit, you have other clients to care for. Yet, you know Mrs. Fasikas has very few family or friends who visit.

What do you say to Mrs. Fasikas?

_____

_____

_____

What might you say/do to avoid this kind of situation in the future and still respect Mrs. Fasikas's needs?

_____

_____

Have you ever been in a situation where you gave in to another person's requests, even though you didn't want to? Perhaps you did this to avoid conflict. Did you feel angry about this afterward? Perhaps you got angry after another person continually put his or her needs before yours, and you "dug your heels in" about an issue you didn't really care about. You might have felt guilty afterward. Assertiveness training can help you to avoid these situations.

Assertiveness is a behaviour that can be learned and practised. It has been described as a technique that helps you to:

- Respect each person in the communication.
- Consider your needs and express them clearly.
- Consider the other person's need and respect it.

It can also help you to more easily resolve issues and problems.

Assertiveness *doesn't* mean always getting your own way. It helps you to balance your needs with those of the other person. Table 11-1 describes the relationships among assertiveness, passivity, and aggression.

TABLE 11-1	Are You a Pansy, a Partner, or a Porcupine?	
Pansy	**Partner**	**Porcupine**
Passive "Whatever you want"	Assertive "What do we both want?"	Aggressive "My way or the highway!"

As we said earlier, assertiveness is a behaviour. Table 11-2 describes some of the characteristics associated with passive, assertive, and aggressive behaviours.

TABLE 11-2	Characteristics of Passive, Assertive, and Aggressive Behaviours		
	Pansy	**Partner**	**Porcupine**
Behaviour	▪ Lets others make decisions ▪ Doesn't express feelings, ideas, wants ▪ Gives in ▪ Hedges ▪ Apologizes ▪ Hopes someone will guess what he/she wants	▪ Appropriately honest ▪ Expresses wants and feelings directly ▪ Chooses for him/herself ▪ Exercises his/her rights ▪ Respects rights of others ▪ Listens, uses direct language ("I" statements)	▪ Inappropriately honest ▪ Puts others down ▪ Ignores others' rights ▪ Chooses for others ▪ Is sarcastic ▪ Blames ▪ Overreacts
Reasons for the behaviour	Wants to avoid conflict, upsetting other people	To get a win-win situation if possible; to know he or she has done his or her best to meet needs	To get what he or she wants at all costs; may only see things in terms of "I win only if you lose"
Feels this way about his or her behaviour	Guilty, helpless, hurt, powerless Can feel angry or resentful afterward	Confident, relaxed, good	Hostile, defensive, righteous
How others feel	Guilty, angry, disrespectful, frustrated	Respected, respectful, sometimes threatened	Hurt, humiliated, defensive, angry

WHAT IS ASSERTIVENESS TRAINING?

Assertiveness requires two things:

- That you know your soft spots—the people or situations in which you find it difficult to be assertive.
- That you develop a sense of comfort in your right to express your needs and what you want.

It's not uncommon to be more assertive with certain people or in certain settings. You might be very assertive with your co-workers, but not at all with your clients. You could be a real partner to your sisters, but a real pansy when it comes to your brothers.

Take a few minutes to think about how assertive you are in the following settings.

STOP AND REFLECT ((11-5))

Where/with whom are you:

A Pansy?

_____

_____

_____

_____

A Partner?

_____

_____

_____

_____

A Porcupine?

_____

_____

_____

_____ ■

Developing a sense of comfort in your right to express your needs and wants is often difficult. As caregivers, we're taught to put others' needs first. The key word here is practise. Start by stating your wants with something simple, perhaps in a discussion of what movie to see or where to go for dinner. When you've become comfortable with that, go on to something more difficult. Don't worry; it will take time. Be sure to savour the good feeling that comes with having expressed yourself.

Remember, it is not disrespectful to state your own needs and desires, so long as you state them in a way that does not deny others their right to do the same thing. Rights always come with responsibilities. Table 11-3 lists some common rights and their respective responsibilities. Assertiveness becomes easier with practice. It sometimes helps to "think through" how you might respond assertively in a situation. Use Stop and Reflect 11-6 to plan your communication.

TABLE 11-3	Rights and Responsibilities
If you have this right...	**You also have this responsibility...**
To Speak Up	To Listen
To Take	To Give
To Have Problems	To Find Solutions
To Be Respected	To Respect

STOP AND REFLECT ((11-6))

Answer the following questions. Your answers will help you plan to become a more assertive person.

One situation in which I'd like to become more assertive is:

_____

_____

_____

_____

I can become more assertive in that situation by doing/saying:

_____

_____

_____

_____

I need to practise becoming more assertive in that situation by:

_____

_____

_____

_____

You may also want to practise a difficult situation with a friend. Have your friend take on the role of the person with whom you find it difficult to be assertive. You can then practise responding assertively.

PROBLEM SOLVING

Sometimes, despite our best efforts, we come across a situation that must be worked through. Perhaps the communication wasn't as clear as we thought it was. Perhaps the interests of the people concerned just don't seem to match up.

There are three types of problems: those that aren't worth bothering with, those that are minor and require only a quick answer, and those that are serious and require work.

Recall a situation in which you spent a lot of effort (perhaps worrying or deciding what to do) on a problem that you realized later simply wasn't worth it.

How did you feel?

_____

_____

_____

In Chapter 4, you learned not to "sweat the small stuff" when you manage stress. This saying also applies to problem solving. When you commit time and effort to a problem that is not worth it, you're really wasting your resources. Before you decide to spend a great deal of effort on an issue, ask yourself the following questions:

1. Is it really a threat?
2. Is it worth the worry?
3. Even if I want to, can I change the outcome?

Is the problem really a threat? Is the problem really affecting you? Or is it just that you're reacting to the change it might bring? Ask yourself what the problem really threatens. If it's simply that it's different, go no farther. It's not worth the effort.

If it does threaten something you hold dear, ask yourself: is the problem worth the worry? If your answer to this question is no, and the problem is not a major one for any of the parties, spend a few minutes generating ideas about what to do. Then make a quick decision (or let others make it) and get on with things.

If your answer to Question 2 is yes, ask yourself: even if I want to, can I change the outcome of the problem? If your answer to this question is no, put your efforts toward adapting to the decision you'll have to live with.

However, if you answered yes to all three questions, you will need to do some problem-solving. Exactly what type of problem-solving you should do will depend upon two more questions:

- Do you and the others involved all agree that the problem is minor or routine?
- Is this a problem where there are good solutions that everyone involved would accept?

If the answers to these two questions are yes, make the decision based upon the information you have. You may discuss the issue and solutions with others, particularly if this is a new problem. If it's a routine issue, you may be able to simply apply a good solution you've used before.

If the problem isn't minor or routine, or those involved have significantly different views and desires so that there's no clear good answer, you will have to use a problem-solving technique to attempt to resolve the issue.

Problem solving involves five processes: sharing information, clarifying each person's views, identifying priorities, brainstorming options and negotiating.

Sharing information requires you to share your views and needs and to listen and try to understand the views and needs of the others involved. **Clarifying** involves describing things clearly so that others understand or asking questions and checking back with the others to make sure you understand them. Identifying priorities refers to listing criteria that a good solution must meet and ranking these criteria in order of importance to those involved. Brainstorming is a technique in which you and the others involved list all the possible solutions. **Negotiating** refers to the give and take used to solve a problem.

Using the following questions may help you to work through the process more effectively. With the others involved, answer the following questions:

1. What is the real problem?
2. What information do you need to deal with it?
3. Who else (if anyone) needs to deal with it?
4. What criteria (needs) does a "good" solution have to meet?
5. What possible solutions could be used?
6. Which solutions best meet the parties' criteria?
7. Which solution will be tried first?
8. What will we try next if the first solution fails?

It's very important to resist the temptation to act too quickly to resolve a serious problem. We often feel the pressure to fix things but with a serious problem, acting too quickly may only address the symptoms, leaving the underlying cause unresolved. If so, the problem will return. If at all possible, take the time (and make the time) to get the answers to the above questions.

Communication skills are essential to problem solving. At each step in the process, you need to take the time to explore how the other person sees things as well as explain your view. Only if you know how the other person sees things will you know how much you have in common.

SPOTLIGHT 11-1 HOW DO WE LEARN TO SOLVE PROBLEMS?

Most of us learn to solve problems by watching others and by trying things out to see how well they work. Usually, we rely a great deal upon skills that work for us. Because we develop them from our experience, they are heavily influenced by our personal culture. This is also true of our co-workers and clients. For example, you might strongly feel that it's really inappropriate for a younger person to disagree with an elder. Another person might strongly feel that all people in a situation have an equal right to be heard.

What skills do you rely upon to solve problems? How did you learn and develop these skills?

It can be challenging when you must resolve an issue with a person whose approach to solving problems is different from yours. In a sense you have to resolve two things: the issue and the way you try to work it out.

Can you recall a situation where your way of solving a problem was very different from the other person's? How did you deal with the difference in method? What did you learn from this experience?

Table 11-4 outlines an effective procedure to use when you want to find out how the other person sees things (Adapted from Tom Rusk, *The Power of Ethical Persuasion*).

TABLE 11-4	Exploring the Other Person's Opinion

1. Agree that your first task is to understand each other's opinion, not to immediately solve the problem.
2. Ask the person how he or she sees the issue and how she or he would like to see it change.
3. Ask the person to help you understand his or her view. DO NOT argue with the person or defend your position.
4. Once the person shares his or her view, repeat it in your own words to show that you understand.
5. Ask the person to correct what you said so that you can fully understand.
6. Repeat the process until the person agrees without hesitation that you understand his or her view. Responses like "I guess so" or "sort of" do not indicate agreement.

Always listen to the other person's viewpoint first. When you express your opinion, follow the steps in Table 11-5.

TABLE 11-5	Explaining Your Own Opinion

1. Ask the person to hear you out.

2. Carefully explain your thoughts and opinions as your opinion, not the "way things really are."

3. Ask the person to repeat what you have said. Correct any errors until you can truthfully say that the other person understands.

Once you have explored each other's opinions, look for the similarities. Identify where your view and the other person's view are similar. Even if you disagree on some things, you likely share the same perspective on others. Look for the common ground—the things you see the same way. For example, even though you might disagree with a client's daughter about what you can do during a client visit, you likely both agree that you want the best for that client.

Repeat this technique at each step in the problem-solving process.

It's the Real Thing

STOP AND REFLECT ((11-8))

Consider the following situation.

You have a 17-year-old child. You have set a curfew of midnight on weekends, 9 p.m. on weeknights. Your child constantly breaks curfew, coming in half to three-quarters of an hour later than required.

What is the issue?

_____

_____

_____

_____

_____

_____

If you said something like "She doesn't respect me," you're not alone. But, is that the issue? Or, is it more likely a symptom or a cause?

A *problem* refers to a situation that is not planned and not desired. To resolve it, you've got to know the desired state of things—the real thing—before you can figure out what's gone wrong.

Focus on the behaviours. If your response to the curfew problem was something like "He doesn't listen to me," or "She wants to do her own thing," you're going down the wrong path. What is it that the person is doing that makes you say these things? That's likely the behaviour (or part of it) you need to get at.

Flesh out the issue. When does it happen? Does it always happen that way? Who is involved? Are there causes you can identify?

Whose Issue Is It, Anyway?

Once you've got the issue/problem described, it's time to consider ownership. Ownership refers to who should be involved in dealing with the issue, *not whose fault the issue or problem is.*

Many systems have been developed for identifying who should be involved in resolving a problem. A simple test is to ask yourself the following three questions:

- **Do I need the cooperation and support of others to make this solution work?** If so, involve those people in the decision. Some challenging situations will require you and your client to work together to problem solve.
- **Do I need expertise I don't have?** If so, get it. You may need to contact your supervisor for information and guidance. With your supervisor's permission, you may ask others for help.
- **Do I need both cooperation and expertise?** If so, get the parties together.

What Do We Want? Setting Criteria

CASE EXAMPLE 11-4

The story is told of the two hard bargainers. These two, who are sisters, are staying at a cottage miles from the nearest town. They have supplies but, between them, have just one orange. One sister needs the entire orange for juice; the other needs the rind of the entire orange for a cake. Both want the entire orange. They argue. As neither will give in, they split the orange in half. Neither gets what she wants and neither is happy.

The moral of this story? *The best solutions are those that address your "must haves," not those that give a specific answer.* There may be many ways to satisfactorily address an issue. You help to ensure success by identifying the criteria a good solution must meet, rather than identifying just one right answer.

What Do You Want? What Does the Other Person Want?

When you figure out what the real problem is, you should have developed some idea of what the desired solution might look like. This will give you an idea of the criteria any solution must meet. You may also have criteria set for you, such as any solution must not cost more than a specific sum. These ideas are a start toward developing criteria that solutions must meet.

You may also find that you have two types of criteria: "must haves" and "like to haves." This is fine.

If you're working with others, you may find that your criteria differ from those of others in the group. If the differences are complementary (i.e., they can coexist), include both. If one or more contradicts another, you'll need to negotiate. Use a similar process in the event that one of your "musts" is another's "like." Generally, if one person sees a criterion as a "must have," it's best to simply include it.

CASE EXAMPLE 11-5

Instead of insisting on having the entire orange, the sisters decide to take a moment to decide what each really wants. The first sister determines that she needs only the juice. The other sister decides that she needs only the *peel. The sisters quickly determine that their needs are complementary. Both can get what they want from the single orange. They squeeze the orange for the juice, then grate the rind for the cake.*

Do We Have Everything?

At some time in this process, you may find that you need additional information. Information on how others have approached a similar issue, an expert opinion, and success stories are all useful if you know what you want from them.

Before you search for information, know what kind of information you want to find. Be specific about your needs, and collect only that which is useful in making the decision.

How Can We Get It? Creating the Options

Sometimes setting the criteria will suggest the best option. For example, when the sisters described their needs, the best option to solving their problem was clear.

Sometimes, the answer is not so obvious. The problem may be complex, or one of the parties may feel very strongly that a single answer is the only answer. The most desirable option may not be possible for reasons beyond any of the parties' control.

Consider the situation described in Stop and Reflect 11-9.

There is no obvious solution here. The client's needs seem to differ from yours. Furthermore, some options (such as having additional time at the client's) are impossible. You would have to work with the client to determine her criteria, figure out yours, and then generate options to address the issue.

When you discussed the above situation with your colleagues, did you find that you came up with even more options? Chances are that you did. Each person sees the situation a little differently. This difference in perspective allows us to see other options. The discussion of these different points of view often spawns creativity.

Creativity is at its peak when we are young. Remember when you were a child? Do you remember making up stories about imaginary friends, animals, almost anything? Anything was possible: stories knew no rational bounds. Until you grew up.

As we grow, we learn rules. Research suggests that our creativity at age 40 is 5 percent of what it was at age five. Luckily, regaining the creativity of youth is not like regaining the energy of youth. We can do it, with a little practice.

Brainstorming is perhaps the oldest and best known of all the creative idea generating methods. It is done by having a group contribute ideas in a free-flowing session, without any initial evaluation of the ideas. The function of brainstorming is to generate a wide variety and number of ideas quickly, without censorship, judgment, or premature evaluation. Remember these ground rules:

1. No comments or judgments on the ideas until it is time for discussion.
2. Write down all the ideas you generate.
3. Share all ideas that come to mind, without prejudging.
4. The idea-generating time period can be either specific or open-ended, although a specific time period seems to work best as it helps to keep the group on task.

STOP AND REFLECT ((11-9))

You have just been assigned a new client. The client lives with her son and his family. You are asked to assist the client with a bath, to do her personal laundry, and to do "light" housekeeping.

When you arrive at the client's home, she shows you where her cleaning supplies are kept. She tells you that she is "so glad that you will take on the housework." You review the tasks you are assigned to do. The client becomes upset and says, "My daughter can help me with my bath. I need you to do the housework." She asks you to vacuum, dust, and wash floors in the house. While the client's personal area is part of this, much of the housekeeping is for the areas used by other members of the family.

You contact your supervisor for advice. She tells you that your agency does not have a strict definition of "light" house-keeping—it's worked out with each client. Your supervisor also tells you that she cannot authorize any additional hours of service. However, it's up to you to work it out with the client.

You speak with the client. She tells you that it is very important to her to know that she is not a burden to her son and that you doing the housekeeping she requests will make her feel less a burden.

What are your criteria here?

_____
_____
_____
_____
_____

What do you think your client's criteria are?

_____
_____
_____
_____
_____

What options can you generate that might solve this problem?

_____
_____
_____
_____
_____

Share your answers with your colleagues. Did they generate other options?

_____
_____
_____
_____
_____

Brainstorming can generate an amazing number of ideas in a very short time, if you stick to the rules. This can be difficult because we all tend to examine each idea as it comes along. You may have found this happened when you discussed your responses to the floor-washing situation. If you heard a lot of things like "If you do that, you'll never be..." or "That won't work," you know how difficult it can be not to prejudge an option.

Getting the Best Fit—Evaluating the Options

Once the options have been generated, they need to be ranked against the criteria you generated earlier. Ideally, one or more options will meet all criteria but, if not, you have two choices:

1. Select options that meet as many of your criteria as possible.
2. Go back and generate other options.

It's important to work with your client to attain agreement on the options you'll try first. Consider again the floor-washing situation. What options do you feel would meet your criteria? What options would meet your client's? Which option seems most likely to meet both your needs?

Then, Do It

Once you've determined the first option to try, put it in place. If it doesn't work out, go to the next option.

When You Must Decline a Task

When you must decline a task, you must do so only for the right reasons. Not liking a task or not feeling that it is as important as another are not acceptable reasons to decline. However, sometimes you simply cannot do what another person asks. This may be for many reasons: you may not have time; you may not have the training to do the task; or the task may not be permitted by your agency. In some of these cases, you may need to seek your supervisor's guidance to resolve the issue. In other cases, you may be able to decline the task with your client's understanding.

The Gentle Art of Declining a Task

Following these guidelines will help you and the client to resolve issues when you cannot do what is asked.

1. **Focus on the issue, not the people.** The client is not a "bad person" for asking you to do something that you cannot do. Similarly, you are not a "bad person" for being unable to do what the client asks. You simply have needs and obligations that conflict. Make certain your communication reflects the fact that the issue is no one's "fault."
2. **Your goal is to get mutual understanding, not prove that you are right.**
3. **Be aware of your tone of voice and your body language.** Some situations can easily become emotionally charged. When this happens, the people involved may react mostly to your nonverbal communication. Keep your nonverbal communication caring.
4. **Be creative.** If the issue is insufficient time, is it possible to do the task requested if another, nonessential, task is postponed or done by another? For example, a client whose sister is coming to visit may prefer you assist her with a bath, even if it is not her usual bath day and other tasks must be postponed.

5. **Be gracious.** It's perfectly fine to apologize for the effect a decision has upon the client, although you feel that the decision is appropriate. For example, when responding to the client in Stop and Reflect 11-9, you might say, "I'm sorry that I can't do the family's housekeeping. I know that it would make you feel better. However, I must do the tasks assigned by my agency."

Questions for Review

1. Review the personal goals you set in Stop and Reflect 11-1 on page 156. Write down the steps you must take in order to attain two of these goals.

2. What is an overlapping task? Give an example of a set of overlapping tasks.

3. What three benefits can you attain by planning tasks with your client?

4. Describe assertiveness. What are the three things that assertiveness helps you to do?

5. What is the problem-solving process?

6. What are the four skills involved in problem solving?

7. What five principles are useful when you must decline a task?

Questions for Discussion

1. Review the following case study. How would you use problem solving, assertiveness, and negotiation skills to help resolve this issue?

   You are the client attendant in a seniors' day program. Your agency has planned a bus trip for clients and their spouses. Your supervisor has already left on the first bus, after telling you to take care of everything while she is gone—including solving any problems that might arise.

   Mr. Gray, the husband of a client, approaches you. He is holding his wife's torn coat. He appears very angry as he holds the coat out to you and says, "This should never have happened. The bus driver didn't even look when he closed the door. I told him the coat was caught, but he didn't stop. What are you going to do?" You speak with the bus driver, but he says that he neither saw the coat nor heard Mr. Gray. Furthermore, he says that the bus company isn't responsible for these things, and points to a sign on the bus that says just that.

2. What do you do to make better use of your time? Share your ideas with your colleagues.

3. With a group of your colleagues, review the list of rights and responsibilities listed in Table 11-3 on page 163. Are there other rights and responsibilities you might add?

4. Who and what have influenced your problem-solving skills? Have you had to change the way that you solve problems you encounter as a support worker? If so, how? Are there situations (such as disagreeing with an elder) that are really challenging for you? How do you work through these situations? Do you discuss the issue with another person, or ask for help from another person?

Chapter 12

Contributing to the Client's Support Plan

Learning Objectives

Through reading this chapter, you'll be able to

1. Tell what the purpose of the support plan is.
2. List four common types of support plans.
3. Outline the stages in the support planning process.
4. Explain the role of the support worker in contributing to the client's support plan.
5. Describe the ABCS of observation.
6. List the two main types of reporting and the five guidelines for organizing a verbal report.
7. Accurately record client information in the proper format, using the ten rules for documentation.
8. Use common terminology in documentation.
9. Describe federal and provincial privacy legislation and discuss how it affects how we keep and use client information.
10. Differentiate between privacy, confidentiality, and security of client information, and list some activities a support worker should perform to ensure client information is not inappropriately kept or shared.

Chapter at a Glance

- What Is the Support Plan?
- The Support Planning Process
- The Role of the Support Worker in the Support Planning Process
- Observation Skills
- Respecting Privacy, Maintaining Confidentiality, Ensuring Security
- Reporting Your Observations and Actions
- Guidelines for Recording
- Common Terminology and Abbreviations Used in Documentation

Terms You'll Use

Appearance Observations about body language, dress, and cleanliness.
Assessment The phase of support planning that determines the type of support needed.

Behaviour Observations about actions, awareness and interest in surroundings, and awareness and interest in others.

Communication In reporting, this means observations about messages, including what is said and how it is said.

Confidentiality The obligation to keep the client's personal information private.

Documentation Written reports such as notes, reports, and checklists.

Evaluation The phase of support planning that reviews the client's situation, needs, and preferences.

Goal Setting The phase of support planning in which client goals are identified, along with the methods that will be used to attain the goals.

Implementation The phase of support planning in which the methods identified in the goal-setting phase are put into practice.

Status Observations about a client's condition, function, and any change that was seen.

Support Plan The foundation for all services that a client receives; also called a care plan.

Support Planning Process The process used to identify the goals and preferences of the client.

WHAT IS THE SUPPORT PLAN?

The **support plan** is the foundation for all the services the client receives. The plan provides a central point of reference for information about the client, the client's goals, and the services the client receives. Many different terms are used to describe the support plan, such as care plan, service agreement, bookings, or support agreement.

Most of your clients will have had a support plan developed with them. However, some persons who direct their own care do not develop a support plan. When there is no support plan in place, you must be certain to get clear direction from the client as to the needs and tasks to be done.

The support plan is one of several documents that provide up-to-date information about the client and the client's needs. The other documents can include client assessments, referral forms, progress notes, and reports of any therapy the client receives. Other documents may also be included. Each agency develops its own set of documents, although some agencies in the same area may share certain forms.

The support plan is a *dynamic document*. It changes as the client's needs, condition, or goals change. It is intended to be developed, then reviewed and revised as required.

THE SUPPORT PLANNING PROCESS

The *support planning process* is often a function of the support team we discussed in Chapter 5. The client or the client's representative should *always* be involved in the **support planning process**, during which the goals and preferences are identified.

The support planning process is much like the nursing process. It contains four phases: *assessment, goal setting, implementation,* and *evaluation* (Figure 12-1). Each of these phases is described in this section.

Assessment Phase A client's initial assessment is often done by the person who will be responsible for organizing the support provided. The **assessment** involves

FIGURE 12-1
The phases of support planning

determining what types of support are needed. This person may complete the entire assessment or take the responsibility for organizing assessments from other care providers. In community settings, a case manager is often responsible for the assessment. In a facility setting, a charge nurse often takes the responsibility for coordinating the assessment for a resident of a long-term care facility.

Client situation, needs, and preferences are reassessed on a regular basis. Most provinces have regulations as to how often this assessment must happen. A significant change in a client's situation should always trigger a reassessment.

Goal-Setting Phase Goal setting is usually done at the time of the assessment. Goal setting is essential to the success of the support plan and ensures that the client's goals are identified and that the methods to be used to help the client attain the goals are in line with the client's preferences.

Implementation Phase The implementation phase occurs when the methods identified in the goal-setting phase are put into practice. The actual provision of direct service begins with this phase. Many times, methods are tried and then refined so as to get the best effect. Occasionally, new goals are identified in this phase.

Evaluation Phase Evaluation is not necessarily a distinct phase that occurs after implementation. The evaluation of needs, goals, and methods is ongoing. Nonetheless, a review of the client's overall situation, needs, and preferences is usually done on a predetermined basis.

THE ROLE OF THE SUPPORT WORKER IN THE SUPPORT PLANNING PROCESS

The support worker is often the person who spends the most time with the client. As a result, the support worker is often the first person to identify changes in the client's situation, needs, or preferences. It's also likely that the support worker is the person who is responsible for implementing many of the methods identified in the client's support plan. Thus, the support worker may learn valuable information about the effectiveness of the methods.

The information the support worker obtains must be shared with the other members of the support team. The support worker's role is to make accurate observations and to communicate those observations clearly to the team.

CASE EXAMPLE 12-1

Wai Po is a support worker for an Alzheimer day program. The support team includes the program's director and social worker, each client, and the client's family. When a new client comes to the program, the support team meets to establish the support plan. Wai Po attends the meeting, making note of any information that she may need in her work with the client. She also helps identify the methods to be used to assist the client to attain his or her goals.

Wai Po is often the person responsible for carrying out many of the methods. As she works with each client, Wai Po makes note of any changes to the methods used as well as any other pertinent information.

Wai Po documents in the client's progress notes any new information she learns and any changes in method

she has made. If appropriate, Wai Po discusses the changes with other members of the support team.

Each client's support plan is reviewed monthly. At this meeting, Wai Po informs the team of the information she's learned and of any modifications she has made to the methods identified. In turn, Wai Po makes note of the other team members' observations and changes in approach, including changes in client goals, needs, and preferences. She joins the team in updating the support plan.

What types of observations are important to include in a team conference?

This case example lists some team members who might take part in this conference. What other team members may attend?

OBSERVATION SKILLS

Because support workers tend to have more contact with the client, other members of the support team often rely upon the support worker to be their "eyes and ears." This places a special responsibility upon the support worker to meet three aims when making observations: to be complete, to be sensitive to detail, and to include only significant information.

You will want to pay particular attention to any unexpected condition as well as to any changes in the client's *appearance, behaviour, communication,* or *status.* You must also be careful to provide the *significant information*—the information that other members of the team will need. Do not "pad" your observations with great details about insignificant items. To do so only makes it more difficult for the other members of the team to find the information they need.

Observations should follow the ABCS: appearance, behaviour, communication, and status. We'll discuss each of these in this section:

- **Appearance** includes facial expression, posture, and stance (recall the discussion on body language in Chapter 9). It also includes the client's dress and cleanliness.
- **Behaviour** includes any action the client takes, the level of awareness of his or her surroundings, his or her interest in the surroundings, and interest in others.
- **Communication** includes what the client says and how he or she says it. This includes any feelings or emotional "message" the client sends.
- **Status** includes the client's current condition and how well the client functions.

Table 12-1 lists common types of observations under each of the ABCS. Be aware that you may be asked to observe for specific things with a particular client.

TABLE 12-1	Common Observations of the Client

Appearance

Client's dress, cleanliness

Client's skin condition, presence of swelling, colour of lips, fingers, and toes

Clarity of client's eyes, presence of any discharge from the client's nose or ears

Client's environment: such as too hot, too cold, messy, or odours present

Weight gain or loss

Behaviour

Client's mood

Client's ability to respond appropriately to stimulation (such as picking up the phone when it rings, ability to follow communication, and remembering what has been said to him or her)

Communication

Client's ability to hear, see, and sense touch in communication

Client's ability to start a conversation, to understand what is said to him or her, to appropriately respond to questions, to ask questions, to respond to non-verbal communication

Quality of client's communication: use of complete sentences, ability to form words, use of nonverbal communication

Status

Client's sensory status: ability to see, hear, touch, smell, and taste

Client's cognitive status: orientation, ability to pay attention to stimulus, to organize information, to remember, and to problem-solve

Client's physical status: respiration, heart rate, pain, sleeping habits, movements, appetite, thirst

Client's functional status: ability to bathe, dress, groom, feed him- or herself, to move about, to grasp things

Describing What You Observe

You must be particularly careful to describe the ABCS, not to make an assumption. *Describing* the event means just that—giving a description of what happened or what something looked, sounded, or smelled like. An assumption is a guess that may or may not be correct. Documenting an assumption does not give the reader the facts and may give the reader false information. Table 12-2 describes some common "Do's and Don'ts" of describing.

TABLE 12-2	Describing Do's and Don'ts	
DO Describe	**DON'T** Assume
Mrs. Jones ate all of her lunch: a sandwich, coffee, and small salad.	Mrs. Jones had a good meal.
Mrs. Jones was crying when she talked about her husband's illness.	Mrs. Jones is depressed over her husband's illness.
Mrs. Jones was angry when the taxi came late to take her for her appointment.	Mrs. Jones was aggressive.
Mrs. Jones' skin colour is an unusually pale shade of pink.	Mrs. Jones is ill.

Reporting Opinions

At times, you may be asked to give an opinion about what you have observed. Opinions are drawn from the observations you have made and usually include possible "cause-and-effect" relationships. For example, you might observe that every time a client eats peanut butter, the client has trouble swallowing. Your observation as to the possible cause of the client's problem could be most useful in resolving the problem.

Opinions are not the same as assumptions. An opinion asks you to draw a conclusion from what you have observed. An assumption is a guess. While opinions can be useful, assumptions can be dangerous. Always make sure your opinion is based on a valid observation.

For example, if your client tells you she always feels better after speaking with her sister, she is telling you the cause-and-effect relationship. If you report this, it is a report of your observation. If you notice that the client seems happier after each call from her sister, you may report this as your opinion. You have seen two things happen (a call and a change in the client's behaviour) and drawn a conclusion.

STOP AND REFLECT ((12-1))

Recall the last visit you had with a client. (If you do not yet work in the field, recall your last interaction with a friend or family member.) Describe the person following the ABCS of observation. Write down your description.

_____

_____

_____

Tell your observations to a colleague. When you are finished, ask the colleague to tell you what she or he heard you say. Did you find that you made some assumptions? Were your observations complete? Did you miss any essential details?

_____

_____

_____

RESPECTING PRIVACY, MAINTAINING CONFIDENTIALITY, ENSURING SECURITY

In Chapter 3, we discussed privacy. When you are using, reporting, or documenting client information, it is particularly important to respect a client's right to privacy, to maintain confidentiality, and to ensure security of the information. We'll look at each of these items in this section.

Privacy—It's the Law

Since January 1, 2004, privacy of personal information has been regulated in Canadian provinces. On that date, a federal law, the *Personal Information Protection and Electronic Documents Act* (PIPEDA), was extended to cover certain types of personal information (including health information) in all provinces, unless that province had substantially similar legislation. As of this publication, many provinces have enacted privacy legislation, but only Ontario's *Health Information Protection Act* has been determined by the federal government to be substantially similar to PIPEDA.

The federal legislation is built upon ten principles developed by the Canadian Standards Association:

- **Accountability:** An organization is responsible for personal information under its control and shall designate an individual or individuals who are accountable for the organization's compliance with the remaining principles.
- **Identifying Purpose:** The purposes for which personal information is collected shall be identified by the organization at or before the time the information is collected.
- **Consent:** The knowledge and consent of the individual are required for the collection, use, or disclosure of personal information, except when inappropriate.
- **Limiting Collection:** The collection of personal information shall be limited to that which is necessary for the purposes identified by the organization. Information shall be collected by fair and lawful means.
- **Limiting Use, Disclosure, Retention:** Personal information shall not be used or disclosed for purposes other than those for which it was collected, except with the consent of the individual or as required by the law. Personal information shall be retained only as long as necessary for fulfillment of those purposes.
- **Accuracy:** Personal information shall be as accurate, complete, and up-to-date as is necessary for the purposes for which it is to be used.
- **Safeguards:** Personal information shall be protected by security safeguards appropriate to the sensitivity of the information.
- **Openness:** An organization shall make readily available to individuals specific information about its policies and practices relating to the management of personal information.
- **Individual Access:** Upon request, an individual shall be informed of the existence, use, and disclosure of his or her personal information and shall be given access to that information. An individual shall be able to challenge the accuracy and completeness of the information and have it amended as appropriate.
- **Challenging Compliance:** An individual shall be able to address a challenge concerning compliance with the above principles to the designated individual or individuals for the organization's compliance. (Source: Office of the Privacy Commissioner, Government of Canada, 2007)

SPOTLIGHT 12-1 SOME DEFINITIONS

These definitions adapt federal and provincial privacy legislation definitions to support work:

- Privacy. The fundamental right we all have to control the collection, use, and disclosure of information about ourselves.

- Confidentiality. The obligation of a worker holding personal information to protect and not misuse or wrongfully disclose it.

- Security. The way the worker identifies/learns of risks for misuse or disclosure and the steps he or she takes to keep the information safe.

CASE EXAMPLE 12-2

As you read through this case example, identify the things that might breach the client's privacy. With your colleagues, identify what Cathy should do differently to maintain confidentiality and keep her clients' information secure.

Cathy is a support worker for her community's support services. She has been with the program for a long time and often handles the most difficult cases.

It's Friday—a typical end of the week for Cathy. She starts the day by reviewing her schedule as she eats breakfast with her family. She makes notes on the paper about what she has to do at each client visit. She adds a reminder to herself to pick up her son's skates at the arena between clients and another to get milk at the Northern Store. Midway through breakfast, a neighbour calls. Cathy is on the phone when her son scribbles a question on Cathy's work schedule and passes it to her. Cathy mouths the answer to him and he heads off to school.

After seeing all the family off, Cathy heads to her first clients, Gwen and her son. On her way to Gwen's house, Cathy passes several of Gwen's neighbours. They tell her that she should come to Gwen's house when Gwen doesn't expect her "so that you can see what she's really like." Cathy tells them that Gwen is doing all that she is supposed to do for her son.

Gwen asks about Mrs. Beedle, who has been out of the community for treatment. Mrs. Beedle is Gwen's aunt and she is worried about her. Gwen and Cathy spend a few minutes discussing the how Mrs. Beedle is doing. Cathy finishes her tasks. During the visit, she learns that Gwen has just had a call from her son's occupational therapist in Winnipeg. The therapist has been

able to get her son's surgery moved up to mid-December. As a result, he will have a bandage on his leg and will have special exercises to do. Cathy makes a mental note to tell her supervisor. At the end of the visit, Cathy, with Gwen's permission, uses Gwen's phone to call her next client.

Between clients, Cathy meets another worker at the community centre for lunch. They both provide support for a client, Mr. Poreaux. Over lunch in the common room, they discuss changes in Mr. Poreaux's needs.

After lunch, Cathy heads to her car. She checks her appointment book (left open on the front seat of her car) for the information on her next client, Mrs. Marsden. Cathy's supervisor has given her a form to give to Mrs. Marsden to complete. Cathy tosses the book in her purse.

Cathy arrives at Mrs. Marsden's home. She pulls out her appointment book, opening it on the table. She gives Mrs. Marsden the form. She leaves Mrs. Marsden to complete the form as she makes a phone call. When Cathy returns to the room, she takes the completed form from Mrs. Marsden and places it in her book. When she leaves, Cathy gathers up the book and the form, putting them in her purse.

Cathy picks up her son at school. He has to go to hockey practice. The coach wants to know if Cathy can make snacks for the team's away games next week. Cathy pulls out her appointment book and makes a note to do this.

How many privacy issues did you identify in Cathy's day? If you work in the field, have you ever done some of the things Cathy did? Why? Which of the situations Cathy experienced would be most difficult for you to handle? Why?

Respecting Privacy

As a support worker, you will learn a great deal about your client. This is normal. After all, you generally spend a great deal of time together. Much of this information may be necessary for the support you provide. Some, however, may not be significant for the client's support.

You must always be careful to respect the boundaries of your relationship with the client. In particular, it's important to avoid asking for information that does not relate to the client's care. This is not as easy as it sounds—you do not want to appear uninterested in the client as a person, but you must be careful not to pry or discuss information that is beyond the bounds of your relationship. If you are uncertain about whether certain client information is important, discuss the issue with your supervisor.

Maintaining Confidentiality and Security

There are five areas to which you must pay particular attention: when you receive client information (such as an assignment or a referral), when you report information (such as when you leave information on your supervisor's voice mail or complete a summary report), when you share information with another member of the client's support team, when you are asked for information by someone who is not part of the client's support team, and when you must keep client information in your possession.

Keeping Assignment and Referral Information Confidential

You must be cautious when you receive client information or updates. Many community support workers receive client assignments and information through messages left on their voice mail. If you receive information in this manner, make sure that you retrieve those messages in a private spot so that the message cannot be overheard and any notes you make are not seen by people who are not authorized to see them.

Some community workers access or print information from their agency's website. If you do this, be certain to follow your agency's guidelines for where you may access the website. Do not use public computers unless your agency gives you permission to do so. Public computers include computers in a library or Internet café or other location where members of the general public may use them. The information you access is often still held in the computer's memory or temporary files, even if you have closed the program or even turned off the machine. Someone else might be able to recall the client information.

As well, make certain that no unauthorized person can read the screen when you are accessing the information. "Shoulder-surfing"—reading information over someone's shoulder without the person realizing it—is much more common than you might think.

Finally, print off information only if you must. If you must print client information, print the minimum amount of information. For example, if all you really need is the client's address, do you need to print off a screen that contains additional information? It may be best to simply note the address in a secure binder or notebook.

Many facility support workers receive client updates and information through a report at the beginning of each shift. Always take care to receive this information in a secure area so that other residents, family, and other visitors to the facility do not overhear confidential information.

SPOTLIGHT 12-2 WHO CARES ABOUT CLIENT INFORMATION?

You may be asking yourself "Why would someone want to access client information? Why would they be interested in the service my client receives?"

The information you receive could tell a person much more than the fact that a client uses support services.

Information on the client's age, address, phone number, and diagnosis may be of interest to a thief or fraud artist who is interested in taking advantage of people who seem vulnerable.

Keeping Information You Report Confidential

When you report client information by telephone, make sure that you are in an area that is secure (i.e., where you cannot be overheard by persons who should not hear the information). You must also make certain that you keep confidential any notes you have used to organize your thoughts.

In a facility, it can be very tempting to share client information when you see another member of the health care team. Always make sure that your communication cannot be overheard by others (Figure 12-2).

FIGURE 12-2
Sharing too much?

Written reports must be completed and handled so as to be kept out of view of unauthorized persons. When you write a note or report, make sure that your work is not left where others can see it. For example, facility support workers should not leave written reports on the ledge of the nursing station. Community support workers who must complete reports at home should not leave reports on the kitchen table or in other places where unauthorized persons can see them.

If you have difficulty completing a report, speak with your supervisor. Never ask a family member, a friend, or even a colleague to help you.

Sharing Information with Other Members of the Client's Support Team

It's essential to share information needed by other members of the client's support team. How and where you share information may determine whether unauthorized persons hear the information.

Make certain you cannot be overheard. Even if you think other persons cannot hear you, you may be wrong. You may not see the person around the corner in the hall, but the person may well be able to hear you.

Share only the information that the other person needs. Discussing the other information about the client's personal life breaches the client's privacy. For example, it may be important to share that a client is upset over a family matter and may not have as much interest in taking part in household activities. It's likely not important at all to share details of the family matter, even if you know them.

SPOTLIGHT 12-3 AREAS WHERE INFORMATION IS OFTEN OVERHEARD

These are some of the areas where support staff and other professionals sharing information are at risk for being overheard. Are there others you can think of?

Elevators	Staff room
When shopping	When out to lunch or on breaks
Hallways	In class
Washrooms	In the parking lot

Responding to Requests for Information from People Who are Not Members of the Client's Support Team

Consider the following situation. You are leaving a client's home at the end of a visit. The client's neighbour sees you and asks how the client is doing. What do you say? What can you say?

Many people who ask for this type of information have a genuine interest in the client. Even so, you cannot share information without the client's permission. You also do not want to be needlessly hurtful to someone. What do you say? The best answer will depend upon the needs and wishes of your client, but one of the following may work well:

- You might suggest that the person call or visit the client.
- You might advise the client that the person was asking about him or her and ask the client how you should respond.
- You might tell the person that you cannot say, for confidentiality reasons.

Did you have other ideas? Discuss them with your colleagues.

Keeping Information in Your Possession Confidential

Many community support workers are required to carry client information with them. If you must keep client information in your possession, you must be extremely careful to keep it secure. Do not leave the information where others can see it. Most community agencies have policies about how this information is to be kept. For example, it is best that you not keep client information in your personal appointment book. Consider the following scenario:

A support worker records her visits in her personal appointment book. She is careful to write only the client's address and phone number and never to write the client's name in the book. She is at the dentist. When she opens her book to schedule an appointment, the dental assistant notices the phone number and address on a specific date. "Why do you have my aunt's address and telephone number?" she asks. "Is she ill? Why is she needing support services?" At the very least, this is an uncomfortable position for you to be in. How do you respond? It's best to simply keep personal and client information separate.

Client information should be kept out of sight when not in use. This means using a tote bag or satchel that securely closes. It also means keeping information secure when you must leave it unattended. For example, your agency might ask that you lock your satchel in the trunk of your car when you make a visit.

Facility support workers often handle client information. In some facilities, duty rosters are printed out and given to support workers. Support workers often make notes about specific requests or changes in routine. Because many people who are not staff members may be in the facility, you must also take care to keep confidential any information in your possession. Ask for and follow your agency's procedure for handing in or destroying these notes when they are no longer needed.

In most cases, there is no need for facility workers to keep client information with them when they are not on duty. Never take client information out of the facility without your supervisor's approval. Follow your agency's procedures for handling any confidential information accidentally taken out of the facility.

REPORTING YOUR OBSERVATIONS AND ACTIONS

Your observations are of little use unless you report them to the appropriate person. No one will know if the client is receiving proper care unless you report on your actions. These written reports and transcripts of verbal reports are part of the client's record. A client's record is a legal document and may be subpoenaed for an inquest or other legal proceedings. It is important that any documentation be complete and give an accurate picture of the client's situation and the service provided.

Each agency has policies for reporting information. These policies cover the ways that information must be reported, to whom it must be reported, and when it must be reported.

Observations and Actions

When you report, you must include your actions, as well as your observations. You should also include any questions you have about the client's service. Table 12-3 discusses a simple method for organizing your information into a concise format.

Verbal and Written Reporting

There are two types of reporting: verbal and written. Within each type, there are many variations. Each agency develops its own forms. Make sure you are familiar with the forms your agency uses and with the procedure for completing each form.

Verbal reporting can take the form of a face-to-face communication, a telephone conversation, or a message left on voice mail or relayed through a third party (such as an answering service or a ward clerk).

Written reporting can take the form of a progress note, a completed checklist, a note written in a communication log, or a telephone message transcription.

TABLE 12-3	One Method of Organizing Your Information

This method of organizing information is easy to use. It organizes information into four categories: the event, the action, the result, and the client response.

Event
Can be an observation:
- Client is flushed, crying
- Client is not dressed

Can call attention to more detailed instructions found elsewhere:
- Client has new diet—details in progress notes

Can be a change in schedule:
- Client must change visit date, as has conflicting medical appointment

Can be an issue or problem

Action/Plan
The action you:
- take as a result of the event
- record that someone else took as a result of the event (based upon the report made to you)
- record to advise another to follow up on the situation

Result
What you expect (or hope) will come of the actions you take

Response
The client's response to the actions taken

No matter what type of reporting you use, you must be objective, accurate, complete, and clear when you report observations or your actions to others. Your reporting should also be organized so that the most important observation or action is presented first. You must also make sure that the person receiving your report knows the name of the client about whom your report is made, as well as the time of your observations or actions and the time of your report.

Organizing Your Report

No matter what type of report you are making, always take the time to organize the information you will be reporting *before* you report. This ensures that all your information is in order and will be presented clearly. This is particularly important if you are reporting your observations for more than one client at the same time.

Organize your observations by client. For each client, use the following procedure:

1. State the client's name.
2. State the date and time of your visit.
3. State the *most important* information first.
4. State the next most important information.
5. Repeat step 4 until all information has been recorded.

Making a Verbal Report

Each agency has its own policies and procedures for making verbal reports. If you are working in a long-term care facility, you will most often give a verbal report directly to another staff member. If you are working in the community, you may find that you make most of your verbal reports by telephone. The information in this section provides general guidelines for making a verbal report.

1. **Be sure you have the correct telephone number and extension (if applicable).** Always keep the correct telephone numbers handy. You must also keep handy any extensions (voice mail numbers) you require to report information. Remember that many agencies do not have a live receptionist to forward after-hours calls. You may not be able to leave a message if you do not have the proper extension number.
2. **Let the person you are speaking to know who you are.** If you are reporting by telephone or voice mail, make sure to state your name.
3. **State the day, date, and time of your call.** Make sure to state this information *before* you report your observations.
4. **If you need a return call, be sure to leave the telephone number at which you can be reached.** Make sure that the number you leave is the one at which you can be reached *when the person you are calling is likely to return your call.*
5. **Report the information about each client as described in** *Organizing Your Report.* Verbal reports are much harder to follow than written reports. Make sure your information is well organized.
6. **Know what kinds of information your agency requires you to report to a live person.** Certain types of information (for example, client emergencies) cannot be left on voice mail or on an answering machine. Always follow your agency's policies and know how to contact the on-call supervisor.

STOP AND REFLECT 12-2

Review this transcript of a report left on a supervisor's voice mail.

> *Hi, it's me. I saw Mrs. Rose today. Boy, is she fussy! Nothing I could do would please her! Did you know that her whole house is filled with antiques? I could hardly get the sweeper through the living room. I did notice that you've scheduled me to go back next week. I can't, because I have a doctor's appointment and won't be finished in time to get there. Oh, while I think of it, Mrs. Zaheer has to reschedule her visit for Friday because she has a doctor's appointment. Anyway, Mrs. Rose finally settled down, although she wouldn't let me do half of the things I was scheduled to do. Let me know if I should reschedule next week's visit with Mrs. Rose, OK?*

What information is missing? What information should not be in the message at all? How could you restate this message to make it more clear, concise, and easily understood?

_____

_____

_____

_____

_____

Written Reporting

Written reporting is called documentation. There are several types of documentation, such as checklists, progress notes, summary reports, and incident reports.

Checklists Checklists require you to place a check mark in a box. Checklists provide little space for writing any information. These forms are commonly used to record routine events, such as whether a bath was given or if vacuuming was done. Many agencies refer to these forms as "tick sheets." A sample form is shown in Figure 12-3.

When recording on a checklist, you must be particularly careful to make sure you have the right client's form and that you are placing a check mark in the proper box. It is easy to accidentally place a check mark in the wrong row or column. This may change the information dramatically and result in improper client care.

FIGURE 12-3
Sample tick sheet

Task / Day	M	T	W	T	F	S	S
Client Name — **Activity Log**							
Dates: _____ to _____							
Assist with bath							
Mouth/Skin Care							
Intake/Output							
Client Safety							
Ambulate/Mobilize							
Meal Prep							
Next Day Meal Prep							
Special Diet							
Shopping							
Feeding							
Light Cleaning							
Laundry							
Clean Fridge/Stove							
Cupboards							
ADL							
Children ADL							
Socialization							
Take to Drs. Office							
Pick Up From Hospital							
Caregiver Relief							
Other							

Progress Notes Progress notes usually contain information about the client's status and changes over time. Some agencies have separate notes for each discipline. Others use a common note—a form on which all members of the team record.

Summary Reports Summary reports are reports that summarize a client's service over a period of time. Some agencies require support workers to complete monthly reports for each client to which they are assigned. In other agencies, support workers join the other members of the team to complete a summary report when the support plan is reviewed.

Incident Reports Incident reports are completed when an accident or unexpected event involving a client occurs. In some cases, incident reports must be sent to the governmental department that regulates the agency.

GUIDELINES FOR RECORDING

How you write your progress notes is also important. An illegible, messy note will not convey the information you want to share. In fact, it could mislead others who read the note incorrectly or who have problems deciphering your handwriting.

Observing the following ten rules will help to ensure that your notes are clear and accurate.

1. **Write legibly.**
2. **Write accurately.** Use specific words that mean what you intend to say.
3. **Record concisely.** Do not add information that is not useful. This can sometimes cause the person who reads your note to miss essential information.
4. **Record events chronologically.** Make sure that you record Monday's activities before Tuesday's activities, for example. This way, the reader can follow the events as they happened.
5. **Leave no spaces between notes.**
6. **Record information as soon as is practical.** Information is always best recorded when it is fresh in your mind.
7. **Sign or initial your notes according to your agency policy.**
8. **Write in ink—do not change pens in the same note.** Changing ink colours gives the impression that the note was written at two different times.
9. **Use terminology and short forms of words according to your agency's policy.**
10. **Correct errors openly and honestly.** Draw a line through the error and write the word "error" above it.

COMMON TERMINOLOGY AND ABBREVIATIONS USED IN DOCUMENTATION

Abbreviations

Each agency has its own list of approved terms and abbreviations for common words and phrases. Make sure that you know the terminology and short forms your agency has approved. Table 12-4 lists some common abbreviations.

Health Care Terminology

Have you ever listened to a physician and a nurse talk about a health condition? It's often difficult to understand—almost like another language. If you've been tempted to say, "It's all Greek to me," you might be right. Many health care terms are based on Greek or Latin. However, by learning a few word parts and simple rules, you can often figure out the meaning of many health care terms. Most health care terms contain at least two of the following:

- The Root, which refers to the body part.
- The Prefix, which describes the root in some way.
- The Suffix, which describes the root in some way.

Table 12-4	Common Abbreviations Used in Documentation
Word or Phrase	**Term or Abbreviation**
People	
client	cl
resident	res
case manager	cm
homemaker	hm
patient	pt
Verbs	
ambulates	amb
complains of	c/o
increase	≠
decrease	∅
leading to	→
change	D
Descriptive Words	
full-time	FT
part-time	PT
with	c̄ or w/
plus	+
without	w/o or s̄
by mouth	po
nothing by mouth	npo
topical	top
Service	
morning care	am care
evening care	hs care

▶▶▌

Table 12-4	Common Abbreviations Used in Documentation *(continued)*
Word or Phrase	**Term or Abbreviation**
Frequency	
once a day	q1d or 1xd or od
twice a day	2xd or bid
three times a day	tid
every two days	q2d
every 2 hours	q2h
every 4 hours	q4h
as required, as needed, as the client prefers	prn
Nouns	
wheelchair	w/c
oxygen	O2 or O_2
bowel movement	bm
temperature, pulse, respiration	tpr
blood pressure	bp

For example, the term *bradycardia* is made up of the root, *cardia*, which means heart. The prefix *brady* means slow. The suffix *ia* means condition or state. Thus, bradycardia means an abnormally slow heart rate.

Not all terms have all three components. Some add a vowel (usually an o) when two roots are combined. An example of this is *cardiopulmonary*, which combines *cardi*, meaning the heart, and *pulmonary*, meaning the lungs. These two parts are joined with the vowel o. Thus cardiopulmonary refers to the heart and lungs.

Table 12-5 lists common roots, prefixes, and suffixes used in health care terminology.

TABLE 12-5	Common Roots, Prefixes, and Suffixes Used in Health Care Terminology				
Prefix	**Definition**	**Root**	**Definition**	**Suffix**	**Definition**
a, an	without; absence of	arteri	artery	ac, ar, eal, ic, al, ary, ial, ous	pertaining to
				algia	pain
ante	before	arthr	joint	ectomy	cutting out; excision or surgical removal

TABLE 12-5	Common Roots, Prefixes, and Suffixes Used in Health Care Terminology *(continued)*				

Prefix	Definition	Root	Definition	Suffix	Definition
anti	against	aur	ear		
bi	two	axill	armpit	ia	condition or state
brady	slow	cardi	heart	ism	state of
de	from; down from; lack of	cerebro	brain	itis	inflammation
dis	to undo; free from	coron	heart	logy	study of
dys	difficult; painful; abnormal	derma	skin	oid	resembling
ecto	outside; outer	enter	intestines	ology	study of
endo	within	gastr	stomach	opia	vision (condition)
hemi	half	glyc	sugar	opsy	to view
hyper	too much	hem	blood	ostomy	creation of an artificial opening
hypo	too little	kinesi	movement; motion	paresis pathy	slight paralysis disease
mal	bad	nephro	kidney	pnea	breathing
meta	after; beyond; change	neuro	nerve	scope	instrument
patho	disease	opt	vision	sepsis	infection
peri	surrounding (outer)	opthalmo	eye		
poly	many; much	oste	bone		
tachy	fast; rapid	pulmon	lung		

Try It Out *12-1*

For each of the following terms, identify the root, the prefix and/or the suffix. Then, list the meaning of the term.

Term	Root	Prefix	Suffix	Meaning
Biology				
Hematology				
Colostomy				
Apnea				
Bronchitis				
Pathology				

Questions for Review

1. You have been assigned to a new client. What information would you expect to find in the client's support plan?

2. What is your role in the support planning process?

3. What four types of observations should you make?

4. What do we mean by privacy? By confidentiality? By security?

5. Does your province have privacy legislation? If so, what is it called? How does it protect health information?

6. What is the difference between a description and an assumption? Why should you avoid documenting an assumption?

7. What is the difference between an opinion and an assumption? When should you document an opinion?

8. Why is it important to organize your information prior to making a verbal or written report?

9. Review the note to the right. Identify the errors in it. What information is unclear? What information is missing? What information is unnecessary? How would you rewrite the note?

10. Why is it important to use standard abbreviations in documentation?

11. What are four common types of written reports? What kinds of reports does your agency use?

Tuesday, 9:25:
Mrs. Jones was really agitated. She just wouldnt settle. Says something is wrong with her leg. Checked and looked OK to me.
Says dtr is coming to take her to store. I wonder if she'll be here for tomorrow's visit. Told her to call the office.
Harriet

12. For each of the following terms, identify the root, the prefix, and/or the suffix. Then, list the meaning of the term.

Term	Root	Prefix	Suffix	Meaning
carditis				
nephritis				
hemiplegia				
dermatitis				
hypertension				
hypoglycemia				

Questions for Discussion

1. A resident, Mrs. Grant, asks you if you can keep a secret. She then tells you that she has been incontinent four times in the last week and is very frightened. What do you do? Should you keep the information to yourself? Why or why not? What are the possible consequences of sharing this information? What are the possible consequences of keeping it to yourself? Are there people with whom you feel you should share this information?

2. You are one of three support workers assigned to work with Mr. Rodriguez, a particularly challenging client. He requires a great deal of help and reassurance. You sometimes feel that you aren't sure just how to best provide the emotional support he needs. Today, in the grocery store, you see one of the other support workers assigned to Mr. Rodriguez. You very much want to talk to her about his support. Is this an appropriate setting to share information? Why or why not? What are the possible consequences? What might you do to share information and maintain confidentiality?

3. You work in a long-term care facility in a small town. Everyone seems to know everyone else. Today, one of your neighbours asks you about a resident, Mrs. Claire. "I know that she's been ill," the neighbour tells you, "How is she feeling now?" What do you say to the neighbour?

Chapter 13

Safety

Learning Objectives

Through reading this chapter, you'll be able to

1. Define safety.
2. Identify common risks related to clients, related to where support is provided, and related to the type of support.
3. Explain the chain of infection and infection control.
4. Demonstrate the appropriate handwashing technique.
5. Demonstrate the application of standard precautions.
6. Tell what the Workplace Hazardous Materials Information System is and how it applies to work in a client's home and in a long-term care facility.
7. Describe fire prevention and the steps to take in the event of a fire emergency.
8. List the general procedures to follow in the event of a client emergency.
9. Discuss the use of physical restraints as a temporary safety measure.
10. Identify risks associated with the use of restraints.

Chapter at a Glance

- Safety
- Risks Related to Your Client
- Risks Related to Where You Provide Support
- Risks Related to the Type of Support Provided
- Health and Safety Legislation
- Infection Control
- How Infection Is Transmitted
- Reducing the Transmission of Infection
- Workplace Hazardous Materials Information System
- Fire Safety
- Client Emergencies
- Restraints

Terms You'll Use

Antibacterial An agent that destroys bacteria and/or prevents bacterial growth.

Antibiotics Medications that treat bacterial infections.

Bacteria Microscopic organisms that we commonly call germs.

Chain of Infection The process of transmission of an infection.

Clean Technique A method of destroying many pathogens to prevent transmission of infection; also called medical asepsis.

Disinfection The process of destroying pathogens.

Fire Hazards Things in the environment that pose a risk of fire or could make a fire spread.

Fungi A microscopic plant that lacks chlorophyll and must rely on a host to survive.

Infectious Agent Microorganism capable of causing disease. These are also called pathogens.

Isolation Precautions Techniques used to prevent transmission of serious or highly contagious diseases.

Means of Transmission The method of transfer of a causative agent from a reservoir to a susceptible host.

Medical Asepsis The destruction of many pathogens to prevent transmission of infection; also called clean technique.

Microorganisms Organisms that cannot be seen without a microscope, including bacteria, viruses, protozoa, and fungi.

Nosocomial Infections Infections acquired after admission to a facility.

Parasitic Worms Multicelled organisms that live within the human body and obtain nourishment from this host.

Pathogens Microorganisms that cause infection.

Polypharmacy The use of more than one medication.

Portal of Entry The path into the body through which the infectious agent enters the host.

Portal of Exit The path by which the infectious agent leaves the reservoir.

Protozoa Single-celled microorganisms considered to be more complex than bacteria. Only some may cause disease.

Reservoir The place where the infectious agent survives.

Rickettsia Specialized bacteria that live like a virus and are parasitic. Rickettsia are almost always transmitted by insects, such as lice, fleas, and ticks.

Standard Precautions A set of procedures used to prevent the spread of a communicable or contagious disease.

Susceptible Host A person lacking resistance to a particular infectious agent.

Viruses Microscopic organisms that grow in living cells and use the cells to sustain themselves. Also commonly called germs.

WHMIS The Workplace Hazardous Materials Information System used to provide information about the proper use, handling, and storage of hazardous materials.

SAFETY

As we discussed in Chapter 7, safety is a basic need and is closely linked to our need for security. We all need to feel safe and secure, whether we are at home, at work, or elsewhere.

We usually think of our homes as safe. We usually consider long-term care facilities to be safe. In fact, accidents can—and do—occur in both settings. According to Statistics Canada, 60 percent of the injuries older adults sustain happen at or near their homes. Twenty percent of injuries to people aged 20 and under happen at home (Statistics Canada, *National Population Health Survey,* 1999).

Safety encompasses many factors: the client, the environment, equipment, supplies, and procedures.

We cannot eliminate all risk of harm. However, no one wants to experience a needless injury. Most injuries can be prevented. Taking proper precautions can save your client—or you—pain and frustration. Your clients entrust their safety to you when you are providing support. You must always look out for both your own and your client's safety. Remember that a safe environment promotes a sense of security.

RISKS RELATED TO YOUR CLIENT

Many clients are at increased risk for injury. This can be due to the client's age, health status, or medications he or she is taking. Let's take a look at each factor.

Types of Risks

One of the most common risks is the risk of tripping or falling. Children can be seriously injured in a fall (for example, falling from a counter). A fall can result in significant injury or even death to an older person. Burns and injuries from fires claim over 500 victims in Canada each year (Statistics Canada, *National Population Health Survey,* 1999). Food poisoning (usually due to improper food handling or storage) also poses a hazard.

Age

Infants, children, and older adults are at greater risk for injury than are adults. Infants and children are not aware of many risks. They are naturally curious and want to touch, taste, and manipulate the things around them. A child may want to touch what's on top of the stove and may not know that the stove is hot and will burn the skin. Furthermore, an infant or young child may not be physically able to avoid a risk. For example, an infant or toddler left in a car seat in the hot sun is not able to move to avoid sunburn or heat stroke.

Older adults are also at increased risk for injury. An older client may well know that the stove is hot, but, due to a diminished sensitivity to temperature and pain, may not know that he or she can be burned by accidentally touching the stove. Similarly, an older client may not see a fold in a scatter rug, catch his or her foot on the fold, and fall.

Additionally, older adults are often very aware that they do not see, hear, or feel things as accurately as they once did. Any of these changes can make a person more susceptible to injury. This can cause the older adult to become very anxious or even fearful about doing things. Sometimes this loss of security can become disabling—for example, by preventing a person from going out of the house.

Health Conditions

A health condition can put a person of any age at greater risk for injury, particularly if the condition is new and the person is still adjusting to any changes it has caused.

Health conditions may alter a person's balance, affect the person's ability to walk, or make the person tire more easily and be less aware of what is around him or her.

Some health conditions affect a person's cognitive ability. The person may become less aware of his or her surroundings, may not be able to perceive things properly, and may not be able to make sound judgments or to problem-solve. A person whose cognitive ability has been affected may pose a danger to himself or herself and to others around him or her.

Medications

Medications may affect a person in many ways. They may alter vision or balance, make a person drowsy, or even affect how a person thinks. Some medications can make a person fearful or suspicious. A medication does not have to be a prescription medication in order to produce these types of side effects. For example, many over-the-counter cold and allergy medications can make a person drowsy.

Additionally, polypharmacy (the use of more than one medication) may pose particular problems. Some medications produce different side effects when combined with other medications. Sometimes, an effect becomes much more pronounced. For example, a medication that causes mild drowsiness may cause extreme drowsiness when mixed with another medication.

RISKS RELATED TO WHERE YOU PROVIDE SUPPORT

Your client's physical surroundings may pose risks that must be addressed. Some of these risks may be related to the actual structure. Others may be related to where the building is located or to the number of other people who use the building.

Risks Related to a Client's Private Home

Many private homes you will visit will be older. Some may not be in good repair. Staircases may be very steep or not well lit, making it easy to fall. Bannister spindles may be placed too far apart, making it possible for a young child to slip between them and fall into the staircase opening. There may be loose stair treads or missing railings. A client may draw water from an unsanitary well or may not have the space to properly store food. Clients may have old electrical equipment that has frayed or damaged cords.

Risks Related to a Long-Term Care Facility

Long-term care facilities may have equipment or supplies that could be harmful if used improperly. They may have elevator and stairway access that could allow a person to leave unescorted. Hallways may have shiny floors and be too brightly (or unevenly) lit, making it difficult for the client to see where he or she is going. Noise from other activities in the facility may distract the client, making it difficult to pay attention to the risks around him or her.

Risks Related to Location

Workers providing support in the community must be aware of any risks related to the location of their clients' homes. Some clients may live in neighbourhoods that were once residential but are now commercial. There may be fewer people around, particularly in evening hours. The worker must be cautious of personal and client safety if travel after dark is required.

Caution must also be taken when travelling to and from the client's home, particularly late at night or early in the morning, when you are not familiar with the location of the client's home, or during months when weather is severe.

Most agencies have policies governing these issues. Always follow your agency's procedure. Discuss the issue with your supervisor if you feel that your own or your client's safety is at risk.

RISKS RELATED TO THE TYPE OF SUPPORT PROVIDED

There are two types of support activities that pose a significant risk to clients and support workers alike: the risk of physical injury and the risk of infection.

The Risk of Physical Injury Support workers frequently provide physical assistance to clients who may not be able to support their own weight or move independently. Good body mechanics and proper technique are essential for both your own and your client's safety. Chapter 18 discusses the fundamentals of safe physical assistance.

The Risk of Transmitting Infection Infection poses a significant health risk, particularly to a client who is frail or whose immune system is compromised. Remember that an infection that produces a brief illness in a strong and healthy adult may produce a life-threatening illness in a person who is frail. Some infections are perilous to all.

The nature of personal support will require you to be in very close physical contact with clients. You must be certain to reduce the opportunity to transmit infections to a client, to transmit infections from one client to another, or to pick up an infection from a client. The risk of transmission is present in both individual homes and in long-term care facilities. Nosocomial infections are infections acquired in facilities. This term is not used to describe infections acquired in a client's home. We'll discuss infection control following the next section.

HEALTH AND SAFETY LEGISLATION

Each province has its own health and safety legislation. This legislation usually covers employer responsibilities for safe procedures and equipment, employee responsibilities to work safely, as well as what to do if an emergency or an unsafe condition arises. This legislation usually applies to work done in a long-term care facility, but some portions of the legislation may apply to work done in a client's home.

INFECTION CONTROL

Three groups of people are at risk of infection: clients, staff, and, through exposure to staff and clients, the community at large. Support workers play a significant role in controlling the spread of infection through preventing the spread of **pathogens** (*microorganisms* that cause infection).

Microorganisms

Many agents can cause disease. **Microorganisms** are microscopic organisms that may cause disease. They are divided into four types: bacteria, viruses, protozoa, and rickettsia. Although bacteria and viruses are the most common, any of the four types can cause a serious infection. Fungi and parasitic worms can also cause disease.

Most disease-producing microorganisms produce toxins as a waste product of their activity. The body's immune system tries to fight off these toxins. This results in the common symptoms of an infection: inflamed, reddened, or hot areas; pain; aches; swelling; fever; chills; and discharge (runny eyes, nose, ears, or pus from a wound).

Bacteria   Bacteria are microscopic cells that can multiply quickly. Many people refer to bacteria as *germs*. Most bacteria thrive in an environment that is warm, moist, and dark, has plenty of oxygen, and some form of nourishment. Bacteria can survive on living or dead material, as long as nourishment is available. Not all bacteria are harmful. In fact, some are necessary for our bodies to break down food.

Some bacteria are harmful only if they enter certain areas of the body. For example, the bacteria *Escherichia coli* is found in the intestinal tract where it helps break down food particles. When *E. coli* enters other areas of the body, such as the urinary tract, it can cause an infection.

A healthy person is usually able to fight off many mild bacterial infections. Many medications, called **antibiotics**, have been developed to treat more severe bacterial infections. Antibiotics work in one of two ways: by killing the bacteria directly or by stopping bacterial growth so that the body's own immune system can effectively fight the infection. You may have taken an antibiotic for strep throat or to treat another type of infection.

Remember that antibiotics are developed to treat specific bacteria. An antibiotic effective against one type of bacteria may not be effective against another type. Additionally, bacteria can adapt so as not to be affected by antibiotics developed for the initial strain. Many researchers have linked antibiotic use to the development of antibiotic-resistant bacteria.

Viruses   Viruses grow in living cells and use the components of the cell to sustain themselves. They are extremely small and are harder to treat because any medication must kill the virus *without* killing the cell in which the virus lives. Antibiotics are not effective against viruses. However, some viruses (e.g., measles, polio, and many strains of influenza) can be prevented by vaccines.

As with bacteria, a healthy person may be able to fight off weak viruses. However, some viruses may actually make it easier for the person to catch other infections (viral or bacterial).

Protozoa   Protozoa are single-celled organisms. Some are parasitic and may thrive in areas with poor sanitation. Malaria is the most common disease caused by a protozoan. Toxoplasmosis is another protozoan-borne infection that is carried by cats and can be contracted by humans through the improper handling of cat feces. Some strains of protozoa that cause infections are resistant to medications.

Rickettsia **Rickettsia** are bacteria but are similar to viruses in that they can multiply only inside cells. Rickettsia are almost always transmitted by insects. Many rickettsia are not harmful to humans. Some common human infections caused by rickettsia are Rocky Mountain Spotted Fever and typhus. Most rickettsia-transmitted infections can be treated effectively with antibiotics.

Fungi **Fungi** are microscopic plants without chlorophyll that require a host to survive. Fungi can be found in air, soil, and water. Fungi are not a major cause of infection. One of the most common fungal infections is athlete's foot. Many fungal infections respond well to antifungal medication.

Parasitic Worms **Parasitic worms** are multicelled organisms that live within the human body and obtain their nourishment from this host. One of the most common of the parasitic worm diseases is trichinosis, which can occur when raw or under-cooked pork is eaten. *Beef tapeworm* can be contracted by eating insufficiently cooked beef from a cow that was infected by the tapeworm. Another common but lesser known parasitic infection is *hookworm*, which can be transmitted from dogs and cats to humans through poor pet care and poor hygiene. There are a number of medications that can treat parasitic worm infections.

HOW INFECTION IS TRANSMITTED

Six things must be present for an infection to be transmitted. These six items are often called the **chain of infection**. The chain represents the process as well as the cyclical nature of infection transmission.

The Chain of Infection

The chain of infection has six components: the infectious agent, the reservoir, the portal of exit, the means of transmission, the portal of entry, and a susceptible host (Figure 13-1). Each component is defined in this section.

Infectious Agent **Infectious agents** are the organisms capable of causing disease. These are also called pathogens.

Reservoir The **reservoir** is a place where the agent survives, such as on or in a client, support workers, other caregivers, equipment, or the environment. Remember that the reservoir need not be a living thing. The agent simply must have access to the nutrients required to survive. These conditions do not have to be plentiful. For example, an agent can live on moisture and deposits left by a handprint on a door handle. Others can live on a person's skin, a telephone, or any other item where the nutrient supply is present.

Portal of Exit The **portal of exit** is the path by which the infectious agent leaves the reservoir. This is usually through blood, wound drainage, respiratory secretions, feces, or other body substances.

FIGURE 13-1
The chain of infection

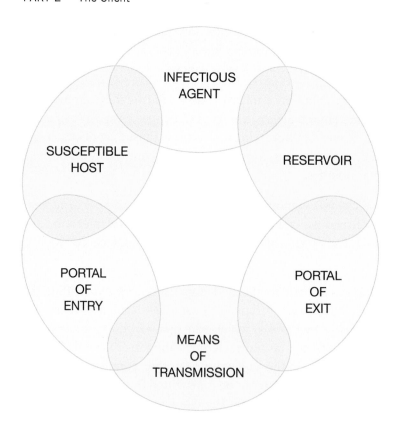

Means of Transmission The **means of transmission** is the method of transfer of a causative agent from a reservoir to a susceptible host. This includes physical contact, bites or stings, breathing in airborne pathogens, or ingesting pathogens. Unclean hands are among the most common means of transmission.

Portal of Entry The **portal of entry** is the path into the body, such as a break in the skin (a cut or other wound) or through a mucous membrane (such as the eye, mouth, vagina, rectum). For example, a person who contracts an agent on his or her hand may transmit the agent to a mucous membrane by touching his or her mouth, eye, or other membrane.

Susceptible Host A **susceptible host** is a person lacking resistance to a particular pathogenic agent. Host factors that influence susceptibility include underlying disease, immune status, medications, nutrition status, as well as certain types of treatments (such as chemotherapy or immunosuppressive medications).

Nosocomial Infections

Clients who are receiving support come in contact with many people. They may receive treatments and services from many different people (formal caregivers and family members). They may also have visits from friends or neighbours. Clients who live in long-term care facilities are often in very close contact with other clients who have illnesses.

We use the term **nosocomial infections** to describe infections acquired after admission to a facility. Clients receiving services at home are also at increased risk for infection as a result of this increased contact. In fact, clients at home may come in contact with many people who are not aware of the need to take the proper precautions. As a result, clients in home settings may be exposed to more infections than one might expect.

Drug-Resistant Infections

Drug-resistant infections are types of infections that cannot be treated by the medications usually prescribed. These infections are caused by organisms that are sometimes called *antibiotic-resistant microorganisms* or AROs. You may have heard of methicillin-resistant *Staphylococcus aureus* (MRSA), vancomycin-resistant enterococci (VRE), or drug-resistant tuberculosis. These are examples of drug-resistant infections. They are discussed in greater detail in Chapter 20, "Common Conditions."

Some people who have drug-resistant infections don't know it and may harbour the infection for a long time. Although they may be unaware of their infection, they can transfer the infection to others. People who have an infection but do not have symptoms are called carriers.

Many microorganisms adapt and develop resistance to the antibiotics used to treat them. There is also evidence that overuse of antibiotics contributes to increased resistance to treatment. Some drug-resistant infections respond to different medications while others do not. Many of these infections clear up over time if the person is otherwise healthy. Even so, it can take months for an infection to heal.

Assisting the Person with a Drug-Resistant Infection

It is important to follow standard precautions if you are assisting a person with a drug-resistant infection. This is essential even if you are not handling materials containing the client's blood. Fecal material and other body fluids can harbour the infection.

Clients with drug-resistant infections are not always isolated. If the person has been in a hospital, he or she will likely return home, have visitors (if the visitors are healthy), and do the things he or she feels able to do. However, clients and caregivers should practise good handwashing technique to reduce the risk of spreading the infection. You should review, with your supervisor, the specific precautions to take when caring for a person with a drug-resistant infection.

Photo 13-1
Handwashing is the simplest and most effective method of infection control a support worker can use.

REDUCING THE TRANSMISSION OF INFECTION

In order to reduce the transmission of infection, you must break the chain of infection. The primary method by which a support worker can break the chain is by destroying pathogens before they can be transmitted to other people. We use the term **disinfection** to describe the process of destroying pathogens.

One of the most effective ways the support worker can destroy pathogens is by practising **clean technique** (also called **medical asepsis**). Clean technique does not remove all pathogens, but it does reduce the number of pathogens.

Handwashing is the most important component of clean technique (Photo 13-1). Proper handwashing helps eliminate microorganisms that can cause disease.

Microorganisms on human skin are grouped into two types: resident microorganisms that live within the skin and transient microorganisms that are acquired through routine activities. Handwashing is very effective in eliminating transient microorganisms and (with *antibacterial* soap) can be effective against resident microorganisms. Antibacterial soap contains an **antibacterial** agent that destroys bacteria and prevents bacterial growth.

In order for handwashing to be effective, it must be done correctly and as often as practical. The best handwashing technique is of no use if it is not performed when necessary. You should wash your hands:

- before and after giving care to a person
- before putting on gloves
- after removing gloves
- when you have been in contact with any body fluid or substance, whether it is your own or that of another person
- after you have coughed, blown your nose, or sneezed
- before you handle, prepare, or eat food
- after you handle money
- after you have touched any surface that is unclean
- after using the washroom
- before breastfeeding
- before and after providing first aid

Studies indicate that people think that they wash their hands more consistently than they do. Other studies link the lack of proper handwashing to the potential for illness, many of which are serious and potentially deadly.

Table 13-1 describes three types of handwashing and the times when each is most appropriate. Procedure 13-1 describes the method of proper handwashing.

TABLE 13-1	Types of Handwashing
Type	**Best to Use:**
Plain soap and running water	After most activities requiring handwashing. Properly done, this process will remove dirt and transient microorganisms. This remains the best method of preventing the transmission of microorganisms.
Antibacterial soap and running water	In situations where risk of transmission is high (such as caring for a client whose immune system is depressed or who is very frail). In addition to removing dirt and transient microorganisms, this process inhibits the growth of resident microorganisms. Remember that these soaps are not required in most instances, and their overuse may contribute to antibiotic-resistant bacteria.

▶▶|

TABLE 13-1	Types of Handwashing (*continued*)
Type	**Best to Use:**
Alcohol hand-rub products	When handwashing is not possible, but **only** when hands are not soiled with dirt, blood, or other matter. These products kill or inhibit the growth of transient and resident microorganisms, but do not remove them. Alcohol hand rubs do not remove dirt. Alcohol hand-rub products are relatively new items. As they are alcohol based, excessive use may cause excessive skin dryness and increase the risk of skin cracking. Care must be taken in their use.

Procedure 13-1
Proper Handwashing

Liquid soap is preferable to bar soap, as bar soap often harbours microorganisms. If you must use bar soap, rinse it off under the running water before you use it. Be aware that liquid soap dispensers (particularly those found in many homes) can also be dirty. Take the time to wash off the plunger of the dispenser if necessary.

1. Make sure that your arms are bare at least 10–12 centimetres above your wrists. Push up your sleeves and your watch.
2. Remove rings.
3. Turn on the tap and adjust the water to a comfortable, warm temperature.
4. Wet your hands and wrists thoroughly under the running water. Be sure to keep your hands lower than your elbows, so that dirty water does not run up your arm.
5. Apply soap. Work up a lather by weaving your fingers together and moving them back and forth.
6. Continue this motion for 10–15 seconds, longer if your hands are very dirty or if obvious signs of dirt remain.
7. Wash sides and backs of each hand.
8. Wash under fingernails by rubbing the fingertips of each hand against the palm of the other. Use a nailbrush or orange stick if necessary. You will find it easier to keep this area clean if your nails are kept short.
9. Wash your wrists.
10. If you are using bar soap, *drop* the soap back onto its dish. Avoid touching the dish or any soap residue in it.
11. Rinse your hands thoroughly.
12. Using a clean paper towel, dry your hands.
13. Using another paper towel, turn off the taps. Avoid touching the taps with your hands.
14. Dispose of the paper towels.

EQUIPMENT

Soap

Clean paper towels

Orange stick or nail brush

Wastebasket

Standard Precautions

Standard precautions are a set of procedures used to prevent the spread of a communicable or contagious disease. There are many such diseases. Some of the more common ones are influenza or chicken pox. Human immunodeficiency virus (HIV), hepatitis B, and tuberculosis are communicable diseases that can have serious consequences. Standard precautions were formerly called universal precautions.

Standard precautions are focused on establishing barriers to prevent contact with body fluids. They were first established by the Centers for Disease Control and Prevention (CDC) in the United States. These guidelines were updated in October 2002. The CDC suggests that standard precautions be used with all clients. Many agencies have policies on the use of standard precautions. Make sure that you are aware of your agency's policy.

Most Canadian agencies follow the CDC's standard precautions. Table 13-2 describes these precautions.

TABLE 13-2   Standard Precautions

1. Protective, disposable gloves should be worn:

   - when touching any client's blood, body fluids, mucous membranes, or non-intact skin;

   - when you have broken skin;

   - when you come in contact with surfaces soiled with blood or body fluids (such as a bathroom floor, soiled linens, or incontinence briefs);

   - when changing diapers if visible blood or diarrhea is present; or

   - when handling clothes, bed linen, or equipment that has been soiled by body fluids.

2. Gloves should be disposed of after each contact. Never wash disposable gloves for reuse.

3. Hands should be washed with warm, soapy water before gloves are put on, immediately after gloves are removed, and any time hands are soiled.

4. Gowns, aprons, and, if needed, eye protection, should be worn during procedures that are likely to generate splashes of blood or other body fluids (such as vomit or urine).

5. Masks may be worn when working with a client who is coughing excessively.

6. Precautions should be taken when disposing of needles and other sharps. To prevent needlestick injuries, needles should not be recapped, purposely bent or broken by hand, removed from disposable syringes, or otherwise manipulated by hand. After they are used, dispose of syringes and needles in an approved container. Cover the can with a lid. When the can is full, place it in a plastic garbage bag. Dispose of this bag as directed by your agency. Similar procedures should be followed when disposing of razor blades.

▶▶|

TABLE 13-2	Standard Precautions (*continued*)

7. Wear gloves when collecting specimens of body fluids (such as urine, feces, or sputum). Tightly close the container so it will not leak and place it in another, larger container for transportation.

8. If you accidentally get contaminated body fluids on a mucous membrane or broken skin, or are stuck by a contaminated needle, you should:

   - immediately wash the contaminated area thoroughly with soap or antiseptic cleanser and warm water. It is not necessary to use a hard brush, as this may irritate skin and result in an open sore;

   - contact your supervisor to report the exposure; and

   - be prepared to consider having your blood tested and periodically retested during the following year.

9. If you have a skin lesion or weeping dermatitis, you should not provide direct client care or handle client-care equipment until the skin condition is cleared up.

Procedure 13-2
Cleaning Spills of Blood and Body Fluids

1. Protect yourself by wearing disposable gloves. If there is a risk of the fluid splashing, wear protective eyewear and/or a gown.
2. Remove as much of the spill as possible using disposable absorbent material such as paper towels. Place used material in a plastic bag, tie it shut, and deposit in the garbage.
3. Wipe the floor or any contaminated surfaces with a disinfectant solution. This can be easily made by mixing one part household bleach to ten parts of water. This type of bleach solution should be freshly made up as it loses its strength over a period of time. Use a disinfectant or household germicide to clean soiled carpets or upholstery that may be damaged by the bleach solution.
4. Soak mops or brushes that have been used for cleaning in a disinfectant for 20 minutes.
5. When you are finished, wash your hands thoroughly with soap and water.

EQUIPMENT

Disposable gloves

Paper towels or other absorbent material

Soap

Disposable gloves

The Use of Gloves

Using gloves is an important part of the standard precautions. Gloves help to reduce transmission of infectious agents. Procedure 13-3 outlines the way to apply, use, and remove gloves.

Procedure 13-3
Applying, Using, and Removing Gloves

EQUIPMENT

Disposable gloves

Soap

Towels

Disposable gloves

Applying and Using Gloves

1. Use a new pair of gloves for each client. Replace the gloves if you touch unclean surfaces.
2. Wash your hands before applying gloves.
3. Pull your gloves over your wrists. If you are wearing a gown, pull the glove over the cuff of the gown.
4. Remove gloves before touching surfaces not part of the client's care (such as answering the phone or door). Put on a fresh pair of gloves when you return to the client's care.
5. If your glove develops a hole, rip, or tear, remove both gloves immediately, wash your hands, and put on a fresh pair. Remember that jewellery and long or ragged fingernails can easily puncture a disposable glove. Trim nails and remove jewellery before applying gloves.
6. If your gloves become contaminated, remove and replace them before completing your client's care.

Removing Gloves

1. Remove one glove by grasping it just below the cuff (Figure 13-2a).
2. Pull the glove down over your hand, making sure that the glove is inside out (Figure 13-2b).
3. Hold the glove you have removed in your gloved hand.
4. Slide two fingers of your *ungloved* hand between your skin and the glove on your other hand. Do not touch the outside of your gloved hand.
5. Pull the glove down over your hand and over the other glove.
6. Holding the gloves by the *inside*, dispose of the gloves.
7. Wash your hands.

FIGURE 13-2A
Removing gloves

FIGURE 13-2B

Isolation Precautions

Isolation precautions are frequently used when a client has a disease that is serious and highly contagious. Isolation precautions can also be used when a client is so frail that the risk of infection must be minimized. Table 13-3 describes the major components of isolation technique.

TABLE 13-3	Isolation Technique

1. Isolation procedures may require you to wear gloves, a gown, a mask, or eye protection. You may have to use special procedures (such as double-gowning or double-bagging contaminated items). Make sure you know what specific precautions are to be followed.

2. Collect all necessary equipment before you enter the room. This reduces the number of trips in and out and reduces the potential for drafts and other irritants. It also means that you can spend more time with the client.

3. Remember that anything that falls to the floor is considered to be contaminated.

4. Use paper towels to handle contaminated items. If your gloves or hands become contaminated, do not handle clean items.

5. Do not touch your eyes, nose, mouth, hair, or other body parts when caring for your client.

6. Remove and dispose of gloves, gowns, and other protective garments properly.

7. Wash your hands after removing any protective garments.

Isolation can have devastating effects on the person. A person with a serious and highly communicable disease may worry that he or she will infect others. The person may feel unclean, untouchable, and unwanted. The person can become very lonely as visits are often limited and the ability to receive real, caring touch is severely restricted.

Remember that it is the disease the person has that is undesirable, not the person. Make sure to treat the person with respect and to preserve his or her dignity. If possible, provide things in the person's room that interest him or her and help occupy the person's time, such as a telephone, radio, television, magazines, or books. Whenever possible, spend a few minutes visiting with the person. Make sure that your body language, as well as your words, shows the person that you care for him or her.

Cleaning Equipment

Equipment must be kept clean to reduce the potential of transmitting harmful microorganisms. In most cases (particularly in a client's home), a thorough washing with soap and water is all that is needed. A thorough cleansing washes microorganisms away.

In some cases, there is a need to disinfect items to further reduce the risk of the transmission of microorganisms. Disinfection either kills microorganisms or inhibits their growth. Most commercial items sold as chemical disinfectants are not effective against all microorganisms.

Sterilization kills virtually all microorganisms. Boiling is the most common method of sterilization.

FIGURE 13-3
Remember that disinfection and sterilization do not remove dirt. You must clean first.

You must realize that disinfection and sterilization by themselves do not remove dirt. Dirt can harbour microorganisms. Thus, the best disinfection or sterilization procedure will not be effective if the area is dirty (Figure 13-3). A good rule of thumb is "Clean first, then disinfect or sterilize when necessary."

You always must be careful when cleaning or disinfecting with chemicals. In the next section, we'll discuss a labelling system that helps you to identify the proper procedure for handling and storing chemicals.

Clean first!

Then disinfect or sterilize.

WORKPLACE HAZARDOUS MATERIALS INFORMATION SYSTEM

The Workplace Hazardous Materials Information System (WHMIS) was created by the Government of Canada in 1987. The legislation governing WHMIS and how it is used is governed by both federal and provincial legislation.

WHMIS's purpose is to make sure that employers and workers have the information they need about hazardous materials so as to handle, use, and store these materials safely. There are three components to the WHMIS system: product labels, material safety data sheets (MSDS), and worker education. These three components apply to all long-term care facilities. Provincial regulations govern how WHMIS applies to work done in clients' homes, but in most cases, provincial legislation requires that workers be educated in the handling, use, and storage of hazardous materials they may be expected to use.

WHMIS groups hazardous materials under three general headings: flammability, reactivity, and health risk.

Flammability

Flammable substances are things that can ignite and burn easily. Many things other than open flame can ignite a flammable substance. Sparks from electrical equipment and heat from a source such as a stove, toaster, or dryer can ignite flammable substances.

Reactivity

Reactive substances are things that can react with another substance to form a hazardous material. It's important to note that substances that are relatively harmless alone can react with other substances to become very toxic. For example, vinegar is a common item in many homes and is often used for cleaning. Used alone, it is quite safe. When vinegar is mixed with bleach, it produces a toxic gas.

Health Risk

Many common substances can pose a health risk if used improperly or for too long a period of time. For example, many cleaners (including bleach) can irritate skin if the substance is left in direct contact with the skin. Even shampoos and other personal care substances can irritate mucous membranes. Some substances (such as household bleach) can irritate the airway if inhaled.

Labelling of Hazardous Products

WHMIS legislation does not require that household products be labelled. However, many of the six WHMIS symbols are commonly used to label household products, as well as materials found in long-term care facilities. Each label and its meaning is presented in Figure 13-4.

Flammable   Corrosive   Explosive   Chronic Hazard   Biohazard   Reactive

FIGURE 13-4
WHMIS symbols
Source: © Her Majesty the Queen in Right of Canada, represented by the Minister of Health (2005).

While consumer products are generally exempt from WHMIS labelling requirements, products must indicate the presence of certain hazardous substances. There are four labels you might see, as illustrated in Figure 13-5.

FIGURE 13-5 *Health Canada Consumer Hazard Labels*

Source: © Her Majesty the Queen in Right of Canada, represented by the Minister of Health (2005)

 CORROSIVE
The product can burn your skin or eyes. If swallowed, it will damage your throat and stomach.

 FLAMMABLE
The product or its fumes will catch fire easily if it is near heat, flames or sparks. Rags used with this product may begin to burn on their own.

 EXPLOSIVE
The container can explode if heated or punctured. Flying pieces of metal or plastic from the container can cause serious injury, especially to eyes.

 POISON
If you swallow, lick, or in some cases, breathe in the chemical, you could become very sick or die.

Always read the label (and, if available, the Material Safety Data Sheet) when using cleaning and other household substances. Make particular note of any protective equipment you need to safely work with the substance, as well as the proper procedure for use. Ask your supervisor if you are unsure how to properly use a substance.

Not all substances must be labelled. Cosmetics, plants, and medications are not required to be labelled, yet can be harmful if used improperly.

FIRE SAFETY

When we speak about fire safety, we are actually describing two things: *fire prevention* and *safety in a fire emergency.*

Fire prevention refers to the steps that you take on a day-to-day basis to prevent a fire emergency from occurring. Many of these steps are much like those you would do to keep your own home safe, such as not smoking in bed, checking for frayed electrical cords, or not leaving items on the stove unattended. Some procedures are different, though. We'll discuss specific approaches in this section.

Safety in a fire emergency means the steps that you take to respond to a fire. These steps are broken down into two parts:

1. The actions that you take if you are the first person to discover the fire.
2. The actions that you take if you hear a fire or smoke alarm.

In each case, **the main purpose is to ensure the safety of the clients, visitors, volunteers, yourself, and other staff.**

The material in this section is intended to introduce you to the basic ideas about fire safety. You'll find that your agency has a specific fire safety procedure that must be followed.

The Main Components of Fire Prevention

There are two main components of fire prevention: reducing or eliminating *fire hazards* and reducing or stopping *hazardous behaviour.*

Fire Hazards

When we speak about **fire hazards**, we mean the things in the environment that pose a risk of fire or that could make a fire spread more quickly. Clients may not be able to easily identify these hazards due to poor vision or sense of touch or, possibly, confusion. Some of the more common hazards are discussed in this section.

Ashes from Cigarettes, Cigars, or Pipes **The most careful smoker can accidentally dump** hot ashes in a wastepaper basket or onto furnishings. As well, some ashtrays are shallow and allow cigarettes and ashes to easily fall off their edge. A person with impaired vision may not realize that he or she has placed a lit cigarette on a combustible surface.

You should make sure that all ashes are dumped into a metal can after the smoker is through. Be sensitive to the smell and sight of smoke—if you see or smell something, check it out.

Damaged Electrical Cords Often, people unplug an item by pulling on the cord instead of the plug. This can break the wiring, even if the covering is not broken. As well, items, including cords, wear out. If the cord or plug is frayed or broken or feels warm to the touch, it is a fire hazard. The cord should be unplugged until it can be checked by a qualified person.

Overloaded Extension Cords Extension cords present two potential hazards: fire and falls. Many older homes do not have the number of electrical outlets required to power the quantity of electrical appliances we use. Sometimes, the location of the outlet is inconvenient. Your client may use extension cords without thinking about whether the circuit is overloaded or whether the amperage rating for the cord has been exceeded (Photo 13-2). It's good practice to use only one appliance per cord and to unplug the appliance when it is not in use.

Photo 13-2
Overloaded electrical outlets can overload circuits, creating a fire hazard.

Damaged Electrical Equipment As with cords, equipment itself wears out or breaks. Damage due to a drop on the floor or getting wet, for example, often can't be seen. Unplug any electrical equipment you observe not functioning properly or from which you get a shock.

Flammable Materials Many chemicals we use on a daily basis are flammable, meaning that they can easily burn. It is often confusing because, in the English language, both the words flammable and inflammable are used to refer to these items. Any chemical or material labelled as flammable, that carries the WHMIS symbol for flammable materials, or that you know to be flammable should be properly handled and stored. You should read, understand, and follow the use and storage instructions for flammable chemicals. Properly dispose of cloths or papers soaked in the chemical. If in doubt about how to handle a particular chemical, ask your supervisor.

Hazardous Behaviour

Long-Term Care Facilities

One of the greatest hazardous behaviours in any facility is careless smoking. Though even the most careful smoker poses a risk, cognitively impaired or physically disabled smokers are at much greater risk, both to themselves and others. Cognitively impaired smokers may no longer understand why it is not safe to smoke in bed. They may drop ashes in wastebaskets. A physically disabled smoker may not be able to pick up a lit cigarette from his or her lap, a couch, or carpet.

Most nursing homes, homes for the aged, and retirement homes have set policies about smoking: where (and possibly at what times) residents can smoke, whether residents can smoke without supervision, and whether they can carry their own cigarettes, matches, etc. Make sure that you know the smoking policies of your own facility. If you do encounter a hazardous situation, report it to your supervisor.

Community Settings

Clients living in their own home or apartment can unknowingly have unsafe behaviours. Sometimes, the client simply doesn't realize that something is a hazard. At other times, the client may not have realized that a situation has become unsafe (such as not noticing that an electrical cord is frayed). Occasionally, the client cannot see, hear, smell, or feel things accurately enough to know that there is a potential problem.

Clients should be provided information on fire hazards, including smoking, overloading electrical wiring, and improper use of the stove. Many fire departments provide brochures on fire safety free of charge. Remember that your client has a great deal of control over how he or she will use this information and whether he or she will follow the advice given.

Be the eyes, ears, hands, and nose for your client. Identify fire hazards you see, and talk them over with the client. Most clients will want to change a situation that is hazardous.

Safety in a Fire Emergency

The other component of fire safety has to do with handling a fire emergency. This component has two parts:

1. What to do if you are the person discovering a fire.
2. What to do when you hear the fire alarm.

If You Discover a Fire

No matter where you work, in a fire emergency there are two important points to remember:

1. **The sooner the fire department is called, the sooner they will arrive.** You are not trained to fight fires—the fire department is. Make sure that the fire department is called as quickly as possible. Once they arrive, they will give you instructions as to what to do.
2. **Fire itself is not often the killer—smoke is.** Make sure that you do what you can to prevent smoke from spreading, such as closing doors or windows of the room that has the smoke.

Long-Term Care Facilities

Each long-term care facility has its own procedure to handle fire emergencies. In general, though, the procedure requires you to:

1. Pull the fire alarm or call the fire department.
2. Remove anyone in immediate danger, if possible.
3. If the fire is in a room or contained area, close the door to contain the fire and smoke.
4. Move residents out of the fire area, usually to an area protected by fire doors.
5. Close all other corridor and room doors.
6. If the fire is small, and you feel you can safely do so, try to put the fire out.

It is of extreme importance that you know and follow your agency's procedure for a fire emergency. This ensures that you are working as a team in the most effective manner.

Please note that most long-term care facilities do not immediately evacuate the entire building when the fire alarm sounds. These homes generally do what is called a four-stage evacuation.

Stage 1   Removal of anyone in immediate danger, if possible
Stage 2   Horizontal Evacuation (like step 4, page 212)
Stage 3   Vertical Evacuation (move residents to a lower floor)
Stage 4   Premises Evacuation (move residents out of the building)

You would perform a Stage 3 or 4 evacuation when the fire marshal (the person on staff who is in charge in a fire emergency) or the fire department tells you to do so.

Community Settings

A fire emergency procedure should be tailored to each client's home. A fire evacuation plan should be developed, identifying the emergency exit for each room. As many fires start at night, any fire plan should include escape routes from rooms in which people sleep.

Many people live in apartment buildings. Often, the local fire department has specific recommendations as to the steps to take if a fire erupts in a client's unit. These recommendations often include the seven steps listed here:

1. Remove anyone in immediate danger, if possible. Assist your client to leave the building if able, or to wait in a stairwell landing, **with the fire door closed,** if not able to leave.
2. Close room or apartment doors to contain the fire.
3. Pull the nearest fire alarm or call the fire department.
4. Close all other corridor and apartment doors, if possible.
5. If possible, return to apartment to fight fire. Do this only if the fire is small, is not fed by gas or flammable liquid, and is reasonably safe to attempt.
6. If necessary, move others out of the fire area, usually to a stairwell landing protected by fire doors.
7. Never use elevators in a fire emergency.

Remember that the procedures in some buildings may require you to assist clients to get out as a first step. Often, these are buildings where all apartments have wheelchair access to the outside (they are all on the first floor, for example). It is essential to read and follow the procedure established for the client's setting.

Using a Fire Extinguisher

You may decide that it is safe to fight the fire with a fire extinguisher. If so, the following guidelines can help you minimize the risks. **Never put yourself at risk by trying to fight a fire that is too large or smoky.**

1. Only try to extinguish small fires. If the fire is too large, get out and close all doors behind you.
2. Bear in mind that while some extinguishers work on all kinds of fires, some are only effective on certain types. The classification of the extinguisher tells you what fires it is designed to fight:

   Class A   Ordinary combustibles such as wood, paper, cloth, and rubber
   Class B   Flammable liquids such as fuel oil, gasoline, cooking grease, and solvents
   Class C   Energized electrical equipment such as wiring, fuse boxes, and electrical motors
   Class D   Combustible metals such as magnesium, sodium, and zirconium

Photo 13-3
*Aim the extinguisher
at the base of the fire
and use a sweeping
motion.*
Source: Prentice Hall, Inc.
Photographer:
Tom Boschler

3. Use the PASS method to fight the fire:
   Pull the pin
   Aim the nozzle at the base of the fire
   Squeeze or pump the handle
   Sweep from side to side at the base of the flame
4. Make certain that you are between the exit and the fire so that you can escape if the fire does not go out.
5. Know where the extinguisher is kept and how to use it.

If You Hear the Fire Alarm

Long-Term Care Facilities

These procedures vary from facility to facility. In general, though, the procedure asks you to:

1. **Report to the fire location**, bringing, if possible, wheelchairs to assist in transporting residents.
2. **Follow the directions of the person in charge** (the fire marshal) with regard to evacuating residents, closing doors, and/or helping in other ways.
3. **Unless instructed to do so, don't use the telephone to call** other floors, the switchboard, etc. You may prevent important calls from the fire department from getting through.

Community Settings

Clients living in apartments should respond to a fire alarm, even if the fire is not in their units. If you are visiting a client when the fire alarm sounds, you must assist the client. As with long-term care facilities, each apartment building (particularly buildings catering to older adults or persons with physical disabilities) has specific guidelines. In general, the following steps are often included:

1. **Call the fire department.** Meet the fire department in or near the lobby with a list of clients. If you can't leave the apartment, let the fire department know and provide the list by phone, if necessary.
2. **Reassure the client.**
3. **If a client cannot leave the building without using the elevator, instruct the client to remain in his or her apartment, unless told otherwise by the fire captain or other person in charge.**

4. **Close the apartment door, but leave it unlocked.** This allows the fire department to quickly enter should they need to do so.
5. **Block door with wet towel if smoke begins to seep in.** If smoke begins to enter heating or other vents, block them off with wet towels pinned or taped to the vents.
6. **If smoke enters the apartment, keep low to the floor.** Move the client to a balcony, if available.

CLIENT EMERGENCIES

You should be prepared to provide emergency assistance to a client. It is strongly recommended that you take a first aid and cardiopulmonary resuscitation (CPR) course offered by a recognized safety organization in your province. Life-saving techniques such as CPR or clearing the airway of an unconscious victim should be learned and practised under the guidance of a trained professional. Speak with your supervisor to find out which organizations offer courses in your area.

This section provides basic information on responding to client emergencies. Some clients may have specific instructions to follow in the event of an emergency. As well, your employer will have specific instructions to follow in an emergency. It is important to know what the specific instructions are and to follow them if the situation arises.

In the absence of specific instructions, use the following as a guide:

1. Remember that the two purposes of emergency care are to prevent death and prevent additional injury.
2. Remain calm. You are of no use to your client if you become so upset that you cannot assist.
3. Assess the situation. Is it safe for you to assist the client? Are there hazards, such as fire or live electricity, that must be controlled before you can assist? Can you deal with the situation or do you need to call for help to do so?
4. If possible, remove any hazards. Avoid moving the client unless you have no other alternative.
5. Practise standard precautions. You may have to adapt your approach if proper supplies are not readily available. For example, if gloves are not readily available, you may cover your hand with a plastic bag in order to apply pressure to a bleeding wound.
6. Check for signs of life-threatening conditions: no breathing, no pulse, or profuse bleeding.
7. Call for help or have someone else in the room do this for you. Table 13-4 outlines the information to have ready to provide the emergency personnel answering the call.
8. Keep the client warm. Use blankets, towels, coats, or sweaters.
9. If the client is conscious, ask if he or she has pain or discomfort. Discourage the client from moving as it may make an injury worse.
10. Reassure the victim that help is on the way.
11. Do not give a victim any food or liquids.
12. Assist the person, if possible. Table 13-5 provides accepted methods of treating common emergencies. **Never attempt a procedure you have not been trained to perform, unless you are following the step-by-step instructions of trained emergency personnel.**
13. Stay with the person until help has arrived. You may be asked to accompany the person to hospital. If so, advise your agency.

TABLE 13-4	Emergency Information

Contacting emergency services is commonly called *activating emergency medical services* or *activating EMS*. In many areas of Canada, you activate EMS by dialling 9-1-1. Some areas do not yet have this service, so make certain that you know the number for your area.

When you call emergency services, make certain you have the following information:

1. Your location: street name and number, unit or apartment number, if applicable. In a rural area, it's often helpful to know the nearest main intersection or landmark.
2. The telephone number from which you are calling.
3. What has happened. Be sure to tell the emergency personnel if the person has a life-threatening condition: no pulse, no breathing, or profuse bleeding.
4. Description of injuries.

EMS personnel may ask you specific questions or give you instructions to carry out while help is on the way. Provide the required information and follow any instructions to the best of your ability.

TABLE 13-5	What to Do If…

This table describes accepted methods for responding to common emergencies. Be certain to:

- activate EMS for any serious emergency unless specifically directed to do otherwise; and
- follow your agency's procedure for handling emergencies.

Problem	Solution
The person is not conscious.	Lean close to the person's ear and loudly say, "Are you OK? Wake up!"
The person appears to not be breathing.	1. Open the person's airway by placing two fingers under the person's chin and pulling the chin forward. 2. Place your ear near the person's mouth. Listen and feel for breathing. 3. If the person is not breathing, pinch the person's nose, place your mouth over the victim's and slowly blow air into the victim's mouth. 4. If the air does not cause the person's chest to rise, reposition the head and try again. 5. If the person's chest still does not rise, the airway may be obstructed. Attempt to clear the airway using abdominal thrust if the person is conscious. Use the procedure below if the person is not conscious or becomes unconscious.

▶▶|

TABLE 13-5	What to Do If... *(continued)*
Problem	**Solution**
The person's airway is obstructed.	1. Attempt to clear the airway using abdominal thrust if the person is conscious. 2. If the person is unconscious, locate the proper spot for compressions by running your finger up the person's rib cage to the point where the ribs join. Position your two fingers below this point, with your fingers pointing toward the person's head. Deliver quick upward thrusts to clear the airway.
The person is bleeding profusely.	1. Use standard precautions. Wear gloves if possible. 2. Use clean material (washcloth, clothing, etc.) to cover the site. 3. Apply pressure directly over the site with your hand. 4. Leave your hand in place until the bleeding is controlled.
The person appears to be having a seizure.	1. Lower the person to the floor. 2. Cushion the head by placing a towel under the head or by cradling the head in your lap. 3. Loosen tight clothing. 4. Push furniture or other objects out of the way so that the person will not hit them and injure him- or herself. 5. Do not place any object in the person's mouth. 6. Do not restrain the person's movement.
The person is burned.	1. Stop the burning process. Extinguish flames by wrapping the person in a heavy blanket or coat to smother flames. Cool heat burns by running cool water over the site. Disconnect or unplug (if possible) any electrical appliance that is causing a burn by using an object that does not conduct electricity (dry rope or wood, for example). 2. Cover the burn with a clean, wet covering. DO NOT apply ointments, oils, or fats to the burn.

RESTRAINTS

Restraints are devices that restrict a client's movement. There are three main types of restraints: environmental, chemical, and physical.

Environmental restraints include things like locked areas or units. Some types of this restraint, such as a well-designed "secure" unit that is large enough to provide areas for walking, opportunities for interaction and stimulation, and support the person to function as well as he or she can, are useful and beneficial. A locked area that is too small to provide for these opportunities would be harmful.

Chemical restraints are medications given to clients to control behaviours. Chemical restraints usually include medications such as sedatives or antipsychotic medications. It is generally agreed that it is not acceptable to use these medications to control behaviour that is bothersome but not unsafe. People who are given medications as a form of chemical restraint may also be unable to interact or to perceive things in their environment as a result. If the chemical restraint is used long enough, the person's ability to interact and perceive may be permanently lost, even if the medication is discontinued.

Physical restraints alter a client's ability to move. Examples of these restraints are wheelchair lap belts, vest restraints, bed rails, geriatric chairs with tables, or even recliner chairs that prohibit a person from getting up and out of the chair.

For many years, restraints were seen as a way of keeping a client safe. For example, clients were restrained so as to keep them from falling or to keep them from entering unsafe areas of a building. Some research now shows that people who are restrained are actually at greater risk of falling and injury (D. Evans, J. Wood, and L. Lambert (2003). Patient injury and physical restraint devices: A systematic review. *Journal of Advanced Nursing*, 41(3), 274–282). As well, restraints lessen a person's independence and diminish self-worth. In some cases, such as when the client has a cognitive impairment, restraints can actually provoke aggression.

STOP AND REFLECT ((13-1))

Imagine that you are in a long-term care home. Now, imagine that a person you don't know has made you sit in a chair and has placed a table in front of you so that you cannot get up. No matter what you do, you can't move the table and can't get out of the chair.

How do you feel?

_____

_____

_____

What do you do?

_____

_____

_____

Did you feel upset? Angry? Perhaps you would try to get out of the chair. If so, you've demonstrated the common reactions a person with cognitive impairment may have to a physical restraint. The restraint may well make the situation worse.

We now know that restraints can be very harmful or even deadly if improperly used. The effects of restricted movement can result in decreased muscle and bone strength, pressure sores (decubitus ulcers), incontinence, and constipation. An improperly applied restraint can cause a resident to slip and possibly asphyxiate. In March 2007, Health Canada issued a warning about the use of waist and torso restraints, in response to reports of asphyxiation related to the use of these restraints (http://www. hc-sc.gc.ca/dhp-mps/medeff/advisories-avis/prof/2007/restraints_dispositifs_ nth-aah_e.html). Clients who are restrained may become agitated, depressed, or angry as a result of the restraint.

Restraint use has decreased since the 1980s, largely because of increased awareness of the risks of restraint use, increased awareness of other ways to prevent falls, and the development of safer alternatives and less restrictive restraints. Most facilities, professional organizations, and even legislatures have adopted a policy of "least restraint." Some provinces have passed legislation that defines the use of restraints. The purpose of British Columbia's *Patient Restraints Minimization* Act, 2001 is to "minimize the use of restraints on patients and to encourage hospitals and facilities to use alternative methods, whenever possible" (*Patient Restraints Minimization Act, 2001*, S.O. 2001, Chapter 16, Section 3). Newfoundland and Labrador has included a "least restraint" policy in its 2005 standards for long-term care facilities. In 2001, Ontario passed legislation that included a "least restraint" policy.

STOP AND REFLECT ((13-2))

Does your province have legislation or policies about restraints? If so, what does the legislation or government policy say? Do other organizations (such as the association of long-term care facilities or home care agencies) in your province discuss restraints? What are their views?

_____

_____

_____

_____

_____

_____

Table 13-6 lists several alternatives to restraints

TABLE 13-6	Alternatives to Restraints

Many clients and long-term care facilities have found that the following alternatives can reduce the use of restraints.

1. Using positioning devices to assist a client to keep his or her balance in a chair. (Instead of a lap belt or vest restraint.)
2. Using lower beds, or placing a bed directly on the floor. (Instead of using bed rails that a client tries to climb over.)
3. Removing rugs and other items that present a risk for falls. (Instead of restraining a client's freedom to walk.)
4. Assisting the client to perform strengthening or balance exercises to make walking safer.
5. Finding activities that engage the client and provide respite from boredom or an outlet for energy.

As you have seen in this section, the decision to use restraint of any type must always take into account the potential harm and possible benefit to the client. A problem-solving approach should always be taken before a decision to use a restraint is made. Table 13-7 describes a problem-solving approach, based upon one used by the Alzheimer Society of Canada to address issues that might result in the use of a restraint. **Restraints are never to be used simply to make it easier for a caregiver to provide support.**

TABLE 13-7	A Problem-Solving Approach

1. Identify the problem: Take a step back and objectively pinpoint the problem. What are the real risks? What are the fears? Can you get information that will help you decide if a fear is valid and help you make an informed decision?
2. Analyze the problem: Is the person trying to communicate something? What factors might be contributing to the person's reaction? What is happening and why? Could the person be reacting to something or someone in the environment?
3. List possible strategies: Think of all the ways to possibly solve the problem. Discuss the issue with your supervisor, other caregivers and the client if possible.
4. Choose a strategy: Weigh the pros and cons of each strategy. Select one.
5. Take action: Put the chosen strategy into effect.
6. Assess the results: Did the chosen strategy work? If not, why not? Should another strategy be tried?

Sometimes the first strategy is not successful. Or, it may work the first time, but not with subsequent attempts. Can you identify reasons and perhaps change them? Were there reasons that the approach worked at one time, but not another?

Source: Adapted from "A problem-solving approach," Alzheimer Society of Canada, 2007

There are times when a specific client's condition can benefit from a properly applied restraint. An example of this is a client's use of a Velcro® leg strap to assist him or her in keeping his or her legs properly positioned in a wheelchair. The client can open or reposition the Velcro belt to maintain comfort, yet make use of the benefits of the strap to maintain his or her legs in the position the client desires.

When a Restraint Must Be Used

A restraint is the option of last resort. It should be used only after all other options have been examined and efforts have been made to try alternatives. In most parts of Canada, restraints used in long-term care homes must be used only when ordered by a physician. (In some provinces, a nurse practitioner or other designated professional may also make this order.) There are often specific requirements for how often the restraint must be checked and how often the client must be repositioned.

Each restraint has a proper method of application. You must know and follow the procedure for the restraint, as well as know where and how to attach the restraint. The client must be checked regularly (this is a legal requirement) to ensure that the restraint remains properly applied. The restraint must also be removed on a regular basis to allow the client to move and, when necessary, to attend to bodily needs.

Each facility should have a policy covering the use of restraints. You must follow the policy set by your facility. The following list provides some general guidelines for the proper use of restraints. You must always remember that any restraint is used for specific purposes, not for the caregiver's convenience or comfort.

1. **Restraints should be used only after a thorough assessment of all other options.** Assessment of the client's need for the restraint should continue after the restraint is used. A client may not always need to use a restraint simply because one was once necessary.
2. The restraint applied should be the correct type and size and be in good repair. Do not use any restraint that is damaged or so worn that it is unsafe.
3. Apply the restraint according to the manufacturer's instructions.
4. Adjust the restraint so that it is comfortable for the client. If at all possible, the client should be able to adjust the restraint.
5. Document the use of the restraint according to your agency's guidelines.

Questions for Review

1. What are the three types of risk encountered in support work? Give two examples of each type.
2. Describe the chain of infection.
3. Describe two things you can do to reduce the risk of transmission of pathogens.
4. Describe the three methods of handcleaning. When is it appropriate to use each type?
5. When should you wash your hands?
6. What are the two purposes of emergency care?

7. What does PASS stand for when using a fire extinguisher?

8. What are the three types of restraints?

9. What approach should be used before considering any type of restraint?

10. Do restraints actually help prevent falls?

11. What are the five general guidelines you should follow when a client in your care uses a restraint?

Questions for Discussion

1. Consider these two case studies. Discuss:
   a. whether each client should be restrained; and
   b. what other measures might be taken.

Case 1
Mr. Greave is a resident in a long-term care facility. He spends most of the day wandering through the halls on his floor. He usually stays in the hall, but recently he has been entering other residents' rooms. The residents whose rooms he enters have become a bit upset. As well, Mr. Greave has recently had the flu and, as a result, is a bit unsteady on his feet.

Case 2
Mr. Lee is a resident of a long-term care facility. He is recovering from a fractured hip and has just begun to bear weight. Mr. Lee often forgets that he is not supposed to walk and tries to get up. He has been receiving physiotherapy, and the therapists feel that he will soon be able to walk with a walker. The therapists do not feel Mr. Lee is able to walk alone.

2. Your client, Mrs. Ross, has chicken pox. As a result, she must keep away from pregnant women and others who have not had the disease. Mrs. Ross's daughter is pregnant with twins. As a result, Mrs. Ross has had to move to her son's home. Even at her son's home, she must remain away from the family because only her son has had chicken pox before. What are some of the effects this type of isolation might have on Mrs. Ross? How might these effects be lessened?

3. As a support worker, you may be called upon to work with clients who have incurable and communicable diseases. How do you feel about working with clients in these situations?

4. You arrive at your client's home to find her unconscious on the floor. There is a small amount of blood on the floor behind her head. What do you do? What would you do if the client was living in a long-term care facility?

Chapter 14

Fundamental Terms and Concepts in Personal Support

Learning Objectives

Through reading this chapter, you'll be able to

1. Define health, health condition, impairment, disability, participation, and handicap.
2. Describe prevention and how the concept applies to a client situation.
3. Describe habilation and rehabilitation and how each concept applies to a client situation.
4. Define palliation and describe how the concept applies to a client situation.
5. Give two reasons why it is important to involve the client in his or her support.
6. List the nine levels of involvement a client may have in his or her support.
7. Outline six methods you might use to involve the client in his or her support.
8. Identify the actions a support worker should take when the support required is beyond the support worker's training or authority.

Chapter at a Glance

- The Concept of Health
- Health Conditions, Impairment, Disability, Participation, and Handicap
- Fundamental Concepts of Support Work
- Applying the Four Concepts in Your Work with Clients
- Working with Your Client to Determine His or Her Involvement in the Support You Provide
- When Your Client's Needs or Requests Exceed the Bounds of Your Role

Terms You'll Use

Disability A limitation to a person's functioning, caused by an impairment, that affects things the person needs or wants to do.

Habilitation A process by which a person chooses to gain or regain function, or to adapt to a change in function in order to attain self-fulfillment.

Handicap Commonly used to refer to a disability or activity limitation; not as widely used as it once was.

Health "A state of complete physical, social, and mental well-being, not merely the absence of disease or infirmity" (WHO, 1998).

Health Condition Something that causes a change in a person's health status.

Impairment A change in a person's functioning that differs from that expected of others of the same age or sex.

Palliation Providing care, support, and comfort to a client whose condition cannot be cured.

Prevention Avoiding the creation of unnecessary illness, impairment, or disability.

Rehabilitation A process that helps people regain desired activities and levels of participation when these things have been affected by an impairment.

THE CONCEPT OF HEALTH

We often assume that the term *health* refers to not being ill. Though part of the concept of health refers to physical function, health is a much broader concept that takes into account many aspects of well-being. In this text, we'll use the definition developed by the World Health Organization (WHO). The WHO defines **health** as "A state of complete physical, social, and mental well-being, not merely the absence of disease or infirmity" (World Health Organization, *Health Promotion Glossary*, 1998).

The WHO goes on to define health as a "resource for everyday life, not the object of living" that emphasizes an individual's social and personal resources as well as the person's physical capacities. In this sense, health is a means to an end in that it allows us to do what we need or want to do.

STOP AND REFLECT ((14-1))

Consider the WHO definition of health. Would you describe yourself as healthy? What factors do you consider when you consider your own health?

_____

_____

_____

_____

_____

_____ ■

Did you find that you tended to define your health in terms of how well you were able to do the things you need or want to do? If so, you are not alone. When asked if they are healthy, many older adults will respond that they are well enough to do what they want to do (Photo 14-1).

HEALTH CONDITIONS, IMPAIRMENT, DISABILITY, PARTICIPATION, AND HANDICAP

Health Condition

Support workers frequently work with people who have some condition that affects their ability to do what they need or want to do. The World Health Organization defines a **health condition** as something that causes a change in a person's health status. Many things can cause this change: injury, disease, distress, or a condition such as pregnancy.

Impairment

An **impairment** occurs when the health condition results in a change in the person's functioning in relation to what is expected for people of the same age or sex. An impairment could be due to a loss of a body part, an injury or abnormality of a body part, or a change in psychological functioning.

It's important to remember that although an impairment results in a change in functioning, it may not be a change that affects the person's everyday life. Even if it does, the person may be able to use a device that helps him or her to overcome the effects of the impairment. For example, nearsightedness is an impairment whose effects can usually be overcome by the use of eyeglasses or contact lenses.

Disability

Disability occurs when a person's functioning is limited by an impairment in a way that affects things the person needs or wants to do. Disability can be defined only in the context of the individual because the extent to which an impairment affects a person's activities will vary by the activities the person wants to do. As Case Example 14-1 illustrates, it is quite possible for the same impairment to cause great disability for one person and very little disability (if any at all) for another person.

CASE EXAMPLE 14-1

Jasmine Rajpaul is 34 years old. She experienced significant hearing loss at age seven. She has no functional hearing. Jasmine can remember when she was able to hear. However, she has not been able to hear for many years and has grown quite accustomed to the impairment. As a statistical analyst, she finds that the absence of noise actually helps her in her work. "I can focus on what I'm doing without interruption," she says. Jasmine does not see her activities as being limited or see herself as a "disabled person."

Carrie Weatherall is 38 years old. She experienced significant hearing loss at age 24. Like Jasmine, Carrie has no functional hearing. Unlike Jasmine, Carrie's activities are dramatically affected by the impairment. Carrie has had to leave her job as a recording technician (a person who mixes the sounds you hear on a compact disc) as the result of her impairment. She underwent a period of retraining and now works as a researcher for a university. Carrie misses her career in music and feels that her activities have been significantly limited by her impairment.

Would you react to hearing loss in the same way as Jasmine or Carrie did? Why or why not?

The term disability is often replaced by the phrase *activity limitation*. Activity limitation is seen as being a more accurate description of the changes affecting a person.

Carrie's and Jasmine's levels of disability are very much different despite the similarity in their impairments. Their experience is not unusual.

Remember that experiencing disability is not something that the person can completely control. Three things, the degree of impairment, societal attitudes, and physical barriers, affect the experience of disability.

Significant impairments may result in changes in ability that are impossible for a person to completely overcome. As with Carrie, the nature of the impairment may result in dramatic changes.

Secondly, societal perceptions and stereotypes can also create disability. For example, a person may be disabled by an employer's perception that a person who uses a wheelchair cannot possibly perform a specific job, or by a family that believes that a person in a wheelchair could not make a suitable spouse for their son or daughter.

Thirdly, physical barriers may impose disability upon a person. For example, a person's ability to obtain a job may be restricted by how accessible the building is to a person with a particular impairment. Though many physical barriers can be removed, some cannot be easily resolved and may impose a disability upon a person.

As a support worker, you must take particular care to not impose disability upon your client through your attitude or the way you provide support. You must always take particular care to ensure that your attitude does not convey assumptions about what your client can or cannot do based upon his or her impairment.

Don't forget that small things can pose a real barrier for a person with impairment. A glass of water left just outside the client's reach, or a load of laundry left in the washer when the client cannot lift it out and place the laundry in the dryer can be just as disabling as an inaccessible building. Make sure that all your activities reduce or eliminate barriers and don't create them.

Participation

Participation in the context of health refers to the ability to participate in all activities: social, occupational, and interpersonal, as well as physical and psychological. Ability to take part in life (i.e., to participate) is affected by the degree of disability experienced by the person.

Participation is closely linked to life satisfaction in the sense that satisfaction with one's level of participation is a key component of satisfaction with one's life. Remember that more participation does not always equal more satisfaction. One person may be very satisfied with a lesser degree of participation than might satisfy another person.

Take the time to learn how your client prefers to participate in activities. Support the level of participation he or she desires. Avoid encouraging your client to participate in ways the client does not prefer simply because you feel that it might be good for him or her. This does not mean that you should not provide encouragement to a client who needs a bit of support to take part in an activity, but do not impose your preferences on your client.

Handicap

The term handicap has been used in several different ways. The term is considered by many people to have a negative meaning. It is less often used now than in years past. In the 1950s and 1960s, *handicap* was often used to describe what we would now call a disability or activity limitation. We still see some use of this meaning of the term in legislation.

Also, you might still see the phrase "handicapped parking" to designate parking spaces for use by persons with physical impairments. Handicap is also used to describe a disability created by society, either through physical barriers or attitudes.

FUNDAMENTAL CONCEPTS OF SUPPORT WORK

As we discussed in Chapter 1, the purpose of support work is to assist clients to accomplish the tasks of everyday living so that they can get on with their lives. This chapter is concerned with four concepts that guide how you work with your client to provide that assistance.

These four concepts are *prevention, rehabilitation, habilitation,* and *palliation.* They are based upon the ethical principles of autonomy, beneficence, and nonmalificence we discussed in Chapter 3. All four principles are based on respect for the client's right to take risks and make decisions, to not cause harm, and to promote that which is good. These principles are also based on the holistic approach discussed in Chapter 7.

Prevention

Prevention refers to avoiding the creation of unnecessary impairment or disability. Support workers practise prevention in many ways, such as by encouraging a client to maintain activities he or she enjoys, by assisting a client with exercises to maintain muscle tone and movement, or by providing personal care in a way that minimizes the risk of skin breakdown. Case Example 14-2 illustrates one type of prevention.

CASE EXAMPLE 14-2

Mrs. Hopkins has several serious health conditions. She has lung cancer and chronic bronchitis. She also has a chronic liver condition. As a result of these conditions, she is too weak to walk or even to sit in a chair. She spends all her time in bed.

It's important for Mrs. Hopkins to be able to sit up in bed a few times each day. Not only does the change in position help prevent skin breakdown by changing the pres-

sure points on her buttocks and legs, it provides Mrs. Hopkins with a sense of accomplishment and a way to feel "more like her old self" again. Mrs. Hopkins relies upon her support workers to assist her to sit up in bed, using a procedure laid out by an occupational therapist.

How does the support worker's care support prevention?

Rehabilitation

Rehabilitation refers to a process that helps people to regain desired activities and levels of participation when these things have been affected by an impairment. Rehabilitation includes two general aims: the regaining of function that has been lost and the learning of new skills or abilities to provide a more effective way of attaining desired activities and participation. Many people take part in rehabilitation as part of their recovery from a stroke or to regain function after having broken an arm or a leg.

Some professionals feel that rehabilitation includes assisting a client to retain function. The phrase "If you don't use it, you'll lose it" is an example of this view.

In this sense, many of the activities we do to keep fit can be seen as rehabilitative as well as being preventative. On the other hand, many professionals feel that the use of the term rehabilitation in this manner places too much emphasis on everyday activities as therapy.

STOP AND REFLECT 14-2

What sorts of things do you do to maintain your abilities? For example, do you do crossword puzzles to help keep up your mental skills and your vocabulary? Do you exercise to maintain muscle tone and range of motion?

_____

_____

_____

_____

_____ ∎

It's likely that you do many activities that could be seen as rehabilitative. It's also likely that you don't think of these things in this way. Most of us think of these activities as helping us attain a desired goal, such as feeling better or taking some time to relax with an activity we enjoy.

This is probably the way that your client thinks about the things that he or she does—in light of what he or she wants to accomplish, not as a specific activity he or she wants to be able to perform. As we discussed earlier in this chapter, health is a means to an end, not an end in itself. Keep this in mind when you assist your client: activity must have a purpose that is meaningful to the client, and that purpose is more likely centred around what a particular ability lets the client do, as opposed to having the ability to perform the activity.

Habilitation

Habilitation can be defined in two ways. The most common definition describes habilitation as the process by which a person attains his or her optimal function when the person has had a lifelong impairment or acquired an impairment at an early age. Habilitation differs from rehabilitation in that it is concerned with acquiring ability—not regaining ability lost to an impairment.

Another, newer definition of habilitation describes it as a process by which a person chooses to gain or regain function, or to adapt to a change in function in order to attain a sense of self-fulfillment. This concept of habilitation includes the adaptation of the person's surroundings (both the people and the setting), if necessary, to assist the person to attain his or her optimal level of functioning. This concept can be particularly useful when the client cannot or chooses not to gain or regain function. Case Example 14-3 describes one such situation.

CASE EXAMPLE 14-3

Anna Reese has Alzheimer Disease. She lives with her son and his family. Mrs. Reese has always enjoyed being a homemaker and hostess. In years past, she enjoyed preparing and serving meals to her family and guests.

Now, Mrs. Reese's condition makes it impossible for her to safely use a stove without help. Her condition makes it impossible for her to regain this ability. So, Mrs. Reese's daughter-in-law and grandson adapt. They
assist Mrs. Reese in preparing some dishes while taking on the aspects of the meal that are now too difficult for Mrs. Reese to perform. Her family's adaptations assist Mrs. Reese to participate in activities that are meaningful for her.

> **Can you apply the concept of habilitation to your life? How?**

Palliation

Palliation refers to providing care, support, and comfort to a client whose condition cannot be cured. Palliation is often referred to in the context of terminal (or life-threatening) illness. In fact, palliation can be appropriately provided at any time that a condition cannot be cured, whether or not the condition is terminal. For example, osteoporosis cannot be cured, yet measures can—and should—be taken to prevent excess disability, maintain client comfort, and preserve function.

APPLYING THE FOUR CONCEPTS IN YOUR WORK WITH CLIENTS

As a support worker, you will regularly apply the concepts of prevention, rehabilitation, habilitation, and palliation in your work with clients. You may even apply all four concepts to your work with a single client. Consider the following example.

CASE EXAMPLE 14-4

Su Ping works with Mrs. Leung. Mrs. Leung has diabetes and arthritis, and has recently undergone a knee joint replacement. Su Ping applies the concepts of prevention, rehabilitation, habilitation, and palliation to her work with Mrs. Leung in the following ways.

Because Mrs. Leung's diabetes requires her to follow a strict diet, Su Ping makes sure to adhere to any dietary guidelines when she prepares meals for Mrs. Leung, so as not to introduce foods that will affect her client's condition (prevention). At first, this was difficult, as Mrs. Leung did not like the dietary restrictions and asked for foods she should not eat. Su Ping felt uncomfortable when she could not meet her client's requests. She discussed this with her supervisor and after a case conference, Su Ping became more comfortable with maintaining the diet prescribed for Mrs. Leung.

Su Ping regularly assists Mrs. Leung with knee and leg exercises set out by Mrs. Leung's physiotherapist. These exercises are designed to help Mrs. Leung regain the ability she had before her knee deteriorated (rehabilitation).

Although Mrs. Leung's knee is progressing well, and she is physically able, she has decided that climbing the stairs to the second floor is simply too much effort. As a result, Su Ping is now helping her client to reorganize the main floor of her home so that Mrs. Leung will not need to climb stairs (habilitation).

Finally, Su Ping assists Mrs. Leung with specific activities designed to minimize the pain of her arthritis. Although these activities will not cure Mrs. Leung's arthritis, they do provide relief from pain and discomfort (palliation).

Although Su Ping applies all four concepts to her work with her client, she does not organize her thoughts and activities into four distinct categories. She provides the support the client requires in response to her client's goals and preferences. She is able to change her focus from rehabilitation to palliation to habilitation to prevention as her client's needs require.

Always attempt to apply these concepts as appropriate to your client, even if you do not feel that you would make the same decision as your client has made. For example, your client may make a decision to cease playing cards at the seniors' centre as it requires too much effort for the benefit he or she receives. You may feel that the activity is worthwhile, and, if you were the client, you would maintain the activity. You may feel that the client should maintain the activity because it is good for him or her to get out. Despite your feelings, you must support the client's decision. For example, if your client decides to cease participating in the seniors' centre, you might work with him or her to find and make use of alternate ways to interact with others.

In some specific cases, you may not be able to support your client's decisions. This may be because the client no longer has the ability to make sound decisions (for example, as the result of a dementia) or when the client's decision requires you to do something that is prohibited by law or by your employer's policies (for example, the client asks you to drive her or his car or to witness a legal document). Often, the client's support plan provides information on how to respond to these situations. In other cases, you may need to speak with your supervisor or other members of the support team to determine the best response.

WORKING WITH YOUR CLIENT TO DETERMINE HIS OR HER INVOLVEMENT IN THE SUPPORT YOU PROVIDE

As you learned in the previous section, the activities you perform with a client must be placed in the context of the client's goals. Two clients may have very different desires and goals in response to the same health condition. By discussing your client's goals, needs, and preferences with your client, you will be able to put your activities in the proper context (Photo 14-2). You will also understand each activity's significance to your client.

In addition, working with your client involves your client in the process. Most of us respond more fully and are more satisfied when we are involved in the decisions that affect us. Your client is likely no different.

Although most clients want to have some level of participation in planning or helping to provide the support they receive, the exact type and extent of participation each person wants is unique. One client may want to assist with as many activities as possible. Another client may simply want you to know what is important to him or her. Moreover, your client's level of participation may increase or decrease depending upon the activity. For example, your client may be very interested in participating in grocery shopping but have no interest in how you do the laundry.

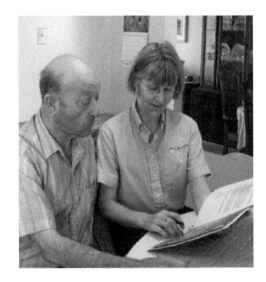

Photo 14-2
Worker and client discussing an issue.
Source: CHATS

Levels of Client Participation

As Figure 14-1 illustrates, there are nine general levels of participation (adapted from Zgola, *Doing Things*, 1987). Remember that an individual client's level of participation may be a combination of one or more levels, and that any client's level of participation may vary over time.

Techniques to Involve Clients in Their Support

It's often the support worker's responsibility to discuss preferences and client participation with the client. If you are working with a client for the first time, you will need to take a few minutes to go over this information.

When you do, bear in mind that the client has the right not to participate at all in his or her support (unless the client has agreed to participate as part of the support plan). You should never attempt to coerce a client into participating in a manner or to an extent with which he or she is uncomfortable. On the other hand, you should always try to make use of a client's willingness to participate. Try the following ideas to involve your client:

FIGURE 14-1

General levels of participation

Source: Adapted from Jitka M. Zgola, Doing Things: A Guide to Programming Activities for Persons with Alzheimer's Disease and Related Diseases, *p. 35, 1987. © Reprinted with permission of the Johns Hopkins University Press.*

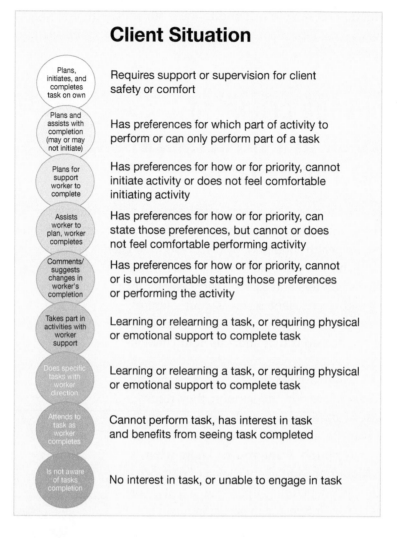

Client Situation

Level	Client Situation
Plans, initiates, and completes task on own	Requires support or supervision for client safety or comfort
Plans and assists with completion (may or may not initiate)	Has preferences for which part of activity to perform or can only perform part of a task
Plans for support worker to complete	Has preferences for how or for priority, cannot initiate activity or does not feel comfortable initiating activity
Assists worker to plan, worker completes	Has preferences for how or for priority, can state those preferences, but cannot or does not feel comfortable performing activity
Comments/suggests changes in worker's completion	Has preferences for how or for priority, cannot or is uncomfortable stating those preferences or performing the activity
Takes part in activities with worker support	Learning or relearning a task, or requiring physical or emotional support to complete task
Does specific tasks with worker direction	Learning or relearning a task, or requiring physical or emotional support to complete task
Attends to task as worker completes	Cannot perform task, has interest in task and benefits from seeing task completed
Is not aware of tasks completion	No interest in task, or unable to engage in task

1. **Ask the client what he or she would like to do.** For example, you might say, "I'm happy to do the laundry, Mrs. Green, but are there parts of this task you would like to do, or that you would like us to do together?"

2. **Accept and encourage client interest in taking part.** If necessary, break the task into manageable components that the client can perform. If the client requires a great deal of time to complete a component of an activity, consider starting that part earlier. Your client can then work on that component as you do other things. For example, a client may be able to (and interested in) dressing herself or himself if you lay the clothing out in the order it will be put on.

3. **Recognize that a client "complaint" about how something is done may simply indicate the client's interest in being involved.** If your client says something like "That's not how I would do it," or "Why would you do it that way?" don't become defensive. Take a few minutes to ask the client how he or she would do it. You may be able to use your client's technique. You may also find that the client's approach is easier and quicker. At the very least, your client will feel that you have taken his or her needs into account.

4. **Recognize that, for some clients, observation is participation.** Your client may benefit greatly from watching you do a particular activity. Encourage the client to talk with you (if possible) as you complete the activity.

5. **Modify your approach to take into account your client's "good" and "bad" days.** Your client's level of participation may change in light of many factors: stress, health

conditions, and the number of other things going on at once. If your client is not up to a task she or he customarily enjoys, be prepared to adapt your approach to accommodate the tasks.

6. **Support and encourage your client's efforts.** Your client may not perform a task perfectly, but you must support and encourage his or her efforts. Be aware that the performance of the task may be more important to the client than the actual degree of perfection.

WHEN YOUR CLIENT'S NEEDS OR REQUESTS EXCEED THE BOUNDS OF YOUR ROLE

Occasionally, a client will have needs or requests for support that you cannot fulfill. This may be because the request exceeds the bounds of your role or because you are not trained to perform the specific task. Your agency may not allow you to perform tasks that you have not been trained to do.

If your client does make such a request, explain the situation to the client. Many times, clients are not aware of the boundaries of your work. They will understand if you tell them why you cannot fulfill their request.

If you cannot resolve the situation with the client, speak to your supervisor. Your supervisor will work with the client to resolve the issue.

Questions for Review

1. How does the World Health Organization define health? According to this definition, would you describe yourself as healthy?

2. What is an impairment? How does it differ from a disability or a handicap?

3. How are habilitation and rehabilitation different?

4. Why should you attempt to involve the client in his or her support?

5. What are the levels of involvement the client may have in his or her support?

Questions for Discussion

1. Consider the definitions of impairment and disability. Do you have an impairment? If so, in what ways (if at all) does it limit your ability? Do you consider yourself to be a disabled person? Why or why not?

2. Mrs. Smith asks you to take her to the grocery store in her car. Your agency does not allow you to do this. What do you do?

3. How would you apply the concept of a holistic approach to the fundamental concepts discussed in this chapter?

4. When might it be a good idea to do something for a client that the client is able to do for himself or herself? When might it be a bad idea?

Chapter 15

Working in the Client's Home

Learning Objectives

Through reading this chapter, you'll be able to

1. Describe a client's home.
2. Identify three common needs that can be affected by having support services in the home.
3. Outline the importance of home management in terms of client safety, comfort, and well-being.
4. List three benefits that can result from involving the client in the management of his or her home.
5. Discuss six ways that you can assist your client to maintain a sense of home.
6. Identify the appropriate procedures for common household tasks.
7. Describe the common precautions to be taken when shopping or banking for a client.
8. Discuss specific considerations when helping the client who lives in a long-term care facility.

Chapter at a Glance

- The Client's Home
- The Purposes of Home Management: Safety, Comfort, and Well-Being
- When Support Services Are Provided in the Client's Home
- Performing Household Tasks Effectively and Safely
- Caring for the Client's Clothing
- Shopping and Banking
- The Client in the Long-Term Care Facility

Terms You'll Use

Biodegradable A material that is easily broken down into chemicals that do not harm the environment.

Home Management The process of taking care of the client's home.

Laundry Symbols Symbols that indicate the type of care a garment should receive.

Sense of Home The feeling that a person has about where he or she lives.

THE CLIENT'S HOME

STOP AND REFLECT ((15-1))

How would you describe your home? How does your home provide you with a comfortable place to live?

_____

_____

_____

_____

Are there things about your home (such as what it looks like, specific possessions, where it is located) that provide you specific comfort?

_____

_____

_____

_____

Have you ever heard the phrase "A man's home is his castle"? We all need a place where we can feel safe, at ease, and in our own domain. We look forward to having a place where we can relax and get away from the pressures that face us.

STOP AND REFLECT ((15-2))

Recall a particularly hectic day you have had. Did you look forward to going home?

_____

_____

_____

If you did look forward to going home, why did you?

_____

_____

_____

If you did not look forward to going home, why not?

_____

_____

_____

Did you find that your home took on a special significance when you had a hectic day? If so, you may have some idea of how important home can be. In Chapter 7, we discussed the needs for territoriality, privacy, and control. Homes have traditionally been the site of family events, a place where we feel that we belong, where we have a sense of familiarity. We often look to our home as a setting in which we can meet these needs.

CASE EXAMPLE 15-1

Ada helps Mrs. Stein. Usually, she helps with personal care and Mrs. Stein's laundry. However, in the spring, Ada helps Mrs. Stein prepare for the Jewish Passover. Mrs. Stein is no longer able to make all the preparations herself and now goes to her son's home for the Seder (dinner on the first night of Passover). However, she does observe some rituals, such as removing all leavening and leavened bread from her kitchen. She also wants to put away her "regular" dishes, utensils, and pans and bring out special ones kept just for Passover. Although this is not Ada's usual role, she understands the importance of these tasks to Mrs. Stein and performs these tasks for her.

As you can see, these household tasks contribute to the client's well-being, as they allow her to maintain religious practices and traditions. Even though Mrs. Stein no longer makes all the preparations she once did, the preparations Ada helps her to do are very important.

In what ways do your traditions affect how you maintain your home? Perhaps you use special dishes or make certain meals for certain celebrations. You might decorate your home or have family or friends over. Have you ever had to change your traditions? How did this make you feel?

In a very real sense, a home is more than the building itself. Whether the home is a house, an apartment, or a room in a long-term care facility, it has special significance to the client.

SPOTLIGHT 15-1 A SPECIAL SIGNIFICANCE OF HOME

It's likely that many of your clients will have taken great pride in keeping their homes. You may have clients who were homemakers (and possibly mothers) all their lives.

They may well have very strong feelings about how a home should be kept. They may also have strong feelings about not being able to keep up their homes as they once did.

THE PURPOSES OF HOME MANAGEMENT: SAFETY, COMFORT, AND WELL-BEING

The purpose of *home management* is determined with the client when the service is planned. For clients receiving community services, this information may be listed in the referral information you receive. This information may not always be identified when a client moves into a long-term care facility. In these cases, you may be able to identify some things that are important by talking with the client or with the client's family.

In general, **home management** meets three purposes: client safety, comfort, and well-being.

■ *Client safety* is attained through the management of pathogens and pests, proper cleaning and storage of foodstuffs, and the prevention of falls.
■ *Client comfort* is attained through many tasks, such as providing clean and wrinkle-free clothing, towels, and linen; maintaining a dust-free environment; or by having clean floors.
■ *Client well-being* is attained through the satisfaction of having a clean and neat environment.

Be aware that there may be other purposes as well. For example, a client who is recovering from a stroke may want you to assist him or her in relearning certain household tasks, such as making a bed.

As a support worker, you must always remember that the household tasks you perform for a client may be as important to the client as any personal care you provide. In fact, these tasks can contribute greatly to your client's well-being.

SPOTLIGHT 15-2 JUST A HOMEMAKER

Why don't we value homemaking? Perhaps you've heard a client say, "I was just a homemaker." Perhaps you've heard a friend say, "I don't work, I stay home with my children." You might even have heard a colleague say, "I am a support worker, I'm not cleaning someone's kitchen."

A clean, safe, and comfortable environment is essential to all of us. Yet, many people don't seem to value homemaking, or value it as much as other tasks. Why do you think this is? How might you respond when you hear comments like the ones in this passage?

STOP AND REFLECT 15-3

Have you ever had someone visit you for a long period of time? If so, did you find that you began to crave a bit of privacy even though you enjoyed the person's visit?

_____

If that person tried to help out with the household chores, did you find that he or she did things differently than you would do them? Did you have mixed feelings about the help—for example, grateful but a little frustrated that he or she did things differently?

_____
_____
_____
_____

How a support worker might assist the client in meeting these purposes and maintaining a sense of home will vary according to where the client lives. In the next section, we'll discuss the support worker's role when the client lives in the community. The following section will discuss the role of the support worker when the client lives in a long-term care facility.

WHEN SUPPORT SERVICES ARE PROVIDED IN THE CLIENT'S HOME

If you found yourself answering the preceding questions with something like, "I really like her, but we just do things differently," you have experienced some interference with your control over your domain. If you have had the help of support workers (perhaps when you were recovering from an illness), you probably experienced loss of your privacy as well.

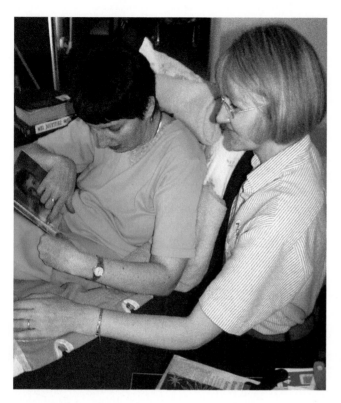

Clients who receive the help of support workers experience many significant changes in how they live in their homes. Support workers may perform tasks the client once enjoyed and took pride in doing "just so." Support workers may be handling items that have particular significance to the client, yet the client may not feel that he or she can tell the worker about the item's importance (Photo 15-1). The client who receives help frequently may feel a loss of privacy and control.

Helping the Client to Maintain a Sense of Home

As a support worker, you will often be the person who is with the client most frequently. You can do a great deal to help the client maintain a sense of home, no matter where that home may be. A **sense of home** is the feeling that a person has about where they live. Make use of these six techniques when assisting your client:

Photo 15-1
A client's possessions are important and must be respected. Handle them gently to prevent damage.
Source: CHATS

1. **Always work in a manner that shows that you know you are a guest in the client's home.** Keep to the tasks you are assigned to do. Do not assume that you should be involved in any of your client's affairs beyond those tasks.
2. **Be aware that people differ in their standards for cleanliness.** One client may thrive in a somewhat disorganized or cluttered environment. Another may require a very organized and clean environment in order to attain a sense of comfort and well-being. You will have to adapt your approach to take into account the client's standards. Speak with your supervisor if you are concerned that a client's safety is at risk due to severe clutter.
3. **Learn your client's preferences and keep them in mind as you assist the client.** Remember that the client may well have done the tasks you are now doing. Ask how your client prefers you to do these tasks. As far as possible, try to follow the client's preferences.
4. **Support your client's control over things that happen in his or her home.** A client may not be able to perform all of a certain task but may want to and be able to perform some of it. Work with the client to find out what the client prefers to do. For example, a client who is very particular about how precious figurines are displayed may be able to return them to their proper spot after you dust.
5. **Realize that items need not be of obvious value to be significant to the client.** Many items have sentimental value. Treat all client items as though they are significant.
6. **Always respect the client's territory.** We all need personal space. (For example, you probably have a favourite room or space in your home that is "your" space.) Respect the client's preferences about what areas of the home you may enter and what you may do in those areas.

The Tasks of Home Management

STOP AND REFLECT 15-4

Put yourself in this situation.

You have just returned home after a particularly hectic day. You walk into your home to find that your children have left your living room in a mess. Pop cans, potato chip bags, and magazines are all over. A note on the hall table tells you that your children have gone to the recreation complex.

You decide to go to the kitchen to make yourself dinner. When you get to the kitchen, you find that there are no clean dishes. The dishwasher is full, yet no one turned it on. You find a microwave meal in the freezer. You pop the package in the microwave, wash a mug, and put the kettle on for tea. You clear a spot at the breakfast table and sit down to have your meal. As you sip your tea, you notice that the floor hasn't been cleaned in some time. There's a spill on the floor under the table and dirty footprints on the floor near the back door.

You decide to take a bath and relax. Once in the bathroom, you find that the tub has not been cleaned and there are no fresh towels.

How would you feel in this scenario? Defeated? Discouraged? Out of sorts? Angry? Most of us would not be happy. In general, all of us are happier when our surroundings are clean and neat.

As we said earlier, the tasks of home management may be as important to the client as any support that you may provide. Assigned tasks such as dusting, cleaning, and doing the laundry are not "add-ons" to the client's support—they form an essential *part* of the client's support (Photo 15-2).

Photo 15-2
Caring for a client's clothing, towels, and linens is often a part of support.
Source: Leisureworld Inc.

PERFORMING HOUSEHOLD TASKS EFFECTIVELY AND SAFELY

There are six principles to remember when cleaning any area:

- Work from top to bottom.
- Work from far to near.
- Work from cleanest to dirtiest.
- Put clean items in clean areas; put dirty items in dirty areas.
- Change cleaning solutions, rinse water, and cloths before they become dirty to avoid spreading dirt and microorganisms.
- Unless instructed to do otherwise, rinse all washed surfaces.

Working in this manner helps to avoid contaminating a clean area. For example, if you are wiping down a refrigerator door, starting at the top and working your way down allows the dirty water to run down over dirty areas.

Similarly, if you are mopping a floor, you would start from the corner farthest from the entrance to the room and work toward the entrance. This avoids having to track over the freshly cleaned areas to clean the rest of the floor.

There are three major exceptions to the principle of working from cleanest to dirtiest. You should:

1. Blot or mop up large spills before cleaning any area.
2. Treat first any dirt that has the potential to stain.
3. Spot-clean an area first when you know the area will require a second cleaning.

The Supplies You'll Need

Most clients will have the necessary cleaning equipment and supplies for the cleaning they need to have done. At a minimum, the client should have a broom and dustpan, clean water, cleaners, clean rags, a mop, a pail, and a brush. Speak with the client or your supervisor if the client does not have the necessary equipment.

Most clients have preferences for the cleaning products they use. Many clients prefer to use environmentally friendly cleaners when possible. Do not ask your client to use a cleaner you prefer. Speak with your supervisor if the client uses cleaners that you feel are unsafe.

Using Cleaning Products Safely

You may hear of environmentally friendly cleaners. There are generally two types of these cleaners: those that are formulated by a manufacturer to be **biodegradable** (easily broken down into chemicals that do not harm the environment) and those that are made from common household chemicals. Remember that some common household chemicals can become hazardous when combined. For example, mixing vinegar and baking soda can cause foaming. If you mix these substances in a jar with a lid, the jar may explode. Mixing bleach and ammonia can produce a poisonous gas. Always use caution when combining chemicals, even if the instructions come from a known and reputable source.

Even the safest chemical can be harmful if used improperly. Be sure to observe the following guidelines:

1. Always read the directions for use on the product label. Follow the instructions, paying particular attention to the amount to be used. Note any hazard labels and follow the precautions listed.
2. Do not mix chemicals unless you have been instructed to do so by someone who is knowledgeable. Improper mixing of chemicals can produce toxic gases or cause damage to surfaces.
3. Always check with a knowledgeable person before using a strong or abrasive cleaner on a surface to make sure that the chemical will not harm it.
4. Do not leave cleaners on any surface for a long period of time as this can cause discolouration, etching, or other damage.
5. Use caution when scrubbing a surface. Excessive rubbing or pressure can mar the finish.
6. Do not use products in unlabelled containers. If you must use a container to store a cleaner, make sure to use a clean container and clearly mark the contents on the container with permanent marker.
7. Store all cleaning products according to the manufacturer's directions. Ensure that all products are kept out of the reach of children and pets.

Care of Cleaning Equipment

You cannot clean properly if your equipment is not clean. Before you start any cleaning job, make sure that you have a clean mop, dustmop, broom, pail, sponge, and cloths. Keep your equipment clean by doing the following:

1. Shake your dustcloth and dustmop frequently to remove accumulated dust. To avoid spreading dust in the client's home, shake the cloth or mop outside. If you cannot get outside to shake the equipment, shake it out an open window.
2. Wash cleaning cloths and dustcloths after each use. Wash mop heads and dustmop heads as required. Do not put these items in the washer or dryer if you have used them with a flammable solvent because fire can result.
3. Change wash water before it becomes dirty. If necessary, wash out the pail.
4. Store equipment properly after use.

Operating Electrical Equipment Safely

It's likely that your client will have a vacuum cleaner or other electrical cleaning equipment. When you use electrical equipment, you must be careful to:

1. Ask for help if you are unsure how to use a particular piece of equipment. Read the instruction manual (if available) to learn how to use the equipment.
2. Check the equipment for frayed cords and loose parts. Do not use equipment that has a frayed cord or that works only when the cord is in a certain position. Unplug any equipment that gives you a shock when you operate it or that causes a fuse to blow (or a circuit breaker to trip) when it is operated.
3. Do not operate electrical equipment with wet or damp hands or when standing in a wet or damp spot.
4. Do not use a vacuum to pick up any liquids unless the vacuum is a "wet-dry" vacuum. Even "wet-dry" vacuums must have special preparation to be used to pick up liquids.
5. Do not use objects such as a screwdriver or knife to attempt to clear a jam in any appliance.
6. Unplug any appliance before you disassemble any part of it, such as replacing the vacuum cleaner bag or opening the crumb door on the bottom of a toaster.
7. Unplug any appliance before you wipe it off. Use a damp cloth to wipe off the equipment. Never place electrical equipment in water or any other liquid.

General Cleaning Procedures

General cleaning includes dusting; spot-cleaning; washing dishes; washing counters, bathroom fixtures, and other surfaces; emptying garbage; and cleaning floors. Your specific assignment may include cleaning kitchen appliances or washing windows. In general, you should dust, empty garbage, spot-clean, wash surfaces, and then wash floors. Always observe the principles of infection control when cleaning.

Dusting

Use a clean, lint-free cloth or duster when dusting. If possible, spray the cloth with a commercial dusting spray or mist the cloth lightly with water to trap and hold dust.

Turn the cloth frequently so that you are using a clean part of the cloth to dust. If you are using a duster, make sure not to move the duster too quickly as that can spread the dust.

Some clients may have specially treated cloths to use for dusting. Be sure to follow the instructions for caring for these cloths.

Dust can aggravate a client's allergies. You may have to dust more frequently or use a vacuum cleaner to pick up dust.

Spot-Cleaning

Blot up excess liquid and matter before attempting to clean the spot (Photo 15-3). Use a butter knife to scrape off excess sticky or dried material if this will not damage the underlying surface. An ice cube can harden some sticky materials and make them easier to remove.

Once all excess material has been removed, apply the appropriate cleaning solution to the stain. Follow the directions for applying the solution. You may need to leave the solution on the spot for a few moments.

Avoid scrubbing the spot, as this may mar the surface or alter its colour. Gently blot the spot, or carefully rub the spot, working from the outside of the spot to its centre. Some spots will require a second application of cleaner. Once the spot is gone, allow the surface to dry. Use caution when using heat to dry an article with a stain. Heat can set stains, making them very hard to remove. If you cannot remove the stain, or are concerned that you will damage the surface, consult your client or your supervisor.

Photo 15-3
Blotting a spill helps to prevent the spread of the material and makes cleanup easier.

Washing Dishes and Other Small Washable Objects

Hand Washing

Use dish detergent to wash dishes and small washable objects. Wear rubber gloves to protect your hands. Use moderately hot soapy water to wash items and moderately hot clean water to rinse items. Wash the least dirty items first.

If possible, place the items on a dish rack to air-dry. Be sure to use a tray under the dish rack to collect the water running off the items. If it is not possible to air-dry items, use a clean tea towel to dry them before storing. Damp or hot dishes can mar wooden shelves.

Using the Dishwasher

Load the dishwasher so that dishes do not touch one another. Make sure that all items placed in the dishwasher are dishwasher safe. Scrape excess food off plates before placing in the dishwasher. Rinse the dishes off before placing in the dishwasher if your client prefers or the dishwasher's operating guide advises you to do so.

If possible, run the dishwasher only when full to save water and energy. Use the recommended amount of dishwasher detergent. Never use *dishwashing* detergent as it will foam excessively.

Unless you are instructed to do otherwise, never place anything but dishes, cutlery, and glasses in the dishwasher.

Washing Kitchen Counters and Other Surfaces

Remove all items from the counter or the surface before you wash it. Place these items in a safe area. If you must set them on an area that has been cleaned, make sure to wipe the items off first.

Wash the counter or surface, starting with the area furthest from you. Work from farthest to closest until the counter is cleaned. Let the counter air-dry or wipe dry with a clean cloth before replacing the items. Clean and dry off all items before replacing.

Cleaning Bathroom Fixtures and Surfaces

Many newer homes have bathroom fixtures made of acrylic. These fixtures can easily be scratched by the use of scouring powders or abrasive pads. Use a bathroom cleaner designed for use on acrylic surfaces, following the directions carefully. As an alternative, you can use laundry detergent on a cloth. No matter what cleaner you use, rinse the surfaces well.

Clean the toilet with a brush or cloth used *only* for that purpose. Wipe down the tank and outside of the bowl. Raise the seat and clean the rim of the bowl. Clean the bottom of the seat. Use a separate cloth to wipe down the top of the seat.

Use a toilet bowl cleaner to clean the bowl. Follow the directions carefully. Brush down the sides of the bowl with a brush. Be sure to brush under the rim. Flush the toilet to remove the solution. Rinse the brush in the flushing water. Hang the brush to dry.

Emptying Garbage

If possible, empty dry garbage (such as that found in bedrooms or living rooms) first. Empty wet or messy garbage last. Use plastic garbage bags for this purpose if the client uses them. If the client uses garbage cans, empty the garbage into the can.

If possible, line garbage pails or wastebaskets with the appropriately sized plastic bag. Empty the garbage by removing the bag and placing it with the garbage.

Make sure that the garbage bag is tied or the can lid is securely attached when you are done. Garbage can attract insects and animals. Some clients have containers to keep bags of garbage or garbage cans secured. If your client has one of these containers, make sure to use it. If animals getting into the garbage is a problem and the client does not have a container, try pouring 125 mL (1/2 cup) of ammonia into the can or bag. This smell will discourage many rodents and animals from chewing through the garbage.

Cleaning Floors

High-traffic areas (halls, entrances, and frequently used rooms) must be swept or vacuumed regularly to keep dust, dirt, and other particles from accumulating. Some clients will have a vacuum that is suitable for use on noncarpeted floors. If so, be sure to use the correct nozzle. Always sweep a floor before you wash it.

Wash floors with the proper cleaner, prepared according to the instructions on the label. Some "no-wax" floors require a special cleaner. Wood floors usually require a special cleaner. Make sure you have the proper cleaner before you start. Wring out the mop each time you dip it into the pail so that you do not put too much water on the floor. Be aware that too much water can loosen tiles or ruin a wood finish.

Discuss with your supervisor before performing heavy cleaning tasks such as stripping wax from floors or cleaning carpets.

Cleaning Appliances

You should always wipe up spills in the refrigerator or on the surface of the stove. This helps to keep the appliance free from microorganisms and helps to keep other items from becoming dirty.

Remember that your assigned duties may also include cleaning the client's refrigerator or stove. Speak with your supervisor if your client asks that you perform these tasks.

Refrigerator

Cleaning a refrigerator does not usually require special cleaners. Working from the top, remove items from the fridge one shelf at a time. Remove the shelf (if possible) and wash and dry it. Be careful not to use very hot water to wash a glass shelf as it may cause it to crack. Wipe down the sides of the interior and replace the shelf.

Wipe off containers with a clean damp cloth and replace on the shelf. Take a moment to organize the items if possible. Ask your client about disposing of stale or old items. Repeat this procedure until all shelves are done. Clean the door bins in the same manner. When you have finished, wipe off the outside of the appliance.

Stove

There are many types of stoves and stove surfaces. Using a damp cloth to clean a surface (such as when you are wiping up a spill) is usually safe. It's usually safe to remove the drip pans (the removable metal plates below each burner) for cleaning. Do not line drip pans with aluminum foil as this may cause the burner to overheat. Some clients have a glass or ceramic cook top that has burners below the surface that cannot be removed. The glass or ceramic surface may easily scratch. Ask for direction as to how to properly clean this type of cook top.

Cleaning the oven may require cleaners specifically formulated for the client's stove. Do not attempt to clean an oven unless you are certain that you have the proper cleaner and know how to use it.

CARING FOR THE CLIENT'S CLOTHING

STOP AND REFLECT ((15-5))

Do you have a favourite piece of clothing? What makes it your favourite?

_____

_____

Do you have clothes you wear specifically for certain occasions? Perhaps you have a specific outfit that makes you feel particularly good. Are you fussy about how these clothes are cared for?

_____

_____

Have you ever had someone do your laundry improperly? How did you feel when your clothes were not washed properly?

_____

_____

Chances are that you are particular about your clothes. You might have specific outfits you wear only for certain occasions, or articles of clothing that are only worn with other articles. You might have specific ways of caring for your clothing. Most of us see our clothes as a way of expressing who we are. How our clothing looks (and thus makes us look) is important to us.

It's very likely that your client has preferences as to how his or her clothing is cared for. It's also very likely you will have to do your client's laundry. A few moments taken to properly care for your client's laundry will avoid damage to clothing and make the laundry tasks much easier.

Canada has implemented laundry symbols that indicate the type of care a garment should receive. These symbols cover washing, bleaching, drying, ironing, and dry-cleaning, and use the colours of the traffic lights (red, amber, and green) to indicate how you should proceed. Figure 15-1 presents these symbols in black and white and gives their meaning.

General Laundry Procedures

Use the following guidelines to clean washable clothing safely.

Preparing Items for Washing

1. **Sort clothing by colour, fabric type, and washing requirements.** Group loads into similar colours, weights, and washing requirements. Avoid washing clothing that is heavily soiled with clothing that is lightly soiled, even if they are the same colour, type, and have the same washing requirements.
2. **Close zippers, button buttons, and snap up snaps before washing.**
3. **Empty pockets and repair small splits in seams or tears.** If you cannot easily repair the garment, advise your client.

Washing Items

1. **Do not wash items that have been soaked in or spotted with gasoline or other flammable liquids.** Such items can ignite in the washer.
2. **Follow the manufacturer's instructions for loading the washer. Load articles loosely.** In general, top-loading washers may be filled to the top of the agitator. Make sure to place clothing evenly around the drum so as to keep it balanced. Front-loading washers should be loaded so that the drum is no more than half full.
3. **Adjust the water level to the amount of laundry to be washed.** Articles should have enough water to move about without rising above the water line.
4. **Adjust the water temperature appropriately to the clothing being washed.** Make sure that the detergent you use is appropriate for the water temperature.
5. **Use the appropriate washer cycle.** Special wash cycles (such as permanent press) have been developed to best care for specific types of items.
6. **Never pour detergent or fabric softener directly on clothing.** This can cause spotting and colour changes. If the washer has no detergent dispenser, fill the washer with water, add the proper amount of detergent, and then load the clothing.
7. **Remove clothes from the washer as soon as possible after the cycle finishes.** Clothes left in the washer too long will develop a musty odour and wrinkles. If this happens, the items must be washed again.

Laundry Symbols

Washing

 Wash in commercial machine in water not exceeding 95°C, at normal setting.

 Wash in commercial machine in water not exceeding 95°C, at permanent press setting.

 Wash in domestic or commercial machine in water not exceeding 70°C, at normal setting.

 Wash in domestic or commercial machine in water not exceeding 60°C, at normal setting.

 Wash in domestic or commercial machine in water not exceeding 60°C, at permanent press setting.

 Wash in domestic or commercial machine in water not exceeding 50°C, at normal setting.

 Wash in domestic or commercial machine in water not exceeding 50°C, at permanent press setting.

 Wash in domestic or commercial machine in water not exceeding 50°C, at delicate/gentle setting.

 Wash in domestic or commercial machine in water not exceeding 40°C, at normal setting.

 Wash in domestic or commercial machine in water not exceeding 40°C, at permanent press setting.

 Wash in domestic or commercial machine in water not exceeding 40°C, at delicate/gentle setting.

 Wash in domestic or commercial machine in water not exceeding 40°C, at normal setting.

 Wash in domestic or commercial machine in water not exceeding 30°C, at permanent press setting.

 Wash in domestic or commercial machine in water not exceeding 30°C, at delicate/gentle setting.

 Wash gently by hand in water not exceeding 40°C.

 Wash gently by hand in water not exceeding 30°C.

 Wash in domestic or commercial machine at any temperature, at normal setting.

 Do not wash.

Bleaching

Use any bleach when needed

Use only non-chlorine bleach when needed.

Do not bleach.

Professional Textile Care

(P) Dry-clean, normal cycle. Any solvent except trichloroethylene.

(F) Dry-clean, normal cycle. Petroleum solvent only.

Do not dry-clean.

Drying

 Tumble dry at high heat (not exceeding 75°C) at normal setting.

 Tumble dry at medium heat (not exceeding 65°C) at normal setting.

 Tumble dry at medium heat (not exceeding 65°C) at permanent press setting.

 Tumble dry at low heat (not exceeding 55°C) at permanent press setting.

 Tumble dry at low heat (not exceeding 55°C) at delicate cycle.

 Tumble dry any heat.

 Tumble dry no heat/air dry.

 Do not tumble dry.

 After extraction of excess water, line dry/hang to dry.

 Hang up the soaking wet article to "drip" dry.

 After extraction of excess water, dry the article on a suitable flat surface.

 Dry in the shade (symbol added to line dry, drip dry, or dry flat).

 Do not dry. To be used with "Do not wash" symbol.

Ironing/Pressing

 Iron with or without steam by hand, or press on commercial equipment, at a high temperature (not exceeding 200°C). Recommended temperature for cotton and linen textiles.

 Iron with or without steam by hand, or press on commercial equipment, at a medium temperature (not exceeding 150°C). Recommended temperature for polyester, rayon, silk, triacetate and wool textiles.

 Iron with or without steam by hand, or press on commercial equipment, at a low temperature (not exceeding 110°C). Recommended temperature for acetate, acrylic, modacrylic, nylon, polypropylene and spandex textiles.

 Do not steam.

 Do not iron or press.

Dots for Defining Water Temperature

⠿	95°C (near boil)	•••	50°C (hot)
⠿	70°C (extremely hot)	••	40°C (warm)
⠿	60°C (very hot)	•	30°C (cool)

Supplementary Care

 Do not wring.

 Wet-clean.

 Do not wet-clean.

FIGURE 15-1

Laundry care symbols

Source: Canadian General Standards Board, 2008, CAN/CGSB-86. 1-2003.

Drying

1. **Avoid drying articles with fresh stains that have not been completely removed.** The heat from the dryer can set these stains and make them impossible to remove.
2. **Don't overload the dryer.** This can cause wrinkling and heat damage to clothing.
3. **Use the cycle most appropriate for the load.** Use the shortest time possible to dry the items to avoid possible damage and wrinkling.
4. **Remove items from the dryer as soon as they are dry.**
5. **Empty the lint trap after each load.** If you cannot find the lint trap, ask for help. Lint build-up can cause a fire.
6. **Never dry foam rubber, rubberized items, or any items that have been soaked in gasoline or other flammable liquids.** These can ignite and cause a fire.

SHOPPING AND BANKING

You may be asked to shop or do banking for a client. Most agencies have specific procedures to follow when these tasks are done. These procedures usually govern the amount of the client's money you may handle and how you must account for the purchases you are asked to make or the banking you are asked to do. Realize that these procedures are in place for the protection of both you and your client. Always follow the procedure established by your agency, no matter how well you know your client.

THE CLIENT IN THE LONG-TERM CARE FACILITY

A client who lives in a long-term care facility often experiences a very strong sense of loss of control. The move to the facility usually means many changes—in surroundings, in the number and type of possessions, and in routine. If the client shares a room with another person, the client may experience a very real sense of loss of privacy.

It's likely that the facility's housekeeping department will be responsible for most cleaning of client rooms. However, you, as a support worker, can do much to ensure that your client's personal space is respected.

You must always be aware that the client's room is his or her home. It is the only personal space the client has in the setting. Treat the client's space as his or her home by adhering to the following guidelines:

1. **Help the client to have a sense of personal space by respecting the person's territory.** Knock before you enter a client's room, or ask before you approach the client's area in a shared room. Avoid walking through a client's personal area unnecessarily.
2. **Respect the client's possessions.** It's likely that the client has brought his or her most cherished items to the facility. Thus, each may have special significance. Be careful when you must move the client's items. Don't set extra laundry or other items down on a client's bed or furniture.
3. **Encourage the client to do what he or she can and wants to do to maintain personal space.** For example, a client might be able to make his or her bed or put away some of his or her clothes. Encourage the client to do tasks that give the client satisfaction, even though the result may not be perfect.

4. **Encourage the client (or the client's family, if the client is unable) to bring permissible items that help the client to feel at home.** Remember that some things, such as electrical appliances, must be approved before the client can use them.

5. **If you are assigned to tidy the client's bedside table or cabinet, remember to place items where the client can easily find them.**

Questions for Review

1. How might a client's need for privacy, territoriality, and control be affected by having support services in his or her home?

2. Why is home management important to a client's sense of well-being?

3. What are six ways that you can assist your client to maintain a sense of home?

4. You must clean your client's kitchen counter. On this counter, there is a coffee maker, a set of canisters, a blender, this morning's dirty breakfast dishes, and a plant. A large jar of grape jam has been spilled on the counter. Apply the six principles of cleaning an area to this task.

5. What seven guidelines should you follow when using cleaning products?

6. What seven guidelines should you follow when operating electrical equipment?

7. You have a sweater that can be washed in warm water (below 50°C) on a gentle cycle. What does the laundry symbol for this type of care look like?

8. Why shouldn't you pour detergent or fabric softener directly on clothes?

9. What five things can you do to show a long-term care facility resident that you respect his or her home?

Questions for Discussion

1. Some people don't feel that household tasks are as important as personal care tasks. They feel that support workers should not have to do these tasks. How do you feel? Why do you feel this way? If you were a client, how might you feel?

2. Your client, Mrs. Berg, has always been particular about how household tasks are done. You have been assigned to assist her with household tasks. As you plan your work with her, you find that Mrs. Berg's expectations of how you are to dust and do laundry are very high. For example, Mrs. Berg wants each figurine on her shelves washed and dried by hand each week. She also asks that you wash her clothing by hand. If you follow all of her requests, you will not have time to do all your assigned tasks. When you discuss this with your supervisor, she asks that you try to work out something with the client. How do you attempt to resolve this situation with Mrs. Berg?

3. Imagine that you were moving into a long-term care facility. What possessions would you like to have with you? How do you think you would feel about sharing your room with other people? How would you feel about having staff members in your room?

4. What are some of your traditions that involve making special preparations in your home, such as having a family dinner at holidays, etc.? If you had a broken leg, how might these traditions be affected? What help might you need to prepare your home?

Chapter 16

Meal Planning, Preparation, and Assistance

Learning Objectives

Through reading this chapter, you'll be able to

1. List the five reasons we need to eat a balanced diet.
2. Explain *Canada's Food Guide* and give examples of balanced meal plans.
3. Describe changes in nutritional needs across the life span.
4. Outline the components of common special diets.
5. Describe four ways of making meals more appealing to clients.
6. Identify the steps to take when planning a menu with a client.
7. Discuss the factors to consider when shopping for food for a client.
8. Describe safe food practices.
9. Explain the twelve principles and proper techniques you should follow when assisting a client to eat.
10. Describe swallowing problems and list six steps that can minimize the risk of a swallowing problem.

Chapter at a Glance

- Food and Nutrition
- *Canada's Food Guide*—2007 Version
- Nutritional Needs across the Life Span
- Client Preferences
- Special Diets
- Planning Meals
- Making Meals Appealing to Clients
- Safe Food Practices
- Assisting the Client with Eating
- Choking

Terms You'll Use

Canada's Food Guide A guide that is based on nutritional needs and provides an easy way to ensure that people obtain the nutrients required to build and maintain a healthy body. *Canada's Food Guide* was revised in 2007.

Carbohydrates Substances formed of starches and sugars that provide energy.

Fat The substance that allows fat-soluble vitamins to be used by the body. Fat forms adipose tissue in the body and serves as an energy reserve.

Minerals Inorganic materials that the body requires.

Nutrients Vitamins, minerals, proteins, fats, carbohydrates, and water that your body needs to be healthy.

Protein The substance essential for growth and tissue repair.

Vitamins Organic compounds that provide elements that the body needs to function.

FOOD AND NUTRITION

Food provides the nutrients (vitamins, minerals, proteins, fats, carbohydrates, and water) your body needs to become and remain healthy. These nutrients give the body energy, help to maintain strong bones and build muscle, help the body to repair and grow new cells, and help to fight off infections and disease. Each nutrient has a unique purpose. Table 16-1 identifies the recommended ranges of carbohydrates, proteins, and fats for various age groups. Table 16-2 identifies the function and common sources of these nutrients.

TABLE 16-1	Nutirent Ranges For Various Age Groups		
Age group	Percentage of total calories from		
	carbohydrate	protein	fat
1–3 years	45–65%	5–20%	30–40%
4–18 years	45–65%	10–30%	25–35%
19 years and over	45–65%	10–35%	20–35%

Source: http://www.hc-sc.gc.ca/fn-an/pubs/res-educat/res-educat_2_e.html, accessed 2007 Vitamins

Vitamins

Vitamins are organic compounds that provide elements that the body needs to function. Our bodies manufacture some vitamins but usually cannot manufacture them in large enough amounts to meet our needs. The bulk of vitamins must come from food. It's important to note that many of the body's functions require several vitamins at the

TABLE 16-2	Common Nutrients, Their Functions, and Common Sources	
Nutrient	**Function**	**Common Sources**
Water	Helps water-soluble vitamins to be absorbed by the body. Brings nutrients to cells and carries away waste products. Regulates body temperature.	Drinking water, beverages, and fruits are common sources. Almost all foods (except fats and sugars) contain some water.
Protein	Essential for growth and tissue repair.	Complete proteins (come from animal sources): meat, fish, eggs, cheese, poultry, and milk Incomplete proteins (come from plant sources): soybeans, nuts, grains, beans, peas, and other legumes
Carbohydrates	Provide energy and fuel for the body to generate heat.	Cereal grains and products made from these items (pasta, bread), potatoes, vegetables, and nuts Milk sugars (lactose) found in milk products Fruit sugars (fructose) found in fruits
Fats	Provide fatty acids, which are required for growth. Provide medium for body to use fat-soluble vitamins.	Many foods, even vegetables, contain some amount of fat. Some products are primarily fat: lard, butter, margarine, vegetable oils, many salad dressings.
Minerals		
Calcium	Essential for healthy bones and teeth. Helps to regulate heart action and maintain nervous system.	Milk, milk products (except butter), canned salmon and sardines, and most dark green vegetables
Iodine	Essential for proper thyroid gland function.	Iodized salt, sea-caught fish, some foods grown in iodine-rich soil, and many canned or processed foods
Iron	Essential in forming hemoglobin (the part of blood that carries oxygen to cells).	Meat, organs such as liver and kidney, eggs, potatoes, dark yellow and green vegetables, dried fruits, and whole-grain products
Phosphorus	Essential to proper formation of nerve tissue. With calcium, helps to form strong bones and teeth.	Found in many foods: legumes, whole-wheat products, oat products, meat, fish, poultry, nuts, and cheese

▶▶▏

TABLE 16-2	Common Nutrients, Their Functions, and Common Sources (*continued*)

Nutrient	Function	Common Sources
Vitamins		
A	Essential to eye function, especially night sight. Essential to healthy skin, hair, and mucous membranes. Contributes to some types of infection resistance.	Apricots, cantaloupe, milk, cheese, eggs, organs (liver, kidney), dark green and dark yellow vegetables
B Complex	The B-complex vitamins include four common vitamins: thiamine (B_1), riboflavin (B_2), niacin, and B_{12}. In general, the B complex is essential for the proper functioning of nerves, digestion, oxidization, and metabolism.	Organs (liver, kidney), whole grains, milk, cheese, leafy green vegetables
C	Helps cells to work together. Essential for sound condition of bones, teeth, and gums.	Fresh, raw citrus fruits and vegetables
D	Essential for the body to make proper use of calcium and phosphorus.	Vitamin D–fortified milk, fish-liver oils, eggs, and one non food source: sunshine
E	Helps maintain healthy body cells and muscles. Many claims have been made about vitamin E, but it is only now being studied to determine its actual effects.	Dark leafy vegetables, nuts, seeds, beans, vegetable oils
K	Required for proper clotting of blood	Green leafy vegetables

same time: the function is disrupted when not all of the necessary vitamins are present. There are two types of vitamins: fat-soluble and water-soluble.

Fat-Soluble Vitamins

Fat-soluble vitamins are vitamins A, D, E, and K. They are absorbed with help from fats found in the diet. Fat-soluble vitamins can remain in the body for long periods of time.

Water-Soluble Vitamins

Water-soluble vitamins are vitamin C and the many B vitamins. Water-soluble vitamins cannot be stored in the body for very long. Good sources of these vitamins should be consumed every day.

Minerals

Minerals are inorganic materials that the body requires. Iron and calcium are probably the best-known minerals. However, there are many others: phosphorus, potassium, sodium, iodine, magnesium, zinc, and copper. Some minerals work best in combination with other minerals. For example, calcium and phosphorus work together to form strong bones and teeth. As almost all foods provide some minerals, it is not difficult to obtain the needed amounts of minerals through a balanced diet.

Proteins

Proteins are the body's second most prevalent substance and are essential for growth and tissue repair. Proteins are made up of amino acids. Some foods provide all the amino acids required to produce protein. Other foods do not possess all the amino acids required and must be combined with other foods to provide a complete protein. For example, bread and butter, when eaten separately, do not provide a complete protein. When eaten together, they do provide a complete protein.

Fats

Fat, the substance that allows fat-soluble vitamins to be used by the body, is made up of four different types of fatty acids:

- Polyunsaturated
- Monounsaturated
- Saturated
- Trans

Some fat is essential for a balanced diet because it allows fat-soluble vitamins to be used by the body. The type of fat eaten is very important, however. Some types of fats are much healthier for you than others.

Saturated fats can contribute to excess cholesterol in the body (a condition linked to cardiovascular disease). Trans fats are found naturally in some animal-based foods, but are also formed when liquid oils are made into semi-solid fats such as shortening and hard margarine. Scientific evidence has shown that dietary trans fats can increase the risk of developing heart disease.

Monounsaturated and polyunsaturated fats can actually lower risk of heart disease. Olive oil and canola oil are high in monounsaturates. Polyunsaturated fats contain Omega-3 and Omega-6 essential fatty acids. Our bodies don't create these essential fatty acids, but they are essential to good health. We must get them from our diet. Corn oil, sunflower oil, and soybean oil are rich in Omega-6 essential fatty acids. Canola and soybean oils (and some fish oils) are rich in Omega-3 essential fatty acids.

Carbohydrates

Carbohydrates are formed of starches and sugars and provide energy. Carbohydrates make up most of the diets of people around the world. Be aware that starches and sugars do not provide the same benefit to the body. Starches provide nutrients and are often found in foods that also contain amino acids. Sugars provide no nutrients, only calories.

Water

Water is the most common element in the body. Over half of the human body is water. This water is required by the body to make use of water-soluble vitamins and for the body's chemical reactions to take place.

CANADA'S FOOD GUIDE

While it's possible to develop your own menu plan to include all essential nutrients, it would be time consuming. For this reason, Health Canada has developed *Canada's Food Guide*. Based on nutritional needs, Canada's Food Guide is a summary of the nutrients that people require to build and maintain a healthy body.

The *Guide* groups foods into four categories: grains; vegetables and fruit; milk and milk products; and meats and meat alternatives. Table 16-3 shows sources of common nutrients among the food groups

TABLE 16-3	Some Important Nutrients in the Food Groups			
Key Nutrient	**Vegetables and Fruit**	**Grain Products**	**Milk and Alternatives**	**Meat and Alternatives**
Protein			X	X
Fat			X	X
Carbohydrate	X	X	X	
Fibre	X	X		
Thiamin		X		X
Riboflavin		X	X	X
Niacin		X		X
Folate	X	X		
Vitamin B6	X			X
Vitamin B12			X	X
Vitamin C	X			
Vitamin A	X		X	
Vitamin D			X	
Calcium			X	
Iron		X		X
Zinc		X	X	X
Magnesium	X	X	X	X
Potassium	X	X	X	X

Source: Health Canada

The *Guide* was revised and updated in 2007. Though it still uses the familiar rainbow format (see Figure 16-1), it has been updated to include foods that represent Canada's diverse ethnic makeup. You'll now find recommendations for servings of tofu, soymilk, polenta, couscous, and other foods as well as those found in previous versions.

Specific recommendations for the number of servings are included in the *Guide* and are presented in Table 16-4.

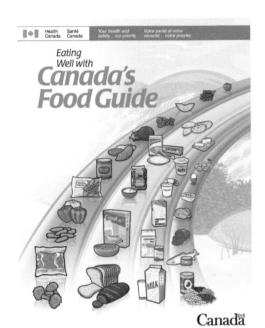

FIGURE 16-1

Canada's food guide to healthy eating

Source: Eating Well with Canada's Food Guide (2007), Health Canada.

TABLE 16-4	Recommended daily servings

Recommended number of Food Guide Servings per day

	Children			Teens		Adults			
	2-3	4-8	9-13	14-18 Years		19-50 Years		51+ Years	
	Girls and Boys			Females	Males	Females	Males	Females	Males
Vegetables and Fruit	4	5	6	7	8	7-8	8-10	7	7
Grain Products	3	4	6	6	7	6-7	8	6	7
Milk and Alternatives	2	2	3-4	3-4	3-4	2	2	3	3
Meat and Alternatives	1	1	1-2	2	3	2	3	2	3

The eating pattern also includes a small amount (30 to 45 mL or about 2 - 3 tablespoons) of unsaturated fat each day.

Source: Eating Well with Canada's Food Guide (2007), Health Canada. Reproduced with the permission of the Minister of Public Works and Government Services Canada, 2007.

Spotlight 16-1 identifies the principles used in the *Food Guide* to help people choose food wisely. As you can see, the *Guide* encourages people to eat whole grains, avoid processed foods, and limit fat, salt, and sugar intake.

SPOTLIGHT 16-1 CHOOSING HEALTHY FOODS

Healthy food choices are easy if you just follow *Canada's Food Guide*'s recommendations.

Remember to:

Eat at least one dark green vegetable and one orange vegetable each day.

Choose vegetables and fruit prepared with little or no added fat, sugar, or salt.

Have vegetables and fruit more often than juice.

Make at least half of your grain products whole grain each day.

Drink skim, 1%, or 2% milk each day. Drink fortified soy beverages if you do not drink milk.

Have meat alternatives such as bean, lentils, and tofu often.

Eat at least two *Food Guide* servings of fish each week.

Select lean meat and alternatives prepared with little or no added fat, sugar, or salt.

Include a small amount of unsaturated fat each day.

Satisfy your thirst with water.

Limit foods and beverages high in calories, fat, sugar, or salt.

Source: Health Canada

STOP AND REFLECT 16-1

Record what you eat each day for a one-week period. Then, compare your daily portions to those recommended by *Canada's Food Guide*, represented in Table 16-4.

How well do you eat?

_____

_____

How easily could you change your habits?

_____

_____

Did you find that your eating habits are in line with the *Guide*'s prescriptions? If not, how easily could you change your eating habits?

NUTRITIONAL NEEDS ACROSS THE LIFE SPAN

Although we generally need the same nutrients all our lives, the amounts we need may change with our age, condition, and size. In Table 16-4, you can see how serving sizes vary by age and gender. In general, older adults usually require fewer calories than they did when they were younger.

Other factors affect nutritional needs and recommended intake. For example:

- A pregnant woman will require more calcium than a woman who is not pregnant.
- A pregnant woman needs more folic acid than one who is not pregnant.
- A person with severe burns may require two to three times the number of calories than does a healthy person of the same age.
- A tall and stocky male will usually require more nutrients and calories than a petite woman.

Your client will have specific needs, based upon his or her age, size, condition, and any medications he or she is taking (Photo 16-1). Some lifestyle choices, such as smoking or use of carbonated beverages, affect how the body absorbs certain nutrients. Finally, peer pressure can affect the food choices some people (especially teenagers) make. You must be prepared to adapt your meal preparation to accommodate these differing needs.

CLIENT PREFERENCES

You likely will find that your client has specific food preferences. These preferences are the result of many things, including religious prescriptions, cultural practices, tradition, taste, appearance, smell preferences, and habit. These preferences are very hard to change, even if we are motivated to do so.

We often prefer certain types of foods in certain circumstances. For example, you might prefer a certain soup when you have a cold. The term *comfort foods* has been used to describe these foods that benefit us emotionally. Sometimes these foods are also nutritious, such as a well-prepared and hearty soup we may eat when we have a cold. Others such as ice cream and cake may be less nutritious, and must be eaten sparingly.

Photo 16-1
If possible, you should plan menus with your client. Here, a support worker and client review a grocery store ad before deciding on the menu and shopping list.
Source: CHATS

You must respect your client's food preferences. You may have to learn how to make new dishes or to use ingredients with which you are unfamiliar. You may prepare familiar foods for the client to eat at times that seem unusual to you (for example, cereal and eggs as an evening meal). Do not force your client to eat meals that he or she does not prefer simply because you are more familiar with their preparation.

You may find that your client does not eat a balanced diet. If so, you must not demand that the client change his or her diet. You might be able to talk with your client about other food choices and perhaps introduce a new food or two. You might find that your client does not eat a particular food because it was too difficult for him or her to prepare. The client may try this food if you are preparing it. With your client's agreement, you might be able to substitute healthier choices for some ingredients (for example, using low-fat milk instead of whole milk).

Eating foods that are healthy and that we like makes it easier to eat well. Recall your answers to Stop and Reflect 16-1 on page 256. How easy would it be for you to change your eating habits? Would you avoid giving up favourite foods and snacks? You'd probably find it easier to slowly change your habits rather than to make many changes all at once.

SPOTLIGHT 16-2 A CUSTOMIZED FOOD GUIDE

Confused about where your favourite foods fit in the new *Food Guide*? Health Canada has introduced a new feature for Canadians wanting to develop their own personal food guide. *My Food Guide* is available on Health Canada's website. It allows you to select foods that you prefer to create a food guide that describes the amounts of each that you require at your age for good nutrition. The guide takes about 10 minutes to complete and can be printed or saved on your computer. You can find it at: http://www.hc-sc.gc.ca/fn-an/food-guide-aliment/myguide-monguide/index_e.html.

However, keep in mind that your client may not wish to change his or her habits. Discuss the issue with your supervisor if attaining a balanced diet is one of the reasons you have been assigned to assist a client and your client does not wish to alter his or her diet.

STOP AND REFLECT ((16-2))

How have your dietary needs and preferences changed over time?

_____

_____

Did you eat differently as a child? As a teen?

_____

_____

What factors influenced these needs and preferences?

_____

_____

Do you have certain foods you customarily eat at certain times?

_____

_____

Do you have certain foods that you prefer when you are ill?

_____

_____

SPOTLIGHT 16-3 TRACK YOUR EATING AND ACTIVITY HABITS

The Dietitians of Canada has launched an interactive website that allows you to keep a daily log of your eating and activity patterns. It then compares your patterns to recommendations in *Canada's Food Guide* and to validated activity recommendations. You can access this internet resource at www.eatracker.ca.

Source: Dietitians of Canada, 2007.

SPECIAL DIETS

Some clients will have a special diet that they follow. There are many types of special diets. Table 16-5 lists some common diets and their purpose. Be aware that your client's specific diet may not be identical to any of the diets listed in Table 16-5. Some clients have a diet that combines two or more of these diets, such as a diabetic and mechanically soft diet.

If your client has a special diet, you must take the time to learn about it and how it affects the food choices and cooking methods.

PLANNING MEALS

Planning meals includes determining preferences, planning combinations for a period of time, determining supplies the client has on hand, and, possibly, shopping for food items. It is very important that you work with your client to determine dietary, cultural,

TABLE 16-5	Common Special Diets			
Diet Type	Characteristics	Purpose	Foods Often Excluded	Foods Often Recommended
Normal or Regular	Well-balanced diet	General purpose (regular diet is often listed on support plans)	None	Full range of items included in *Canada's Food Guide*
Mechanical Soft or Dental Soft	Same range of foods as regular diet, but chopped, diced, or otherwise tenderized to make them easier to eat	Clients with difficulty chewing or swallowing	None	As for regular diet
Low Salt Low Sodium No Added Salt	Limited amount of foods containing sodium; no added salt (e.g., no salt at the table)	Clients with water retention, heart, kidney, or circulatory problems	Canned vegetables, processed meats, dried meats, hot dogs, many "convenience foods"	Fresh vegetables, most meats bought raw and prepared, fruits
Diabetic Sugar-Free	Balance of proteins, fats, and carbohydrates as the client's needs dictate; not just a sugar restriction	To match intake with bodily needs	Sugared foods or beverages	Fresh fruits and vegetables, low-sugar or sugar-free products
High-Protein	Regular diet supplemented with high-protein foods	To assist the body in recovery from illness or injury	None	High-protein foods

or religious requirements, as well as the foods that he or she prefers to eat in a meal. You should use this information, the information in *Canada's Food Guide,* and the hints contained in this section and the section on presentation (later in this chapter) to develop a meal plan for a one- or two-week period.

It is vitally important that your client be involved (if possible) in the planning of the meals, even if only to state preferences. A lovely meal, prepared and served beautifully, is of no use if it contains foods the client will not eat.

Key Considerations in Menu Planning

In addition to requirements and preferences, there are four other items to be considered when planning meals: budget, volume, storage, and brand preferences.

Budget

You must consider a client's budget, even if you are not shopping for a client. You do not want to use up an item in a week when the client cannot afford to replace it for two weeks. Make sure any menu you plan is affordable.

Volume

Purchase amounts that can be used before they spoil. This may vary by the type of storage the client has. A client with ample freezer space may be able to purchase larger amounts of some items that can be frozen for a period of time.

Storage

If you shop for a client, make sure that you have sufficient appropriate storage for the items you purchase.

Brand Preferences

Many clients have specific brand preferences. Follow these preferences. Do not substitute another brand for the client's preferred brand unless the client has given you permission to do so.

Smart Shopping

Even though your client may have strong brand preferences, limited storage, and a limited budget, you can still shop "smart." The following suggestions can help you get the most for your client's money:

- **Check unit pricing.** If your client's budget, storage, and needs will allow the purchase of a larger package, compare the unit prices of the different sizes of the same brand (Figure 16-2). One size may be a better buy. Unit pricing can also help you compare the value of two similar products (if your client does not insist on a particular brand).
- **Check labels.** There's a great deal of information on the package label. You can use this information to compare different brands and varieties to select the best choice for your client's needs.

FIGURE 16-2

A unit pricing label provides information useful for comparison shopping. Comparing the price per unit of measure (shown at the right of the label, just below the item name) can help you to determine which brand or size is the best value.

Source: Aurora IGA

CARMIT SUGAR FREE WAFERS LEMON

2.39 $1.195/100GR
200 GR

PK 12

01550502012

Ingredients

By law, ingredients must be listed in descending order of proportion. This means that the most plentiful ingredient must be listed first, followed by the next most plentiful, the third most, and so on. This allows you to compare the ingredients to see which brand has the order of ingredients your client prefers. For example, you may compare two brands of sweetened shredded wheat. Brand A may list wheat as the first ingredient, followed by a sugar. Brand B may list sugar first, then wheat. This tells you that Brand B has more sugar in it than any other ingredient.

Nutritional Labelling

Nutrition labelling became mandatory for most prepackaged foods in 2005. Standard *Nutrition Facts* labels have been established for use on products. Figure 16-3 shows an example of the new labels.

CONTENTS:

1. Nutrition Facts Table
2. Specific Amount of Food
3. % Daily Value
4. Core Nutrients
5. Nutrition Claims
6. List of Ingredients

Nutrition Facts[1]
Per 0 mL (0 g) [2]   [3]

Amount	% Daily Value
Calories 0	
Fat 0 g	0 %
Saturates 0 g	0 %
+ Trans 0 g	
Cholesterol 0 mg	
Sodium 0 mg	0 %
Carbohydrate 0 g	0 %
Fibre 0 g	0 %
Sugars 0 g	
Protein 0 g	

Vitamin A	0 %	Vitamin C	0 %
Calcium	0 %	Iron	0 %

[4]

[6] **Ingredients:** Whole wheat, vegetable oil shortening, salt

[5]

Low fat, cholesterol-free, source of fibre

FIGURE 16-3
Nutrition labelling required by Health Canada

Source http://www.hc-sc. gc.ca/fn-an/label-etiquet/ nutrition/interactive/ inl_main_e.html

© *Reproduced with the permission of the Minister of Public Works and Government Services 2007.*

Nutritional Claims

Canada regulates nutritional claims. Table 16-6 lists Health Canada's criteria for specific nutritional claims.

Expiry or "Best Before" Dates

These dates appear on many products. The product can safely be used before the date stated if stored properly. Always check dates, and select the package with the latest date. As many stores put their oldest stock on the front of the shelf or cooler, you may have to look further back to get a package with a later date. Don't buy anything that your client will not use before the "best before" date. Bear in mind that "best before" dates only apply to *unopened* products. Opened product must be used quickly, despite any "best before" date.

TABLE 16-6	Health Canada criteria for Health-Related Claims
Keyword/Phrase	What it means
Free	an amount so small, health experts consider it nutritionally insignificant
Sodium free	less than 5 mg sodium*
Cholesterol free	less than 2 mg cholesterol, and low in saturated fat (includes a restriction on trans fat)* not necessarily low in total fat
Low	always associated with a very small amount
Low fat	3 g or less fat*
Low in saturated fat	2 g or less of saturated and trans fat combined*
Reduced	At least 25% less of a nutrient compared with a similar product
Reduced in Calories	At least 25% less energy than the food to which it is compared
Source	always associated with a "significant" amount
Source of fibre	2 grams or more fibre*
Good source of calcium	165 mg or more of calcium*
Light	when referring to a nutritional characteristic of a product, it is allowed only on foods that are either "reduced in fat" or "reduced in energy" (Calories) Explanation on the label of what makes the food "light"; this is also true if "light" refers to sensory characteristics, such as "light in colour." Three exceptions that do not require an explanation are "light maple syrup," "light rum" and "light salted" with respect to fish. Note that a separate provision is made for the claim "lightly salted" which may be used when a food contains at least 50% less added sodium compared with a similar product

*per reference amount and per serving of stated size (specific amount of food listed in Nutrition Facts)

Source: http://www.hc-sc.gc.ca/fn-an/label-etiquet/nutrition/educat/te_background-le_point-08-table1_e.html

MAKING MEALS APPEALING TO CLIENTS

Many things can affect how we eat. Busy schedules can cause us to rely on fast foods or to eat snack foods instead of more nutritious choices. Cooking for just one person may seem like a great deal of fuss. We may get tired of the "same old thing" for lunch. Smoking, illness, and medications, or changes in vision, taste, and smell may make food less attractive to us. It's important to make meals as appealing as possible to your client.

Eating as a Social Event

Have you ever insisted (or wanted to insist) that your family be together for meals? For most of us, eating is a social event. We see meals as a time to share what has happened in our day, not just a time to eat.

It's quite likely that your client has lost many opportunities to enjoy the social aspect of meals. Your client may say to you things like, "It's no fun just cooking for myself," or "I just eat in front of the TV for company." If your client misses the social aspect of meals, try to prepare a meal (or suggest that the client eat his or her meal) when you are there. You may still be able to complete other assigned tasks as your client eats, as well as provide company to him or her. Consider Case Example 16-1.

CASE EXAMPLE 16-1

Ginger is a support worker for Mr. Baraki. Mr. Baraki lost interest in eating when his wife died last year. Ginger makes a point of preparing a nutritious meal, using recipes that Mr. Baraki's wife used so that they are familiar. While Mr. Baraki eats, Ginger folds laundry in the same room. This way, Ginger keeps Mr. Baraki company and completes her assigned tasks.

Is mealtime a social event in your home? Why or why not?

Remember that each person has his or her own preferences for the amount of conversation during a meal. Also, clients whose vision or hearing impairments make it difficult to eat and converse at the same time may prefer you to simply be around when they eat. Some clients may prefer to be alone. They may simply like to be by themselves or may feel less self-conscious about how they eat. Take the time to find out what level of social interaction your client prefers during a meal.

Attractive Presentation

Do you ever recall being in an elegant restaurant? How was the meal presented? Chances are, it was visually pretty as well as tasty. Meal presentation has a lot to do with how interested a person is in eating. Meal presentation has several factors such as portion size; variety of colour, tastes, textures, and temperatures; placement on the plate; and the table setting.

Portion Size

Make sure that the size of the portion is appropriate to the client. Many clients are put off by portions that are too large. Ask your client how much of a food is enough. If you are asked to encourage the client to eat, offer second helpings rather than putting a large portion on the client's plate at one time.

Variety

Try to include foods of a variety of colours, textures, and temperatures in the meal you prepare. Place the items on the plate so that the colours are most appealing. For example, combining servings of fish, butternut squash, and a spinach salad provides variety and visual appeal.

Table Setting

Take a few minutes to set the table as the client likes it (Photo 16-2). Some clients prefer the use of a tablecloth while others prefer a placemat. If possible, try to use colours that complement the meal.

Incorporate Food Preferences

Always prepare meals in accordance with your client's dietary, religious, or cultural requirements. If possible, incorporate your client's other food preferences into each meal. Ask your client about preferred foods and dishes and the ways he or she prefers they be combined.

Don't Get into a Rut

Work with your client to keep the menu as varied as the client wishes. Be aware that some clients prefer the same breakfast each day but may want much more variety in their lunch or supper. Try to combine enough preferences to result in the variety the client prefers.

Photo 16-2
An attractive place setting can make mealtime more enjoyable.

SAFE FOOD PRACTICES

Safe food practices include five things: shopping, storing, handling, preparing, and serving. You can keep food safe (and your client safe from food-borne illnesses) by practising a few techniques.

Shopping

Buy food that is in good condition. Do not buy canned food in cans that are rusted, bulging, or otherwise damaged. Do not buy fresh meat, fish, or poultry that is not cold to the touch, or meats, fish, or poultry that are sold as frozen and yet are soft to the touch. Do not buy foods that appear spoiled or smell "off."

Try to buy frozen and fresh foods last. Don't put them in your shopping cart first—they may sit at room temperature for half an hour or more while you shop. Also, if you're running many errands for your client, do the food shopping last. A car's trunk can reach unsafe temperatures for food storage, even on a cold, sunny day.

Storing Food

Refrigerate ASAP

Make sure that you refrigerate fresh food as soon as you get to the client's home. A good rule of thumb is that the client's refrigerator should be as cold as possible without freezing the milk and other liquids. Put packages of fresh meat and other "juicy" items on plates so that the juices do not drip onto other items. In addition to ruining the taste of the foods the juices drip on, these juices often contain bacteria.

Freezing

Place any frozen item in the freezer unless you are thawing it for immediate use. Do not refreeze any item that was frozen but thawed before you got it to the client's home. Check the labels of any non-frozen food products before you freeze them. Previously frozen products must not be refrozen.

It's always a good idea to write on the package the date you put the item in the freezer with a grease pen or a marker. This helps to keep food from being frozen too long and becoming unsafe.

Shelf Storage

Make sure that the item can be safely stored without refrigeration. If your client has some of the same item that you have purchased (for example, a partial box of the cereal you have just bought), position the old box so that it is used first. It's always a good idea to write the date you bought the item on the box. Follow any special instructions for storage, such as storing in a dark or cool area.

Make sure that any opened packages are securely sealed when stored to keep out flying insects and rodents. You may have to use a glass jar (with lid) or a plastic tub with lid. Be aware that some items must be refrigerated once opened.

Handling

No matter when the food was bought, check it before you use it. If you're not sure that it's OK, don't use it. Mould, a bad smell, or a "slimy" texture are all signs that the product has spoiled. Even food that is not obviously spoiled but looks "funny" should be discarded. Remember: "When in doubt, throw it out."

Cutting out an obviously spoiled part and using the rest may expose your client to unseen microorganisms. Cooking will not fix food that has spoiled.

Always wash your hands before preparing food. This helps to prevent the transmission of microorganisms to the food.

Wash your hands after handling any raw poultry, meat, or eggs. When uncooked, these items can harbour harmful bacteria. Do not wipe your hands on a towel without washing them as this simply transmits any bacteria to the towel where they can easily spread. Similarly, wash utensils and any cutting boards that have been used to prepare eggs, uncooked poultry, or meat before you use them for any other purpose.

Cooking

Thaw food in the refrigerator, oven, or microwave—never at room temperature. Marinate food in the refrigerator. Defrosting or marinating at room temperature allows the food to host harmful bacteria.

Cook foods thoroughly. If possible, use a meat thermometer to determine when meat or poultry is done. Make sure to insert the thermometer carefully and properly, according to the manufacturer's instructions. An improperly inserted thermometer can give a false reading. If you don't use a thermometer, follow these guidelines:

- Cook red meat until it is brown or grey inside.
- Cook poultry until the juice is clear.
- Cook fish until it flakes easily.

Remember that a microwave does not cook foods evenly. Some parts of a dish may be well done while others are barely warm. Stir contents, and rotate the dish (if the microwave does not have a turntable) to make sure foods heat evenly. Also, microwaved food continues to cook during the "standing time" (the time after food is removed from the oven before serving). Serving food too soon may mean that it's not fully cooked.

Although Canada has used metric measures for more than 20 years, many recipes still give imperial measures. Table 16-7 lists some of the common conversions used in cooking.

Serving

Never leave food out at room temperature for more than two hours. Bacteria multiply rapidly at room temperature and can quickly render a dish harmful.

Use clean utensils to serve food. For example, never put cooked chicken on the plate that held the raw chicken unless you have washed the plate. Bacteria present on an unwashed utensil will contaminate the cooked food.

Divide leftovers into small dishes when storing. Small dishes allow the food to cool more evenly and quickly, minimizing the opportunity for bacteria to multiply. Separate out warm dishes in the refrigerator to speed cooling. Containers should ideally be metal.

Make sure that you fully heat leftovers before serving. Cooked food can harbour harmful bacteria just as easily as uncooked food. Make sure the leftovers are heated thoroughly and completely to a minimum temperature of 77°C (170°F).

ASSISTING THE CLIENT WITH EATING

Some clients may require assistance with eating a meal. There are several reasons the client may require assistance: physical conditions (such as weakness, paralysis, or vision loss) as well as cognitive conditions (such as the loss of the ability to sequence events due to a dementia).

TABLE 16-7	Common Conversions Used in Cooking
Standard Cup (250 mL)	**Tablespoon (15 mL)/Teaspoon (5 mL)**
1 cup	16 tablespoons + 2 teaspoons
$1/_2$ cup	8 tablespoons + 1 teaspoon
$1/_4$ cup	4 generous tablespoons

Imperial	Metric	Metric	Imperial
1 oz	28.35 g	100 g	3.53 oz
2 oz	56.7 g	200 g	7.06 oz
3 oz	85.05 g	300 g	10.59 oz
4 oz	113.4 g	400 g	14.12 oz
5 oz	141.75 g	500 g	17.65 oz
6 oz	170.1 g	1 kg	35.27 oz
7 oz	198.45 g		
8 oz	226.8 g		
1 lb	453.6 g		

Temperature Conversion

Fahrenheit	Celsius
225° F	110° C
250° F	130° C
275° F	140° C
300° F	150° C
325° F	170° C
350° F	180° C
375° F	190° C
400° F	200° C
425° F	220° C
450° F	230° C
475° F	240° C

Principles of Assistance

The assistance you will provide each client is unique. Some clients will require only prompting. Others may require total assistance. All clients need the meal to be a pleasant experience that is not rushed. Keeping the following twelve principles in mind will help to ensure that the meal is as pleasant as possible.

1. **Take steps to avoid embarrassing the client.** If the client tends to spill foods, suggest that he or she wear a smock or apron that can be washed. Even men may not mind donning a chef's apron for the meal. Avoid using children's bibs or towels.
2. **If the client wears dentures,** make sure that they are clean and in place.
3. **Set a proper place setting, even if the client does not use all of the utensils.** Having the right cues may assist the client to be more independent. An attractive place setting simply may make the experience more pleasant.
4. **Make sure that foods are served at the proper temperature.** Cold peas or runny gelatine do not stimulate one's appetite!
5. **Cut, dice, or purée the food before taking the meal to the client.** It can be very embarrassing for the client to have his or her entrée cut while he or she watches.
6. **Use dishes that are appropriate to the consistency of the food being served.** One support worker found that her client was much more likely to eat puréed foods if they were served from a soup bowl.
7. **Season the food according to the client's preferences.** Be sure to avoid any forbidden seasonings.
8. **Follow the order the client prefers.** For example, some clients eat salad before their meal; others eat it with their meal. Additionally, some do not want a hot beverage until after the meal. Find out your client's preferences. If necessary, ask a family member.
9. **Do not mix foods on the fork or spoon.** This can make the best food unpalatable. If you must moisten or thin a food, use broth, milk, or water.
10. **Assist the client to eat at a relaxed pace.** Rushing the client will not allow time for him or her to be as independent as possible and may cause choking.
11. **Never force-feed a client.** If the client does not want to eat or closes his or her mouth when the food comes in contact with the lips, stop. A person who is not eating well may have ill-fitting dentures, sores, or abrasions in the mouth. Report the situation to your supervisor.
12. **Quietly clean up any spills.** Do not call attention to any mess caused by the client.

Assisting the Client with a Tray or Table Meal

1. **Prepare your client for the meal.** Many clients prefer to be toileted before a meal. Assist the client to wash his or her hands.
2. **Assist the client to the table, if appropriate.** If the client is remaining in bed, position the client in an upright position. If the client is not able to sit up, place the client in a side-lying position.
3. **Be sure there are no unpleasant odours in the room,** as they can interfere with the client's desire to eat.
4. **If the client receives a tray,** ensure that the name on the food tray matches the client's.

5. If the client is served a tray, open cartons, remove covers, and cut food (if it cannot be done beforehand).
6. Add salt and pepper according to the client's preferences.
7. Assist the client as necessary.
8. Allow the client time to finish the meal before removing the tray or plates.

Feeding the Client

1. **Prepare your client for the meal.** Many clients prefer to be toileted before a meal. Assist the client to wash his or her hands.
2. **Assist the client to the table, if appropriate.** If the client is remaining in bed, position the client in an upright position. If the client is not able to sit up, place the client in a side-lying position.
3. **Be sure there are no unpleasant odours in the room,** as they can interfere with the client's desire to eat.
4. **If the client receives a tray,** ensure that the name on the food tray matches the client's.
5. **If the client is served a tray,** open cartons, remove covers, and cut food (if it cannot be done beforehand).
6. **Add salt and pepper according to the client's preferences.**
7. **Position the client appropriately.** A client who can sit up should be assisted to do so. A client who cannot sit up should be positioned with his or her head and shoulders at a 60° angle. Photo 16-3 shows proper positioning to assist a client.
8. **Wash your hands.**
9. **Use a fork or dessert spoon to feed the client.** Do not use a soup spoon. Unless specifically prescribed, do not use a syringe or plastic utensils.
10. **Sit close to the client so that he or she can see you and you can properly assist.** Do not stand, as this can cause you to scrape the roof of the client's mouth with the utensils. Figure 16-4 shows what can happen if you stand to assist the client.
11. **Tell the client what is on the tray.**
12. **Test the temperature of the food by testing a few drops on your wrist before giving to the client.**
13. **Serve the food in bite-sized pieces.** Offer each piece slowly so that the client has time to swallow each bite.
14. **Offer a sip of fluid after a few bites.**

Photo 16-3
If possible, a client should be seated in a chair for meals. If this is not possible, make certain that the client is in as upright a position as is possible.
Source: CHATS

FIGURE 16-4
Feeding a client from a standing position can scrape the roof of the client's mouth.

15. Stop when the client indicates he or she has had enough.
16. Note the amount of food, and calculate the fluid intake if required.
17. Remove the tray or plates.
18. Assist the client to wash his or her hands and face.
19. **Assist the client to a comfortable position.** It is wise to leave the client in the upright position or side-lying position for 15–20 minutes. (This helps to ensure that the food is out of the esophagus and prevents aspiration or the accidental intake of food into the respiratory tract.)
20. **Provide mouth care.**

Special Considerations When Assisting a Client to Eat

Paralysis

A client with paralysis affecting her or his ability to swallow should have an assessment by a qualified professional, such as a physician or speech pathologist. This assessment will indicate the foods the client can tolerate, how they must be prepared, as well as any special methods of assisting. In general, a client with hemiparesis (paralysis on one side of the body) can be assisted by putting small bites in the unaffected side of the mouth. You must be careful to allow sufficient time for the client to chew and swallow the bite before offering another. The client's mouth should be checked for food before you leave to ensure that no food is left for the client to choke on later. If the client begins to cough during feeding, he or she may be aspirating food into the lungs. If the client has difficulty breathing or cannot stop coughing, call for help.

Visual Impairment

Most visually impaired clients can eat independently if they are told what food is on the plate and where the food is located on the plate. Describe the location of each food item as if the plate was a clock. Take the client's hand and direct it to each item and then assist as necessary. Figure 16-5 illustrates a meal described by the clock method.

FIGURE 16-5

Describing the location of food using the clock method

Description	Location
Your meatloaf is at 8 o'clock.	
Canned baby peas are at 2 o'clock.	
Steamed diced carrots are at 4 o'clock.	
A buttered slice of whole-wheat bread is at 11 o'clock	

Swallowing Problems

Some clients may experience swallowing problems. Swallowing problems can result from a stroke and can have serious consequences. A person with swallowing problems may fear choking or inhaling food particles (aspirating) and, therefore, may limit foods or fluids. This, in turn, can lead to malnutrition and dehydration.

A client who complains of food sticking in his or her throat, who coughs during meals, or who seems to make great effort to swallow may have a swallowing problem. You should report any signs of swallowing problems to your supervisor. A health professional should evaluate the needs of a client with swallowing problems. The following approaches may be useful to reduce the chance of having difficulty:

1. Keep the client upright at a 60–90° angle.
2. Try smaller, more frequent meals.
3. Give small amounts (1/2 to 1 teaspoon) of food or fluid.
4. Encourage the client to swallow twice after each bite.
5. If the client complains of food sticking, encourage a cough to clear the throat.
6. Encourage the client to remain in an upright position for two hours after the meal, if possible.

CHOKING

Have you ever taken too big a bite of something or had something "go down the wrong way" and begun to choke? It's a frightening feeling, isn't it? Any client can be at risk for choking. A client who requires assistance eating is at additional risk.

Helping to Prevent Choking

Many clients with swallowing problems will show four common signs: drooling, chewing for a long time without swallowing, coughing when swallowing, or choking. You should always observe for these signs and report any difficulty swallowing that you suspect or observe. Following the guidelines for assisting a client, presented in this chapter, will also assist the person with swallowing problems and help avoid choking.

A client who has known swallowing problems may have specific techniques or routines that must be followed. Make sure that you are aware of any specific instructions for assisting your client. The following measures can also help prevent choking:

1. Arrange the client in an upright position. Place a pillow behind the client's shoulder blades to help keep the torso upright.
2. Encourage the client to keep his or her chin down when swallowing.
3. Avoid very sticky foods such as dry toast, peanut butter, or similar foods.
4. Discuss with your supervisor the use of a thickening agent to thicken clear liquids such as tea, coffee, or water. Do not use thickening agents without your supervisor's approval.
5. Discourage the client from talking while eating.

If Choking Occurs

The actions you take in the event your client is choking depend upon whether or not the client can cough.

A client who can breathe, speak, cough, or make loud noises should be assisted to bend forward at the waist and lower his or her chin as close as possible to the chest. The client should be instructed to cough while in this position to clear the airway.

FIGURE 16-6

Proper positioning of hands for abdominal thrusts

A client who cannot cough or who can only make high-pitched noises has an obstructed airway. In this case, the food has lodged in the larynx, blocking the passageway completely or almost completely. You must assist the client by performing abdominal thrusts. The procedure for this is as follows:

1. Reassure the client. Tell him or her that you will help.
2. Move behind the client, standing directly behind the client, facing the client's back.
3. Bring your arms around the client's waist, clasping your hands together just above the client's navel. (See Figure 16-6.)
4. Give thrusts in a quick upward motion until the obstruction is ejected.

Questions for Review

1. What are the benefits of a balanced diet?

2. What is a nutrient? What types of nutrients are there?

3. What are the four food groups defined in *Canada's Food Guide*?

4. What are five age- or condition-related changes in nutritional needs?

5. Why is it important for you to respect a client s food preferences?

6. What tasks are included in planning a week's meals?

7. Does the order in which ingredients are listed on a food item mean anything?

8. What principles should you keep in mind when you assist a client to eat?

9. What are two signs that your client might have difficulty swallowing?

10. What observations might mean that your client is prone to choking?

Questions for Discussion

1. If you had to rely on someone to plan meals, grocery shop, and prepare meals for you, how would you react? What would you say your preferences are? How would you prefer to have your food prepared? How would you feel about someone using your kitchen?

2. The new edition of *Canada's Food Guide* is supposed to include foods that reflect Canada's ethnic diversity. Does it? Does the *Guide* include foods that you eat? If not, what is missing? Compare your observations with those of your colleagues.

3. Your client, Mrs. Chandra, is a diabetic. Her diabetes is controlled by diet. You know that she has a sweet tooth. Despite knowing that she should not have sugar, Mrs. Chandra sweetens fresh fruit with it. She also uses sugar in her tea. She tells you that sugar substitutes do not taste the same as the "real thing." How do you think you would react to this situation? What, if anything, would you do?

4. You are assisting Mrs. Mumm. One of your tasks is to prepare a meal for her to eat while you are there. When you serve her meal, she says, "Aren't you having any? I can't eat alone." You assure her that you'll just be working in the kitchen while she eats and that you can talk with her. She again asks you to join her and eat. What do you do in this situation? How do you feel?

Chapter 17

Understanding the Elements of the Body

Learning Objectives

Through reading this chapter, you'll be able to

1. Identify why a basic understanding of how the body works is helpful for support workers.
2. Explain how the body is organized.
3. Describe the structure and function of the ten systems of the body.
4. Discuss, in general terms, growth and development of the person from birth to adulthood.

Chapter at a Glance

- From Cell to System: How the Body Is Organized
- The Systems of the Body
- Age-Related Changes

Terms You'll Use

Abdomen The portion of the body between the pelvis and the diaphragm.

Age-Related Changes The changes that are part of the aging process that happen to everyone if they live long enough.

Alimentary Canal The structure that links the organs of the digestive system. It is also called the gastrointestinal tract

Anatomy The study of the body's structure.

Blood Assists in nutrition and elimination, regulation, protection, and oxygenation of the body.

Bones Hard, rigid, living structures that provide support for the body.

Cell The basic element of the human body and all living things.

Connective Tissue The tissue that forms bones, tendons, cartilage and other fibrous tissues.

Embolus A mass, such as an air bubble, a blood clot or clump, or a foreign body, that travels through the bloodstream and lodges in a way that blocks a blood vessel.

Epithelial Tissue The tissue that covers the internal and external body tissues.

Integumentary System The system that includes the skin, nails, oil and sweat glands, and hair.

Joints The points where two or more bones meet and may move.

Matrix The substance found between the cells in connective tissue.

Muscle Tissue The tissue that can contract and relax; may be smooth, striated, or cardiac.

Muscles Part of the musculoskeletal system that helps to maintain posture, causes movement, and produces and helps to maintain body heat.

Nerve Tissue The tissue made of nerve cells, or neurons, that transmits electrical signals from the central nervous system to various parts of the body.

Organelles Specialized structures within the cell that carry out particular cell processes that, in turn, carry out the cell's functions.

Organs Groups of tissues working together with a specific purpose.

Physiology The study of the body's functions.

System Group of organs working together with a specific purpose.

Thorax The portion of the body between the diaphragm and the shoulders.

Thrombus A blood clot that forms in a vessel and remains attached to that site.

Tissues Groups of cells linked together by a matrix.

FROM CELL TO SYSTEM: HOW THE BODY IS ORGANIZED

As a support worker, you will be called upon to provide assistance to your clients. It's very likely that a considerable part of this assistance will be physical assistance. As we've discussed, you must always focus on the whole person when providing any assistance to your clients. This is called holistic care. None of us wants to be seen simply as a diagnosis, disability, or procedure.

A basic understanding of anatomy and physiology will help you to understand and appreciate why certain things happen and identify why assistance is best provided in a certain way.

You've likely heard the terms anatomy and physiology. They are often used in the same phrase, but they do not mean the same thing. **Anatomy** is the study of the body's structure. The body is often described in terms of general areas, also called regions. The major regions are the head and neck, the upper limbs, the thorax, the abdomen, the pelvis, and the lower limbs. Two of these regions are located in the trunk of the body. The **thorax** is the portion of the body between the diaphragm and the shoulders. The **abdomen** is the portion of the body between the pelvis and the diaphragm.

Physiology is the study of the body's functions. As a support worker, you likely won't use detailed anatomical and physiological information in your work. However some information about how the body is structured and functions is helpful in understanding normal function as well as the effect of conditions.

The Cell

The **cell** is the basic element of the human body. There are more than 75 trillion cells in the human body. Cells are too small to see with the naked eye, but we can easily see them under a microscope. There are more than 100 types of cells in the human body, and though all cells have the same basic structure, their size, shape, purpose, and life span differ with their function. Some cells have smooth, rounded surfaces, while others seem to have tentacles. Some cells have cilia or flagella—hair-like projections that the cells use to move substances. For example, the ear has tiny cells with these projections whose purpose is to carry sound down the ear canal. Cells in the lung have cilia that help a person to expel foreign particles.

Some cells, such as blood cells, replace themselves, while other cells, such as nerve cells, cannot. This is why a person can give blood and make more, yet cannot recover from severe damage to nerve cells in the brain or spinal cord. Figure 17-1 illustrates different types of cells.

Cells are made up of three main components: the membrane, the cytoplasm, and the nucleus. Figure 17-2 illustrates the basic structure of the cell.

FIGURE 17-1
Common types of cells

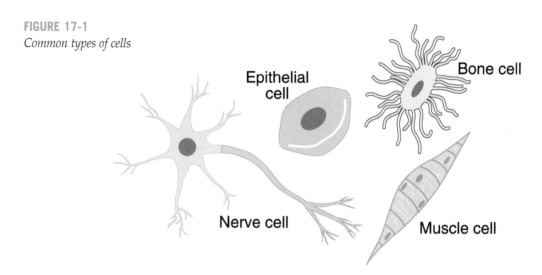

The membrane is the outer covering of the cell. It gives the cell its shape and provides it with protection. This membrane has tiny openings that allow substances such as nutrients, water, and other substances in and out of the cell. Other parts of the membrane allow oxygen and other gasses to move in and out of the cell, such as when blood cells "pick up" oxygen from the lungs to circulate to (and nourish) other cells in the body.

The interior of the cell is made up of the nucleus and the cytoplasm. Some cells, such as striated muscle cells, have many nuclei within a single cell. Others, such as the

FIGURE 17-2
The basic structure of the cell

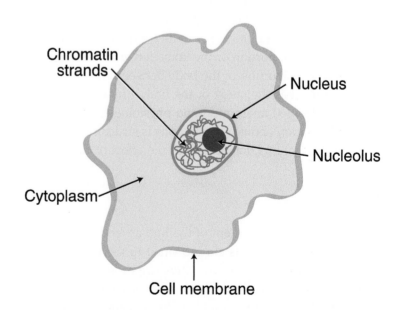

cells in smooth muscle tissue and cardiac muscle cells, have only one per cell. Mature red blood cells have no nuclei.

The nucleus is the centre of the cell. It contains the cell's chromosomes that, in turn, contain genes. Humans have 46 chromosomes. Within them there are many thousands of genes. Genes determine inherited characteristics such as eye colour, hair colour, body type, and, in part, personality and susceptibility to certain kinds of disease.

The *cytoplasm* is the substance that fills the cell and surrounds the nucleus. Within the cytoplasm is protoplasm, a gel-like substance that contains structures called organelles. **Organelles** (the term literally means "little organs") are specialized structures that carry out particular cell processes that, in turn carry out the cell's functions. Metabolism is the term that describes the work of all of the cells, considered together, that carry out the body's functions. However, each cell has its own metabolism; some cells work much more rapidly than others.

Each type of cell has its own life expectancy. Some cells, such as white blood cells, last only a few hours, while other cells, such as nerve cells, are expected to last a person's lifetime. Cells that do not last a lifetime generally divide into new cells in a process called *mitosis*. Mitosis is complete when one cell becomes two cells: the original cell and an exact copy.

Tissue

Most cells are grouped together, linked by a matrix, to form tissues. A **matrix** is the substance found between cells. There are four major types of **tissue**: muscle, nerve, epithelial, and connective. Each type of tissue has its own function with variants within each type. Let's examine them. Most organs contain many types of tissue, as Figure 17-3 illustrates.

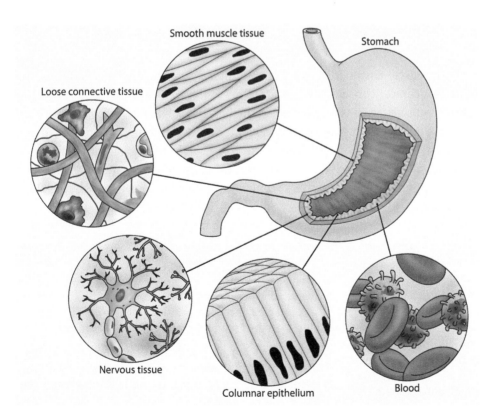

Loose connective tissue

Smooth muscle tissue

Stomach

Nervous tissue

Columnar epithelium

Blood

FIGURE 17-3
Many types of tissue can make up an organ.

Muscle Tissue

Muscle tissue is the only type of tissue that can contract and relax. There are three types of muscle tissue: striated, smooth, and cardiac (Photo 17-1). You may think that muscle tissue is found only in the muscles, but different types are found in all organs.

Striated muscle tissue is the type of tissue found in the muscles that move your bones. These cells form tissue that can expand and contract to a much greater degree (extent) than can the other types of muscle tissue. Because the person controls when striated muscle tissue contracts and expands, the striated muscles are called *voluntary* muscles. This tissue is able to contract and expand and to maintain a particular state for long periods of time.

Photo 17-1a
Skeletal muscle

Source: Dr. Gladden Willis/Visuals
Unlimited/Getty Images

Photo 17-1b
Smooth muscle

Source: Dr. Gladden Willis/Visuals
Unlimited/Getty Images

Photo 17-1c
Cardiac muscle

Source: Dr. Fred Hossler/Visuals
Unlimited/Getty Images

Smooth muscle tissue lines many of the internal organs, and is called involuntary, as the person cannot consciously control it.

Cardiac muscle tissue is found only in the heart. It is considered to be a very strong type of muscle tissue as it controls the movement of the heart. Cardiac muscle looks a bit like striated muscle, but each cell in cardiac muscle tissue has only one nucleus. Like smooth muscle tissue, the person cannot fully control cardiac muscle tissue. However, as Spotlight 17-1 describes, some people are able to control the rate at which their heart beats.

SPOTLIGHT 17-1 CAN WE TELL OUR HEART WHAT TO DO?

In general, our heart beats without our conscious thought or effort. However, some scientists believe that, in some cases, a person can control his or her heartbeat to some extent (Victor, Mainardi, and Shapiro, 1978; De Pascalis, Palumbo, and Ronchitelli, 1991). In particular, some feel that training in yoga will allow some people to slow or speed heart rate at will. Others cite biofeedback methods as useful; and yet other studies identify the positive effect of encouraging the person to control the rate (in effect, cueing the person to consciously change heart rate).

It's likely that our ability to alter our heart rate is limited—that we can change its pattern only slightly. Cases of a person's ability to actually stop his or her heart are extremely rare.

Nerve Tissue

Nerve tissue is tissue made of nerve cells (neurons) and transmits electrical signals (also called impulses) from the central nervous system (the brain and spinal cord) to various parts of the body. Adults have between 10 billion and 100 billion neurons, most of which are in the brain and the spinal cord. Most neurons develop before birth. Some continue for a few years after birth. Nerve cells do not replace themselves, although they can repair themselves to some extent. The most common example of this occurs as a person recovers from a stroke.

The neuron looks very different from other cells as it has a cell body from which many *dendrites* project. Dendrites are designed to receive electrical impulses and are shaped somewhat like branches. At the other end of the cell body is a long fibre called an *axon*. The axon's purpose is to carry impulses away from the cell body. The axon ends in a number of finger-like structures. Photo 17-2 illustrates a nerve cell. Some neurons are very small. Other neurons in the peripheral nervous system, such as those that travel from your spinal cord to your foot, can be more than one metre long.

Photo 17-2
A nerve cell
Source: Shutterstock

Epithelial Tissue

Epithelial tissue forms the covering of all body surfaces, lines body cavities and hollow organs, and is the major tissue in glands. Your skin, the lining of your mouth, nose, and stomach, as well as your hair and nails, are formed of epithelial tissue. It is attached only on one side—to the surface it is covering. There are several types of epithelial cells that, in turn, form the various types of epithelial tissue. The epithelial tissue in the capillaries is only one cell thick, allowing oxygen and nutrients from the blood to be exchanged by the cells for carbon dioxide and waste materials in a very efficient manner. Figure 17-4 illustrates some of the body's epithelial cells.

FIGURE 17-4
Common epithelial cells

Connective Tissue

Connective tissues have many purposes: they bind structures together, form a framework and support for organs and the body as a whole, store fat, transport substances, protect against disease, and help repair tissue damage. They occur throughout the body.

Connective tissue is the kind of tissue that forms the bones, tendons, cartilage, and other types of connecting tissue. Unlike other tissue, connective tissue has cells spaced apart on a matrix. There are many types, but we'll discuss the most common ones here.

Adipose tissue is connective tissue that functions as the major storage site for fat.

Areolar connective tissue (or loose connective tissue) is found in many places in the body. It is found in skin, surrounds the blood vessels and nerves, and is also a part of the mucous membranes found in the digestive, respiratory, reproductive, and urinary systems.

Fibrous connective tissue is another type of connective tissue. It is densely packed and forms structures such as tendons and ligaments.

Blood is also a type of connective tissue. Even though it has a different function than other connective tissues, it has the same matrix.

Photo 17-3a
Areolar connective tissue
Source: Copyright 2008 Educational Images – Custom Medical Stock Photo, All Rights Reserved

Photo 17-3b
Adipose tissue
Source: Copyright 2008 Educational Images – Custom Medical Stock Photo, All Rights Reserved

Photo 17-3c
Fibrous connective tissue
Source: Copyright Keith – Custom Medical Stock Photo, All Rights Reserved

Organs

Tissues with a common purpose group together to form organs. Each organ has a specific function. Some organs are very rigid, such as the bones. Other organs, such as the skin, are very flexible. We'll discuss the various types of organs later in this chapter.

Systems

A group of organs with a similar purpose are grouped together into a system. For example, the digestive system groups together all the organs required to convert food into energy and eliminate solid wastes. This system includes the pancreas, liver, intestines, and other organs. There are ten systems in the human body. The next section of this chapter provides an overview of the structure and purpose of each system.

THE SYSTEMS OF THE BODY

Within the body, there are ten systems, each with its own function. These systems are:

- The Integumentary System
- The Musculoskeletal System
- The Circulatory System (incorporating the lymphatic and immune systems)
- The Respiratory System
- The Digestive System
- The Urinary System
- The Nervous System
- The Sensory System
- The Endocrine System
- The Reproductive System

Although each system has a distinct function, each of these systems relies upon the function of the other systems in order to work to ensure the efficient and effective functioning of the body as a whole. No system can function alone. For example, you could not survive without your integumentary system, no matter how well your other systems could function. In fact, the loss of only one-third of a person's skin may cause death. The inability of a system to function at peak ability may also affect the function of other systems, as you likely will see with your clients. For example, a respiratory system that does not work at peak capacity may well affect the ability of the cardiovascular system to work well. Thus, you may see changes in your client that are caused by a problem that doesn't seem to be related to the person's impairment.

The Integumentary System

The **integumentary system** is the largest system of the body. It is made up of the skin; epithelial, connective, and nerve tissue; oil and sweat glands; nails; and hair.

There are two layers in the skin, the epidermis and the dermis. Figure 17-5 illustrates these layers, as well as the other structures found in the skin. The epidermis contains both living and dead cells; the dermis contains only living cells. The living cells in the epidermis have pigment, which gives the skin its colour.

FIGURE 17-5
The skin

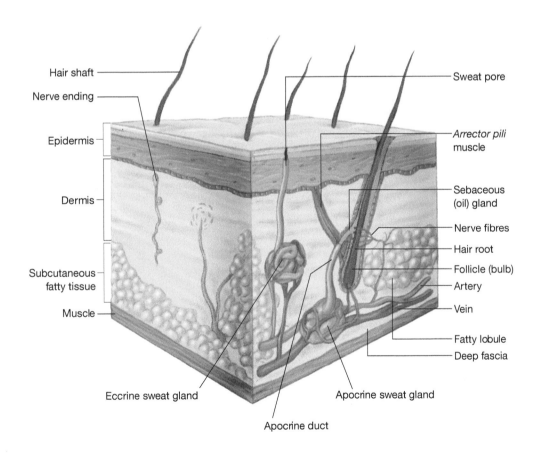

Hair shaft
Nerve ending
Epidermis
Dermis
Subcutaneous fatty tissue
Muscle
Eccrine sweat gland
Apocrine duct
Sweat pore
Arrector pili muscle
Sebaceous (oil) gland
Nerve fibres
Hair root
Follicle (bulb)
Artery
Vein
Fatty lobule
Deep fascia
Apocrine sweat gland

Note that the epidermis has few nerve endings and no blood vessels. The dermis, however, contains many nerve endings and blood vessels. This arrangement provides a barrier layer, preventing us from receiving so many sensations that it becomes overwhelming, and also reducing the potential for blood loss from the wear and tear of everyday activities.

The integumentary system performs many functions. First, it protects the body from bacteria and other potentially harmful substances and protects the internal organs from injury. Second, it prevents excessive water and fluid loss. Third, the system helps the body to regulate its temperature through the evaporation of moisture through sweat glands, or by contracting to reduce heat loss (as in "goose bumps"). Fourth, it provides a way for the body to sense textures, temperatures, pressure, and pain, all of which can reduce the risk of danger.

Care of the skin is one of the most significant aspects of physical support. In Chapter 19, we'll look at common changes in the integumentary system and how these affect the care you provide.

The Musculoskeletal System

The **musculoskeletal** system provides the basic structure of the body and the mechanisms by which the body can move (Figure 17-6). This system contains bones, muscles, joints, ligaments, cartilage, and tendons.

FIGURE 17-6
The human skeleton

Skull — Cranium
       — Face
Hyoid
Sternum
Ribs
Vertebral column
Sacrum

Clavicle
Scapula
Humerus
Radius
Ulna
Pelvis
Carpals
Metacarpals
Phalanges
Femur
Patella
Tibia
Fibula
Tarsals
Metatarsals
Phalanges

Bones

Although **bones** are hard and rigid, they are living structures made of cells. Bones have three main elements: the marrow, the periosteum, the compact bone, and the spongy bone. Figure 17-7 illustrates these four components.

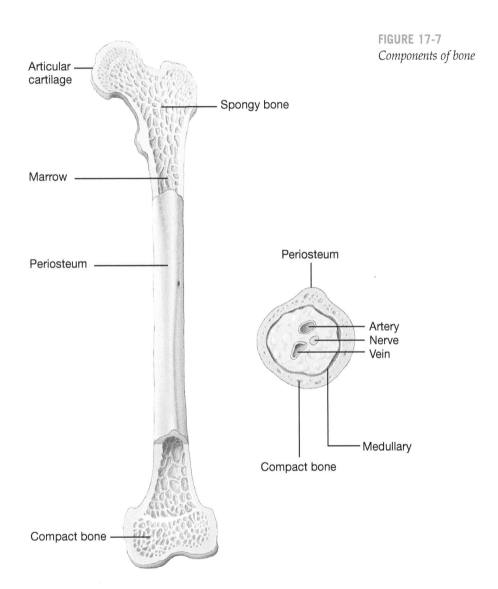

FIGURE 17-7
Components of bone

Marrow exists in the centre of the bone. One of its purposes is to manufacture blood cells. Spongy bone is the tissue that makes up the interior of bones. It's called spongy because it is less dense and resembles a sponge in appearance.

The periosteum is the outer covering of the bone. It contains blood vessels to nourish the bone.

There are 206 bones in the human body. These bones are grouped into four categories: long bones, short bones, flat bones, and irregular bones. Each has a particular purpose, as Table 17-1 illustrates, but in general, bones give structure and shape to the body.

TABLE 17-1	Categories of Bones	
Bone Type	**Purpose**	**Example**
Long Bones	Leg bones bear the weight of the body. These bones permit leverage and gross movement.	Leg bones (femur, fibula, tibia) Arm, forearm (humerus, ulna, radius)
Short Bones	These bones allow for small, precise movement over a wide arc.	Wrist bones Hand bones (carpals and metacarpals) Foot bones (tarsals and metatarsals) Fingers and toes (phalanges)
Flat Bones	These bones protect the organs of the body.	Skull (cranium) Shoulder blades (scapula) Breastbone (sternum) Ribs Pelvis (some)
Irregular Bones	These bones do not fit in the other three categories.	Backbone (vertebrae) Pelvis Facial bones

Pivot joint
e.g., neck

Hinge joint
e.g., elbow

Ball-and-socket joint
e.g., hip

FIGURE 17-8
Three types of joints

Joints

Joints are where two or more bones meet. There are three categories of these joints and these are:

1. the immoveable joints, as seen in the suture lines of the skull
2. the slightly moveable joints, as seen between the adjacent vertebrae of the spine
3. the freely moveable joints, as seen in the neck, the knee, or the hip

Joints allow the body to move in specific ways. In this module, we will study the freely moveable joints. These joints are unique as they are constructed with two specialized protective mechanisms. The first is the cartilage, a living connective tissue that covers and protects the ends of each of the bones where they meet. The second is the synovial membrane that lines the capsule that encloses the joint and produces synovial fluid, a lubricant that allows smooth movement of the bones within the capsule.

The three types of freely moveable joints that we will concentrate on are pivot, hinge, and ball-and-socket. Figure 17-8 illustrates these three types. Pivot joints allow side-to-side movement, such as the movement of the head on the neck. Hinge joints allow movement back and forth in a single direction. A knee joint is an example of a hinge joint. A ball-and-socket joint allows movement in all directions. This joint is made up of a hollowed end of one bone (the socket) into which fits the rounded end of another joint (the ball). Your hip joint is a ball and socket joint, as is your shoulder joint.

Muscles

Muscles perform three essential functions: maintaining posture, moving the body, and producing and maintaining body heat. As we discussed earlier in this chapter, muscles can be voluntary (i.e., moved as the person desires) or involuntary (i.e., moved in response to body processes that cannot be consciously controlled by the person).

The human body contains more than 500 muscles in various sizes. Figure 17-9 illustrates some of the major muscles. Muscles are attached to bones by tendons, a particularly tough form of connective tissue. As the muscle contracts, the tendons move the bones.

The contracting and relaxing of muscles generates kinetic energy or heat. For example, you probably notice that you generate heat when you exert yourself. You may notice that your client may feel cold if he or she cannot move about a great deal. You probably shiver when you are very cold—these muscle contractions are your body's way of generating heat.

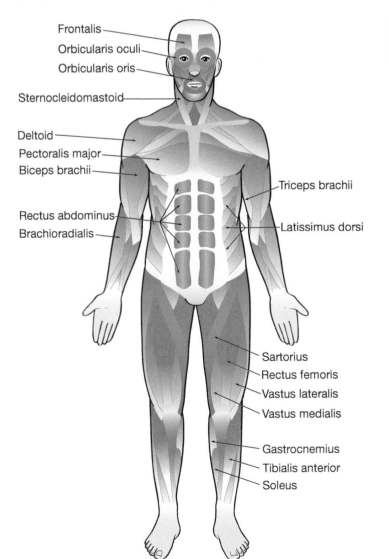

FIGURE 17-9
The major muscles of the body

Frontalis
Orbicularis oculi
Orbicularis oris
Sternocleidomastoid
Deltoid
Pectoralis major
Biceps brachii
Rectus abdominus
Brachioradialis
Triceps brachii
Latissimus dorsi
Sartorius
Rectus femoris
Vastus lateralis
Vastus medialis
Gastrocnemius
Tibialis anterior
Soleus

The Circulatory System

The blood, the heart, and the blood vessels make up the circulatory system (Figure 17-10). This system is also called the cardiovascular system. In this closed system, blood is pumped through blood vessels by the heart to all of the cells throughout the body.

The circulatory system has two components, called circuits. These are called the pulmonary circuit and the systemic circuit. We'll discuss these later in this section.

The circulatory system performs four functions, as listed here:

■ **Nutrition and Elimination.** Blood carries food and other substances to the cells and removes waste products from the cells.

■ **Regulation.** Blood helps to regulate body temperature by carrying heat from muscles to other body parts. Blood vessels help to regulate temperature by constricting (to retain heat) and expanding (to release heat).

■ **Protection.** Some blood cells produce antibodies and other substances that help the body fight off disease.

■ **Oxygenation.** Blood carries oxygen to the cells and removes carbon dioxide.

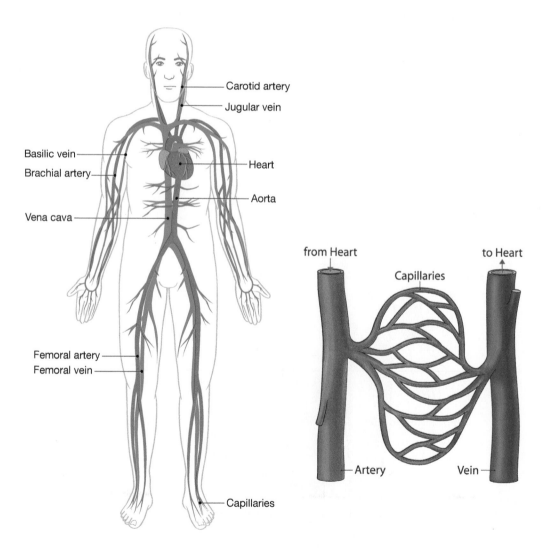

FIGURE 17-10

The circulatory system, showing pathways of circulation throughout the body

Blood

Blood is made up of several components: blood cells, platelets, and plasma, each component having a specific function.

Blood Cells

There are two types of blood cells: red and white.

The red blood cells, or erythrocytes, are created in bone marrow and live for approximately three to four months. There are more than 25 trillion red blood cells in the body. These cells contain hemoglobin, which gives blood its colour. It is a substance that picks up oxygen from the lungs and carries it to the cells, where it is exchanged for the cells' carbon dioxide. Figure 17-11 illustrates the function of red blood cells. As red blood cells wear out, they are destroyed by white blood cells in the liver or spleen.

White blood cells aren't really white. They are colourless. Some of these cells are known as leukocytes. The purpose of these cells is to fight infection and foreign substances. They do this by seeking out, destroying alien bacteria, viruses, and fungi. They also rid the body of dead or dying blood cells as well as foreign matter such as dust and asbestos. They are produced in bone marrow and in the lymphatic system (a subsystem of the cardiovascular system) and live about nine days. White blood cells make up a very small component of human blood: there is only one white blood cell for every 500–1000 red blood cells.

Photo 17-4
Red blood cells
Source: © Micro Discovery/Corbis

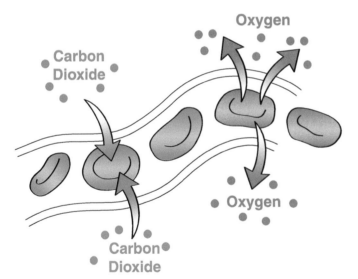

FIGURE 17-11
Functions of the red blood cells

A bruise occurs when a force causes blood vessels under the skin to rupture and leak. The size of the rupture as well as the size of the vessel will determine the size of the bruise. As the vessel wall repairs, the flow of blood is stopped. Gradually, the body absorbs the leaked blood and the bruise disappears.

Platelets, known as cytoplasmic fragments, are substances in the blood that function to assist the blood to clot. This prevents excessive blood loss and attempts to maintain the integrity of this closed system. Platelets are also created in bone marrow. They live only a short time—approximately four days.

Plasma is the fluid transportation medium of the blood. It is colourless, mostly water, and moves the blood cells and platelets to every cell in the body. It makes up about 55 percent of the blood's volume.

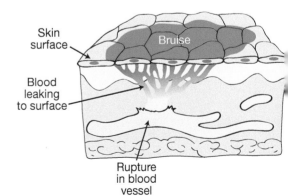

EXHIBIT 17-1
Anatomy of a bruise

Blood Vessels

There are two main types of blood vessels: veins and arteries. Veins carry blood to the heart. Arteries carry blood from the heart. Connecting these blood vessels are the capillaries, blood vessels so small that blood cells must travel through the vessel in single file. Healthy blood vessels are smooth-walled and flexible (much like a new garden hose).

Sometimes due to disease, blood vessels become hardened and their interior walls may become roughened with cholesterol or calcium deposits that can interfere with the smooth movement of the blood through the vessels. When a blood clot forms around a point in this roughened surface and remains there, the clot is called a **thrombus**. Also, pieces of these deposits can break off and travel, causing an embolus. An **embolus** is a mass, such as a blood clot or clump, a foreign body, or even air that travels through the bloodstream and lodges in a way that blocks a blood vessel. This embolus may then travel through the circulatory system until it reaches a point at which is too narrow to allow it to move further. When this occurs, the tissue served by the vessel loses its blood supply and can die. If the clot stops the circulation in cardiac tissue, then a myocardial infarction or heart attack occurs. If the clot occurs in an area of the brain, a cerebral vascular accident (a CVA or a stroke) occurs. If the clot obstructs a vessel in the lung, then this pulmonary embolism may cause part of the lung to die and seriously affect the person's ability to breathe. Any of these conditions may even result in the person's death.

The Heart

The heart is a very strong muscle that is approximately the size of your fist. The purpose of the heart is to pump the blood continuously through the blood vessels with enough force to circulate the blood throughout the body so that each and every cell is nourished and its wastes removed.

The heart is the pump that sends blood through the two circuits that make up the cardiovascular system. These are the pulmonary circuit and the systemic circuit.

The pulmonary circuit includes the heart and lungs. Its purpose is to carry deoxygenated blood from the heart to the lungs to be replenished with oxygen.

The systemic circuit carries oxygenated blood around the body in the arteries to nourish the body. It also returns the deoxygenated blood to the heart through the veins.

In the pulmonary circuit, the blood enters the right atrium of the heart through the superior vena cava. The right atrium contracts and pushes the blood through the tricuspid valve into the right ventricle. The right ventricle then contracts and pushes the blood through the pulmonary valve into the pulmonary artery, which brings it to the lungs. In the lungs the blood cells exchange carbon dioxide for oxygen. This oxygenated blood returns to the heart by way of the pulmonary vein and enters the left atrium.

The left atrium contracts and pumps the blood through the mitral valve into the left ventricle. Then, the left ventricle contracts and pushes the blood into the aorta. At this point, the blood enters the systemic circuit. The aorta branches off into several different arteries that pump the oxygenated blood to various parts of the body. Figures 17-12a and 17-12b illustrates the path of these circuits.

a) Pulmonary Circuit

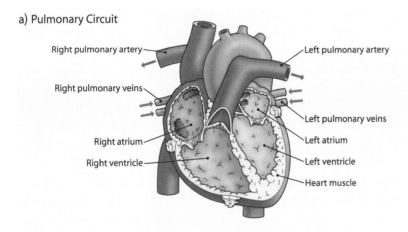

Right pulmonary artery

Left pulmonary artery

Right pulmonary veins

Left pulmonary veins

Left atrium

Right atrium

Left ventricle

Right ventricle

Heart muscle

FIGURE 17-12A
Pulmonary circuit
Source: SEER

b) Systemic Circuit

Head and arms

Superior vena cava

Aorta

Inferior vena cava

Abdomen and legs

FIGURE 17-12B
Systemic Circuit
Source: SEER

The Immune System and the Lymphatic System

STOP AND REFLECT ((17-1))

Have you ever had an infected cut? Perhaps you noticed that the area around the cut was swollen and red. You might even have had some whitish discharge from the cut. These things—the swelling, redness, heat, and discharge—are signs that your immune system is fighting a foreign invader.

The immune system is made up of the circulatory system and the lymphatic system. The purpose of the immune system is to recognize and resist specific foreign substances or the toxins they release. The immune system protects the body from disease and infection whether the threat is internal or external. By recognizing any abnormal and unwanted invaders, specific antibodies are then produced that attack these invaders. The lymphatic system is sometimes called the lymphatic network. The lymphatic system and immune system are actually subsystems of the circulatory system.

The lymphatic system is a one-way system of blind-ended microscopic vessels that originate in the interstitial tissues of the body. These vessels run parallel to the venous circulation and become larger as they move toward the heart, the fluid collected in these vessels re-entering the blood circulation at the subclavian veins just before the blood enters the heart.

The lymphatic system includes the lymph vessels, the lymph nodes, the lymph fluid, the spleen, the thymus gland, the tonsils, and some tissue in the intestinal tract. Figure 17-13 illustrates this system.

There are two main functions of the lymphatic system. The first is to defend the body against internal and external infections by draining lymph fluid through nodes to remove contaminants. The second purpose is to maintain the fluid balance of the body's internal environment by draining excess interstitial fluids from large areas of the body and returning these cleansed fluids to the blood stream. By this method, edema is prevented or reduced.

The lymph is a straw-coloured fluid composed of the fluid collected from the interstitial spaces and from the intestines. The lymph vessels are similar to the veins in structure with semi-lunar valves that help to prevent the backflow of the lymph fluid as it returns to the heart. The lymph vessels also run through muscle tissue that, when it contracts, exerts pressure, also assisting the movement of the lymph upward toward the heart.

The lymph nodes are oval, encapsulated filters that are found throughout the body distributed along the pathways of the lymph vessel, their function being to filter out the pathogens collected by the lymph from the interstitial spaces and intestines of the body.

The thymus is the central organ of the lymph system and is located in the thorax (as shown in Figure 17-13), its main function being to produce T cells that attack pathogens.

The spleen is located in the left upper quadrant of the abdomen and also filters out microorganisms. It stores blood and destroys worn-out red blood cells and platelets.

Figure 17-13 illustrates the lymphatic system. Figure 17-14 illustrates how white blood cells destroy harmful viruses and create antibodies.

FIGURE 17-13
The lymphatic system

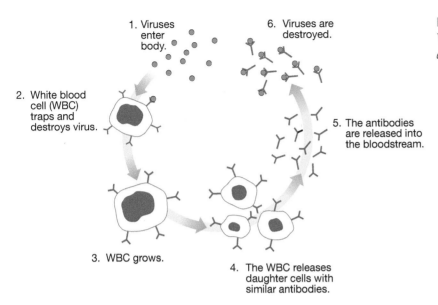

1. Viruses enter body.

2. White blood cell (WBC) traps and destroys virus.

3. WBC grows.

4. The WBC releases daughter cells with similar antibodies.

5. The antibodies are released into the bloodstream.

6. Viruses are destroyed.

FIGURE 17-14
White blood cells destroy viruses

Sometimes, the immune system attempts to defend the body against invaders that are not really harmful. We say that a person has an allergy when the person's body misidentifies a usually harmless substance and attempts to defend the body against it. The runny nose, watery eyes, and sneezing that some people get when they are near dogs or cats is a common example of an allergy. More severe forms of misidentification can cause a person's body to attack vital organs, as is the case in conditions like Guillain-Barre Syndrome.

Sometimes autoimmune reactions can occur. This is when the immune system malfunctions and reacts to the body's natural tissues and, thinking that these are unwanted foreign invaders, attacks them. Examples of this type of condition are diseases such as rheumatoid arthritis, lupus, and Grave's disease. Many researchers now feel that multiple sclerosis may occur when the body attacks the myelin sheath.

The Digestive System

The purpose of the digestive, or gastrointestinal, system is to break down food (physically and chemically) so that the body may use the nutrients from these foods and to eliminate the wastes the body does not use. This process is called digestion. The digestive system of an average person will process between 29 000 and 60 000 kg of food over a lifetime.

The digestive system contains many organs such as the tongue, salivary glands, pharynx, teeth, esophagus, stomach, small intestine, liver, pancreas, gall bladder, large intestine, anus, and rectum. The structure that is formed by all these organs linked together is called the alimentary canal. These organs are usually made up of layers of smooth muscle and are capable of churning the food. The **alimentary canal** is about 8 m long, beginning at the mouth and ending at the anus. Figure 17-15 illustrates the alimentary canal. It is also called the gastrointestinal tract.

Digestion is a process that can actually begin before you start to eat. Has your mouth ever watered when you were thinking of your favourite food? Your digestive system is actually beginning to work in preparation for eating. Saliva in the mouth flows in anticipation of having food to break down.

At the first bite, food is broken or ground into tiny bits by the teeth. The lining of the mouth helps to cool food to a temperature that makes it easy to swallow. The

FIGURE 17-15
The alimentary canal

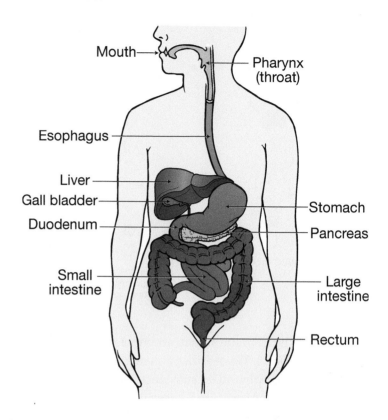

muscles of the cheeks help to mix the saliva, moistening the food, making it easier to continue the process down the canal.

Figure 17-16 shows the major structures used in swallowing. A structure called the epiglottis automatically covers the trachea (windpipe) so that the person does not inhale the food. Sometimes, when a person tries to swallow too fast, the epiglottis cannot close quickly enough and some food enters the trachea and goes into the lungs. You've probably had the experience of food "going down the wrong way." When this happens, you cough, forcing the food back up into the mouth where it can be properly swallowed.

FIGURE 17-16
The structures involved in swallowing

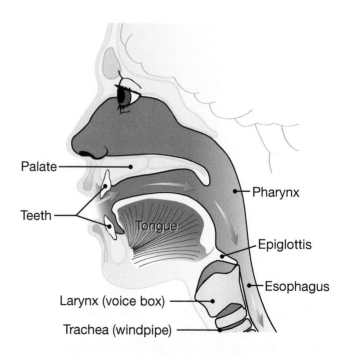

Food moves down the esophagus into the stomach through a process called peristalsis. It takes only a few seconds to move food from your mouth to your stomach. Once in the stomach, the food is churned and tossed to mix with digestive acids and enzymes. These juices help to kill any harmful bacteria and continue to break down the food into nutrients the body can use. Carbohydrates are the easiest substances to break down and pass through the stomach first. Proteins and fats are harder to break down, so they remain in the stomach longer. This is one reason why most of us eat salad (comprised mostly of water and carbohydrates) before we eat other foods (which are usually higher in protein and fats) at a meal.

Material broken down in the stomach passes through a sphincter muscle into the start of the small intestine (duodenum). The sphincter opens and closes, allowing a small amount of matter to pass into the small intestine so that digestion may continue at a rate the body can use effectively.

The small intestine is the longest part of the alimentary canal. In the average adult, it is about 6.4 m long and is divided into three main parts, the duodenum, the jejunum, and the ileum.

The pancreas secretes insulin into the blood stream. Insulin controls carbohydrate metabolism, maintaining the blood sugar within normal limits whenever possible. The liver produces and excretes bile; the gall bladder stores the bile until it is required for the emulsification and easier digestion of fats. Bile is excreted directly into the duodenum. The food continues along the small intestine that is lined by villi—small finger-like projections that substantially increase the absorptive surface of the small intestine. These thousands of villi have a large blood supply that absorbs the available nutrients from the small intestine, immediately circulating these to the cells throughout the body.

Indigestible components of food then pass into the large intestine, or colon, that runs from the cecum in the lower right quadrant of the abdomen, up the right side of the abdomen, across the abdomen just under the diaphragm and goes down the left side, terminating in the rectum. In this part of the digestive system, residual water is returned to the body and the waste is stored in the rectum until defecation takes place. The external sphincter that releases the stool is called the anus.

The Respiratory System

The respiratory system consists of the lungs, the sinuses, the trachea, the bronchi, the bronchioles, and the alveoli. The lungs are housed within the thoracic cavity, between the diaphragm and the shoulders, and encased by the rib cage. There are two lungs, one on each side of the trachea. The right lung has three lobes, the left only two lobes as the heart also shares this space. The trachea branches into the right and left bronchi. These, in turn, branch into bronchioles and, finally, end in the alveoli sacs. Figure 17-17 illustrates the major components of the respiratory system.

The lungs are responsible for the work of *respiration*: the exchange of oxygen for carbon dioxide. The mechanics of respiration are as follows. The respiratory centre in the brain signals the diaphragm to contract downward, and the intercostal muscles to contract, pulling the rib cage outward and thus expanding the thoracic cavity. Then, since the pressure within the lungs is less than the atmospheric pressure outside, air rushes in to fill the lungs.

When the pressure equalizes, the lungs recoil and we breathe out the waste carbon dioxide. The walls of the alveoli sacs, through which this exchange is made, are

FIGURE 17-17
*Major structures of the
respiratory system*

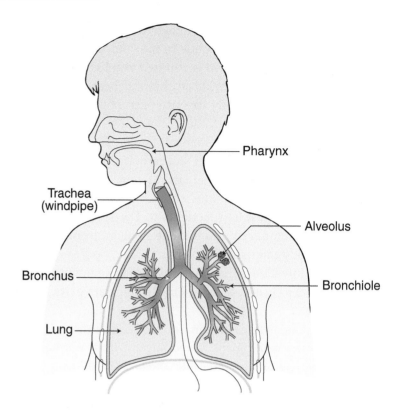

surrounded by tiny blood vessels (capillaries). These vessels contain blood cells laden with carbon dioxide that are returning from the body. This carbon dioxide is then passed through the alveoli cell walls and into the lungs and expelled. The oxygen, which is in the alveoli sacs, passes into the blood stream for circulation throughout the body. Figure 17-18 illustrates this exchange.

FIGURE 17-18
*Gas exchange in the
lungs*

At rest
- Muscles relax
- No air movement

Breathing in
- Muscles contract
- Chest expands
- Diaphragm moves down
- Air is drawn into lungs

Breathing out
- Muscles relax, causing lung recoil
- Diaphragm moves up
- Air moves out of lungs

FIGURE 17-19
The mechanics of breathing

The Urinary System

The urinary system consists of a pair of kidneys, two ureters, a bladder, and a urethra. There are two main functions to the urinary system: to cleanse the blood and to regulate the amount of water and chemical balance in the body. Figure 17-20 illustrates the urinary system.

Kidneys

The kidneys are bean-shaped organs about 13 cm long, which are held in place by connective and adipose tissue and are located on either side of the vertebral column at the level of the twelfth thoracic and third lumbar vertebrae. Each kidney has more than a million tiny filtering nephron units that represent the basic working unit of the kidney.

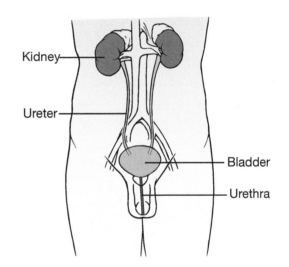

FIGURE 17-20
The urinary system

The ureters connect the kidneys to the bladder. These long slim tubes are about 25 cm in length and by muscular contraction and peristaltic waves pass the urine into the bladder.

The urinary bladder is a hollow, distensible organ that can hold about 500–800 millilitres. The bladder stores the urine until there is an urge to void. In the bladder there are three openings—two for the ureters and one for the urethra.

The urethra allows the urine to flow to the outside. It is shorter in the female than in the male and is controlled by the external sphincter muscle that is voluntarily controlled by a healthy person. When we relax this sphincter, we urinate.

The nephrons in the kidneys have a very rich blood supply that delivers about one quarter of the cardiac output every minute and that, for an adult, equals about 170 litres of fluid daily. As the blood moves through the nephrons, the metabolic wastes are extracted and the remainder of the fluids are returned to the blood stream. In this way the kidneys help to regulate the composition and volume of body fluids to help to maintain vital homeostatic balances.

The Nervous System

The nervous system has been described as the body's switchboard, whose purpose is to transmit messages to and from the various parts of the body. The nervous system is composed of the central nervous system, which includes the brain and the spinal cord, and the peripheral nervous system, which includes all of the nerves outside the central nervous system. The central nervous system is covered by three layers of protective membrane, called meninges. These are called the pia mater, the arachnoid, and the dura mater. To cushion and protect the fragile and vital brain and spinal cord, cerebrospinal fluid flows between the pia mater and the arachnoid meninges. A second protective mechanism for the central nervous system is bone—the skull protects the brain, and the vertebral column protects the spinal cord. Figure 17-21 illustrates the major components of the central nervous system. Figure 17-22 shows the position of the spinal cord in the bony spine.

FIGURE 17-21
The major components of the central nervous system

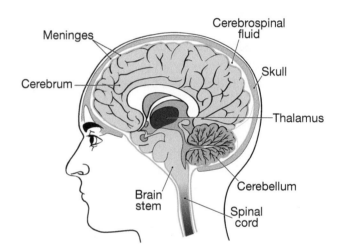

FIGURE 17-22
The spinal cord (cross-section)

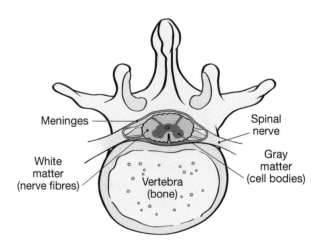

The peripheral nervous system comprises the nerves that emanate from the brain and spinal cord. These nerves have two types of fibres: motor fibres, which control movement, and sensory fibres, which transmit sensory messages of pain, temperature, touch, and vibration. These two types of nerve fibres create the somatic nervous system that is responsible for controlling the body's relationship to the environment by connecting to the skin and muscles.

Another part of the peripheral nervous system is the network of nerves connecting the internal organs. This network is called the autonomic nervous system, as one cannot consciously exert extensive control over it. The brain operates this system through the parasympathetic and the sympathetic nerves. Figure 17-23 shows the peripheral nervous system.

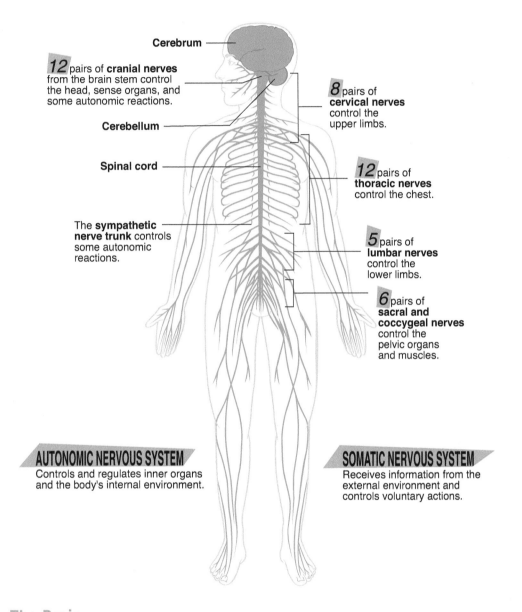

FIGURE 17-23

The peripheral nervous system

Cerebrum

12 pairs of **cranial nerves** from the brain stem control the head, sense organs, and some autonomic reactions.

Cerebellum

Spinal cord

The **sympathetic nerve trunk** controls some autonomic reactions.

8 pairs of **cervical nerves** control the upper limbs.

12 pairs of **thoracic nerves** control the chest.

5 pairs of **lumbar nerves** control the lower limbs.

6 pairs of **sacral and coccygeal nerves** control the pelvic organs and muscles.

AUTONOMIC NERVOUS SYSTEM
Controls and regulates inner organs and the body's internal environment.

SOMATIC NERVOUS SYSTEM
Receives information from the external environment and controls voluntary actions.

The Brain

The brain is the most complex part of the nervous system, and it contains billions of neurons. When you see an image, remember something, or learn a new skill, you are training the neurons in your brain to connect in new ways. Neurons connect without making actual physical contact. Synapse is the term that describes this junction. The connection is completed by a chemical connection, or neurotransmitter, from the axon of one neuron to the dendrite of another neuron. Some of the more familiar neurotransmitters are dopamine, serotonin, and acetylcholine.

As we discussed earlier, neurons cannot be replaced. Because of the number of neurons in the brain and the infinite ways that they can connect, researchers estimate that the capacity of the brain is limitless.

Different areas of the brain control specific functions. We'll discuss the three main areas: the cerebrum, cerebellum, and the brain stem. Figure 17-24 illustrates the major structures of the brain.

FIGURE 17-24

The brain controls all functions that occur within the body, whether voluntary or automatic, motor or sensory

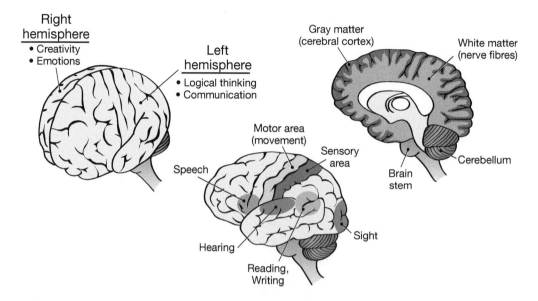

The cerebrum is comprised of two halves, called hemispheres, with nerve fibres connecting them. Each hemisphere is composed of a core of white matter (nerve fibres covered with a protective coating called myelin). A layer of grey matter called the cerebral cortex surrounds this core. The cerebral cortex receives all body sensations and controls all voluntary movements. It is also responsible for the things we call cognitive function, such as learning, judgment, and reasoning. Specific areas of the cerebrum control different functions. For example, the left hemisphere of the brain controls the movements of the right side of the body. Similarly, the right hemisphere controls voluntary movements of the left side of the body. Specific areas in each hemisphere receive sensory impulses.

Some categories of functions are controlled by a specific hemisphere. For example, the right hemisphere is responsible for spatial perception, creativity, emotions, and impulse control, as well as artistic ability and creativity. The left hemisphere is responsible for logical thinking and, for most of us, the use of language in reading, writing, and speaking. (The language centre of some left-handed people may be in the right hemisphere.)

Some functions, such as memory, are probably controlled deep in the brain and likely in more than one area of the brain. Chapter 23 will discuss memory and cognitive ability in greater detail.

The cerebellum sits at the back of the brain near the base. It is responsible for the coordination of movement and plays a significant role in maintaining balance.

The brain stem is found at the top of the spinal column. Special nerve fibres here control such essential functions as heart rate, breathing, and blood pressure.

The Spinal Cord

The spinal cord begins at the base of your brain and extends about two-thirds of the way down your spinal column. Many nerves emanate from this column—some of them more than a metre long, including the nerves that travel down the legs to the feet, allowing for movement and sensation. Similarly, nerves branch out all along the spinal column, controlling sensation and movement throughout the shoulders, arms, and torso.

The Sensory System

The sensory system interprets information from the environment. The eyes see, the ears hear, the tongue responds to various tastes, the nose to various scents and odours, and sensory nerves perceive temperature, texture, pain, and pressure. Without this ability to perceive what is around us, we would certainly fall victim to any number of perils.

The Eye

We are visual creatures. Most of us rely upon our sight to learn, to avoid danger, to help organize our activities (e.g., by colour-coding items), as well as to obtain information from others. Many researchers compare the eye to a camera. Yet, in many ways, the eye is an ultra-sophisticated camera—a natural creation that no technology can yet match.

The eye is a gel-filled organ with an opening at the front (the pupil) and light-sensitive receptors at the back (the retina and the macula). Just in front of the pupil is the cornea, a transparent structure that protects the pupil. Behind the pupil is the lens. Figure 17-25 illustrates the structures of the eye.

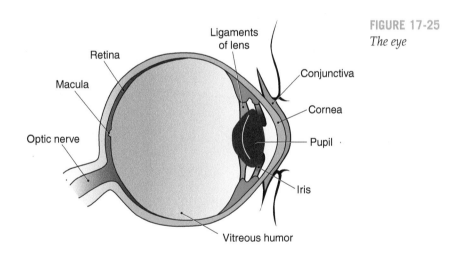

FIGURE 17-25
The eye

In the simplest terms, the eye receives light through the pupil. This light is focused on the back of the eye by the lens. When this image is reflected on the back of the eye, the image is reversed and upside down. The optic nerve receives the electrical impulses from the retina and macula and transmits them to the brain where they are interpreted right side up. Figure 17-26 illustrates this process.

FIGURE 17-26
How the eye "sees"

If a person's retina is too close or far away from the lens, the image on the retina will be out of focus. In this case, a person would wear glasses or contact lenses to correct the problem.

The eye undergoes many changes over the life span. Babies are farsighted and are unable to focus on close objects until they are several months old. The eyesight of a middle-aged person also changes, often requiring the person to use reading glasses to see fine print.

The Ear

The ears perform two major functions. They provide a person's ability to hear and they assist the person in maintaining balance. There are three areas in the ear: the inner ear, the middle ear, and the outer ear. Figure 17-27 shows the major components of the ear. Each has specific functions.

The outer ear collects sound waves and channels them to the eardrum. The eardrum vibrates as these sound waves pound against it.

FIGURE 17-27
The ear

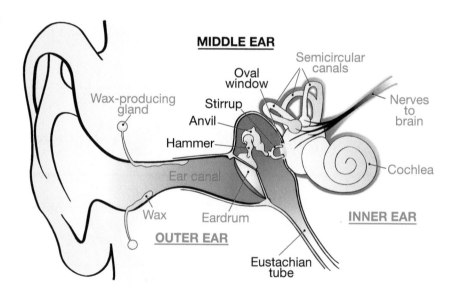

The shape of the external ear structure is designed specifically to collect sounds. Without it, a person would not hear well. You can test the effect of the shape of the external structure by cupping your hand behind one of your ears. Notice how sounds seem to sound different?

The outer ear also has a protective function. The ear produces earwax, which, along with thousands of tiny hairs in the canal, helps to trap dirt and other particles before they reach the eardrum.

The middle ear is responsible for concentrating the vibrations received from the outer ear via the eardrum (tympanic membrane). Within this structure are three bones: the hammer (malleus), the anvil (incus), and the stirrup (stapes) (these bones are named for their shapes). Each bone vibrates when sound waves vibrate the eardrum. These structures are linked to carry and concentrate that sound to the oval window. Also a part of the middle ear is the eustachian tube that leads to the throat. This tube opens when a person yawns or swallows and helps to equalize the pressure on both sides of the eardrum.

The inner ear contains the cochlea, a snail-shaped structure that contains the receptor cells for hearing. When sound vibrations reach the cochlea through the oval window, thousands of nerve cells (that look much like tiny hairs) vibrate, converting the physical movement into electrical impulses that are then transmitted to the brain by the acoustic nerve.

The inner ear also contains the semicircular canals that are fluid-filled structures with receptor cells that report your position to the brain. Because these canals contain fluid, rapid movement (such as spinning or turning one's head suddenly) can cause a person to become dizzy because the fluid doesn't stop moving as quickly as the body does.

The Nose

A human's sense of smell is useful in identifying objects (such as whether a paper bag contains cookies) as well as determining whether danger is present (as in sniffing for the scent of natural gas). Our sense of smell is closely linked to memories—the smell of a favourite food may bring a flood of memories of the meals associated with it.

The nose is the primary organ of scent. It contains olfactory receptor cells that are surrounded by mucus. The mucus traps airborne chemical particles, and these particles stimulate the olfactory receptor cells. The receptor cells then send an electrical message to the brain by way of the olfactory bulb, which is a structure containing nerve cells.

The Tongue

The tongue is the organ that transmits the sensation of taste. The tongue contains thousands of taste buds. These buds contain receptor cells that are sensitive to chemicals that are emitted from substances we chew or swallow. Though there are four main categories of taste—salty, sour, sweet, and bitter—they can be combined in almost limitless ways to form unique taste blends. Some researchers have proposed a fifth "taste"—umami. Umami seems to respond to amino acids (or proteins) and may help us to ensure that we eat enough protein. Specific areas on the tongue are more receptive to different tastes. Figure 17-28 shows these locations.

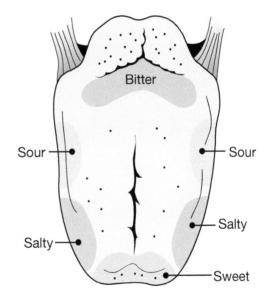

FIGURE 17-28
Taste sensitivity of the tongue

Many things can affect a person's ability to sense tastes. An illness or a medication may coat the tongue, making it harder for the taste chemicals to reach the receptor cells. The number and sensitivity of taste buds declines with age—a fact that may make it more difficult for older people to enjoy foods as they once did.

The senses of taste and smell work closely together. It's often hard to tell which is which. As you've probably realized, when you have a stuffy nose, food doesn't taste the same. This is because some of what your brain thinks is a taste sensation is actually a scent sensation.

The Endocrine System

The purpose of the endocrine system is to regulate many of your body's processes. This system comprises a number of ductless glands, as Figure 17-29 illustrates. Each gland secretes hormones of varying types directly into body fluids. These chemicals help to regulate such metabolic processes as reproduction, growth and development, body defences, electrolytes, water and nutrient blood balances, cell metabolism, and energy balance.

FIGURE 17-29
The endocrine system

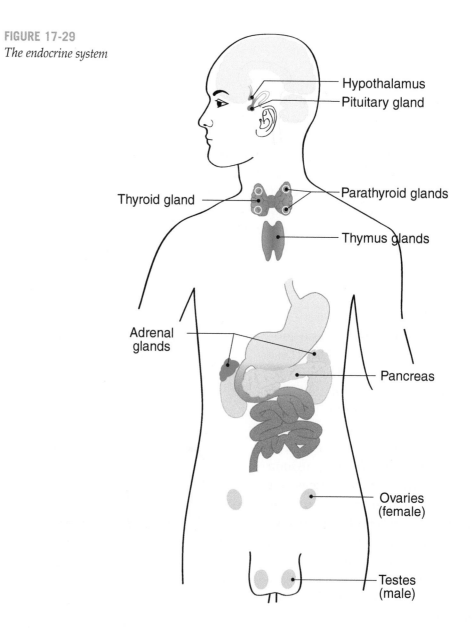

Two glands have tasks of particular importance. The hypothalamus controls the sensations of hunger, thirst, fatigue, and wakefulness. It also helps to maintain homeostasis by regulating many of the involuntary functions of the body such as heart rate, arterial pressure, temperature, and regulation of water and electrolyte balance. The function of the pituitary gland, which is often referred to as the "master gland," is to secrete hormones that interact with and regulate other glands. These include the growth hormone and hormones that affect the thyroid and adrenal glands.

The pancreas secretes insulin, which regulates the amount of sugar in the bloodstream. Insufficient amounts of insulin may lead to diabetes, a condition in which blood sugar rises to dangerous levels.

The Reproductive System

The purpose of the reproductive system is procreation. Unlike all other systems, the structures of this system are different in the male and female.

The Male Reproductive System

The male reproductive system contains two primary (major) organs: the testes and the penis. Figure 17-30 illustrates the organs of the male reproductive system.

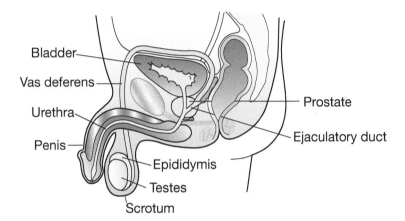

FIGURE 17-30
The male reproductive system

There are two testes that produce sperm, which contains the cells that carry the male's chromosomes and other glandular secretions such as testosterone. Testosterone is responsible for the development and maintenance of secondary male characteristics such as the distribution of body hair and the development of some of the male physical characteristics. The testes are contained in a sac called the scrotum, located at the base of the penis. The scrotum contains smooth muscle tissue that is capable of lengthening or shortening the distance between the testes and the body so as to maintain the correct temperature for the testes to ensure the viability of the sperm.

The penis has two functions: to provide a vessel for sperm to leave the body and to provide a vessel for urine to leave the body. During sexual arousal, the penis becomes rigid with blood, and the opening from the bladder to the urethra closes, allowing only semen to travel down the urethra. This therefore means that a male cannot urinate when sexually aroused.

The Female Reproductive System

The female reproductive system includes the ovaries and the uterus. Figure 17-31 illustrates the major components of the female reproductive system.

The ovaries produce eggs or ova, which contain the female's chromosomes. The uterus provides a host for a fertilized egg. Unlike males, who release sperm at various intervals, the female releases an egg approximately once every 28 days. This is called ovulation and is a part of the menstrual cycle. The uterus develops a blood-rich lining in preparation for nourishing a fertilized egg. If a male's sperm fertilizes the egg, the egg will implant itself into this lining and develop into an embryo.

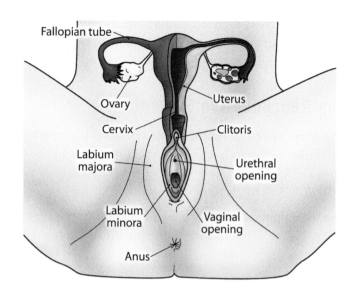

FIGURE 17-31

The female reproductive system

If the egg is not fertilized, or for some reason does not implant in the lining, both the egg and the lining are "sloughed off" from the uterus and out through the vagina. This is called the menstrual period.

AGE-RELATED CHANGES

STOP AND REFLECT ((17-2))

When you think of the phrase "old person," what are some of the characteristics that come to mind?

_____

_____

_____

_____

_____   ■

The body does change as we grow older. The changes that are part of the aging process and that will happen to everyone if they live long enough are called **age-related changes**. However, many of the changes we think are age-related are more likely caused by a lack of proper care of one's body, disease, or other impairment. Look over your answers to Stop and Reflect 17-2. Compare your answers to those in Table 17-2 on page 305.

Each person will experience age-related changes at different times. As well, the effect of any age-related change is often a function of the person's overall fitness level. The person who is extremely physically fit as an older person may be as physically able as a much younger person, even though the older person does not have the ability he or she once did.

TABLE 17-2	Age or Not?
Age-Related Changes	**Changes Caused by Other Factors**
Grey or white hair	Hair loss (inherited or disease)
Decreased elasticity of skin	Excessive wrinkles (exposure to sun, inherited, smoking)
Decreased muscle mass	Arthritis (injury or disease)
Decreased cardiac output	Heart disease
Increased time required to react	Dementia
Decreased ability to hear high frequencies	Decreased ability to hear sound in general (disease, injury, abuse)

Questions for Review

1. What are the four types of tissue? Where is each found?

2. What four functions are performed by the circulatory system?

3. What is the purpose of bone marrow?

4. What organs make up the alimentary canal?

5. What organs make up the sensory system?

6. What are the four types of bones? For each, state its purpose and give an example of the type.

7. What is the function of the urinary system?

8. What do joints allow the body to do?

Question for Discussion

1. Select an older person you know well. How has aging affected his or her ability? Does the person assume that some things are caused by old age? If so, what?

Chapter 18

Mobility

Learning Objectives

Through reading this chapter, you'll be able to

1. Identify three benefits of supporting a client's mobility.
2. Explain the differences between moving objects and assisting people to move.
3. Define and demonstrate good body mechanics and good posture.
4. List the four principles of good positioning.
5. Distinguish between a transfer and a lift.
6. Outline the twelve principles to be used when preparing to assist a client to move from one place to another.
7. Demonstrate the proper procedure for assisting a person to transfer and to pivot and transfer.
8. Identify the principles involved in safely using a mechanical lift to move a client.
9. Describe the eight guidelines when assisting a client with range of motion exercises.
10. List the five main purposes of mobility aids.
11. Describe the proper procedure for walking with a cane, crutches, walker, and rollator.
12. Describe the three general guidelines for assisting a person who is falling.
13. Describe the seven general guidelines for assisting a person who has fallen.

Chapter at a Glance

- Mobility
- Assisting People with Movement
- Good Body Mechanics
- Common Types of Assistance
- Range of Motion Exercises
- Mobility Aids
- Falls

Terms You'll Use

Abduction Moving an arm or leg away from the centre of the body.
Active Range of Motion Exercise Movement completed by the client.
Adduction Moving an arm or leg toward the centre of the body.
Alignment The positioning of the body along a straight line.

Base of Support　That part of the body that is in contact with the supporting surface—the weight-bearing surface most often defined by the position of your feet.

Centre of Gravity　The point where mass is equally distributed.

Contracture　A tightening of muscle, tendons, ligaments or skin that prevents normal movement.

Extension　Straightening the joint.

Flexion　Bending the joint.

Good Body Mechanics　Using your body in a safe and efficient manner to avoid injury and/or repetitive strain.

Lateral　Lying on your side; also refers to body parts away from the midline.

Line of Gravity　The imaginary line in the middle of your body mass where each side is equally balanced.

Mobility Aids　Aids that are designed to improve a person's stability by expanding his or her base of support.

Passive Range of Motion Exercise　Movement done for the client by the caregiver.

Posture　The alignment of the different parts of the body as we change position.

Prone　Lying on your stomach.

Range of Motion　The normal movement a joint can progress through comfortably and safely.

Supine　Lying on your back.

MOBILITY

STOP AND REFLECT ((18-1))

Think back over this past hour. How many times have you physically moved? Perhaps you've gotten up to get a drink or to answer the phone. Maybe you've shifted in your chair to get more comfortable or decided to stretch out on the couch for a bit.

_____

_____

_____

_____ ■

Chances are that you moved frequently in that hour. Why? To meet a need, to become more comfortable, perhaps to take a few minutes to talk to someone. Now, imagine that you could not move independently. How do you think you might feel? Frustrated? Angry? Probably so. It's quite likely that your client, if faced with a reduction in his or her mobility, will have some of the same emotions.

There are physical, social, and psychological benefits to mobility.

Physical Benefits

Mobility promotes improved musculoskeletal strength, circulation, and breathing, which are linked to increased resistance to illness and infection. It helps to maintain muscle mass and muscle tone, as well as overall fitness. Mobility can help to eliminate constipation. It can provide the person with the opportunity to "keep in practice" with walking and other movement, thereby reducing the risk of falls.

Improved mobility can also reduce secondary effects. These are problems that arise because a person cannot easily get from one place to another, such as incontinence due to not being able to get to the bathroom in time.

Social Benefits

Mobility helps us to get out, to see others, to have the opportunity to interact and maintain social skills. It broadens our range of activities.

Psychological Benefits

The satisfaction that comes from being able to go where one wants to go and to move about at will for comfort cannot be underestimated. Mobility supports the client's control over his or her activities and, in turn, promotes a sense of self-worth and confidence. There is evidence that mobility promotes improved cognition. Physical activity can help to reduce feelings of sadness and has been found to elevate the mood of clients with depression.

ASSISTING PEOPLE WITH MOVEMENT

Assisting a person with movement differs from moving an inanimate object. While the principles of good posture and body mechanics are the same, helping a person to move adds two further dimensions to the assistance: the psychological and the physiological.

The Psychological Dimension

Have you ever been afraid of falling or losing your balance? Perhaps you were up on a ladder or step stool. Maybe you were taking your first few steps after you'd been in bed with the flu. If you've been in one of these situations, you can appreciate the psychological dimension of movement. Uncertainty, fear, anxiety, as well as the effect of a previous experience all can affect how we approach movement.

The client who requires assistance with movement may experience many of the same emotions. There are a number of factors that contribute to the psychological dimension:

1. The client may experience emotions associated with having to rely upon another person for help or associated with not knowing how the person helping him or her will assist.
2. The client's desire to move will also affect how he or she responds to assistance.
3. The client's culture may affect the level of comfort she or he has about being touched or about having another person so physically close.
4. Changes in thinking and understanding (such as those associated with stress or with dementia) can heighten anxiety and fear.

CASE EXAMPLE 18-1

The following is the personal experience of a client.

I had not been on my feet since the accident. I was finally allowed to get up [with help] to go to the bathroom. An attendant came to assist me.

My first sensation was of being swept off my feet. I had just begun to try to stand when I was almost lifted by the attendant. I had no time to right myself and became quite dizzy. I found myself leaning on her as she carted me to the bathroom.

The same attendant helped me back to bed. I was a bit stronger that time, yet I still had the sensation of having no control over my movement. I simply hoped that she wouldn't drop me.

The next time I needed to use the bathroom, I crawled there myself.

How would you feel if you were this client? What could the attendant have done differently to provide better assistance?

The Physiological Dimension

This dimension has to do with the client's functioning, the actual degree of control over his or her movement, including strength and endurance, range of motion, ability to bear weight, and balance. There are many factors to be considered in assessing a person's physiological dimension. How much can the client do? What accommodation does the person have to make to address the impairment? Are there contributing physiological factors such as vision or hearing impairment that make it more difficult for the person to follow instruction or assist? Does the client have balance problems that may make it difficult for him or her to remain in one place?

GOOD BODY MECHANICS

Good body mechanics means using your body effectively and in a manner that preserves its physical health. Good body mechanics include proper posture, or alignment, and safe movement.

Good body mechanics are important for both you and your client. They keep you balanced, provide additional stability, and allow you to move about with minimal effort. You should use good body mechanics at all times: sitting, standing, or lying down.

Body mechanics involve maintaining a *line of gravity*, a *base of support*, a *balanced centre of gravity*, as well as the proper use of *leverage*.

Line of Gravity

The line of gravity is the imaginary line that is exactly in the middle of your body mass where each "side" is equally balanced. When you are standing upright, the line passes from your head to your feet. It runs vertically, midway between the front and back of your torso and midway between your shoulders. As the line progresses toward your feet, it passes in front of the centre of your hipbones, in front of your knees and ankles. Figure 18-1 illustrates the line of gravity in a person with good posture.

Good posture is a part of good health. Proper posture maintains the natural curvature of the spine. A person whose mass is not distributed evenly may experience

Line of Gravity

Mid shoulder

Mid torso

In front of
hip bones

In front of knee

In front of ankle

FIGURE 18-1
Good posture

pain and fatigue, as well as risk joint or disc damage. Specifically, poor posture puts your back at risk for injury.

Many of us develop poor posture over a long period of time. The bad habits develop so slowly that our poor posture may feel comfortable. Muscles and ligaments that have stretched or shortened as a result of our body being out of alignment may ache when we correct our posture. It's important to work at attaining and maintaining good posture, even though it will take some time for the correct posture to feel right.

Common examples of poor posture include:

- Asymmetrical body—shoulders, hips, knees are not level
- Flat back—lumbar curve is decreased
- Lordotic back—lumbar curve is increased
- Round shoulders

Good posture is essential in the prevention of back injury.

STOP AND REFLECT ((18-2))

Stand up, keeping your posture as you normally would. Is your body weight equally distributed along the line of gravity? If not, where is your weight unequally distributed?

_____

_____

_____ ▪

Base of Support

STOP AND REFLECT ((18-3))

1. Stand up, placing your feet approximately 30 cm apart (roughly the width of your hips).
2. Sway your body gently from side to side, noticing how stable you feel.
3. Move your feet closer together and sway gently. Do you feel more or less stable than you did when your feet were further apart?
4. Leaving your feet 30 cm apart, rise up on your toes. How stable do you feel?
5. Stand on one foot. How stable do you feel? Stand up with feet close together and shut your eyes. How stable do you feel?

_____

_____

_____

_____ ▪

Chances are that you felt more stable when your feet were flat and 30 cm apart—when you had a wider base of support. A **base of support** is the area upon which an object rests. Generally, the larger the base of support, the more stable the object (Photo 18-1).

Have you ever tried to balance a quarter on its edge? It's very difficult to do because the base of support (the edge that the coin is resting on) is very small. It's much easier for the quarter to rest on its face since the base of support is much wider.

You may have noticed that you felt unstable when you closed your eyes. It's likely that your body started to sway in an effort to maintain your balance. Without the visual input, it's harder for you to maintain balance. This exercise illustrates the importance of other body systems in the maintenance of balance.

Centre of Gravity

The **centre of gravity** is the point where your mass (vertical and horizontal) is equally distributed; it is also the point where all the weight of the object is concentrated. Both your physical mass and the mass of any person or object you are supporting must be included. For example, carrying a heavy backpack on your shoulders moves your centre of gravity toward your back and up to your shoulders.

No matter what you are carrying, your centre of gravity should be between your shoulders and your knees, as close to your line of gravity as is possible. Remember that the higher your centre of gravity (i.e., the closer it is to your shoulders), the harder it will be to maintain your balance.

The centre of gravity is very important in relation to stability. As long as the centre of gravity is directly above some point within the area of support, the system will be stable; if the centre of gravity is outside the base, the object will fall over.

Leverage

Leverage refers to making the most of the effort you expend. In the context of good body mechanics, leverage means two things. First, it means making the larger, stronger muscles (such as those found in the shoulders, upper arms, hips, and thighs) do the work. This allows you to expend less energy to perform a task and to ensure that you are not straining smaller and weaker muscles (such as those in your back or lower arms). Second, it also means keeping the weight closer to the body to reduce the resistance of the weight. When you hold a weight far away from the body, you increase the resistance, making your muscles work harder (Figure 18-2).

Photo 18-1
A good base of support increases stability and safety.
Source: CHATS

FIGURE 18-2
Holding the object closer reduces resistance and the effort required to move it.

Maintaining Good Body Mechanics

Maintaining good body mechanics is a matter of adopting a few simple work habits.

Arranging Your Work

1. **Avoid unnecessary bending and reaching.** If you can, move items that are frequently used from top or bottom shelves to middle shelves, use a good footstool to reach higher items, and sit or crouch down to reach lower items. If you are assisting a person in bed, raise the bed height, if possible, as close as possible to your waist.
2. **Arrange your supplies to avoid excessive twisting and turning.** Put all the supplies in one location. Move your feet to turn your whole body in the direction of your movement.
3. **Position your body to face what you're doing.** This reduces the amount of twisting.

When Moving Objects

1. **Make sure that your body is well aligned.** Fixate your trunk, by contracting your abdominal and buttock muscles and tucking your chin in. This minimizes excessive stress on a body part, maintains the natural curvature of the spine, and helps keep your centre of gravity close to your line of gravity.
2. **Keep your feet approximately 30 cm apart (hip width).** This ensures a good base of support.
3. **Bend your knees to bring your centre of gravity down.** This increases your stability and decreases the resistance of the load.
4. **Use the larger and stronger muscles to lift, carry, or move.** Bend from the knees, not the waist. If you are lifting heavy objects from the floor, bend your hips and knees. Maintain the natural curve of your back. As you raise the object, straighten your hips and knees. This allows you to use your leg and thigh muscles to bear the weight.
5. **Keep objects close to your body.** This keeps your centre of gravity closer to your line of gravity, enhancing your stability.
6. **Use both hands to carry a heavy object.**
7. **Push, pull, or slide a heavy object if possible.** These actions use less effort than lifting. A rug placed under an object may make it easier to slide and may protect the surface on which you're sliding the object.
8. **When pushing an item, move one leg forward.** When pulling, move one leg back.
9. **Use available aids.** Is there a dolly or trolley available for toting larger items? If so, consider using it to carry heavy or awkward items.
10. **Enlist the help of a co-worker if the load is too heavy.**

CASE EXAMPLE 18-2

Nita is a support worker assigned to assist ten clients in a supportive housing unit. One of her many regular tasks is to prepare meals. In order to avoid unnecessary twisting and bending, Nita assembles all the materials required for the meal and places the items on the counter where she is working. In addition to avoiding injury, this approach often saves Nita time. She can then spend more time working with her clients.

Twelve Principles to Follow When Helping a Person to Move

Cooperation is the key to safety.

1. **Make sure that the person knows who you are.** Tell the client who you are and what your role is. Make certain that you allow the person time to recognize you, if necessary.

2. **Make sure that you know the person's level of ability with regard to the movement.** Can the person help? If so, how? Are there issues such as poor balance, poor muscle strength, or lack of range of motion that have to be accommodated? Are there other impairments (such as vision or hearing loss) that affect the person's ability to follow instructions or assist?

3. **Make sure you have help if the person cannot assist.** The client may have equipment (such as a mechanical lift) that enables you to assist him or her. Some clients may require the assistance of two persons. Make sure that you have the proper help.

4. **Explain what you are going to do.** Does the person have a particular way of doing this activity? Can you use the person's technique safely?

5. **Identify the psychological dimension.** Is the person motivated to help? Is he or she fearful or anxious?

6. **Enlist the person's help.** The task will be much easier if you both work together. Plan the task with the client, if possible.

7. **Make sure that you assist the client, not perform the movement for the client.** Too much assistance will foster dependency and perhaps hostility.

8. **Perform the transfer with smooth, even movements.**

9. **Ensure the person's privacy.** Secure clothing so that it does not fall open during the transfer.

10. **Make sure that any catheters, drainage bags, or intravenous lines are moved with the client.** Take care to ensure that any tubing does not get caught on furnishings and that the lines are not kinked.

11. **Ensure that the client has proper shoes.** The best footwear provides a good firm sole that is neither too slippery nor sticky. Avoid flat slippers.

12. **Make sure you know how to safely use any assistive devices the client requires.** Ask your supervisor for guidance if you are unsure of how to use a particular assistive device.

CASE EXAMPLE 18-3

Rebecca assists Mr. Hament, an 80-year-old resident in a long-term care facility. A few years ago, he had a stroke. As a result, he is unable to walk or stand. In addition, he does not hear well and cannot see without his glasses.

When she first started to work with Mr. Hament, Rebecca talked with him about how she could best help him to transfer. She learned what type of help Mr.

Hament needed and was able to adapt her approach to safely assist him. Even so, each time she assists him, Rebecca must make sure that Mr. Hament has his glasses and is able to see her. She must also make sure that Mr. Hament can hear her and understand what she is going to do so that the transfer goes smoothly.

How do the techniques Rebecca uses relate to the physical and psychological dimensions of a transfer?

COMMON TYPES OF ASSISTANCE

There are three general types of assistance with body position and mobility: positioning, moving a person in bed, and transferring or lifting a person from one place to another. Let's take a look at each type in detail.

Positioning

Have you ever fallen asleep in a chair or couch in an awkward position? Chances are that some of your joints and muscles ached when you awoke. This is due to the poor position in which you slept.

Proper positioning (good alignment) is as important to the client as it is to you. There are three reasons why positioning is important. One, proper positioning is essential to body functions such as respiration and circulation. Two, it prevents excess discomfort in joints and muscles. Three, proper positioning can prevent injuries, such as pressure sores (decubitus ulcers) or contractures (a tightening of muscle, tendons, ligaments or skin that prevents normal movement).

There are five common types of positioning for the client who is in bed. These are: Fowler's position, Sims' position, lateral position, prone position, and supine position. Your client may prefer a particular position or may alternate between two or more. A health professional may have prescribed a particular position or advised the client to avoid a particular position. Make sure that you know of any preferences or restrictions before you assist the client. No matter what the position, take care to ensure your client's comfort.

Proper positioning often requires the use of pillows, rolled towels, or positioning aids (such as foam wedges or bolsters). Some positioning devices have a distinct right or left orientation. Make sure you know how these items are used and where they are to be placed.

Fowler's Position

Fowler's position is a semisitting position. It is often used to make it easier for a person in bed to eat, watch television, or visit with other people. It is also used to make it easier for people with heart or respiratory disorders to breathe.

This position raises the back, neck, and head at a 45° to 60° angle. It's important to raise the head of the bed as much as the client can tolerate if they are eating in bed. A 75° angle may be preferable. If the client has an adjustable bed, raising the head of the bed usually does this. If the client's bed is not adjustable, a wedge bolster is often used.

No matter how the angle is attained, it is important to maintain the natural curvature of the client's spine. Many clients will also require a pillow to support their head and, possibly, pillows at each side to support their arms. Your client (or a family member or health professional) may give you instructions as to where any other pillows or supports must be placed. Photo 18-2 shows a person in Fowler's position.

Clients in Fowler's position will tend to slide down in the bed. As well, the client may experience shearing, a condition that occurs when the client's skin remains in place while the client's muscles and bones move in the direction of gravity. This can make the hips and buttocks very sore and can lead to skin breakdown. Figure 18-3 illustrates shearing. You must watch for this and assist the client to reposition as necessary.

Photo 18-2
A person in Fowler's position

FIGURE 18-3
Shearing

Lateral Position

Many people prefer to rest on their sides (laterally). Proper support in the **lateral** position includes placing pillows under the client's head, under the forearm of the upper arm, and under the knee of the upper leg. A pillow is placed behind the client to assist him or her to remain in position. Photo 18-3 shows a client in the lateral position.

Photo 18-3
A client in the lateral position

Sims' Position

In Sims' position, a client is lying on his or her side. The client's upper leg is flexed (bent) so that it is not lying on the lower leg. A pillow supports the leg. The upper arm is also flexed and is placed on a pillow. The lower arm and leg are slightly bent and not supported by a pillow. The client's head is to the side. Photo 18-4 illustrates a client in Sims' position.

Photo 18-4
A client in Sims' position

Prone Position

Prone means lying on one's stomach. A client in the prone position lies on his or her stomach with his or her head turned to one side. To ensure good alignment of the spine, pillows are placed under the client's head and shins. A pillow is sometimes placed under the abdomen if this makes the client more comfortable. Some clients lie in the prone position with their legs over the end of the bed. If so, no pillow is placed under the shins. Photo 18-5 shows a client in the prone position.

Photo 18-5
A client in the prone position

Photo 18-6
A client in the supine position

Supine Position

The **supine** position is also called the dorsal recumbent position. In this position, the client is lying on his or her back. The client's arms are at his or her side. A pillow is placed under the client's head and each arm. A pillow may be placed under the client's knees. Photo 18-6 shows a client in the supine position.

Moving a Person in Bed

Some clients will require some help to move about in bed. Other clients will not be able to move about in bed at all. In addition to positioning, you may need to assist your client to move up in bed, to roll to one side, to move to one side of the bed, or to assist the person in sitting on the side of the bed.

As with any procedure, you must always observe the basic rules of assisting clients to move that we discussed earlier in this chapter.

Assisting a Person with Moving Up in Bed

Every client will slide down in bed if the head of the bed has been raised. This can happen even if the client bends his or her knees or uses a roll at the feet to minimize sliding. As well, some clients will move toward the foot of the bed even if the head is not raised. A client who is too far down in the bed will be uncomfortable and unable to sit up properly. Furthermore, the client's feet may become pinched if they are pressed against the footboard.

If your client can assist, use Procedure 18-1.

Procedure 18-1
Assisting the Client with Moving Up in Bed

1. If the height of the client's bed is adjustable, raise the entire bed to waist height.
2. Lower the head of the bed so that it is as flat as the client can tolerate.
3. Lower the siderail (if any) on the side nearest you.
4. Stand next to the bed, facing the head of the bed. Maintain a good base of support, with your feet approximately 30 cm apart, with one foot ahead of the other in a walking stance.
5. Move the client's pillow to the headboard. This makes it easier for the person to help, as well as protecting the person's head from the headboard.
6. Ask the client to bend both knees and to place both feet flat on the bed.
7. Bending from the hips and knees, and maintaining the lumbar curve, slide one arm under the client's thighs and the other under the client's shoulders.
8. Explain to the client that, on the count of three, you will lift and move the client toward the head of the bed. Ask the client to assist by pushing up with his or her feet and using the side rail to pull with his or her arm toward the headboard. Allow the client time to prepare to assist.

9. Move on the count of three, shifting your weight from your rear leg to your front leg.
10. Assist the person to become comfortable. Assist with positioning, smooth the sheets, and replace the pillow behind the client's head.
11. Lower the entire bed and raise the head of the bed as the client wishes.
12. Place a pillow under the client's knees, if he or she wishes.
13. Raise the side rail (if present and required).
14. Move call bell (if present) to within easy reach.
15. Wash your hands.

Some clients will not be able to assist. In this instance, you will need to enlist the help of another person. You will also require a draw sheet or pad protector.

Procedure 18-2
Moving the Person Up in Bed with a Draw Sheet

1. Follow the basic rules for moving a person.
2. If the height of the client's bed is adjustable, raise the entire bed to waist height.
3. Lower the head of the bed so that it is as flat as the client can tolerate.
4. Lower the side rail (if any) on the side nearest you. Have your partner do the same.
5. Move the client's pillow to the headboard. This makes it easier for the person to move, as well as protecting the person's head from the headboard.
6. Roll the side of the draw sheet or pad protector toward the client's side. (If the client does not have a draw sheet or protector on the bed, install one as per the bed-making procedure in Chapter 19) Have your partner do the same.
7. Stand next to the bed, facing the head of the bed. Maintain a good base of support, with your feet approximately 30 cm apart, with one foot ahead of the other in a walking stance. Have your partner do the same on the opposite side of the bed.
8. Ask your client to cross his or her arms over the chest. Assist the client to do this if required.
9. Grasp the rolled sheet firmly near the client at shoulders and hips.
10. On the count of three, lift the draw sheet and create a sling. Move toward the head of the bed, shifting your weight from your rear leg to the front leg. Ensure your partner does the same.
11. Gently place the client in the new position.
12. Assist the person to become comfortable. Assist with positioning, smooth the sheets, and replace the pillow behind the client's head.
13. Lower the entire bed, and raise the head of the bed as the client wishes.
14. Raise the side rail (if present and required).
15. Move call bell (if present) to within easy reach.
16. Wash your hands.

Moving a Person to the Side of the Bed

Sometimes, a client will need to move to one side of the bed. This could be because the client will be having a bed bath or other procedure. In some cases, the client will not be able to assist. When this is the case, use one of the two following procedures.

Procedure 18-3
Moving a Person to the Side of the Bed, Single-Person Approach

1. Follow the basic rules for moving a person.
2. If the height of the client's bed is adjustable, raise the entire bed to waist height.
3. Lower the head of the bed so that it is as flat as the client can tolerate.
4. Lower the siderail (if any) on the side nearest you.
5. Stand next to the bed, facing the side of the bed. Maintain a good base of support, with your feet approximately 30 cm apart, with one foot ahead of the other in a walking stance. Bend your knees slightly.
6. Ask your client to cross his or her arms over his or her chest. Assist the client to do this if required.
7. Slide your arm under the person's neck and shoulders. Grasp the shoulder farthest from you with your hand.
8. Slide your other arm under the person's middle back.
9. Move the person's upper body toward you by shifting your weight from your front foot to the one in the back. Take care that the person does not move too close to the edge of the bed.
10. Repeat step 9 with your arms under the client's waist and buttocks.
11. Repeat step 9 with your arms under the client's thighs and legs.
12. Assist the person to become comfortable. Assist with positioning, smooth the sheets, and replace the pillow behind the client's head.
13. Lower the entire bed and raise the head of the bed as appropriate.
14. Raise the side rail (if present and required).
15. Move call bell (if present) to within easy reach.
16. Wash your hands.

The following approach is used when the client is too frail or heavy to be moved by the single-person approach, or when the client's spine must be kept straight. This approach requires a draw sheet and is very similar to the approach used to move a person up in bed.

Procedure 18-4
Moving a Person to the Side of the Bed, Two-Person Approach

1. Follow the basic rules for moving a person.
2. If the height of the client's bed is adjustable, raise the entire bed to waist height.
3. Lower the head of the bed so that it is as flat as the client can tolerate.

4. Lower the side rail (if any) on the side nearest you.
5. Stand next to the bed, facing the side of the bed. Maintain a good base of support, with your feet approximately 30 cm apart, with one foot ahead of the other in a walking stance. Bend your knees slightly. Have your partner do the same.
6. Roll the side of the draw sheet or pad protector toward the client's side. (If the client does not have a draw sheet or protector on the bed, place one as per the procedure in Chapter 19.) Have your partner do the same.
7. Ask your client to cross his or her arms over the chest. Assist the client to do this if required.
8. Grasp the rolled sheet firmly near the client at shoulders and hips.
9. On the count of three, lift the draw sheet and create a sling. Move away from the side of the bed, shifting your weight from your front leg to the rear leg. Ensure your partner rocks forward, shifting weight from the rear to the front leg.
10. Gently place the client in the new position.
11. Assist the client to become comfortable. Assist with positioning, smooth the sheets, and replace the pillow behind the client's head.
12. Lower the entire bed and raise the head of the bed as the client wishes.
13. Raise the side rail (if present and required).
14. Move call bell (if present) to within easy reach.
15. Wash your hands.

EQUIPMENT

another person to help you

draw sheet or pad protector

Assisting a Person with Sitting on the Side of the Bed

Assisting a person to sit on the side of the bed is also called dangling. A client might use this procedure when he or she is convalescing and before the client is able to weight bear. Some clients who cannot weight bear are assisted to sit up to vary their position. This procedure is also used when a client is preparing to transfer from a bed to a chair.

Procedure 18-5
Assisting a Person with Sitting on the Side of the Bed

1. Follow the basic rules for moving a person.
2. If the height of the client's bed is adjustable, raise the entire bed to waist height.
3. Raise the head of the bed so that the client is in a sitting position.
4. Lower the side rail (if any) on the side nearest you.
5. Position client in bed so that the client is sitting parallel to the side of the bed, approximately his or her thigh length (the distance from the hip to the knee) away from the side of the bed.
6. Stand next to the bed, facing the far corner of the foot of the bed. Maintain a good base of support, with your feet approximately 30 cm apart.
7. Slide one hand under the person's neck and shoulders and grasp the far shoulder.
8. Place your other hand over and behind the client's thighs, near the knees.
9. Pivot toward the foot of the bed as you bring your client's legs to the edge of the bed.

10. The client's knees should be at the edge of the bed for proper support. DO NOT position client's buttocks too close to the edge of the bed.

11. Ask your client to straighten his or her arms and to make fists and press each of them into the mattress at the client's side. This helps to keep the client balanced.

12. If the client cannot maintain balance or is not used to sitting up, do not leave the client unattended.

13. If the client is not used to sitting up, observe for signs of distress (such as pallor or rapid breathing).

14. If the client is to transfer to a chair, lower the bed so that the client's feet are firmly on the floor but the knees are not higher than his or her hips.

15. Reverse the procedure to assist the client to lie down.

Transfers and Lifts

A transfer is a movement in which the support worker assists the client with the movement. A lift is a movement in which the support worker takes the responsibility to move the client without the client's assistance or when the client can only minimally assist (due to extreme frailty or cognitive impairment).

When choosing a transfer or a lift, ask three questions:

1. Can the client weight bear?
   a. Does the client have sufficient strength and control to maintain his or her weight over his or her legs with assistance?
   b. Does the diagnosis make weight bearing advisable?

2. Does the client cooperate?
   a. Is the client receptive to the move?
   b. Can the move be done without excessive pain on movement?
   c. Does the client have good position sense or visual field?
   d. Can the client concentrate throughout the activity?

3. Does the client understand?
   a. Can the client effectively communicate with you?
   b. Does the client have enough understanding of the task to appropriately participate?

If the answers to these questions are yes, a transfer is appropriate.

The appropriate use of a transfer or lift avoids injury for the caregiver and ensures the safety of the client.

Preparing to Assist

Before you begin the procedure, prepare! Make sure that you do the following:

1. **Review the process with the client.** Even if you are certain that the client cannot understand, this step gives the client some time to adjust to your presence. It may prevent the client from being startled.

2. **Make sure that the area is clear of obstructions.** Move furniture, sheets, and other items that may hinder movement.

3. **Make sure that the equipment you need is in proper position.** Place the wheelchair in the proper spot, with brakes on and foot pedals clear of the client's path. Ensure that you have any necessary assistive devices (such as a transfer board or a transfer belt).

4. **Ensure height of both surfaces are as equal as possible.** For example, drop the height of the bed (if possible) to be level with the chair. The height of some power wheelchairs can also be adjusted.

5. **Make sure that the client has proper footwear.** Make sure that the footwear provides the right amount of grip. Socks and many slippers can easily slide on hard floors. Crepe-soled shoes may be too sticky and cause the person to trip. Ensure that the footwear is the correct size to prevent the person from slipping.

6. **Maintain good posture and body mechanics.**

Transfers

There are two types of transfers: supervised and assisted.

Supervised Transfer A supervised transfer occurs when the client is physically able to complete the transfer but may require redirection or coaching to complete the task. For example, a client who has a dementia may require a supervised transfer.

Assisted Transfer An assisted transfer is used when the client has difficulty getting started but is able to bear weight and perform the remainder of the transfer appropriately. This is most often used to assist clients rising from a chair.

Procedure 18-6
Assisted Transfer

1. Follow the basic rules for moving a person.
2. Stand at the side of the seated client in a walking stance.
3. Ask the client to sit forward in the chair, bending at the hips.
4. Ask client to place his or her feet flat on the floor in a side-by-side position approximately 30cm apart and slightly behind the knees.
5. As the client bends forward, place the palm of your hand (the one nearest the back of the chair) at the middle of the client's upper back, about 6 cm below the neck. Apply pressure to assist the person to move forward.
6. As you are applying pressure, extend your other hand to the client. Allow the client to press down on your hand to assist the client to rise.

Pivot Transfer One of the most common transfers is the pivot transfer. This transfer is used to assist a person to move from a bed to a chair, from chair to chair, or from chair to bed.

Procedure 18-7
Pivot Transfer

1. Follow the basic rules for moving a person. Make sure that the surface to which the client is transferring is at a right angle (90°) to the surface from which the client is transferring.
2. Ask the client to move forward to the edge of the seat. This can be done using a rocking motion, in which each hip is brought slightly forward until the person is at the edge of the seat with his or her feet flat on the floor.
3. Position yourself in front of the client, with your body in a mirror image of the client's. Photo 18-7a illustrates this position.
4. Place your hands around the client's back. Place the palms of your hands on the area of the client's back that will require the greatest support. For example, if the client tends to fall back, place your hands on the client's upper back. If the client has difficulty moving his or her hips, place your hands on the lower back.
5. Ask the client to mirror your hand position and to hold firmly.
6. Ask the client to stand.
7. While holding the client, stand with the client.
8. If the client's feet tend to slip forward, place your foot slightly at an angle in front of the foot to block this movement. Photo 18-7b illustrates this position.
9. Make sure that the client can sense being on his or her feet.
10. Turn with the client toward the surface. Continue until the client can feel the edge of the surface behind his or her knees.
11. Maintain your hands in position as you mirror the client's position as he or she sits down.
12. Avoid gripping both the client's knees with your own, this forces the knees into medial rotation and adduction. It is very difficult to stand up in this position. If it is necessary to block both the knees, do so knee to knee, with a towel or piece of foam between to avoid pain.
13. If the client has one weaker leg and requires some support in standing, the caregiver may grip the one leg with his or her knees or provide blocking knee to knee.

Photo 18-7b
Blocking the client's foot.

Photo 18-7a
Position in front of the client, with your body in a mirror image of the client's.

Lumbar

Scapula

FIGURE 18-4
The pivot transfer

Procedure 18-8
Assisting the Client to Move back in the Chair

1. Stand behind the chair in a walk stance close to the chair.
2. Ask the client to lean forward at the hips with arms crossed over the waist and feet flat on the pedals of the wheelchair.
3. Reach under the client's axillas, grasping the client's wrists.
4. Assist the client back into the chair as the client pushes back but maintains hip flexion.

FIGURE 18-5
Assisting the client to move back in a chair

Procedure 18-9
Assisting the Client into a Shower Using a Shower Chair

If the client has a weak side (for example, as the result of a stroke), the client should have his or her stronger side nearest the tub.

1. Prepare as described earlier in this section. Make sure that the chair is parallel to the tub.
2. Ask the client to push up from the chair, using the armrests, and stand. Provide assistance as per the pivot transfer as required.
3. Ask the client to pivot and sit on the tub seat. Assist as required.
4. Ask the client to slide his or her strongest leg into the tub first.

Photo 18-8
Shower with shower chair
Source: Product shown is the Invacare-I Shower Chair with Back

EQUIPMENT

shower with shower chair

Procedure 18-10
Assisting the Client Out of a Shower Using a Shower Chair

1. Prepare as described earlier in this section. Make sure that the chair is parallel to the tub.
2. Ask the client to slide to the end of the shower chair.
3. Ask the client to lift his or her weakest leg out of the tub first. This will cause the client to pivot in the shower chair. Assist as required.
4. Ask the client to lift his or her strong leg out of the tub.
5. Ask the client to stand. Assist as required.
6. Ask the client to pivot, reach for chair armrests, and sit. Assist as per pivot transfer as required.

EQUIPMENT

shower with shower chair

Procedure 18-11
Assisting a Client to Move from Chair to Toilet

Be aware that the configuration of the client's washroom, the type of assistive devices, as well as the client's degree of mobility will determine the exact procedure used. Adapt the approach to the client's situation while maintaining good body mechanics.

The following procedure assumes that the client can assist and that the bathroom has a grab bar affixed to the wall next to the toilet.

1. Prepare as described earlier in this section. Make sure that the chair is facing the toilet and is approximately 40 cm away.
2. Ask the client to push up, using the chair's armrests. Assist as required.
3. As the client stands, ask the client to grip the grab bar with the hand nearest to the bar.
4. When the client is ready, ask him or her to grasp the bar with the other hand and to pivot around the bar to the toilet. Assist the client by placing your hands on the client's waist to provide support.
5. As the client pivots to the front of the toilet, ask the client to release his or her arm furthest from the grab bar. Support this arm as required.
6. Ask the client to sit on the toilet. Assist as per pivot transfer as required.
7. Reverse the procedure to transfer from toilet to chair.

Procedure 18-12
Assisting a Client Who Uses a Walker to Sit on a Chair or Toilet

1. Prepare as described earlier in this section.
2. Ask the client to get as close to the front of the chair or toilet as is possible.
3. Ask the client to back up to chair or toilet so that back of the client's knees touch the chair or the seat of the toilet.
4. If the chair or toilet has armrests, ask the client to place his or her hands on the armrests and sit down. If the chair or toilet has no armrests, and there are no grab bars, assist the client as required.

Procedure 18-13
Assisting a Client Who Uses a Walker to Rise from a Chair or Toilet

1. Prepare as described earlier in this section.
2. Ensure that the walker is in front of the client and within the client's reach.
3. Ask the client to move as close to the front of the chair or toilet as is possible.
4. If the chair or toilet has armrests, ask the client to place his or her hands on the armrests (or one hand on the walker and the other on the armrest) and to push up to stand. If the chair or toilet has no armrests, and there are no grab bars, assist the client as required.
5. Ask the client to place his or her hands on the walker.
6. Allow the client to get used to standing before attempting to move.

Procedure 18-14
Assisting a Client Who Uses a Walker to Transfer to Bed

1. Follow the basic rules for moving a person.
2. Ensure sheets and blankets are folded away from the area.
3. Ask the client to approach the bed with the walker, stopping about 50 cm in front of the bed. The client should aim for the upper part of the bed.
4. Ask the client to pivot so that the client's back is facing the side of the bed.
5. Ask the client to step backward toward the bed while using the walker.
6. Ask the client to place one hand on the bed and to sit on the edge of the bed, placing one hand on the walker and the other on the bed.
7. Ask the client to move each hip back alternately until both thighs are on the bed.
8. Ask the client to swing his or her legs into the bed. Assist as required.
9. Remove client's shoes before covering with sheets.

Using a Mechanical Lift

Some clients will require the use of a mechanical lift. There are many types available, each with its own specific procedure for use. Be certain you know how to safely operate any lift you are using. Photo 18-9 shows a mechanical lift.

Remember that the experience of being lifted by a mechanical lift is very different than being lifted by people. Clients often feel that they are "hanging" in space and may feel very vulnerable or frightened. Vision and balance problems may make these sensations very uncomfortable. Take the time to reassure the client.

Photo 18-9
One of many lifts used today.
Source: South Lake Village/Lynelle Hamilton

Procedure 18-15
Guidelines for Using a Mechanical Lift

There are many types of lifts in use today. Each has a specific procedure for its use. You must make certain that you know how to use each lift you operate. The following guidelines will assist you in the use of most lifts.

1. Ensure that the lift's legs are situated in the position that offers the best base of support.

2. Ensure the sling is properly attached. Ensure that the hooks are attached so that the person is in the proper position (as per manufacturer's instructions) when the lift is raised.

3. Ensure that sling hooks face to the outside, as shown in Photo 18-10. This ensures that the hooks do not damage the client's skin.

4. Maintain eye contact with the client to decrease fear and anxiety. Reducing anxiety will also help to keep the client from moving in the swing.

5. When you raise the sling, ensure that you raise it to the proper height, as per the manufacturer's instructions.

6. Move the lift to the desired location.

7. Slowly and steadily lower the client to the chair or bed surface.

8. Remove sling, if desired.

Photo 18-10

Two students practise the proper use of a mechanical lift

RANGE OF MOTION EXERCISES

Range of motion, or ROM, is described as the normal movement a joint can progress through comfortably and safely. Usually the amount is similar on each side of the body, but it is often different from person to person. The purpose of ROM exercises is to maintain the normal movement patterns in the joints and muscles, and to aid in prolonging and maintaining functional movements and independence. There are three general types of range of motion exercises.

You may hear certain terms when you are asked to assist a client with range of motion exercises. Abduction is the term used to describe moving an arm or leg away from the centre of the body. The term adduction describes moving an arm or leg toward the centre of the body. The term extension describes straightening a joint. Flexion describes bending a joint.

1. **Active range of motion exercise.** The client can move all joints independently but may require encouragement or cueing.
2. **Assisted range of motion exercise.** Assisted range of motion exercise. The client requires the aid of an assistant to move through ROM for some joints.
3. **Passive range of motion exercise.** Passive exercises are performed completely by an assistant to move the joint through ROM.

Photo 18-11
Assisting a client with range of motion exercises

Many clients perform range of motion exercises independently. However, you may be asked to assist a client who cannot voluntarily move his or her muscles (Photo 18-11). In some cases, a client will have sensation and will be able to tell you if movement has been carried too far and is painful.

In other cases, the client may not be able to sense pain. As a result, neither you nor the client may know that you have moved a joint too far, even if the joint was not moved across the "normal" full range. Bear in mind that you can seriously injure a client by moving joints too far or by moving joints that are injured or inflamed.

The following eight guidelines can help you safely assist clients with range of motion activities:

1. **Follow the exercise plan set out for the client.** A therapist may have established the plan or it may be one used in an exercise class the client attends. Discuss with your supervisor any questions you have about the plan.
2. **Make certain that you know when and how to help.** Are there exercises the client can do independently? With which exercises do you have to help?
3. **Support all joints when exercising.**
4. **Encourage the client to do as much as he or she safely can.** Do not force a client to the point of exhaustion. Also, bear in mind that the client's ability may vary from day to day.
5. **Be gentle.** Sudden or fast movement may cause pain or injure the client.
6. **Never exercise to the point of pain.** Pain is a sign of injury.
7. **Stop exercising the joint if the client complains of pain or discomfort.** Report any unexpected pain to your supervisor.
8. **Never exercise a swollen, reddened, or painful joint.** Report all signs of inflammation to your supervisor.

MOBILITY AIDS

Many clients use mobility aids that are designed to improve a person's stability by expanding his or her base of support. In addition to making it possible for a person to move, aids serve four purposes. They reduce weight bearing; compensate for lost balance, strength, or coordination; reduce pain while walking; and enhance the person's sense of safety and security. Canes, crutches, walkers, and rollators are common types of mobility aids. There are many variations within each type. In this section, we'll discuss the common uses of each type.

Photo 18-12
Types of canes

Photo 18-13
Pronged cane tip: This tip provides grip in slippery conditions.

Canes

There are three types of canes: single point, tripod, and quad canes. Photo 18-12 shows a quad and a single point. Canes can help compensate for mild balance or leg weakness problems. Within this range, a quad cane provides the greatest support and stability; the tripod cane provides somewhat less. The single point cane provides the least amount of support and stability. Many years ago, a client seldom used a cane unless he or she was advised by a health professional to do so. (In England many years ago, one had to have a permit to use a cane!) The person was usually fitted to the proper size and type of cane, as well as given instruction in its use. Today, many people simply purchase canes in the drugstore. As a result, the cane may be too short or tall or not the right type. As well, the person may not know how to use the cane properly.

Adjusting and Using a Cane

The cane should be adjusted to the correct height:

- To measure a cane, turn the cane upside down and put the handle on the floor.
- Have the patient stand with arms at her or his side.
- The tip of the cane should be at the level of the crease in the client's wrist.

To adjust a cane:

- With the cane upside down, mark the cane at the level of the wrist.
- Remove the rubber tip.
- Cut the cane 1.25 cm shorter than where you marked it.
- Replace rubber tip.
- Aluminum canes can be easily adjusted within an inch of the desired height.

Learn to use a cane correctly:

- Hold the cane in the hand opposite the weak leg.
- Hold the cane so that the tip is about 15–25 cm to the side.
- Move the cane and the weak leg together approximately 30 cm forward.
- Bring the strong leg forward and ahead of the weak leg and the cane.
- Going up the stairs: take the first step up with the strong leg. Then move the cane and the weak leg to the same step
- Going down the stairs: Take the first step down with the cane and the weak leg. Then lower the strong leg to that same step.
- Always replace worn rubber tips and attach an ice pick in the winter (Photo 18-13).

Crutches

Crutches provide more support and stability than a cane. Use of a crutch can allow the person to take all the weight off of a leg (for example, if the person's leg was recently fractured and a walking cast was not applied). A person may use two crutches to remove some pressure from both legs. There are many types of crutches. Photo 18-14 shows one type. Some crutches have specific features designed to reduce the stress on arms or hands. Others have hinged tips to better simulate a natural walking rhythm.

Adjusting and Using Crutches

Like canes, crutches must be properly fitted. Crutch tops should be 3–4 cm below the person's armpits when held in the standing position. Crutch grips should be adjusted so that the person's arm is at a 25°–30° angle when holding the grip. A person using crutches should not rest his or her armpits on the crutch tops. This can compress the nerves and blood vessels in the armpit and result in numbness of the arms and hands. This condition is sometimes called "crutch palsy." It almost always disappears when the person stops resting on the crutch tops.

The usual procedure for walking with crutches is as follows:

1. Standing on the "good" leg, move both crutches and the weak leg ahead approximately 30 cm.
2. While bearing weight on the handgrips (not on the crutch tops), swing the good leg ahead of the crutches.
3. Standing on the good leg, move the crutches and weak leg ahead as in step one.

Photo 18-14
Adjustable crutches

Walkers and Rollators

Walkers and rollators are four-point mobility aids. Walkers may have four legs, two legs and two wheels, or (less commonly) four wheels. Photo 18-15 shows two variations. Walkers equipped with wheels usually have a spring mechanism that prevents the wheels from moving when the person is leaning on the walker. This mechanism prevents the walker from rolling out from under the person.

Photo 18-15
Wheeled and standard walkers

Rollators usually have four wheels. Rollators have hand brakes and a platform that can be used as a seat. Some have baskets so that the person may easily carry items about. Photo 18-16 shows a common style.

Photo 18-16
A rollator: This device provides a seat and basket, making it ideal for shopping.

Walking with a Walker or Rollator

To walk with a walker not equipped with wheels, the person lifts the walker and places it down about 15 cm in the direction the person wants to go. While holding on to the walker, the person then walks up to it. The process is repeated until the person reaches the desired location.

Walking with a rollator or a walker equipped with wheels is similar to walking with a shopping cart. The rollator or walker is pushed ahead as the person walks. (The person will have to release the handbrakes on the rollator to allow it to roll.)

FALLS

Falls can happen any time and any place to people of all ages. Falls are the leading cause of fatal and nonfatal injuries in people 65 and over. The Public Health Agency of Canada estimates that nearly 62 percent of hospital admissions due to injuries among seniors are injuries that resulted from a fall. The number of falls and the severity of injury resulting from falls increases as people get older. A person over 65 is nine times as likely to sustain an injury than is someone under that age (Public Health Agency of Canada).

A fall can be a life-changing event that reduces the person's independence. Falls cause more than 90 percent of all hip fractures in older adults. Twenty percent of the people who have a fracture will die within a year of the fracture (Public Health Agency of Canada).

Falls are not natural events. You can help prevent them. Gait, balance, and posture are responsible for keeping us upright and preventing falls.

It is essential to know the fall risk status of each client and to use proper transfer techniques with appropriate mobility aids specific to the client. It's also important to observe for any unsteadiness or difficulty in walking, sitting, standing, or using stairs. A cluttered environment can also put a person at risk for falls. Discuss your concerns with the client and your supervisor.

If a Person Is Falling

If a fall is happening while you are there, assist the client to attempt to minimize injury. The following general guidelines may be useful in assisting a person who is falling. The person's support plan may provide specific instructions; always use these if they are present.

1. Ensure that you maintain the best body position possible to support the fall, guiding the person gently to the ground.
2. Bend your knees, and continue to provide verbal cueing as you lower the client gently to the floor.
3. In most cases, it's best to help the client slide down and land on his or her buttocks.

If a Person Has Fallen

How a person reacts after a fall can cause more injuries than the fall itself. If the person tries to get up too quickly or to get up in the wrong position, he or she may make an injury worse. The following are general guidelines for assisting a person who has fallen. The person's support plan may provide specific instructions; always use these if they are present.

1. Ask the person if he or she is hurt or in pain. Don't move a person who may have an injury until medical personnel have examined him or her, unless you must do so to avoid further injury. If the person is in pain or says she or he is hurt, call for emergency assistance and advise your supervisor.
2. Don't attempt to assist the person without consent. If the person feels strong enough to get up, allow time for the person to take several deep breaths and regain composure.
3. Place a sturdy stool or stable chair nearby so that the person is facing the seat and can place his or her hands on the surface.
4. Using good body mechanics, provide directions and assist the person get to a standing position. Ask her or him to slowly begin to rise and to bend whichever knee is stronger, while keeping the other knee on the floor.
5. Assist the person to turn so that the backs of the legs touch the chair.
6. Help the person lower himself or herself to a sitting position.
7. Contact your supervisor and document the event.

Questions for Review

1. Why is it important to encourage your client to move about?
2. How does moving people differ from moving objects?
3. What are good body mechanics?
4. What is a good base of support? How far apart should your feet be to ensure a good base of support?
5. Describe leverage.
6. How can you maintain good body mechanics when performing any task?
7. Name the 12 principles that should be followed when you are assisting a person with movement.
8. What is Fowler's position? When is it used?
9. With a partner, demonstrate each positioning and transfer described in this chapter. Ask your partner to give you feedback on how he or she feels as you are assisting.
10. What is the general procedure for using a mechanical lift?
11. What is the proper procedure for walking with a cane? With a wheeled walker?
12. What are the three guidelines to use when someone is falling?
13. Should you always help a person who has fallen to get up? When should you not help such a person?
14. What are the seven guidelines to use when you do assist a person to get up after a fall?

Questions for Discussion

1. How do you think you might feel if you had to depend upon the help of another person in order to get out of bed?

2. Consider the following case study. Then, discuss your answers to the questions at the end.

   Mrs. James has recently fractured her hip. She fell on black ice as she was getting her morning paper. Although her hip was repaired, she spent four weeks in hospital as a result of complications from the surgery. She spent eight weeks in a rehabilitation centre after discharge. She is now home and gradually regaining her ability. She now uses a cane "just to make sure" she won't fall. As well, she requires some help to get out of bed in the morning and to rise from a chair.

   One of your tasks is to assist Mrs. James as she again begins to shop and bank. She has not left her home since discharge from the rehabilitation centre. Although you have been gently encouraging her to go out with you, she politely refuses.

   How might Mrs. James be feeling? How might you apply the principles of assistance to this situation?

3. You work in an assisted-living centre. You have a client who requires a great deal of assistance. In fact, the client is just at the point of needing a mechanical lift. The client repeatedly asks you to assist him without using the mechanical lift. What do you do? What factors must be considered? How do you think you might feel if you were in the client's place?

Chapter 19

Providing Physical Care

Learning Objectives

Through reading this chapter, you'll be able to

1. Discuss the four main purposes of physical care.
2. Define RIDICUPS and apply its principles to providing physical care.
3. Describe changes in the integumentary system often associated with age.
4. Relate the purposes of a back rub and demonstrate a basic back rub.
5. List the steps involved in giving a client a bed bath, assisting a client in taking a sponge bath, a tub bath, or a shower.
6. List the steps in perineal care.
7. Define continence and incontinence.
8. Demonstrate continence care.
9. Demonstrate ostomy care.
10. Discuss the signs and causes of pressure sores and the common measures taken to prevent them.
11. Describe the steps involved in performing or assisting a client to perform mouth and hair care.
12. Outline the proper steps for measuring temperature, pulse, and respiration.
13. Outline the method for obtaining a midstream urine specimen.
14. Describe the procedures to follow when applying heat or cold.
15. Discuss cast care.
16. Identify the steps in applying a clean, dry dressing.

Chapter at a Glance

- Purposes of Physical Care
- Care Routines
- The Client's Skin
- Pressure Sores
- RIDICUPS—Principles of Personalizing Physical Care
- Preparing to Provide Care
- Physical Care Procedures
- Special Situations
- Oral Care
- Hair Care

- Shaving the Client
- Foot Care
- Nail Care
- Eye Care
- Ear Care
- Continence Care
- Assisting the Client with the Use of a Bed Pan
- Assisting the Client with Dressing
- Bed Making
- Measurement of Vital Signs
- Measuring Blood Pressure
- Measuring and Recording Intake and Output
- Measuring Client Height and Weight
- Applying Heat or Cold
- Care in Special Situations

Terms You'll Use

Blood Pressure The pressure of the blood within the arteries.

Continence The ability to control bowel or bladder function.

Decubitus Ulcers Skin breakdown caused when tissue is trapped between a hard surface and a bony prominence. Often occur when clients are not repositioned frequently; also called pressure sores.

Incontinence The lack of ability to control bowel or bladder function.

Ostomy A surgical opening in the body.

Pressure Sores Decubitus ulcers.

Pulse The impulse transmitted to arteries by contraction of the ventricles of the heart. Most often measured by feeling the radial arteries.

Respiration The act of inhaling and exhaling air; breathing.

RIDICUPS An acronym describing the eight principles of personalized care: Respect, Independence, Dignity, Individuality, Communication, Understanding, Privacy, and Safety.

Temperature The measurement of body heat.

Vital Signs Measurements of temperature, pulse, blood pressure, and respiration.

PURPOSES OF PHYSICAL CARE

Physical care includes the many tasks associated with cleanliness and good grooming. There are four purposes to physical care: client comfort, self-image, safety, and health.

Client comfort refers to both the physical and the psychological sensation of being clean. Think of how you feel when you've had a bath and are dressed in fresh clothes. You likely feel fresh and good. This is particularly important when the client has drainage from illness or an operation, if the client perspires as the result of the effort required to accomplish tasks, or when the client is in bed for an extended period of time.

A positive self-image refers to how the client sees himself or herself as an attractive person. A positive self-image results from a combination of cleanliness and grooming. Some things may make it more difficult for a client to attain a positive self-image. A client may have an impairment or disfigurement that may make the client feel that he or she is ugly or "not presentable." Some clients may feel that the physical changes of age may make them unattractive. Assisting clients to feel good about their physical image through proper physical care and grooming is essential to client support (Photo 19-1).

Photo 19-1
A happy, well-groomed client.
Source: CHATS

STOP AND REFLECT

Recall a time when you knew that you looked your best.

_____

_____

Remember how knowing that you looked your best made you feel?

_____

_____

_____

Client safety and health are promoted through the removal of dirt and microorganisms that may cause infection or illness. Improper cleansing can introduce microorganisms into areas of the body and promote infection. In order to ensure that this does not happen, you must carefully follow the principles for providing physical care discussed in this chapter.

CARE ROUTINES

STOP AND REFLECT ((19-2))

What are your physical care routines? Do you prefer to shower or to bathe? Do you do this task in the morning or the evening? Do you have a favourite soap, cream, or talc that you use?

_____

_____

_____

_____

_____

In what order do you perform your physical care? Do you brush your teeth before or after you bathe? Do you fix your hair before or after you dress?

_____

_____

_____

_____

Have you ever had to alter this routine? If so, what was your reaction to the change?

_____

_____

_____

_____

Few things are as personal as the routines we each have for bathing, dressing, and grooming. Some of us prefer showers; others prefer baths. Some prefer to bathe in the morning, others at night. Some of us brush our teeth before we bathe; others do so after their bath. These routines are developed over many years of practice and are hard to change. Performing these routines in specific ways often gives us a sense of comfort.

Like you, your client will have preferences based upon his or her culture and past practices. It's important to respect your client's preferences for how physical care is done.

THE CLIENT'S SKIN

The skin forms the body's first defence against infection. It is also the largest organ in the body. The nerve endings embedded in the skin help us to sense pressure, heat, texture, and pain.

Many physical care routines involve cleansing the skin. Cleansing removes harmful microorganisms and can prevent infection. As well, the act of bathing allows for the skin to be massaged (such as when the client is helped to wash, to dry off, or to apply lotion). This, in turn, promotes circulation and helps to reduce the effects of pressure on circulation. Combined with proper positioning and frequent repositioning, skin care can prevent the development of pressure sores or help to heal existing sores.

As a person ages, the skin becomes thinner and less elastic. You may notice that the skin of some very old clients is almost transparent. As a result, an older person's skin is particularly susceptible to abrasions, bruising, or tearing. Observe these four guidelines when you are providing care to the client's skin:

1. **Remove any rings or other jewellery you are wearing to avoid catching and tearing the client's skin.** Make sure that your nails are cut short and filed smooth so as not to tear the client's skin.
2. **Be cautious when using rough sponges or cloths, as they can cause abrasions.** These items are often called loofah sponges or exfoliating sponges or pads.
3. **Never scrub a client's skin.** If a client has a stain that must be removed (such as ink from a pen), soak the area and gently rub it with a soapy cloth. Sometimes, a mark can be removed by applying a lotion on the spot and allowing it to absorb the stain.
4. **Always pat the client's skin dry.** Rubbing the client's skin to dry it can cause irritation and abrasions. It can also remove too much moisture from the client's skin, making it unnecessarily dry.

PRESSURE SORES

Pressure sores (also called decubitus ulcers) form when tissue is trapped between a hard surface (such as a chair seat or mattress) and a bony prominence (such as a hip bone, heel, or elbow). They can also form when braces or other appliances pinch and trap tissue. The pressure on the tiny blood vessels in the trapped tissue causes them to collapse, resulting in the death of the surrounding tissue. A client who is unable to move and readjust his or her position is at particular risk of having tissue trapped. Figure 19-1 illustrates the common pressure points.

Pressure sores develop in stages. In stage one, the area is reddened. In dark-complexioned clients, the area may appear drier instead of red. In the first stage, it may seem as though there is no damage, as the surface skin is intact. However, damage has been done to the underlying layer of the skin. By the time you or the client has noticed redness there is damage. It's important to report this redness immediately. It's also important to not cause further damage by rubbing the reddened area, as Spotlight 19-1 explains.

SPOTLIGHT 19-1 WHY YOU SHOULDN'T MASSAGE REDDENED AREAS OR OVER BONY PROMINENCES

You may be advised to rub a reddened area of a client's skin or rub bony prominences. You should not. Often, the person who asks you to do this believes that rubbing or massaging promotes circulation, but there is no proof that massage promotes circulation in these cases. In fact, according to researchers (Bergstrom et al., 1992), it may cause further damage to the underlying tissue. As well, vigorous rubbing may also cause damage by shearing.

In stage two, tissue death has occurred As well, the break in the skin can allow microorganisms to enter, resulting in an infection.

In stage three, the skin is open and there is damage to the adipose (fatty) tissue and the muscles at the site. There may also be damage to surrounding areas. The risk of infection is very high.

FIGURE 19-1
Pressure points

Heels   Sacrum   Elbows   Shoulder   Back of
Blades   Head

Ankle   Knees   Hip   Shoulder   Side of
Head

Shoulders

Hips and
Sacrum

Buttocks

Feet

In a stage-four ulcer, all soft tissue at the site is gone. There may be damage to the bones or joints as well. As in stage three, the risk of infection is extremely high.

Photo 19-2 shows the development of a pressure sore.

Preventing Pressure Sores

You can do several things to prevent pressure sores. Table 19-1 lists some common methods to prevent sores. Vigilant observation of potential problem areas is also important, as most sores can be reversed if caught at the first stage.

Stage 1

Stage 2

Stage 3

#1279

Stage 4

Photo 19-2
The stages of pressure sore development
Source: Courtesy of the Wound Care Education Institute

TABLE 19-1	Preventing Pressure Sores

- Take the pressure off. Reposition the client to remove the pressure on specific areas. In general, a client should be repositioned at least once every two hours.

- Avoid shearing of the skin by keeping the head of the client's bed at 30° or lower when possible.

- Use proper lift and transfer techniques to avoid shearing and friction.

- Provide good skin care. Make sure that skin is clean and not left wet. If possible, apply talc or cornstarch sparingly to areas that tend to become damp (under the breasts, the axilla, and the groin).

- Dry skin is prone to chapping and cracking. Ask the client or your supervisor about applying a lotion to dry and rough areas.

- Ensure that bedding and clothing are kept dry. Some clients may perspire and require frequent changes of linen.

- Give good perineal care to maintain cleanliness and protect the client's skin.

- Ensure that incontinent clients are kept dry and clean. Promptly change any wet or soiled incontinence briefs.

- Check with the client or your supervisor before using soap on fragile skin. Soap can dry and burn. If you do use soap, be certain to rinse it off thoroughly.

- Do not scrub the client's skin. Use lotion or oil to soften and remove dried material.

▶▶│

TABLE 19-1	Preventing Pressure Sores *(continued)*

- Massage *around* pressure points to promote circulation. Immediately report to your supervisor any reddened areas that do not blanch to the touch.
- Use gauze, cloth, or a layer of clothing to limit skin-to-skin contact. Skin-to-skin contact promotes moisture and can foster bacterial growth.
- Use protective devices as prescribed.
- Immediately report reddened, abraded, or open areas to the appropriate person.
- Encourage clients who can do so to change position frequently.

Aids

There are a number of items that can help to relieve pressure: pads, special mattresses, and cradles.

Pads are usually made of a synthetic sheepskin that can be easily washed. Others are made of foam and usually cannot be washed. Gel-filled pads are commonly found in wheelchair seats and in some bed pads. These pads provide some cushioning to the pressure point, helping to avoid the pressure that causes the blood vessels to collapse. Some pads are made for a specific part of the body, such as an elbow or heel protector. Others are flat pads that cover a larger area of the bed or chair. Photo 19-3 shows one type of sheepskin pad.

The choice of pad is determined by the area to be protected as well as how likely the pad will become soiled and require cleaning.

Many types of air-filled, water-filled, and gel-filled mattresses are also used to help to relieve pressure points. Some of these mattresses are mechanical, cycling air in cylinders to alter the pressure. Others mould to the body and distribute the pressure across a larger area. Photo 19-4 shows an air-filled mattress pad.

Cradles are metal or wooden hoops that raise bedclothes off the client's legs and feet, relieving pressure on these extremities. Cradles are placed under the top sheet and blankets. Photo 19-5 shows a bed cradle.

Photo 19-3
A sheepskin pad
Source: *CHATS*

Photo 19-4
An air-filled mattress pad
Source: *CHATS*

Photo 19-5
A bed cradle
Source: *Maple Health Centre*

RIDICUPS—PRINCIPLES OF PERSONALIZING PHYSICAL CARE

In addition to using proper and safe techniques to provide physical care, you must always personalize the care you provide. It is very important to identify the process your client uses (particularly if you are assisting the client and not performing the task for him or her).

RIDICUPS is an acronym that will help you to remember eight important principles of personalizing physical care. RIDICUPS stands for Respect, Independence, Dignity, Individuality, Communication, Understanding, Privacy, and Safety (Figure 19-2). No matter what procedure you are performing, you must ensure that it meets the requirement of these eight principles. We'll look at each principle in this section.

Respect

Does the procedure you are using demonstrate respect for the client? Does it take into account what he or she is able to do? Does it respect the client's preferences for when, where, and how the procedure is performed?

Independence

Does the procedure promote the client's independence? Does it support the client's ability? Does it allow the client the time necessary to complete portions of the task?

Dignity

Does the procedure help the client to avoid embarrassment? Is it done in a manner that minimizes discomfort?

Individuality

Is the procedure adapted to meet the needs of the person? Are the client's preferences met? It's extremely important to avoid performing the task without thinking about the client's needs, no matter how many times you have performed it before.

FIGURE 19-2
RIDICUPS

Communication

Does the procedure include communicating with the client? Does it include discussing the procedure to be performed and listening to the client's preferences and concerns? As you perform the procedure, do you read the client's body language and listen to the client's words (and adapt your approach as necessary)?

Understanding

Does the procedure demonstrate an understanding of what it must be like for the client to undergo the procedure?

Privacy

Does the procedure protect the client's privacy? Is it performed in an area away from others' view? Does it include proper draping to prevent unnecessary exposure of body parts?

Safety

Is the procedure safe for both you and the client? Is the procedure complete? Does it leave the client in a comfortable state? Does it include proper body mechanics? Are proper infection control techniques used? Have you minimized any risks?

Personalizing care in this way takes practice. It's a lot to keep in mind all at the same time! The more you use the principles, the easier personalizing care will become.

PREPARING TO PROVIDE CARE

In addition to personalizing care, you must also take steps to prepare for the procedure so that it will go smoothly and comfortably. There are four steps to preparing to provide care: knowing the purpose, organizing your approach, assembling the proper equipment, and knowing the basic techniques that are required in any procedure. We'll look at each step here.

Purpose

In addition to the basic purposes of care, are there other purposes the procedure must meet? Is the procedure especially important because of an event (such as assisting a client to dress for a family wedding)? Is the procedure intended to assist the client to practise skills so as to become more independent?

Organization

You must have a thorough knowledge of the steps involved in the procedure, what equipment you will need, and when you will need it.

Equipment

You must assemble all necessary equipment and supplies before you begin the procedure. Make sure all equipment is clean and in good repair and that you know how to operate each item.

Techniques

Always perform the basic techniques with any procedure. There are four techniques: personalizing the procedure, discussing the procedure with the client, washing your hands, donning gloves or gown (if required).

PHYSICAL CARE PROCEDURES

Bathing the Adult Client

Bed Bath

Principles of bathing the client:

1. Always have the client assist wherever possible to increase the client's feelings of independence, to maintain dignity, and to increase self-esteem.
2. Ensure client privacy with proper draping even if you are the only other person in the room.
3. Bathing is also a time to observe the condition of your client's skin. Look for redness, abrasion, bruising, or skin breakdown. Report any concerns to your supervisor.
4. Bathing also provides uninterrupted time for you to communicate with your client.

Before beginning the procedure, be familiar with the following organizational steps:

1. Offer a bedpan or toilet prior to the bath.
2. Position the client. If the client is able to assist, he or she should be in a sitting position. If the client is unable to assist, he or she should be lying on his or her back closest to the side of the bed the support worker is on.
3. Raise the bed to working level (usually waist level).
4. Have clean pyjamas or clothes readily available.
5. Keep the water warm (40.5–42°C or 105–110°F). Test water temperature with your wrist, never your hand, or a bath thermometer.
6. Change water as needed to maintain cleanliness and proper temperature.
7. Use a bath blanket (flannel or top sheet) to keep exposed areas covered during the bath.
8. Fold the facecloth into a mitt for easier bathing. Figure 19-3 illustrates how this is done.
9. Always wash from clean to dirty areas.
10. Wash from distal (furthest from you) to proximal (closest to you) to avoid contaminating clean areas by reaching over them.
11. Always rinse soaped areas well to avoid drying the skin or soap irritation.
12. Wash perineal area last using a clean washcloth. When providing perineal care, work from the front of the person to the back. Do not use a back-and-forth or scrubbing motion. This reduces the possibility of introducing bacteria into other orifices. For example, when you cleanse a female client's anus, be certain to cleanse toward the back, *away* from the vagina and urethra.
13. Wear gloves to wash perineal area or any area of the skin with draining fluid.
14. Wash around areas with wound or skin dressings. If in doubt about how to cleanse near a wound or a dressing, ask for assistance.
15. Always observe the skin for any breaks, redness, swelling, or other abnormalities (e.g., changed moles, skin discolouration). Report any changes you observe to the appropriate person.

FIGURE 19-3
How to make a mitt

Procedure 19-1
Giving a Bed Bath

EQUIPMENT

bath blanket

basin with warm water

2 facecloths,
1 towel

bar of soap

lotion for back rub

clean sheets
(as needed)

clean gown, pyjamas,
or clothes

1. Place the bath blanket over the top linens and unfold it so that the linens are completely covered. Pull the linens from underneath the bath blanket and leave at the bottom of the bed.
2. Remove the client's soiled gown or pyjamas.
3. Place the basin of water on the over-bed table and position close to the bed.
4. Wash the client's face or assist the client by starting with the eyes. Using a corner of the washcloth with no soap, wash from the inner corner to the outer. Use a second corner of the cloth to wash the other eye in the same way.
5. Gently wash the client's face, ears, and neck using soap only at the client's request.
6. Pat dry with the towel.
7. Place the towel lengthwise under the client's arm. Using a soap-lathered washcloth, wash from the hand to the shoulder using long, firm strokes. Rinse and dry well by patting.
8. Wash and dry the axilla (underarm). Repeat for the other arm. See Figure 19-4.

FIGURE 19-4

Washing one arm with a towel underneath

9. Fold the bath blanket down to the client's pubic area. Lay the towel across the client's abdomen. Wash the chest and abdomen. Rinse and dry well.
10. Observe under the female client's breasts for redness or excoriation. Report any unusual conditions.
11. Lift the client's distal leg and place the towel lengthwise under it. Wash the client's leg from the ankles to the hip using long, firm strokes. Rinse and dry well. Repeat with the proximal leg.
12. Wash the client's feet well, especially between the toes. It is often beneficial to soak the client's feet in a basin. (See the procedure for foot care.) Examine each foot for abrasions, redness, and the condition of the toenails. Rinse and dry well.
13. Discard the water and washcloth.
14. Rinse the washbasin and fill with clean, warm water. Select a fresh facecloth, forming it into a mitt.
15. Assist the client into a side-lying position, facing away from the worker, with bath blanket in place.
16. Place the towel lengthwise on the bed next to the client's back. See Figure 19-5.
17. Wash the client's back using long, firm strokes, working from the shoulders to the buttocks. Rinse and dry.

a)   b)   c)   d)

FIGURE 19-5
Giving a bed bath

18. Give a back rub at this time. (See the procedure for giving a back rub.)
19. Return the client to the supine position. Fold bath blanket up to expose the pubic area. Place the towel between the client's legs. Put on gloves.
20. If the client is able to wash the perineal area independently, hand the soaped washcloth to the client.
21. If the client is not able to wash the perineal area, proceed to wash the groin and perineal area. Check folds in the groin and lower abdominal area for redness or excoriation. Report any concerns to your supervisor.
22. Perform peri-care as follows:
    a. Male: Grasp the shaft of the penis and retract the foreskin, if present. Wash the head of the penis in a circular motion and continue down the penis. Rinse. Dry well and replace the foreskin. Rinse the cloth, apply soap, and wash the scrotum, particularly between all folds of skin. Wash the rest of the perineal area around to the anus. Rinse and dry well.
    b. Female: Spread the inner lips (labia minora) with the nondominant hand, directing the facecloth from the pubis to the anus. Wash the outer area (labia majora), moving the washcloth from the pubis to the anus. Continue until the area is clean. Use a fresh corner for each area washed. Rinse and dry well.
    c. Clients with indwelling catheters: Wash the perineal area as above. Using a clean corner of a facecloth, wash the catheter from the urethra entrance (meatus) down the tube. Repeat if necessary with another clean corner of the washcloth. Never put a dirty facecloth near the urethra entrance.
23. The bath is now complete. Apply lotion to elbows and heels, if needed.
24. Help the client put on a clean gown, pyjamas, or clothes.
25. Assist the client up or into a comfortable position if he or she is to remain in bed.
26. Lower the bed to the lowest position. Attach the call bell, if present.

FIGURE 19-6
Male and female peri-care

Tub Bath or Shower

The principles and organization are the same as for a bed bath.

Procedure 19-2
Tub Bath or Shower

EQUIPMENT

2 facecloths,
1 towel

bar of soap

lotion for back rub

clean sheets
(as needed)

clean gown, pyjamas,
or clothes

1. Be sure tub or shower is cleaned and ready for use.
2. If the client shares a bath with others, place an "occupied" sign on the door.
3. Adjust water temperature in the shower or tub to 40.5–42°C (105–110°F).
4. For a tub bath, fill the tub with 30–40 cm of warm water.
5. Place a rubber bath mat in the tub.
6. Place a bath mat next to the tub or shower on the floor. If the client is unsteady on his or her feet, place a waterproof chair in the shower. (Some clients may have a bath seat installed in the tub, along with grab bars for the client to use.)
7. Have the client sit on the edge of the tub and swing his or her legs over the rim as described in Chapter 18. Provide assistance to the client as necessary.
8. If the client is able to bathe or shower alone, stay near the door so as to provide assistance if needed.
9. If the client is unable to bathe alone, bathe the client in the same order as described in the bed bath procedure.
10. Assist the client out of the tub, drain the water first, and follow the procedure outlined in Chapter 18.
11. Assist the client with drying off and dressing.
12. Clean the tub or shower according to client preference or agency policy.

Whirlpool or Hydraulic Tub

Residential Whirlpool Tubs   Some clients may have a residential whirlpool tub. These tubs are often similar to a standard bathtub and the procedure used to assist the client into this type of bath is essentially the same. Remember the following:

1. Take care to ensure that the water level is above the whirlpool jets (the outlets on the sides of the tub that spray water). If it is not, water will spray out of the tub.
2. Ensure that the force of the jets is not too strong for client comfort. Adjust the jets by turning the air intake valves (usually located on the deck of the tub) to provide a comfortable degree of force. Adjust the jets if the client expresses discomfort.
3. Make sure that any bath salts or other bath supplies added to the water are safe for use in a whirlpool tub. Avoid any product that will make the tub surface slippery.
4. Be sure you know how to stop and start the whirlpool.
5. Run the whirlpool for no more than 15 minutes, unless instructed otherwise. Always stay with the client.
6. If the client complains of dizziness or lightheadedness, stop bathing and remove the client from the tub.
7. When the bath is finished, drain the tub before assisting the client to exit the tub.
8. Take particular care when assisting the client from the tub as the whirlpool action may cause the client to be unusually weak.
9. Pat the client dry, apply lotion, and assist with dressing.
10. Clean the tub as per instructions.

Commercial Whirlpool Tubs   Most long-term care facilities have commercial whirlpool tubs. These tubs are usually much higher than residential tubs and often require that clients use a bath lift to enter and exit the tub. Photo 19-6 illustrates this type of tub.

Procedure 19-3
Giving a Bath in a Commercial Whirlpool Tub

1. Fill the tub with warm water and be sure water is covering the jets in the tub.
2. Undress the client and place a towel over client's perineal area. Seat the client in the bath lift.
3. Follow the instructions for using the bath lift. Be sure safety waist belt is in place and is snug over the client's hips. Constantly reassure the client as the hydraulic lift places him or her in the tub.
4. Turn jets on for no more than 10–15 minutes. Always stay with the client. Ensure that you know how to start and stop the whirlpool.
5. If the client complains of dizziness or lightheadedness, stop bathing and remove the client from the tub.
6. When the bath is complete, turn jets off and drain the water out of the tub.
7. Place a towel over the client's back to prevent chilling, and pat dry as soon as possible.
8. Remove the safety belt only when the client is safe to move into chair.
9. Clean floor of water spills and clean tub according to agency policy.

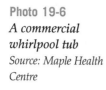

Photo 19-6
A commercial whirlpool tub
Source: Maple Health Centre

SPECIAL SITUATIONS

Possible Problems When Bathing a Client

If the Client Refuses Care

If the client refuses to have a bath, try to find out the reason for the refusal. Perhaps the bathroom is too cold or the client simply doesn't see the need for a bath. You may be able to fix the problem if you know what it is. You could raise the temperature of the bathroom or place towels in the dryer so as to be warm when the client uses them. Sometimes, explaining the use of a bath for refreshment and hygienic reasons will help.

Some reasons are rooted in the client's discomfort with an unfamiliar person assisting him or her. Similarly, the client may feel awkward if the worker is of the opposite sex. Establishing a therapeutic worker–client relationship is the best approach. Make sure that your client knows that you understand his or her discomfort and that you are a professional. Work with the client to find an acceptable solution. You might suggest that the client wash his or her perineal area while you wait at the door. Perhaps a family member could assist in the procedure, particularly if the client is confused or disoriented.

In some cases, a workable solution will not be possible. If all attempts to resolve the issue fail, advise your supervisor of the situation. If the refusal stems from the fact that you are of the opposite sex, perhaps your agency can send a worker of the client's sex to assist with the bath or shower. **Never perform a bath or shower if the client openly refuses.**

If the Client Is Not Able to Tolerate a Suitable Position for the Bath

If the client is unable to sit or lie on his or her back or side for long periods of time due to disease, shortness of breath, or other conditions, you must adapt the procedure to fit the client's needs. There are several possibilities you might explore. A partial bath may be one solution. If another worker is available to assist, you may be able to work more quickly and complete the task before the client's tolerance is exceeded.

You may have to adapt your technique to whatever position the client is most comfortable maintaining. For example, a client having shortness of breath when lying flat could be bathed in a sitting position.

If the Client Is Incontinent of Urine or of Stool While the Bath Is Being Performed

If the client is receiving a bed bath, change the sheets or pads. Use toilet tissue to remove excretions. Change the bath water and facecloths as necessary to prevent contamination. If the client is receiving a tub bath, drain the tub. Place a towel over the client to avoid a chill. Remove excretions with tissue and dispose of in toilet. Assist the client to exit the tub and clean the tub prior to refilling and assisting the client to return to the bath. Use a fresh facecloth to avoid contamination.

If Secretions or Stool Are Hardened on the Perineal Area

Use a commercial perineal wash, unscented back-rub lotion, or petroleum jelly on a dampened facecloth to help remove the hardened secretions without damaging the skin. This procedure may have to be repeated several times. Never rub the skin so hard that it becomes irritated or begins to break down.

If the Male Client Has an Erection While the Penis Is Being Washed

Calmly and casually tell the client you will leave him alone for a few minutes. Stay professional. This is not usually something that the client has control over and it can be just as embarrassing to him as it is to you. By returning in a few minutes and continuing on with the bath, the situation will be easier for both of you.

Bathing a Client Who Has an Ostomy

An **ostomy** is a surgical opening in the body. Gentle washing of the stoma is necessary to maintain cleanliness and prevent bleeding of the surface tissue. Clients and their families are taught how to care for the ostomy immediately after surgery. If you are not permitted to replace the ostomy appliance, try to coordinate the bath with the family so that a family member can change the wafer of the ostomy appliance at the same time.

Initially, the stoma of the ostomy appears fragile and sometimes frightening even to the experienced worker. The stoma is actually mucous membrane, with a consistency much the same as the vagina. There are no nerve endings in the stoma, so the client does not have feelings of pain in the stoma.

There are three types of ostomy. The contents that will evacuate depend on the type:

- colostomy—formed stool contents empty once or twice a day
- ileostomy—loose stool contents may continually drain
- urostomy—continuous drainage of urine

If there is a chance of continuous drainage from the stoma when washing, apply gauze or tampon to the stoma when drying to prevent leakage onto the clean skin.

Procedure 19-4
Bathing a Client with an Ostomy

basin with warm water

2 facecloths,
1 towel

bar of soap

lotion for back rub

clean sheets
(as needed)

clean gown, pyjamas,
or clothes

new ostomy
appliance

A client's ostomy appliance need not be changed at each bath. The following procedure may be used when the appliance is to be changed.

1. Check the service plan or any doctor's orders for bathing. Ask the client or the family (if appropriate) for any instructions they have received. If in doubt as to the procedure to be used, consult your supervisor.
2. Have the new appliance ready to apply.
3. Assure the client that washing around the stoma is as important as any other part of the bathing routine.
4. Remove the old appliance by gently pulling down from one corner and by placing your hand under the appliance as it is lifted. See Figure 19-7.

FIGURE 19-7
Removing the old appliance

5. Use a soaped facecloth and gently wash around the stoma to remove residual glue or stool contents. Repeat until clean. Rinse well.
6. If the area is reddened or excoriated, report to the family or nurse for further treatment.
7. If the client is able to sit in the tub, fill tub up to just below the stoma level to avoid water going in the stoma. If the client is able to shower, ensure that the water is not directed into the stoma.
8. Be sure area around the stoma is dry prior to applying the new appliance.
9. Allow the client or family to assist whenever possible.

Performing a Back Rub

Most clients really look forward to a back rub. It can be performed at bath time or at bedtime or any other time in the day in order to promote relaxation for the client. The back rub has other benefits as well. It promotes dilation of the peripheral blood vessels, which, in turn, enhances circulation. It also rids the surface of dead skin cells. The stimulation of the massaging technique causes relaxation of the muscles of the back and shoulders. It also provides for human contact, and allows you to observe the condition of your client's skin. Figure 19-8 shows the basic motions of a back rub.

FIGURE 19-8
Back rub technique

Principles of giving a back rub:

1. Wash hands prior to and after giving a back rub.
2. Apply lubricant to your hands to reduce the friction created by one skin surface rubbing against another. Many clients have a lotion suitable for this purpose. You may need to apply lubricant several times to the client's back depending on how dry his or her skin is.
3. You may use an unperfumed talc or cornstarch if the client is perspiring and his or her skin is not otherwise dry. Do not allow talc or cornstarch to clump in folds.
4. Explain the procedure to the client.
5. Provide privacy. Ensure that other areas of the client's body are covered.
6. Raise the bed to working level (usually waist high).
7. Ensure that the client is in a comfortable position, preferably prone (on stomach) or side-lying if prone is not possible. If the client cannot lie down, you may be able to provide an upper back rub with the client seated in a chair, leaning forward with his or her arms on a table or other immoveable surface.

Procedure 19-5
Giving a Back Rub

EQUIPMENT

bath blanket or towel

skin lotion or oil

talcum powder
(if needed)

1. Remove the client's gown, loosen ties, or remove pyjama top.
2. Position the client with bedclothes pulled down to the top of the buttocks and bath blanket or towel over top of the bedclothes.
3. Apply a moderate amount of lotion to the your hands and rub hands together to warm lotion.
4. Start in the lumbar region and smooth lotion toward shoulders.
5. Begin the massage with effleurage by stroking with both hands from the buttocks toward the shoulders and back again. Stroke firmly going up to the shoulders and lightly when moving back to the top of the buttocks.
6. Perform long strokes up the back and circular motions around the shoulders at least eight to ten times.
7. Petrissage may be used to knead the superficial tissues between the fingertips of both hands, moving toward the shoulders. Other techniques may be performed if extra training is provided.
8. Complete the massage by changing back to effleurage and stroking the back several more times.
9. Remove excess lubricant with the towel, if necessary.
10. Remove the bath blanket and replace the client's bedclothes.
11. Place the client in a comfortable position. Attach the call bell, if present.

ORAL CARE

Purpose

Oral care is essential to health and to a positive self-image. Whether the client has natural teeth or dentures, oral care must be performed at least four times per day. It is important that oral care be performed even when the client is unconscious. Diseased teeth and gums can make eating painful and even spread infection to other areas of the body.

The mucous membranes of the mouth are made up of delicate epithelial tissues, which are prone to injury and infection, and so must be diligently cared for. If the client is able to move his or her hands and arms, minimal assistance in placing toothpaste on the brush or handing the client mouthwash may be all that is necessary. A client's teeth and oral surfaces should be cleansed after each meal and before bedtime. Oral care may be required more often if the client's mouth is dry due to disease, use of certain medications, or other reasons.

Some clients have specific dental prosthetics such as bridges, full or partial dentures, or dental implants. Some are fixed and others are removable. If your client has dental prosthetics make certain you know how to properly care for the specific prosthetic.

Clients often have strong preferences for how their oral care is provided. It's very important to follow your client's preferences for how oral care is provided and for what supplies are to be used.

Cleaning Teeth

Principles of cleaning teeth:

1. Ensure privacy.
2. Wash hands prior to and after procedure.
3. Use disposable gloves for oral care.
4. Use clean technique when cleaning the oral cavity.
5. Use only the client's personal toothbrush, a fresh toothette, or swab.
6. Allow the client to assist wherever able.
7. Use appropriate solution to cleanse mouth.
8. Gather all equipment.
9. Explain the procedure to the client.
10. Adjust the client to a sitting position if conscious and to side-lying position if the client is unconscious.
11. Identify any problems with full or partial dentures, bridges, or any loose teeth.
12. Be aware that the client may want to leave dentures out at night, so have a denture cup ready.
13. Observe the mouth for bleeding, redness, sores, white patches, or swelling. Report any of these observations to your supervisor.

Different procedures are used for conscious and unconscious clients.

Procedure 19-6
Providing Mouth Care for the Conscious, Alert Client

Figure 19-9 shows mouth care for the conscious and alert client.
1. Place a towel across the client's chest.
2. Assist the client to brush the teeth, including the tongue.
3. Hold basin for the client to spit into.
4. Give several sips of water or mouthwash to rinse.
5. If client's mouth is dry, avoid commercial mouthwashes. Use 5 to 15 mL (1 tsp. to 1 tbsp.) of baking soda to 250 mL (8 oz.) of water to lubricate the mouth. Use as often as needed.
6. Offer the towel. Assist as required to wash and dry the client's face.
7. Remove and wash out the soiled basin.
8. Leave client with fresh water to drink.

EQUIPMENT

toothbrush, tooth-paste, floss (if available) for natural teeth

commercial tooth-ettes, if toothbrush not available

kidney basin or basin

towel, facecloth

mouthwash (if used)

glass of water

FIGURE 19-9
Mouth care for the conscious and alert client

Procedure 19-7
Providing Mouth Care for the Unconscious Client

EQUIPMENT

toothbrush, tooth-paste, floss (if available) for natural teeth

gauze-covered tongue depressor

bulb syringe

towel, facecloth

kidney basin

lubricant for lips (such as petroleum jelly or lip gloss)

Figure 19-10 shows mouth care for the unconscious client.

1. Place the towel and kidney basin under side of mouth while the client is lying on side.
2. Use a gauze-covered tongue depressor to hold the mouth open while brushing teeth. Make certain that the gauze is firmly attached to the tongue depressor. Never put fingers in to the unconscious client's mouth, as he or she may bite down due to the stimulation.
3. Brush the teeth from the gumline down to the tip of the teeth in an up-and-down fashion. Ensure brush angle makes good contact with the teeth.
4. Brush the inside of the teeth and then the outside.
5. Brush the tops of molars.
6. Gently brush the tongue.
7. Rinse the mouth using a fresh gauze-wrapped tongue depressor soaked in fresh water. If directed, you may also use a bulb syringe to rinse the mouth, making sure that no water goes down the client's throat.

FIGURE 19-10
Mouth care for the unconscious client

8. Apply lubricant to the lips. Repeat as needed.
9. Wash and dry the client's face.
10. Observe mouth for bleeding, redness, sores, white patches or swelling.

You may notice that the client's tongue is coated with white patches. This can be due to an infection or to dryness. Report the condition to the appropriate person so that the condition can be properly treated. If the condition is due to dryness, applying an approved solution with a toothette every half hour throughout the day will remove the coating.

Assisting the Client with Cleaning Dentures

Procedure 19-8
Cleaning Dentures

Dentures should be cleaned after each meal. This reduces the possibility of food particles becoming trapped under the plate and causing irritation.

1. Assist the client to a sitting position.
2. Place the over-bed table in front of the client.
3. Place the denture cup or kidney basin close to the client and ask the client to remove his or her dentures.
4. If the client isn't able to remove the dentures, assist by grasping the upper denture with thumb and forefinger and gently wiggling to break the seal. Figure 19-11 illustrates this technique.

EQUIPMENT

kidney basin
or denture cup

denture brush
and paste

mouthwash

glass of water

denture adhesive

towel

FIGURE 19-11
Removing dentures

5. Lift out the bottom denture.
6. Place the dentures immediately into the basin to avoid breakage or dropping.
7. Take the dentures to the bathroom and place the basin in the sink under warm, running water.
8. Using the client's denture brush and paste, clean the dentures from the gumline to the tip of the teeth in an up-and-down fashion. Clean any debris or leftover food out of the crevices. Observe for any broken, rough, sharp, or worn areas. Always brush the dentures over the basin to avoid breakage by dropping.
9. Rinse dentures well.
10. Return the dentures to the client. Before inserting, allow the client to rinse his or her mouth with mouthwash or fresh water. If appropriate, assist client to clean mouth and gums with a toothette soaked in mouthwash. Rinse with water.
11. Assist the client in replacing the dentures if required.

12. The client may want denture adhesive applied. If so, follow the directions for application.
13. If the client is having difficulty replacing the dentures, replace the top denture first. Then, using one finger, open the client's mouth wide and slip the bottom denture in sideways and then turn.
14. Wash client's face and dry with towel.
15. Leave the client in appropriate position.

It is not advisable to leave dentures in an unconscious client's mouth due to the risk of choking or aspiration. Keep dentures stored in water in a denture cup. Advise the family and any other caregivers that the dentures are not in.

HAIR CARE

Purpose

Few things make a client feel better than having clean, well-groomed hair. Often when a client becomes very ill, hair care is neglected. The hair becomes soiled and tangled and may have exudate in it due to excess perspiration or blood (such as from a head injury). This is uncomfortable, negatively affects the client's self-image, and can harbour microorganisms that may be harmful to the client.

After bathing the client, the hair should be combed or brushed into a style that pleases the client. Never cut the client's hair or place in an unfamiliar style without the client's or family's permission. If the hair is badly tangled, apply mineral oil and use a wide-tooth comb to remove tangles. Wash hair after the tangles are removed. Alternately, you can wash the client's hair, apply conditioner, and then use a wide-tooth comb to remove tangles.

Encourage the client to wash his or her hair as often as desired. If the client is able to wash hair independently, provide towels and shampoo. If the client is having a tub bath or shower, assist the client in washing his or her hair. Be sure to dry the client's hair well after shampooing or place a dry towel on the pillow to soak up any additional moisture. Dry shampoos are available in pharmacies if the client cannot have his or her head wet (for example, due to sutures).

Washing Hair Using a Bed Tray

Procedure 19-9
Washing Hair Using a Bed Tray

1. Lay the client flat and place a plastic sheet under the client's head.
2. Place the large bucket on the floor near the bed and underneath the spout of the shampoo tray.
3. Fill the other large bucket with warm water. Test temperature with wrist.

4. Place the client's head in the tray, putting a folded facecloth under the client's neck for added comfort. Figure 19-12 illustrates the proper position.

EQUIPMENT

shampoo tray

2 towels

2 facecloths

2 large buckets

1 small bucket or jug

shampoo and conditioner (per the client's preferences)

FIGURE 19-12
Client properly positioned for a bed shampoo

5. Give the client the other facecloth to hold over his or her eyes.
6. Wet the client's hair with water using the small bucket or jug.
7. Apply a small amount of shampoo to your hands and rub together to form lather.
8. Apply lather to the client's hair, massaging gently in a circular motion to increase the client's circulation. Be sure to wash all parts of the client's head by asking the client to turn his or her head as necessary.
9. Squeeze excess shampoo out of the hair and rinse well.
10. Repeat the shampoo if necessary for very soiled hair; however, check the client's comfort and general condition before going ahead. If the client cannot tolerate lying flat for very long and becomes short of breath or generally distressed, stop the procedure and return the client to a sitting position.
11. Apply and rinse conditioner, if used.
12. Dry the hair well using a large towel.
13. Remove the shampoo tray and plastic sheet.
14. Replace wet towel with another towel and rub hair well to dry. Use a hair dryer if the client has one and can tolerate the heat and airflow. Be sure to set the dryer to a comfortable temperature so as not to burn the client's skin.
15. Comb and style hair according to the client's preference.
16. Clean up and remove the equipment. Clean the shampoo tray with appropriate disinfectant (if required or if it is to be used with another client).

This procedure may be adapted for use where there is no shampoo tray available. Use a firm plastic sheet, such as a vinyl tablecloth, folded in half. Roll a towel lengthwise to form a skinny "rope" and place inside the fold. Place the client's head on the centre of the roll and arrange the plastic sheet to form a trough to drain water from the bed. Figure 19-13 illustrates a homemade shampoo tray.

FIGURE 19-13
Homemade shampoo tray

Washing Hair at a Sink

Some clients prefer to have their hair washed under running water, even if they choose not to wash their hair when they bathe or shower. If the client can sit in a wheelchair or movable recliner chair, he or she may be able to have his or her hair washed at a sink. The client must also be able to hold his or her head forward or backward to accomplish the procedure. Make sure that you check with your supervisor before you wash the client's hair at the sink. An older person may have difficulty holding his or her head back due to neck problems, or may have circulation problems that make holding his or her head back unadvisable.

Procedure 19-10
Washing Hair at a Sink

1. Be sure that the client's chair cannot move before you proceed with the task.
2. If the client is going to hold his or her head forward over the sink, place a towel over the client's shoulders and give the client a facecloth to hold over his or her eyes.
3. If the client is facing away from the sink and is letting his or her head lay backward on the sink, place a folded facecloth on the edge of the sink for comfort.
4. Apply shampoo to your hands and work into a lather.
5. Apply lather to the client's hair, massaging gently in a circular motion to increase the client's circulation. Be sure to wash all parts of the client's head by asking the client to turn his or her head as necessary.
6. Squeeze excess shampoo out of the hair and rinse well.
7. Repeat the shampoo if necessary for very soiled hair, but check the client's comfort and general condition before going ahead.
8. Apply and rinse conditioner, if used.
9. Dry the hair well using a large towel. Use a hair dryer if the client has one and can tolerate the heat and airflow. Be sure to set the dryer to a comfortable temperature so as not to burn the client's skin.
10. Comb and style hair according to the client's preference.
11. Assist the client to a comfortable position.

EQUIPMENT

shampoo and conditioner, per client preference

2 washcloths

comb

2 large towels

hair dryer (if available)

Photo 19-7
A client having her hair washed at the sink.
Source: CHATS

SHAVING THE CLIENT

Purpose

Men are used to shaving daily and when they are unable to do so because of illness or weakness, they do not feel clean or well groomed. Most men prefer to use their own shaving equipment. If the client lives in a facility, the desired equipment can be brought in from home by the family.

Prior to shaving a client, the worker must be aware of the client's general condition. This is particularly important if the client has a bleeding disorder (i.e., bleeding is difficult or slow to stop) or is taking medication to thin his blood (e.g., anticoagulants). You must obtain approval to shave a client who has a bleeding disorder or is taking anticoagulant medication.

Procedure 19-11
Shaving the Client

EQUIPMENT

For shaving with a safety razor:

shaving cream, lather, or soap

facecloth and towel

wash basin with warm water

safety razor

mirror

aftershave lotion, if desired

EQUIPMENT

For shaving with an electric razor:

pre-shave lotion (if available)

electric razor (check that cord is not frayed and that razor is in good working condition)

mirror

aftershave lotion, if desired

If the client is able to shave himself:
1. Assist the client to a sitting position in bed or to a chair with a table in front and a mirror positioned so he can see. Make certain that the lighting is good.
2. Assist as needed.

If the client is unable to shave himself and uses an electric razor:
1. Apply pre-shave lotion if desired by the client.
2. Plug in the razor and begin shaving by moving the head of the razor back and forth over the hair growth. Use your other hand to pull the skin taut as you shave.

If the client is unable to shave himself and uses a safety razor:
1. Apply a damp, hot facecloth to the client's face for five minutes prior to shaving to soften the bristles, especially if the growth is long.
2. Fill the basin with warm water.
3. Position the client in a suitable position to reach all areas of the face.
4. Apply shaving lather, cream, or soap evenly over the face.
5. Hold the skin taut with your nondominant hand and begin shaving using short, even strokes (Figure 19-14).

6. Pull the razor blade lightly but firmly against the direction of the hair growth.
7. Rinse the razor frequently in the warm water.
8. Be sure not to shave off a moustache, beard, or sideburns unless the client or family has given permission.
9. After shaving is finished, wipe face with the wet facecloth and dry well with the towel.
10. If the client desires, apply aftershave lotion.
11. Observe for any nicks or scrapes. If present, apply a pressure bandage and report the occurrence to the appropriate person.

FIGURE 19-14
Shaving the client with a safety razor

FOOT CARE

A client's feet should be inspected daily, especially if the client's circulation to the feet is impaired or the client is diabetic. Observe for any redness, irritation marks from shoes, colour of the feet, and any skin abnormalities. Be sure to check between the toes for any crevices or cracks in the skin. These fissures could lead to infection.

What makes up daily foot care will vary depending upon the client's condition and preferences. If the client has dry skin, bathing the feet every day will excessively dry the feet, eventually cause cracking, and possibly lead to infection. In this case, a foot rub with lotion is soothing to the client. It also gives you a chance to inspect the client's feet.

Clients whose feet smell or are very moist from perspiration may be bathed. In these cases, the client is often advised to wear cotton socks and air his or her feet for some time every day. Moist, damp areas can harbour a fungal infection.

Corns and bunions can interfere with normal walking and should be examined by a podiatrist or chiropodist. You should never attempt to trim a client's corns or to disturb a bunion.

Properly fitting shoes are an important part of foot care. Indentations and reddened or broken areas in the client's foot that indicate that the client's shoes are too tight should be reported to the appropriate person. Decreased circulation may mean that a client does not feel the tightness.

Many clients enjoy a periodic foot soak. Use the following procedure if you are to soak your client's feet. If the client cannot sit in a chair, provide for a foot soak at the end of the bed bath.

Procedure 19-12
Providing Foot Care

If your client can sit in a chair:
1. Assist your client to a comfortable sitting position.
2. Place bath mat on floor in front of client.
3. Place basin on mat.
4. Dissolve soap in warm water of basin.
5. Follow steps 7–15 to complete the procedure.

If the client cannot sit up:
6. Position the basin at the foot of the bed.
7. Place client's feet in basin.
8. Place towel over client's feet to conserve heat.
9. Soak feet for 15–20 minutes. Add warm water as required to maintain proper temperature.
10. At end of soak period, wash feet with washcloth. Note any irregularities in each foot. Rinse feet and pat dry.
11. Using the orange stick, gently clean the toenails. Do not cut toenails.
12. If the client's skin is dry, apply lotion to tops and bottoms of feet. Avoid putting lotion between the toes as this can foster microorganisms. Wipe off any excess lotion to reduce the possibility of the client slipping.

EQUIPMENT

basin with warm water, large enough to hold both of the client's feet

bath mat (on which to place the basin)

foot soap or mild soap (as per the client's preferences)

washcloth

2 towels

orange stick

gloves

13. If the client tends to perspire, apply a light dusting of talcum powder to the feet. Allow feet to air dry, if possible.
14. Assist client to put on socks and shoes or slippers.
15. Report long toenails and other irregularities to the appropriate person.

NAIL CARE

Fingernails and toenails should be inspected daily, when dressing and undressing, and during the bathing routine. Normally, nails are smooth, transparent, and rounded over the edge of the fingers or toes. As a person ages, nails become harder and their care becomes more difficult. Some conditions cause the nails to become discoloured, thick, brittle, or to have different shapes. These conditions should be examined and treated by a specialist.

Your agency may allow you to cut the fingernails of a healthy client. Because of the risk of infection, you must never cut the nails of a diabetic client. Similarly, you should never cut the nails of a client who is taking anticoagulants or has a bleeding abnormality.

Procedure 19-13
Providing Nail Care

EQUIPMENT

nail clippers or sharp scissors

nail file or emery board

orange stick

small basin with warm water and soap

towel

nail polish remover (if required)

nail polish (if required)

1. Position the client so the hands and feet can be soaked in a basin to soften the nails.
2. If the client is on bed rest, place the basin on the bed and soak hands while washing the client's arms and chest.
3. If the client is sitting in a chair, use the procedure defined earlier in this section to soak the client's feet.
4. After soaking, dry the hands and feet well. Inspect the hands, feet, and nails. Report any redness, broken skin, discharge, or other irregularities.
5. Remove old nail polish if necessary. Trim the fingernails if needed (and appropriate) by cutting straight across and avoiding cutting into the corners. Photo 19-8 illustrates proper nail cutting.

Photo 19-8
Cutting nails straight across

6. Clean under the fingernails with an orange stick.
7. File the edges of the fingernails until smooth with an emery board or a nail file.
8. Apply new nail polish if desired by the client.
9. Apply lotion to hands and feet when finished. Rub the lotion in by massaging in a gentle kneading fashion.

EYE CARE

Routine Care

Normally, the eyes do not require any special care other than the routine used in the bathing procedure. You must observe for any drainage, noting the colour, consistency, and where it is coming from, as well as any redness, watering, or signs of irritation. Make note of any complaints from the client (such as itching or dryness) and report these, along with your observations, to the appropriate person.

If your client is very ill, you should watch to ensure that the eyelids are shutting. If they do not, the eye may tend to dry out. Report this observation so that special drops or care may be provided.

Eyeglass Care

Eyeglasses are made of many materials, each requiring a particular type of care. Make sure you know the correct procedure so that the lens will not be scratched or marred.

If there are no special instructions, clean eyeglasses with mild dish soap, rinse with clean water, and dry with a soft cloth. Do not use wipes or hand soap as they will leave a film on the glass. If the client is not wearing his or her glasses, they should be stored in a proper case to prevent damage.

Contact lenses require special care. Make sure you know how to assist the client with lens care and, if you are required to do so, how to insert and remove them.

Artificial Eye Care

An artificial eye is made of glass or plastic and is very close to the actual shape and appearance of the normal eye. You must receive specific instructions on the care of the artificial eye if you are to provide this type of care.

EAR CARE

Routine Care

Most ear care is performed through the bathing procedure. Care must be taken not to introduce any objects into the ear canal. Cotton swabs are a particular hazard as they can puncture the eardrum. A buildup of wax (cerumen) may have to be removed through special procedures if it is affecting hearing capabilities. Report client complaints of pressure or pain in the ear, observations of excessive wax in the ear canal, or observations of diminished hearing acuity to the appropriate person.

Care for the external ear includes gentle washing of the ear lobe, behind the ear, and the folds of the outer ear.

Hearing Aid Care

Photo 19-9
In-the-ear and behind-the-ear hearing aids
Source: Robert Harmon

There are four different types of hearing aids. Photo 19-9 illustrates two types. Although they look different, they all act in the same way. The tiny microphone in the aid picks up sound waves and amplifies them so that sound may be transmitted to the inner ear.

The hearing aid is operated by a battery and has an "on-off" switch. Always turn off the aid when not in use and store in a case to prevent loss or damage. If the client will not be wearing the hearing aid for a few days, remove the battery from the aid and leave it in the storage case.

Clients who use bilateral aids (aids in both ears) have a distinct right ear aid and a left ear aid. Be sure to identify the right and left aids before assisting the client to place the aid in his or her ear. The aid must be properly placed to be comfortable and useful. Ask for specific instruction on how to properly insert your client's aid.

Some aids have an ear mould that is connected to the aid. This mould fits into the ear. You may carefully remove this mould from the aid and wash it with warm soapy water. Dry the ear mould well before connecting it to the aid and replacing it in the client's ear. Do not expose any of the other parts to moisture. Never allow a one-piece aid (sometimes called an in-the-ear aid) to become wet.

CONTINENCE CARE

Continence and Incontinence

Continence refers to the ability to control bowel or bladder elimination. **Incontinence** describes the loss of this control. There are several causes for bowel or bladder incontinence. It's important to remember that a client may be incontinent of bowel or bladder, or both.

Incontinence is often embarrassing to the client and the client's family and can cause significant changes in a client's quality of life. The person may not want to go out or even to have visitors.

A great deal of care is required to assist an incontinent client even if incontinence pads or briefs are used. It can be very difficult for a caregiver to cope. As a result, incontinence is one of the leading reasons given when an application is made to a long-term care facility.

No matter what causes it, incontinence may be resolved, its frequency reduced, or its presence better managed. The underlying cause, as well as the client's ability and motivation, will help to determine whether incontinence can be fully resolved.

Bladder Incontinence

Normal Bladder Function

Normal bladder function depends upon four groups of functions: the urologic, the neurologic, the psychologic, and mobility. These four functions are described as:

- Urologic function: the ability to produce urine and store it in the bladder.
- Neurologic function: the sensation (message) getting to and from the brain.
- Psychologic function: the ability to perceive the sensation and make sense of it.
- Mobility: the physical ability to get to and use a commode or toilet.

Age-Related Changes

Three major age-related changes in the urinary system may affect continence:

- **Thinning of the bladder wall.** Because it is thinner, the bladder can empty at smaller volumes. Sometimes this happens without warning. This thinning usually results in more frequent, less controlled voiding.
- **Reduced bladder capacity.** An older person's bladder may hold only 250–300 mL of fluid—approximately half of a younger person's capacity. As a result, the person will likely have to void more often.
- **Loss of elasticity.** Because of this loss, the bladder can become like an overstretched balloon unable to regain its original shape. This can result in an inability to empty the bladder completely.

Urinary Incontinence

There are six types of urinary incontinence: urge, stress, overflow, total, psychogenic, and mobility-related. Table 19-2 describes each type.

Bowel Incontinence

Bowel incontinence is often called fecal incontinence or incontinence of stool. Like normal urinary function, normal bowel function depends upon four factors: the production of feces; the ability to trigger the need to defecate; the ability to perceive, recognize, and act upon this need; and the ability to physically get to and use a commode or toilet.

Contrary to what we often hear in television advertising, a person does not have to have a daily bowel movement in order to be "regular." Normal patterns of elimination vary from three to four times per week to more than once per day.

Age-related changes may result in reduced muscle tone, making it more difficult for the body to move feces through the intestines. Like urinary incontinence, bowel incontinence can be extremely distressing to the client, family members, and caregivers.

There are four major types of bowel incontinence. These are listed in Table 19-3.

TABLE 19-2	Types of Urinary Incontinence	
Type	**What It Is**	**Possible Causes**
Urge	Sudden, urgent need to void	Urinary tract infection; medications; obstruction of urine flow
Stress	Leakage when a person laughs, coughs, sneezes, stands up, strains, or lifts a heavy object	Urinary sphincter weakness; in women, physical changes caused by childbirth or surgery; in men, removal of the prostate
Overflow	Urine buildup in bladder that becomes too much for the sphincter to hold; urine leaks periodically and without warning	Weakened bladder muscles; obstruction of urine flow; nerve malfunction; medications
Total	Continual leakage as sphincter does not close	Injury to bladder neck
Psychogenic	Loss of control for psychological reasons	Dementia; depression
Mobility-Related	Inability to reach commode or toilet or to do so in time	Mobility problems; physical barriers; communication problems

TABLE 19-3	Types of Bowel Incontinence	
Type	**What It Is**	**Possible Causes**
Physiologic–chronic	Physical inability to control defecation	Loss of sphincter muscle tone; rectal prolapse; tumours; medications; long-term laxative use; injury to sphincter
Physiologic–acute	Physical inability to control defecation in response to an acute condition	Intestinal disorders; diarrhea; impaction
Psychologic	Inability to recognize the need to defecate	Dementia; depression
Mobility-Related	Inability to reach commode or toilet or to do so in time	Mobility impairments; physical barriers; communication problems

Maintaining Bowel and Bladder Continence

Many types of incontinence can be avoided or minimized. You will be much more successful in assisting your client if you first try to identify the cause of the incontinence. You may find one or more of the following ideas helpful.

- Identify and follow the client's bowel and bladder patterns. The client, the client's family, and/or other caregivers can often identify times the client routinely voids or has a bowel movement. Follow the client's established pattern whenever possible.
- Note patterns of incontinence. Toilet the client prior to times of incontinence.
- Keep the routine consistent. Consistency helps establish a pattern. It can also help avoid constipation.
- Encourage the person to try to void or move the bowels at the established times, even if the urge isn't immediately present. Running water in the sink and encouraging the client to bend forward (putting pressure on the bladder) may also help to trigger urge.
- Ensure the client privacy. Voiding and/or having a bowel movement are very personal and private. Remain in the room only if necessary or if the client requests that you do.
- Use a commode or toilet instead of a bedpan. Sitting on a commode or toilet is a more natural position. It makes use of gravity as well as increased abdominal pressure to promote bladder or bowel evacuation. If the client must use a bedpan, make sure the head of the bed is raised as upright as possible.
- Recognize agitation as a possible symptom of the client's need to void or have a bowel movement. Clients with a cognitive impairment or a communication disorder may become more upset when incontinent or because of the fear of being incontinent.
- Periodic agitation, constant requests for toileting, or a change in normal bowel/bladder patterns may signal an infection. Report any observations to your supervisor immediately.

Retraining

It is often possible for a client to re-establish bladder or bowel continence. This works best when the client is cognitively intact and motivated. The rewards are significant: increased client comfort and self-esteem, reduced risk of skin breakdown, and reduced need for personal care.

A registered nurse usually establishes the retraining plan. The plan is developed only after any factors affecting continence are addressed, including the treatment of any underlying infection and the ensurance of adequate food and fluid intake.

Retraining involves a number of people: the client, the client's family members, and other caregivers. Each person's involvement in setting and carrying out the retraining schedule is identified.

An acceptable schedule for toileting is set based on the client's patterns of elimination. In some cases, this schedule allows for increasing periods of time between toileting.

The Support Worker's Role in Retraining

Your participation and support to the client are essential to his or her success. You can assist your client by following a few simple guidelines:

- Learn the client's schedule. Identify whether the schedule is fixed or whether it is set to promote increasing periods of time between toileting.
- Observe for and respond to signs that the client needs to void or to have a bowel movement, whether or not it's at the scheduled time. Unfamiliar foods, a change in food or fluid intake, illness, or medication may affect a client's pattern of elimination.
- Assist the client promptly. Do not make the client wait.
- Make certain that the time provided is sufficient and that the client has privacy. Rushing the client will result in failure and embarrassment.

- Assist the client to maintain good hygiene. Provide or assist the client with peri-care as required. Assist the client to wash his or her hands. Make certain that you wash your hands after assisting the client.

- Be consistent and encouraging. Retraining takes time and patience. Encourage the client and offer praise appropriately when things go well. Offer encouragement if incontinence occurs. Never reprimand or criticize the client for incontinence.

Supporting Good Bowel and Bladder Function

The Fibre-Fluid Balance

Good bowel and bladder function is the result of:

1. Adequate fluid intake
2. Adequate fibre intake

Fibre is essential to the body's ability to easily move wastes through the intestines and bowel. Fibre requires fluid to moisten it and ease its movement. Adequate fibre and fluid can help to reduce the need for laxatives or enemas.

Fibre comes from many sources: fruits, vegetables, grains, and bran (see Photo 19-10). Sometimes, a commercial fibre additive is prescribed to increase fibre intake. Many long-term care facilities provide special high-fibre meals and snacks to residents.

Photo 19-10
Fruits, whole grains, and vegetables provide good natural sources of fibre.

Constipation and Impaction

Insufficient fibre or fibre without adequate fluid can produce constipation. When this happens, the client may experience abdominal discomfort and flatulence (gas).

Long-term use of laxatives can make the body dependent upon them to move waste. When laxatives are discontinued or reduced, the person becomes constipated. The client's doctor should treat constipation related to laxative use. You may be asked to assist a client in carrying out a routine set by the client's doctor to address this problem.

In extreme cases, insufficient fibre or fluid can result in impaction (a condition in which feces becomes "stuck" in the intestines). Impaction can be life threatening. A client who cannot move his or her bowels or passes only small amounts of very thin diarrhea may have an impaction. You should immediately report any observations to your supervisor.

Diarrhea

Diarrhea describes bowel movements that are loose, runny, or almost liquid in consistency. Diarrhea can cause a client to become dehydrated. It can also be a symptom of laxative overuse, a food intolerance, an illness, or an impaction. Any observation of diarrhea must be immediately reported to your supervisor so that the underlying cause may be identified and treated.

Urinary Tract Infections

Urinary tract infections (UTIs) pose great risk to the client. A client with a urinary tract infection can become incontinent or confused. The pain from the infection can range from distracting to disabling. Left untreated, the infection can progress into more serious conditions.

The symptoms of a urinary tract infection are often overlooked. You should observe for any of these symptoms:

- increase in frequency of voiding or incontinence
- increased agitation
- complaints of burning or pain when voiding
- cloudy, strong-smelling urine

Immediately report any observations to your supervisor.

Reducing the Risk of Urinary Tract Infections

Following a few simple steps will help to reduce your client's risk for developing a urinary tract infection.

Encourage your client to drink six to eight glasses of fluid each day. Many older adults reduce the amount of fluids taken so as to reduce the number of times they need to void. Actually, reduced fluid intake results in an increased need to void. This is because reduced fluid results in concentrated urine that irritates the bladder wall. This irritation results in increased sensation and stimulation to void. In addition, concentrated urine may produce a burning sensation when voiding.

Adjust the timing of the fluid intake (not the amount per day) if the client has to void or is incontinent during the night. Encourage the client to drink more during the day and less after dinner.

Immediately report any change in bladder routine or function: in the amount, colour, or clarity of urine; or any complaints of pain or urgency. Any of these could signal a urinary tract infection.

Continence Products

As a support worker, you will become familiar with three types of continence products: briefs and pads, catheters, and ostomy appliances. Properly used, these products can make it easier for a client to live comfortably. Improperly used, they can create unnecessary dependence and diminish a client's self-esteem.

Briefs and Pads

There are many types of absorbent briefs and pads available. Pads range from wafer-thin pads that are attached to a person's underpants to thicker pads (often filled with super-absorbent material) that can hold a substantial amount of urine. Photo 19-11 shows a common pad. Briefs are available in wrap-around and pull-on styles. Photo 19-12 shows a common type of brief. Personal preference as well as the type and degree of incontinence will determine the best product for an individual.

You may hear others speak of these briefs as diapers. Do not use this term. Diapers are used for infants, not adults. Calling briefs diapers can make the client feel like an infant.

Assisting a Client Who Uses Pads

Pads are placed on the crotch of the person's underwear. Some pads have an adhesive strip that attaches them to the underwear. Others require a brief designed to hold the pad.

Photo 19-11
Common incontinence pads

Photo 19-12
Closed incontinence brief

Pads should be checked every two hours unless more frequent checking is ordered. They should also be changed whenever wet or soiled. Your client may be able to tell you when the pad needs to be changed. Dispose of soiled pads as instructed by your client or supervisor.

Assisting a Client Who Wears Briefs

Like pads, briefs should be checked every two hours unless more frequent checking is ordered. Many briefs have an indicator that changes colour when the brief is wet or soiled.

Briefs come in two types: wrap around and pull on. Wrap-around briefs are hourglass shaped when open as shown in Photo 19-13. The top of the hourglass is the back of the brief. The bottom portion of the hourglass is the front of the brief. The narrow section is placed between the client's legs. There are usually three tabs that attach the back of the brief to the front.

Most wrap-around briefs cannot easily be opened and reclosed as the adhesive tabs often tear the outer protective covering. Many have a bar on the outside that indicates whether the brief is wet so that it is not necessary to remove the tabs.

Pull-on briefs are similar to underpants. They are put on in the same manner as underpants, but care must be taken to avoid tearing the waterproof liner and plastic outer covering. As there are no tabs to open and reattach, these briefs can be removed as required. Dispose of soiled briefs as instructed by your client or supervisor.

Photo 19-13
Open incontinence brief

Catheters

Urinary catheters are devices that allow the bladder to drain into a collection bag. There are two categories of catheters: internal and external. Internal catheters are sterile devices that must be inserted by a health professional. If they are not cared for properly, they can put the client at risk for infection. Support workers should never attempt to insert, reposition, or remove an internal catheter.

Internal Catheters

There are two main types of internal catheters: indwelling and straight.

Indwelling Catheter This catheter is usually placed in the bladder for a period of two to four weeks. A balloon at the internal end of the catheter prevents the tube from slipping out. The external end is attached to a draining bag.

Indwelling catheters can be used for men or women. Figure 19-15 shows placement of the catheter in a female bladder. Figure 19-16 shows placement in a male bladder.

Straight Catheter The straight catheter is used when a client's bladder does not drain completely. The catheter is inserted to drain the bladder and then is immediately removed. This procedure may be done several times a day. Some adults with paraplegia use this form of catheter to periodically drain the bladder. The procedure is called intermittent catheterization. Many clients are taught to perform this procedure. As a support worker, you should never attempt to perform this procedure without specific training and approval from your agency.

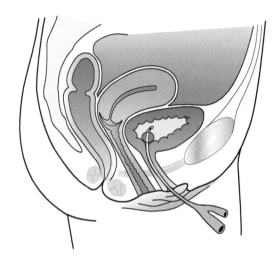

FIGURE 19-15
Indwelling catheter placement in a female

FIGURE 19-16
Indwelling catheter placement in a male

Some male clients use an external catheter. These are sometimes called condom catheters because they resemble a condom with a tube attached to the end. Figure 19-17 shows a condom catheter in place. The tube is attached to a drainage bag. This tube drains urine that flows from the penis into the condom portion.

FIGURE 19-17
Condom catheter in place

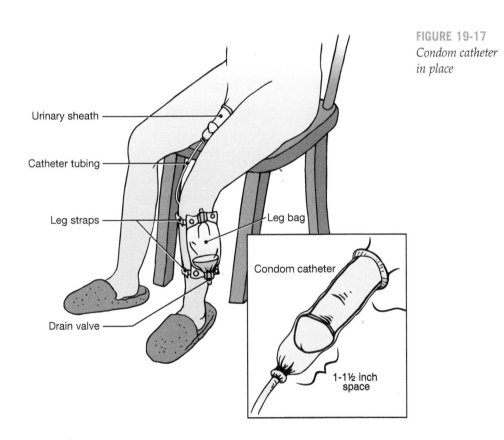

Procedure 19-14
Applying a Condom Catheter

EQUIPMENT

condom catheter
and collection bag

Velcro® band

materials for
perineal care

disposable gloves

small plastic bag

1. Explain what you are going to do.
2. Wash your hands.
3. Provide privacy.
4. Help the client to lie on his back.
5. Put on gloves.
6. Cover the client with a sheet or bath blanket as for perineal care.
7. If a condom catheter is present, remove it gently and place in plastic bag.
8. Give perineal care.
9. Attach the collection bag to leg or bed frame.
10. If using a self-adhesive catheter, apply protective coating, as prescribed, to the skin of the penis.
11. Hold penis firmly. Roll the condom catheter onto the penis with drainage opening at the urinary meatus.
12. Secure the edge of condom catheter in place with Velcro band. Be careful not to constrict the penis.
13. Connect catheter tip to drainage tubing.
14. Make sure tubing is in correct position, is not kinked or twisted, allows for movement, and that the tip of the catheter is not twisted.
15. Make sure client is safe and comfortable.
16. Discard used supplies in plastic bag.
17. Remove and discard gloves.
18. Wash your hands.
19. Document as required by your agency. Report any unusual observations to your supervisor.

Caring for the Client with a Catheter

Using a catheter can be uncomfortable and embarrassing for a client. If not properly cared for, it can also pose a risk to your client's health. You must carefully monitor any client with a catheter to make certain that the client's skin integrity is maintained. Observe for any redness, broken areas, or leakage around the catheter. Immediately report observations of any of these to your supervisor.

The following guidelines can also help a client using a catheter to feel more comfortable:

- **Check collection bag position.** The bag must be placed lower than the bladder in order to prevent urine from flowing back into the body.
- **Make certain urine is draining freely into the collection bag.** Check for kinks in the tubing, punctures in the tubing, or loops that restrict urine flow.
- **Be sure tubing is connected to both condom and collection bag or leg bag.**
- **Empty the collection bag according to the support plan or when full.** Follow the procedure prescribed for the client.

- **Document your actions.** Record the amount, colour, odour, and clarity of the urine.
- **Provide perineal and catheter care daily (more frequently if prescribed in the support plan).** Keep external areas of the catheter and tubing clean.
- **Report unusual observations immediately.** Report leakage of urine around the catheter, holes in tubing, appearance of a dirty catheter tube or bag, or any client complaints of pain, burning, irritation, or feeling the urge to void.

Procedure 19-15
Emptying a Catheter Collection Bag

It is quite likely that you will be asked to drain the catheter collection bag. Use the following procedure.

1. Introduce yourself to the client and tell the client what you are going to do.
2. Wash your hands and put on clean disposable gloves.
3. Position the collection bag drain in the opening of the collection container. Avoid touching the container with the drain.
4. Open the drain at the bottom of the collection bag and completely drain the bag into the container.
5. Close the drain. Wipe with an alcohol swab or disinfectant pad.
6. Note the colour, consistency, clarity, and odour of the urine. Report any concerns to your supervisor.
7. Reposition collection bag if necessary.
8. Ensure client is comfortable.
9. Accurately note amount of urine collected and record it on the intake and output form.
10. Dispose of urine in toilet.
11. Wash and dry collection container.
12. Dispose of gloves, swab, or pad in appropriate container.
13. Report and document as required by your agency.

EQUIPMENT

collection container large enough to hold the contents of the collection bag (Use a graduated container if output is to be measured.)

clean vinyl gloves

alcohol swab or disinfectant pad

Ostomies

An ostomy refers to a surgical procedure that creates an opening (a stoma) in a person's abdomen to allow for urine or feces to be expelled. The bowel, ureters, or urethras are brought out to the surface of the skin of the abdomen and attached to an opening at the surface (the stoma).

Openings in the bowel are called ileostomies or colostomies, depending upon the location of the stoma. Urinary ostomies are called urostomies.

An ostomy appliance snugly fits around the stoma and is securely attached to the abdominal skin with adhesive. A bag is attached to the appliance that collects the drainage. Figure 19-7 (page 352) illustrates the removal of an ostomy appliance. Procedure 19-16 describes how to drain an ostomy pouch. There are two categories of ostomy appliances—one-piece and two-piece. A one-piece ostomy appliance has the bag and the appliance in one unit. The two-piece ostomy appliance has an adhesive appliance and a separate bag. Two-piece appliances allow the bag to be changed

Photo 19-14
A variety of ostomy appliances

without removing the whole appliance from the skin. The type of appliance worn depends a great deal on the wishes of the client and the advice of the physician and ostomy nurse. Photo 19-14 shows a variety of ostomy appliances.

As a support worker, you are responsible to ensure that the drainage is monitored for amount and character; that the bag is emptied as per the client's support plan; that the skin around the appliance is kept clean and dry; and that you report observations and document as required by your agency. Procedure 19-17 outlines the cleaning of the ostomy pouch.

Procedure 19-16
Draining the Ostomy Pouch

EQUIPMENT

plastic container

bed protector

toilet tissue

gloves

basin with warm water

soap

washcloth

towel

container of water (if bag is to be rinsed and reused)

The pouch should be emptied when one-third to one-half full. If the pouch is allowed to fill completely, its weight can cause the pouch to pull away from the body and leak.
1. Introduce yourself to the client and explain what you are going to do.
2. Wash hands and put on clean vinyl gloves.
3. If possible, have the client sit on the toilet or commode. Assist the client as required to remove or reposition garments.
4. If possible, assist the client to hold the pouch and place it between the legs.
5. Remove any urine or feces on the stoma with toilet paper. Discard in trash or flush in toilet.
6. Wash the skin around the stoma gently and thoroughly with soap and warm water. Rinse well and pat dry.
7. Note any redness, irritation, or broken areas. Report any observations to your supervisor.
8. Remove the bar clamp and empty the contents into the toilet. Some clients find it easier to empty the contents into a container first, then into the toilet.
9. Smooth the pouch between your fingers, using a downward motion toward the drain to remove as much urine or feces as possible.
10. If the client has a two-piece appliance, follow the procedure for cleaning the pouch.
11. If the client has a one-piece appliance, follow your supervisor's directions for cleaning.
12. Replace the clamp.
13. Assist client to reposition clothing.

A pouch does not need to be replaced each time it is drained. In general, most pouches are odour-proof if cleaned properly, and may be reused. The following procedure is used when a client has a two-piece appliance.

Procedure 19-17
Cleaning the Ostomy Pouch

1. Remove the pouch from the appliance attached to the skin.
2. Empty any remaining contents into the toilet.
3. Rinse the inside of pouch with warm water.
4. Wipe the last 10 cm (about 2 inches) of pouch with toilet tissue to remove any urine or feces.
5. Replace the clamp.
6. Replace the pouch according to appliance directions.

ASSISTING THE CLIENT WITH THE USE OF A BED PAN

There are two common types of bed pans: standard pans and fracture pans. Photo 19-15 illustrates both types of pans. Fracture pans are used with clients who are recovering from a fractured hip. However, some clients without fractures may prefer a fracture pan.

Photo 19-15
A standard bed pan and a fracture pan

Procedure 19-18
Assisting a Client with the Use of a Bed Pan

1. Provide privacy.
2. Identify what the person can do for himself or herself. Decide with the person what assistance you will provide.
3. Explain what you are going to do.
4. If you are using a stainless steel bed pan, warm it first by holding it under running hot water.
5. Put on gloves.
6. Position the pan according to type. If you are using a fracture pan, place the smaller end under the buttocks. If you are using a standard pan, place the pan with the open end to the front.

EQUIPMENT

bed pan

towel

toilet tissue

disposable gloves

7. Position the person on his or her back with the bed flat. If able, ask the client to flex both knees. Place your hand under the person's lower back and assist him or her to raise the buttocks. Press the pan down into the bedding as you slide the pan under the person. Figures 19-18a and 19-18b illustrate this procedure.

FIGURE 19-18
Placement of the bed pan

a)

b)

8. If the person is unable to assist, turn the person onto the side away from you. Figure 19-19 illustrates the steps in positioning the pan.
9. Place the bed pan firmly against the buttocks while remaining aware of the position of the pan.
10. Push the bed pan down and toward the person. Hold the bed pan securely and turn the person on his or her back.
11. Raise the head of the bed if possible. Positioning the person as close to upright as possible helps in elimination.
12. When the person is finished, lower the head of the bed.
13. Provide tissue to the person if he or she is able to cleanse. If the client is unable, wipe the perineal area from front to back, taking care to gently remove all fluid and fecal matter. Drop used tissue into the pan.
14. Ask client to raise buttocks and remove the pan. If the person is unable to raise the buttocks, hold bed pan securely, turn person away from you, and remove the pan.

FIGURE 19-19
Placing a bed pan when the person cannot assist

15. Clean the genital area from front to back to remove any residual material. Give complete perineal care if necessary.
16. Empty the bed pan and clean it. Make sure the area under the rim is clean.
17. Return equipment to its proper place.
18. Make sure person is comfortable.
19. Remove gloves and wash your hands.

ASSISTING THE CLIENT WITH DRESSING

How we dress is a reflection of how we see ourselves. Remember how you felt when you were well dressed? At other times, casual clothes may be the most appropriate.

Like you, the clothes your client wears depend mostly on his or her environment and preferences. Some clients will dress in casual clothes if their situation allows. Others may need to dress for work. Some clients always wear jewellery; others do so rarely. Health status affects the choice of clothing. If the client is not well, he or she may change into a clean gown or pyjamas after bathing and remain in bed. The client should always have the opportunity to choose the clothing she or he wears. If, due to cognitive impairment, the client cannot make an appropriate choice (for example, selecting a shirt and sweater and nothing else), you can still offer appropriate choices (such as two appropriate dresses) from which the client can choose. Figure 19-20 shows the steps involved in dressing and undressing a client.

Whether it is due to disease, illness, or a physical impairment, the client may need assistance from the worker to get dressed. Assisting the client is much like dressing oneself. However, there are a few hints to help when there is physical impairment of limbs.

If the Client Is Unable to Move a Limb

1. Allow the client to help wherever he or she can to increase the client's feeling of self-worth.
2. Always remove the soiled gown or pyjamas from the mobile limb first.
3. Always replace the new garment's sleeve or leg on the immobile limb first.
4. Be sure to hold the immobile arm by the wrist or elbow or the immobile leg by the knee or ankle to prevent pressure or strain on the muscles.

a)

b)

c)

d)

FIGURE 19-20
Dressing and undressing

FIGURE 19-20
Dressing and undressing (continued)

Elastic Stockings

A client may be instructed to wear special elastic stockings for many reasons. A client on prolonged bed rest, recovering from surgery, or who has poor peripheral circulation may benefit from the long-term use of elastic stockings. The worker should be familiar with the period during which the client is to wear the stockings.

Procedure 19-19
Removing Elastic Stockings

1. Gently pull down the stocking from the upper leg and roll it off of the foot.
2. Turn the stocking right side out and lay it flat over a chair.
3. Repeat for the other leg.
4. Sometimes, the client will have two pair so that one pair can be washed every day. Allow the skin to be exposed to the air for 10 to 15 minutes. This is a good time to bathe and observe the skin for any redness, irritation, etc.

Procedure 19-20
Replacing Elastic Stockings

Before applying the stocking, make certain that it is the correct size.

1. Grasp the stocking and gather it in your hands.
2. Raise the client's foot by holding it at the heel.
3. Start by placing the stocking toe over the foot.
4. Gradually pull the stocking up over the heel, ankle, and the leg.
5. Be sure the stocking is placed evenly along the leg to maximize the distribution of the pressure. Ensure that the stocking does not bunch up in any area and that the top does not roll down. Bunching or rolling will impair circulation. Report any problems with rolling or bunching to your supervisor.
6. Repeat for the other leg.
7. If the client's leg tends to perspire, a slight coating of talcum powder will allow easier replacing of the stocking.

BED MAKING

Strictly speaking, bed making is not a component of physical care. However, it is an essential skill when the client is unable to leave his or her bed for extended periods of time.

Principles of making a bed (occupied or unoccupied):

1. Wash hands prior to and after making a bed; wear gloves if linen is soiled by body fluids.
2. Change only soiled linen or according to agency policy.

3. Bring only the required amount of clean linen into the room to avoid contamination.
4. Do not let soiled linen touch your clothing.
5. If possible, have laundry cart close to bed; do not put soiled linen on the floor.
6. Stack clean linen on a chair or the over-bed table in the order you will use it.
7. Always raise the bed to working level. Use proper body mechanics at all times.
8. Lower the siderail on the side you are working on.
9. Do not shake sheets. Shaking can distribute dust and microorganisms into the air.
10. If you are making an occupied bed, explain to the client what you are doing.
11. Always keep the client covered.
12. Always attach the call bell (if available) when finished making the bed.
13. Leave the over-bed table within the client's reach when finished.

Procedure 19-21
Making an Unoccupied Bed

1. Loosen all soiled linen by pulling it away from the mattress.
2. If the top sheets are clean, remove them by folding top to bottom and place on a nearby chair.
3. If linens are soiled with body fluids, put on gloves.
4. To remove soiled linen, take from top to bottom and roll into a ball. Place in laundry cart or hamper or take directly to client's washer.
5. Remove gloves.
6. Before placing clean linen on the bed, make sure that the mattress is pulled up toward the top of the bed as far as it will go. This will allow for better positioning of the client when the head of the bed is raised.
7. Apply a clean bottom sheet (or previous top sheet) by folding it in half lengthwise on the bed.
8. Tuck one side in and repeat on the other side, making the bottom sheet snug. If a fitted sheet is not available, mitre the corners as in Photo 19-16.

EQUIPMENT

flat or fitted sheet
to cover mattress

pillowcases

flat or top sheet

drawsheet

bedspread

blanket (optional)

laundry cart or
laundry hamper

gloves (if required)

Photo 19-16
Mitred corners

9. Place the drawsheet on the centre of the bed, keeping the top edge at approximately the client's axilla. This will allow easier positioning of the client using the drawsheet as a lift sheet. Photo 19-17 illustrates proper placement.

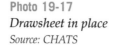

Photo 19-17
Drawsheet in place
Source: CHATS

10. Add the top sheet, blanket, and bedspread in the same fashion, going from side to side.
11. Smooth the top linens over the bed and tuck the ends under the mattress at the foot of the bed. Mitre the corners as in the previous diagram. Omit this step if your client prefers that the linens not be tucked in.
12. Fold back the top linens to make a 15 cm (about 6 inches) cuff at the head end.
13. If the client will be returning to the bed immediately, fan fold the top linen to the bottom of the bed.
14. Add a new pillowcase, and position the pillow for the client's use.
15. Attach the call bell if present.
16. Remove the laundry cart and tidy the rest of the client's room.

Procedure 19-22
Making an Occupied Bed

EQUIPMENT

flat or fitted sheet to cover mattress

flat or top sheet

pillowcases

drawsheet

bedspread

blanket (optional)

bath blanket (to cover client if in bed)

laundry cart or laundry hamper

gloves (if required)

1. Loosen the soiled linens as for the unoccupied bed.
2. Place a bath blanket over the client.
3. Ask the client to hold the top edge while you reach underneath and pull the bedspread down to the bottom of the bed and off.
4. Fold the bedspread in half if you are going to reuse it.
5. Repeat for the blanket and top sheet. If no bath blanket is available, leave the top sheet on the client to cover him or her during the bed change.
6. Have the client roll over to the side away from you. If the client is too ill, obtain help or position the client using pillows.
7. Lift the bottom sheet and the drawsheet from the side edge and tuck under the client.
8. Unfold the clean sheet lengthwise and place it on the bed.
9. Lay the sheet so that there are 2.5 cm (about one inch) over the edge of the mattress at the foot at the bed.
10. Unfold the sheet so that half is on the bed and the other half is tucked under the client.

11. Repeat with the drawsheet, positioning it so the top edge will be under the client's axilla.
12. With the client covered with the top sheet or bath blanket, have him or her roll over to your side.
13. Explain to the client that he or she will have to roll over a lump of linen.
14. Grasping the siderail will make the client feel more secure. If the client is unable to roll, obtain help or raise the siderail and go to the other side of the bed.
15. Lower the rail and roll the client towards the other siderail and position with pillows.
16. Pull the soiled linen out from underneath the client and roll it into a ball.
17. Place the soiled linen in the laundry cart or hamper. Make sure you do not leave the client with the siderail down.
18. Find the edges of the clean linen and pull toward you. Smooth and straighten them.
19. Tuck the bottom sheet under the head of the bed and mitre the corner if necessary.
20. Tuck the rest of the sheet and the drawsheet under the length of the bed.
21. The client may prefer to roll back onto his or her back at this point to finish the bed.
22. Unfold the clean top linen over the client and remove the bath blanket.

Most long-term care facilities have laundry carts with separate containers for client clothing and dirty and soiled linen. Be certain to put client clothing and linen in the appropriate container.

MEASUREMENT OF VITAL SIGNS

Temperature, pulse, respirations, and blood pressure are important measurements of overall body status and are called **vital signs**. Often, when a client is ill, one or more of these signs will not be within a "normal" range. For example, if the client has the flu, his or her temperature may be raised. If the client's heart has an irregularity, the pulse may be irregular. If the client has pneumonia or another chest infection, respirations may be rapid and shallow. It is important for you to understand the normal range of these signs and how to measure them correctly. However, be aware that these are only the basic measurements. There are many more ways to determine the client's condition, particularly observing and listening to the client.

Temperature

Measurement of the total amount of body heat is called temperature. The temperature is maintained by a delicate balance of heat generation and heat loss. In a 24-hour period, it's normal for temperature to fluctuate slightly. Between midnight and 6 a.m., it drops slightly and is at its highest between 4 p.m. and 8 p.m. Table 19-4 gives normal temperature ranges for temperatures taken from various sites on the body. Fever is a prolonged increase in temperature. Fever often accompanies illness or infection.

Taking a Temperature

There are four sites used to take a temperature: under the tongue, the outer ear, the axilla, and the rectum. You must use the most appropriate site for each client. For

TABLE 19-4	Normal Temperature Ranges	
	Normal Range	
Location	Celsius (°C)	Fahrenheit (°F)
Oral	36.5 to 37.5	97.6 to 99.6
Rectal	37.0 to 38.1	98.6 to 100.6
Axillary	36.0 to 37.0	96.6 to 98.6
Tympanic	36.5 to 37.5	97.6 to 99.6

example, an axillary temperature or outer ear temperature may be more appropriate when the client:

- is a baby or young child and cannot hold a glass thermometer in his or her mouth;
- is a confused or elderly client who may bite down on a glass thermometer;
- has just swallowed a hot or cold fluid; an oral temperature will not be accurate.

Some clients or facilities may have only certain types of thermometers. Table 19-5 lists three common types.

TABLE 19-5	Types of Thermometers
Type	Characteristics
Glass Mercury	<ul><li>takes 3 minutes to work</li><li>is breakable</li><li>comes in oral and rectal types (rectal has a short "bulb" at one end)</li><li>can be difficult to read for some people</li><li>at home, is cleansed in cold water, wiped with alcohol, and stored in a clean container</li></ul>
Electronic	<ul><li>gives the temperature reading in a few seconds</li><li>is a probe that is attached to a portable machine</li><li>provides a digital reading in Celsius or Fahrenheit</li><li>has a sound or light to indicate reading is done</li><li>has disposable plastic covers for each client</li><li>usually used in outer ear (tympanic); some can be used orally or rectally</li><li>may need regular maintenance to stay accurate</li></ul>
Chemical Probe	<ul><li>disposable, single-use device</li><li>series of dots change colour as temperature increases</li></ul>

Principles of taking a temperature:

1. Wash hands prior to and after taking the temperature.
2. Assess which method of taking temperature will be most accurate and safe for the client.
3. Avoid touching the end that goes into the body.

Procedure 19-23
Taking an Oral Temperature Using a Glass Thermometer

1. Take a clean glass thermometer and shake the mercury down until it is at the bottom of the scale on the thermometer. It may take several shakes to get it down. Be careful not to shake where you may hit something.
2. Place the thermometer under the tip of the client's tongue and ask the client to close his or her mouth, being careful not to bite down on the thermometer.
3. Leave in place for three minutes, or according to instructions.
4. Remove the thermometer after the correct time and wipe the end with a tissue.
5. Hold the thermometer at eye level, read immediately, and record.
6. Wash the thermometer according to instructions.

EQUIPMENT

clean glass thermometer

tissues

Procedure 19-24
Taking a Rectal Temperature Using a Glass Thermometer

1. Take a clean glass thermometer and shake the mercury down until it is at the bottom of the scale on the thermometer. It may take several shakes to get it down. Be careful not to shake where you may hit something.
2. Lubricate the end of the thermometer with petroleum jelly for easier insertion.
3. Put on gloves.
4. Assist the client into a side-lying position.
5. Explain the procedure to the client.
6. Lower the pyjamas and arrange the bed linens so the buttocks only are exposed.
7. For an infant, grasp both legs and raise up to expose the anus.
8. Place the tip of the thermometer to the anus and tell the client to take a deep breath.
9. Insert the thermometer gently into the anus, pointing it toward the client's umbilicus and sliding it along the rectal wall. Insert about 2.5–5 cm (about 1–2 inches) for adults and 1 cm (about 1/2 inch) for infants.
10. Hold it in place for three minutes or according to agency policy. Never let go of the thermometer when it is in the anus.
11. Remove the thermometer after the time limit and wipe from fingers to bulb with a tissue.
12. Read the thermometer.
13. Remove any extra lubricant from the client's anus and reposition his or her pyjamas.
14. Record the temperature promptly.
15. Wash the thermometer as per instructions.

EQUIPMENT

clean glass thermometer

petroleum jelly

gloves

tissues

Procedure 19-25
Taking an Axillary Temperature Using a Glass Thermometer

EQUIPMENT

clean glass
thermometer

towel

1. Take a clean glass thermometer and shake the mercury down until it is at the bottom of the scale on the thermometer. It may take several shakes to get it down. Be careful not to shake where you may hit something.
2. Position the client laying on the back or sitting up. If using this method for an infant, hold the infant on your lap.
3. Remove the client's clothing on the arm so it is easy to access the axilla.
4. Raise the client's arm and dry with a towel.
5. Place the bulb of the thermometer into the centre of the axilla.
6. Lower the client's arm and hold in place for five minutes or according to instructions.
7. Remove the thermometer.
8. Read and record.
9. Clean the thermometer according to instructions.

Procedure 19-26
Taking a Tympanic Temperature Using an Electronic Thermometer

EQUIPMENT

tympanic thermometer

probe covers

The electronic thermometer is most often used to take a tympanic temperature (in the outer ear). They are most often found in long-term care facilities, but some versions are becoming more common in clients' homes. In some facilities, electronic thermometers may be used for all types of temperature-taking. Be sure to know the policy for your agency. Photo 19-18 shows a typical electronic thermometer.

1. Take the probe handle out of the portable device.
2. Place a probe cover over the end.
3. Remove hair from around the client's ear if it is in the way.
4. Place the probe in the outer ear, making sure the probe is in contact with the skin.
5. Hold in place until the signal alerts that the temperature has been taken (usually three seconds or less).
6. Check the digital display.
7. Remove the probe from the ear and press the release button to allow the probe cover to be discharged.
8. Discard the probe cover.
9. Reconnect the probe to the portable device, if necessary.
10. Record the temperature immediately.

Photo 19-18
Tympanic thermometer
Source: Maple Health Centre

Keep in mind that electronic thermometers can fail. If the reading is at all in doubt, repeat it and, if still concerned, report and have the thermometer checked. Be careful not to drop the device, and store it carefully.

Pulse

Each time the heart beats, it is ejecting a volume of blood from the left ventricle into the aorta and arteries. The **pulse** reflects the impulse transmitted to arteries by contraction of the ventricles of the heart. The pulse is indicative of metabolic conditions; the state of emotions; physiological responses to stress, exercise, blood loss; and other general conditions.

Health care workers can actually feel this push by feeling the pulse of the client. To feel a pulse, you must push an artery against a bone and feel with your fingertips the pulsing sensation. Each time a pulse is taken, it has a rate, a rhythm, and a quality—all of which can be evaluated.

The rate is the number of times the heart beats in one minute. The normal rates are:

- Newborn infant—120 to 140/min
- Child—80 to 110/min
- Adult—60 to 100/min

Many factors determine the pulse rate. Each individual has a rate that is normal for him or her. A higher or lower than normal rate for the client should be reported.

The rhythm of the pulse tells us about the electrical impulses that stimulate the heart muscle to contract. Normally, the rhythm of the pulse is regular. A pulse that has an irregular beat, or multiple beats and then long intervals in between, may indicate a problem with the electrical system in the heart and should be reported as irregular.

The quality of the pulse is measured by how the pulse feels. A weak, thready pulse would indicate that there is a problem with the volume of blood being pumped. A bounding pulse could indicate such things as strenuous exercise, anger, or infection.

Where to Take a Pulse

There are several sites to take a pulse, but you are most likely to take the radial pulse. This pulse is the most common of all the areas and relatively easy to obtain. It is found on the inner aspect of the wrist on the radial bone below the base of the thumb.

Procedure 19-27
Taking a Pulse

1. Wash hands.
2. Explain to the client the procedure.
3. Place the first two fingers of your dominant hand on the client's radial artery. Never use your thumb to take a pulse.
4. Locate the pulsing artery.
5. Do not press down too hard as this may give an inaccurate result.
6. Feel the sensations for a few seconds, noting the rhythm and quality.
7. Count the rate of the pulse by watching the watch for 60 seconds.
8. Once you get comfortable with the procedure, you may count the pulse for 15 seconds and multiply by 4, or 30 seconds and multiply by 2. **However, if there is any concern about the rate, rhythm, or quality of the client's pulse, always count for 60 seconds to be accurate.**
9. Record your findings immediately.
10. If you have any concerns about your findings, report them to the appropriate person.

EQUIPMENT

a watch with a second hand (The face of the watch must include all the numbers to make it easier to count the rate of the pulse.)

STOP AND REFLECT ((19-3))

Find your own pulse. How would you describe its rate, rhythm, and quality?

_____

_____

_____ ∎

Respiration

Respiration is a complex cycle that results in the delivery of oxygen to the cells by inspiration and the return of carbon dioxide to the air by expiration. A breath or respiration is made up of one inspiration and one expiration.

Normally, one breathes quietly and without effort. This can change with exercise, ambient temperature, metabolic changes, and disease. Respiration is monitored for rate, depth, pattern, and quality.

Rate of Respiration

Rate is the number of breaths or respirations the client makes in one minute. The usual adult rate is 14 to 18 respirations per minute. An infant's normal rate is 35 respirations per minute. A particular client's normal rate may vary somewhat. You should be familiar with the client's normal rate.

Infections, stress, and exertion can alter this rate. For instance, a person with a mild chest infection may have 22 respirations per minute, but a person with severe pneumonia may have more than 40 respirations per minute. Some medications can actually depress the rate of respirations. It's important to have a measurement of the client's normal rate to be able to compare when the client is not well.

Depth of Respiration

To observe the depth of respirations, watch the client's chest. Normally, the chest moves slightly. If the chest barely moves at all, the respirations are called shallow. If the chest moves significantly, these respirations are called deep.

Pattern of Respiration

By watching respirations over a minute, you will notice that the rhythm and rate likely form a pattern. There are specific patterns that can occur, as follows:

hypoventilation	decrease in rate and depth
hyperventilation	increase in rate and depth
apnea	complete absence of respiration
Kussmaul's	increase in rate and depth with audible sighs or gasps
Cheyne-Stokes	a repeating cycle found in terminally ill clients in which there is decreasing rate and depth followed by a period of apnea

Quality of Respirations

The quality of respirations is determined both by the client and the worker. How much effort is required by the client to breathe, and the sounds made while breathing, make up the quality. Increased movement of the chest with conscious effort by the client is called laboured breathing. A client who complains that he or she can't get his or her breath or has discomfort when breathing is having dyspnea. A person who has to sit in an upright position to breathe comfortably is having orthopnea.

There are several sounds that can be readily identified. Stridor is a high-pitched crowing sound during inspiration, usually occurring when there is an upper airway obstruction. A wheeze is a high-pitched whistling sound that occurs when the airways are partially obstructed, as in asthma.

Procedure 19-28
Measuring Respirations

1. Hold the client's wrist over his or her chest and pretend to take the client's pulse.
2. Observe the rise and fall of the client's chest, making note of the depth, pattern, and quality.
3. Count the number of breaths in thirty seconds. Count for a full minute if there is concern as to the pattern. Never tell the client you are counting the respirations, as he or she could consciously alter the rate.
4. Record data immediately.
5. Always take the temperature, pulse, and respirations at the same time. Often, the results are relative to each other and are more significant when reported together.

EQUIPMENT

a watch with a second hand

MEASURING BLOOD PRESSURE

You may be asked to measure and record your client's **blood pressure** (BP). This reading tells how much pressure is exerted on vessel walls when the heart is pumping blood (beating) and when it is resting (between beats). The most common way to take a blood pressure is to use a manual sphygmomanometer with a pressure cuff and a manometer. Photo 19-19 shows a common type of pressure cuff and manometer. Clients with hypertension may have a blood pressure machine in their home to monitor pressure.

Blood pressure is usually measured at the brachial artery in the client's upper arm. The cuff is placed on the client's upper arm and is manually inflated by the bulb pump to compress the brachial artery. A stethoscope is placed on the brachial artery. The air in the cuff is then slowly let out. As the pressure is decreased, the examiner can hear sounds through the stethoscope.

The pressure against the vessel wall when the heart is pumping is called the systolic pressure. The pressure against the vessel wall when the heart is between beats is the diastolic pressure. Blood pressure is recorded with the systolic measure over the diastolic measure. When written, the figures are separated by a forward slash. For example, a pressure of 110 systolic and 80 diastolic would be written as 110/80.

Photo 19-19
BP cuff and manometer
Source: Maple Health Centre

The average blood pressure for a normal adult should be no higher than 120/80. Any reading above this should be considered high and should be reported immediately. The person may require tests for hypertension (high blood pressure). Blood pressure can change throughout the day. It is often lower in the morning. As well, blood pressure changes as stress levels change throughout the day. When measuring blood pressure, it is important to take several readings over a specified period of time to indicate the person's normal reading and changes in a trend.

Some people live with a low blood pressure such as 90/60. A lower than average pressure that is normal for the person is not a problem. However, anyone whose blood pressure is constantly falling from his or her normal value over a period of a few hours could be considered hypotensive and may be at risk for shock and other conditions.

Measuring a client's blood pressure can be extremely difficult. An incorrect reading can put the client in jeopardy. You must be taught the procedure by a person familiar with measuring that client's blood pressure.

MEASURING AND RECORDING INTAKE AND OUTPUT

It is often important to know what the client is eating and drinking, as well as how much of this material is being eliminated. You may be asked to measure and record client intake and output because your client has (or may have) a kidney problem or a digestive problem. Sometimes a client's fluid balance is critical to maintain health. For example, having too much fluid could be hard on the heart of someone with congestive heart failure. Conversely, having too little fluid could cause dehydration in a child with the flu.

Items that must be measured when the client drinks or eats them include:

- All fluids including milk, juice, coffee, tea, pop, water
- All thick fluids such as gelatin, porridge, cream of wheat, ice cream, milkshakes
- All intravenous fluids

The following types of output must be measured: urine, liquid stool, emesis or vomit, and fluid draining from a wound.

Each agency or facility has a special form to use on a daily basis for each client. You must be familiar with the form and what each agency uses for measurement. Many long-term care facilities have standard measurements for foods and liquids based upon the serving size each uses. Figure 19-21 illustrates a sample intake and output recording form. If you are measuring intake and output in the client's home, you must be careful to use clearly marked measuring cups for intake. Often, output is measured with a container provided specially for that purpose. A "hat" is a container placed in the toilet and used for collecting urinary output.

Intake and output are usually recorded for a period of a few days for adults. Infants are monitored hourly as they can quickly become dehydrated. The health professional requesting the measurement will observe the daily pattern over the period to detect a trend.

In a healthy person, intake usually equals output. If this balance changes, a client can quickly become ill. It is very important that the worker be accurate and consistent in measuring the client's intake and output so that correct information is provided.

FLUID BALANCE /

IV THERAPY RECORD

LIONS GATE
H O S P I T A L

INTAKE ☐   OUTPUT ☐

DATE: From 07:00 _____ to 07:00 _____

INTAKE											OUTPUT							
INTRAVENOUS								ORAL			URINE			OTHER FLUID LOSS				
														GASRIC			TUBE (Specify)	
START TIME	STOP TIME	SOLUTION VOLUME	RATE	INITIAL	TOTAL IV IN	TOTAL BLOOD IN	TIME	ORAL	TUBE	TIME	VOID	CATH.	EMESIS	N/G	BOWEL			
SUBTOTALS																		

12-H TOTAL:	IN:										OUT:							
START TIME	STOP TIME	SOLUTION VOLUME	RATE	INITIAL	TOTAL IV IN	TOTAL BLOOD IN	TIME	ORAL	TUBE	TIME	VOID	CATH.	EMESIS	N/G	BOWEL			
SUBTOTALS																		

12-H TOTAL:	IN:	OUT:	
24-H TOTAL:	IN:	OUT:	24-H BALANCE + or –

A601 10M-S-TS
Rev. (03/91)

FIGURE 19-21
Sample intake and output recording form

Procedure 19-29
Collecting a "Clean Catch" or Midstream Urine Specimen

EQUIPMENT

midstream urine
specimen kit
from agency

disposable gloves

bed pan, urinal,
or commode

small plastic bag
(sandwich bag size)

small paper bag
(lunch bag size)

1. Explain what you are going to do.
2. Wash your hands and put on clean vinyl gloves.
3. Open the specimen kit. Remove contents. Label container with the client's name.
4. Assist the client to bathroom or commode, or offer the bedpan or urinal as required.
5. Give perineal care. If the kit contains special towelettes, use them.
6. In female clients, keep labia separated until specimen has been collected so that urine will not flow over skin surfaces. Ask male clients to retract the foreskin until the specimen has been collected. Assist as required.
7. Ask the client to begin voiding into urinal, bed pan, commode, or toilet.
8. Instruct client to stop voiding, if possible.
9. Hold specimen container under urinary meatus, but do not allow it to touch the skin surface. Do not touch the inside of the container with your hands.
10. Ask client to start voiding again, if the client stopped.
11. Catch enough urine to fill the container about half way.
12. Ask the client to stop voiding.
13. Remove the container.
14. Ask client to finish voiding.
15. Put lid on specimen container. Be careful not to touch the inside in order to keep the specimen clean.
16. Place container in a plastic bag then into a paper bag.
17. Assist client to complete toileting, if necessary.
18. Clean materials and store them in proper location.
19. Remove and discard gloves.
20. Wash your hands.
21. Assist client to chair or bed. Make client comfortable.
22. Store the specimen as directed.
23. Document as required by your agency.
24. Report observations of anything unusual to your supervisor.

MEASURING CLIENT HEIGHT AND WEIGHT

It's often important to measure the client's height and weight. As children are growing, these measurements are an indicator of growth and development. In adults, weight gain or loss is often associated with disease or illness is an indicator of the client's general well-being. For example, a client who has lost a lot of weight and is scheduled for major surgery may not recover as well as someone who has maintained his or her normal weight. Also, a change in height in adults may indicate a problem in the spine. You must be able to accurately measure your client's height and weight.

Measuring Your Client's Weight

The equipment you use to weigh your client is usually determined by where he or she lives. Long-term care facilities have different types of scales, as Photo 19-20 illustrates.

Photo 19-20
Scales used in long-term care facilities (clockwise from top left): wheelchair scale; standard scale; lift scale (two views).
Source: Newmarket Health Centre

Many different types of scales are used by clients living in the community. Make sure that the scale you are using works properly. Use an item of known weight (such as a 2 kg bag of sugar) to check the accuracy of the scale. If the scale does not seem to weigh properly, contact your supervisor.

Each time, before you weigh your client, check the scale to be sure it is balanced. If required, adjust according to the manufacturer's instructions. Most scales measure in both kilograms and pounds. Be sure to always use the same measurement. As well, always compare the weight you recorded with the previous two or three weights. If there is any discrepancy, reweigh the client or have the scales checked.

Procedure 19-30
Weighing Children and Adults

EQUIPMENT

scale

1. Weigh the client at the same time every day. Make sure that the weight time is recorded in the support plan so that other workers involved will weigh the client at the same time.
2. Ask the client to wear the same type of clothes each time (such as pyjamas or a gown) to make the weight more accurate. Remember that shoes can add over 0.5 kg to a client's weight. If the client is weighed wearing shoes one day and is weighed in stocking feet the next, the recorded weight will not be a true reflection of the client's weight.
3. Follow the instructions for using the particular scale. No matter the type of scale, assist the client to stand on the centre of the scale or wheel the client's chair to the centre of the scale.
4. Read the client's weight.
5. Assist the client off the scale.
6. Record the client's weight.

Procedure 19-31
Weighing Infants

EQUIPMENT

scale

1. Undress the infant and weigh prior to a feeding.
2. Hold the infant steady with one hand while reading the scale. Never take your hand off of the infant, but take care to not alter the scale's weight.
3. Remove the infant.
4. Record the weight.

APPLYING HEAT OR COLD

Heat packs are often used by clients or ordered by a physician or therapist. We often think of heating pads or heat packs (such as those heated in a microwave) as comfort measures. Bear in mind that heat packs pose a serious burn risk to your client. In particular, diabetics, infants, older adults, and people with limited mobility are at greater risk of burns related to heat packs. Hot or cold packs should never be used on an unconscious client.

As a support worker, you must follow your agency's policies and procedures regarding the application of hot and cold packs. You should not apply a heating pad at the request of your client unless the support plan specifically allows you to do so. The support plan should also specify where the packs are to be placed and the length of time they are to be kept in place. Procedure 19-33 identifies the steps involved in applying a hot water bottle. Procedure 19-34 outlines the use of a hot/cold pack.

Procedure 19-32
Measuring Height

1. Ask the client to remove shoes or slippers. Assist the client as required.
2. Raise the bar on the scale to well above the client's head (Photo 19-21).
3. Have the client stand straight on the scale platform and then lower the bar so that it just touches the client's head.
4. Note the measurement.
5. Raise the head bar and assist the client off of the scale.
6. Lower the head bar back to its original position.
7. Record the measurement in inches or centimetres, depending on the agency policy.

Photo 19-21
Height bar on stand-on scale
Source: Maple Health Centre

EQUIPMENT

scale with height bar

Procedure 19-33
Applying a Hot Water Bottle

1. Explain what you are going to do.
2. Wash your hands.
3. Provide privacy.
4. Fill the hot water bag.
5. Secure it with the stopper. Turn the bag upside down to check for leaks.
6. Remove stopper and empty bag.
7. Fill bag one-third to one-half full with water that is no warmer than 115°F or 45°C.
8. Compress bag to remove excess air. Place stopper in bag while it is still flat.
9. Cover bag with a soft cloth or towel and apply to the prescribed area.
10. Document the time the bag was applied, the area to which it was applied, and the temperature of the water in the bag.
11. Refill the bag when it becomes cool.
12. Check the client's skin every ten minutes for signs of redness, numbness, mottling, or discomfort.
13. When finished, remove stopper, empty bag, and hang bag upside down to dry.
14. Place towel or cloth in laundry hamper to be washed.
15. Wash your hands.
16. Document the removal. Report any unusual conditions to your supervisor.
17. When the bag is dry, use a hairdryer to blow air into it. With air inside, replace the stopper. This helps to prevent the insides of the bag from sticking together. Store in proper location.

EQUIPMENT

hot water bottle

soft cloth or towel

cooking thermometer (if available)

pencil

paper

Procedure 19-34
Applying a Hot/Cold Pack

EQUIPMENT

hot or cold pack

soft cloth, towel, or cover

pencil

paper

1. Explain what you are going to do.
2. Wash your hands.
3. Provide privacy.
4. Place the hot pack in the microwave and heat according to manufacturer's directions or remove the cold pack from the freezer.
5. Cover pack with a soft cloth or towel and apply to the prescribed area.
6. Document the time the pack was applied and the area to which it was applied.
7. Check client's skin every ten minutes for signs of redness, numbness, mottling, or discomfort.
8. Remove the pack when the prescribed time is up.
9. Report any unusual observations to your supervisor.
10. Store pack as directed.
11. Wash your hands.
12. Document removal.

CARE IN SPECIAL SITUATIONS

As a support worker, you may be asked to assist clients with casts or who require a clean dressing. If so, you should receive specific instructions as to the procedure you are to follow. The procedures in this section provide general guidelines for these types of care.

Cast Care

You may be asked to assist a client who has injured a limb and has a cast. Casts are rarely completely comfortable, particularly in the first few days after they are applied. The support plan should list specific instructions for cast care. The following guidelines may help promote comfort for a client with a cast.

- Keep the cast up and supported comfortably. An arm cast may be in a sling when the client is standing or raised on a pillow when the client is sitting or lying down. A client with a leg cast should keep his or her foot on a chair or stool when sitting.
- Keep the cast dry at all times. Water makes a plaster cast crumble so it is no longer effective. A wet fibreglass cast can irritate the skin and cause blisters, which can lead to infection.
- Follow the support plan with regard to showering or bathing. Wrapping the cast in towels covered by two large garbage bags held in place with waterproof tape may prevent water from seeping in. Assist the client with a sponge bath, if you are uncertain as to whether you can keep the cast dry in the tub or shower.

Discourage the client from altering the cast or putting things down the cast. Doing so could scratch the client's skin and lead to infection. To help relieve itchiness, use a hair dryer on the lowest (cool) setting to blow air inside the cast.

Signs of Cast Problems

The following signs indicate a problem with the cast and should be reported immediately:

- Tingling or numbness in the affected fingers or toes. This can mean that there is swelling or that the cast is too tight.
- Cold, painful, swollen, or blue fingers or toes
- Pain not relieved by medication
- Soft, cracked, or loose casts
- A foul smell. It is quite normal for cast to smell of perspiration.
- An object is put, or falls into, the cast.

Application of a Clean, Dry Dressing

A client who requires a clean, dry dressing has had a break in the skin and is at increased risk of infection. You must carefully observe clean technique when changing a dry dressing to ensure that no further damage is caused to the already compromised area. Procedure 19-35 outlines one method of applying a clean, dry dressing.

Procedure 19-35
Applying a Clean, Dry Dressing

1. Introduce yourself and explain the procedure to the client.
2. Position and drape the area to provide privacy and keep the client warm. Wash your hands.
3. Put on clean vinyl gloves.
4. Remove the old dressing and place it in the disposal bag.
5. Remove gloves, and put them in the same bag. Wash your hands.
6. Put on fresh gloves.
7. Cleanse the wound using the solution prescribed. Gently pat dry.
8. Apply a clean dressing and secure with tape.
9. Remove all supplies.
10. Discard the soiled dressings as directed.
11. Remove gloves.
12. Reposition client as required.
13. Clean equipment.
14. Wash hands.
15. Document as required by your agency.
16. Report any unusual observations or concerns to your supervisor.

EQUIPMENT

clean dressing

bag to hold old dressing

clean gloves

draping as required

Try It Out *19-1*

You will need a microwave-heatable heat pack and a meat thermometer for this activity.

Heat the pack according to the instructions it came with.

Remove the pack from the microwave. Fold the pack in half and place the thermometer in the fold.

Wait two minutes and read the temperature.

Chances are that the temperature exceeds 65°C (150°F). This is hot enough to cause a serious burn.

Questions for Review

1. What are the purposes of personal care?

2. Describe RIDICUPS and explain each component.

3. How does age affect a person's skin? What precautions should you take when caring for the skin of an older client?

4. Why is it good to give a back rub? How can you give a simple back rub?

5. What are the stages of a pressure sore?

6. How can you help prevent pressure sores?

7. What are eight ways to help a client avoid or minimize incontinence?

8. What two factors support good bowel and bladder function?

9. What are four symptoms of a urinary tract infection?

10. List three ways that you can help a client reduce the risk of a urinary tract infection.

11. Following what seven guidelines can help make a client with a catheter feel more comfortable?

Questions for Discussion

1. How do you think you might feel if you required someone's help to have a bath? If you bathed each other as part of a skill lab, recall how you felt. How would you feel if the person bathing you was of the opposite sex? What could the support worker do to make the procedure a positive experience for you?

2. You are assisting a client with morning care. The client complains that her toenails are too long and catch on her stockings. She asks you to cut them for her. What do you do?

3. Apply RIDICUPS to how you would prefer to be assisted with a bath. Compare your answers to those of your colleagues. In what ways are you similar? In what ways are you different?

Chapter 20

Common Conditions

Learning Objectives

Through reading this chapter, you'll be able to

1. Define functional change and relate it to the concept of disability described in Chapter 14.
2. List the six common ways in which function can change.
3. Discuss the role of the support worker in assisting the client to address common conditions.
4. Explain the eight questions that are useful to ask when observing how a client performs tasks.
5. Describe basic approaches that are useful in assisting the client with any common condition.
6. Discuss, in general terms, the causes of common conditions, the body system each affects, the most frequent functional change each can create, and any specific techniques used to assist clients with the functional change.
7. Describe common acute conditions and illnesses and list the steps a support worker may be asked to take to address them.
8. Describe the steps to follow to obtain information when a client has a condition with which you are unfamiliar.

Chapter at a Glance

- Functional Change and Disability
- Assisting the Client to Minimize the Effects of Conditions
- Approaches Common to Any Assistance
- Common Conditions
- Acute Conditions
- What to Do When You Encounter a New Condition

Terms You'll Use

Acquired Immune Deficiency Syndrome A condition caused by HIV in which the person experiences opportunistic diseases.

Arthritis A condition that causes pain, stiffness, and sometimes swelling in or around joints. It can also affect other tissues.

Cancer A disease in which cells grow abnormally and out of control.

Cerebral Palsy A condition that results from an anomaly or injury to the brain as it develops.

Chronic Obstructive Pulmonary Disease A group of irreversible lung diseases.

Diabetes A disease resulting from the pancreas's inability to produce enough insulin or to properly use the insulin that is produced.

Functional Change The way in which a particular condition affects a client.

Hemiplegia Partial or total paralysis of one side of the body.

Human Immunodeficiency Virus The virus that causes AIDS (Acquired Immune Deficiency Syndrome).

Huntington's Disease An inherited neurological disease characterized by progressive physical and cognitive decline.

Illness An acute or short-term condition of poor health.

Multiple Sclerosis A central nervous system disease caused by the inflammation and scarring of the myelin sheath that protects nerve fibres.

Muscular Dystrophy A condition that causes muscle tissue to degenerate and be replaced by fatty and connective tissue.

Osteoporosis A condition in which bones become less dense, brittle, and weak.

Parkinson's Disease A neurological disorder that affects the ability to initiate movement.

Post-Polio Syndrome A condition that can occur in people who have had polio; causes further weakening of the muscles injured by the virus.

Spinal Cord Injury A condition caused by damage to the spinal cord, usually as a result of injury to vertebrae.

Tuberculosis A bacterial disease most often affecting the lungs.

SCOPE OF THIS CHAPTER

This chapter provides an overview of the more common conditions that you may encounter. It cannot and does not list all the possible conditions a client might experience. It is not an exhaustive guide to all that might be done to support a client with a particular condition. It also cannot take into account the ways an individual reacts to a particular condition and the ways you must personalize your support. It also can't list the resources that may be available in your community to assist a client.

Bear in mind that new developments may provide improved ways of supporting a client. As a support worker, you must keep abreast of changes in technique that will allow you to better assist your client. You are encouraged to contact local associations and use other resources for current information. Many associations have Internet websites with comprehensive information. Many clients, their families, and caregivers have tremendous knowledge about their condition and how support can best be provided.

FUNCTIONAL CHANGE AND DISABILITY

Functional change refers to the way in which a particular condition affects a client. This term means the same as the term *disability* we discussed in Chapter 14. The phrase *functional change* is frequently used in health care and rehabilitation settings. Sometimes, it's called functional impairment, but this term is becoming less common. Generally, functional changes can be organized into six categories:

- Changes in mobility
- Changes in fine motor skill

- Changes in stamina
- Changes in one or more of the senses
- Changes in motivation or interest
- Changes in cognition

This chapter will discuss the effects of the first four categories. Cognitive impairment will be discussed in Chapter 23.

Functional Change

It's important to remember that functional change is not illness. It is a change in how the person does things. These changes can come from an illness, a disease process, an injury, or by something that happened before the person was born. They can even come from how capable or energetic a person feels.

Changes in function can result in disability, but they don't necessarily have to. Much depends upon two factors:

- whether the change in function changes a person's ability to do something, or to do it easily, or in a way that the person did it before; and
- whether the person can compensate for the change in function.

Recall the discussion of vision problems in Chapter 10. If the vision problem doesn't affect your day-to day living, you may well not even notice it. Even if you have significant problems seeing, chances are that you don't feel disabled if you wear glasses or contact lenses. Similarly, the disability or functional change a particular client experiences is directly related to the effects of the change (such as diminished stamina) and the extent to which the client's lifestyle is altered by those effects. Thus, the functional change arising from the same cause will vary from client to client.

It's also important to keep in mind that many conditions can cause the same or similar disability. For example, diminished endurance (tiring easily) can be the result of a stroke, multiple sclerosis, cancer, or a heart condition. How you might assist the person will also be quite similar, despite the differences in the impairment that produced the disability.

Mobility includes the vast number of movements that allow us to move from one place to another. Many things can cause mobility impairments: fractures, nerve or spinal cord damage, amputations, and neurological conditions.

Fine motor skills include the ability to use our hands and other body parts for fine movement. Examples include the ability to hold a pen or to turn a page. A person's ability to do this may be impaired by arthritis, polio, a stroke, or spinal cord injury, among other conditions.

Stamina describes the ability to maintain an activity over a period of time. As described above, many conditions can affect a client's stamina.

Conditions and Illness

As stated earlier in this chapter, the fact that a person has a particular condition does not necessarily mean that she or he is *ill*. **Illness** is a very broad concept, and there are many definitions of the term, but in this text we'll use the definition adopted by the Centers for Disease Control (CDC): "An acute or short-term condition of poor health." Thus, a person with a spinal cord injury would not see the condition as causing him or her to be ill, although the person may have to take special precautions because of any functional change she or he experienced. However, the same person may well see him- or herself as ill if he or she has a cold or the flu.

CASE EXAMPLE 20-1

Salima is a 60-year-old woman. She had polio as a child and as a result, has limited use of her right leg and some loss of respiratory capacity. She was not significantly affected in any other way by the illness and does not now see herself as "ill." Because of the mobility and stamina problems caused by the polio, Salima has to take particular care to pace her activities so as to not become overexerted. As well, her reduced respiratory capacity puts her at greater risk of complications, should she catch a cold. Last month, Salima had the flu and was ill for two weeks. Now fully recovered from the illness, Salima has resumed her regular routine.

Consider the Whole Person

Recall the concept of a holistic approach discussed in Chapter 7. It is essential to consider the whole person when observing responses to impairments. A condition is not the only thing that can affect the client's ability to function. Consider Case Examples 20-2 and 20-3.

CASE EXAMPLE 20-2

Gareth Winter is a retired stockbroker. In years past, he was an avid photographer. His photos have twice won national awards, and he spent many years travelling the world to take pictures.

Two years ago, he had a stroke. Although he has recovered a great deal of function, he is not able to take pictures as easily as he once did. His anguish at the change in his ability is obvious to anyone who works with him. As a result of the stroke, he no longer wants anything to do with photography. He does not like to have photographs around him, and has replaced all photos in his home with paintings. Even his daughter's portrait is a pastel drawing. He tells you that part of his joy in living was lost when he gave up photography.

CASE EXAMPLE 20-3

Meg McBride is a retired textile artist. In her 45-year career, she helped to design patterns for carpets and upholstery fabrics. She often designed patterns by working them out in petit-point (a very fine form of needle point).

Two years ago, she had a stroke much like the one Gareth Winter had. As a result, she has some difficulty holding and manipulating small objects and has begun doing needlework on a much larger canvas so that she can see the stitches and easily handle the needle. "At least I can still make beautiful designs," she tells you.

> **How do Mr. Winter's and Ms. McBride's responses to their impairment differ? What factors might affect each person's reactions?**

Notice how the same impairment affects the two people differently. In these cases, one person has adapted a previous activity to accommodate impairment and, as a result, experiences little disability. The other is not able to adapt (although it would be physically possible to do so) and, as a result, has experienced greater disability.

There are many things that can influence how (or if) a person experiences disability as the result of a condition. Psychological response, the availability of resources to help overcome the effects of the condition (such as the ability to remodel one's home to be accessible to a person using a wheelchair), the number of people the person has who provide support, as well as the number of changes and other conditions the client is experiencing can all influence the client's experience.

A person's psychological response to a condition can help to determine the degree of disability experienced. This does not mean that a "good" attitude will enable a person to overcome the effects of any condition. It simply means that the significance a person attaches to the condition can affect the degree of disability the person experiences.

Remember that psychological responses can be very difficult to change, even if the person wants to change his or her response. It is extremely important to accept the client as he or she is, even if you feel that the client could see the condition differently.

Culture and Response to Conditions

We know that members of different cultures may see having a condition and/or needing health care or assistance in different ways. As well, traditional patterns of accessing and using health services may not be as effective. Consider the following:

- A woman who is from a culture where it is traditional that her husband speaks for her may find it difficult when a health professional insists on speaking directly to her.
- A man who was raised to never make eye contact with the person to whom he is speaking may find it difficult when attempting to talk to a health professional who wants to make eye contact.
- A person who has traditionally made decisions only after talking things over with her family may find it difficult when expected to make a decision alone.

Language may also pose a barrier, as some health care terms do not easily translate. It's important to avoid stereotypes when supporting the person. What a person does is a unique product of what he or she has learned and experienced over time— only a portion of this is from the person's ethnic background. As well, some people may disagree with certain aspects of their traditional culture (just as you might not agree with your family about how certain things should be done). However, it's not uncommon to have differences in the following areas: ways of making decisions, concept of time, use of facial expressions (particularly making or not making eye contact), and roles of men and women. It's usually more useful to observe how your client does things, asking questions when you're not certain what to do.

ASSISTING THE CLIENT TO MINIMIZE THE EFFECTS OF CONDITIONS

As a support worker, you will be called upon to assist the client to perform many routine functions. To do so effectively, you must know the client's priorities, his or her preferred methods of assistance, and appreciate how the client does the things he or she needs to do. Bear in mind that, in many cases, the client has lived with the condition for a long time and has likely developed ways of adapting that work best for her or him. As well, a client may need to conserve energy for activities that are most important. As a result, you may find that your client prefers that you do things that he or she is able to do. Your client has valid reasons for these preferences. You should not refuse to perform these tasks (unless your agency does not permit you to do them) or make the client feel bad that he or she does not do them.

There are eight questions you should always ask yourself when you are assisting a client. (Questions are based upon the work of Jitka Zigola, *Doing Things*, 1988.)

1. WHAT tasks does the client see as important to do?
2. WHAT does the client enjoy doing?
3. WHAT is the client able to do?
4. HOW does the client do those things?
5. WHEN is it easiest for the client to perform the task?
6. WHICH parts of a task is the client unable to do?
7. WHY is the client unable to do those parts?
8. HOW does the client want you to assist?

APPROACHES COMMON TO ANY ASSISTANCE

Because many conditions result in similar impairments, there are some approaches that are often useful regardless of the impairment.

1. **Talk with your client.** Communication is essential to any approach that you take. Approaches 2 to 7 below provide specific examples of ways in which you can communicate.
2. **Take the time to learn the client's needs, preferences, and methods of doing things.** Use the eight questions listed in the previous section to help obtain this information.
3. **Follow the client's cues for pacing any task you do, or that you assist the client to do.** Keep in mind that your client may find it difficult if you do tasks in too much of a hurry. Make sure that your body language does not indicate that you are impatient with your client's pace.
4. **Allow time for rest.** Alternate activity and rest as the client's needs require. This is particularly necessary when the client is practising a task for the first time, when you are helping the client for the first time, or when the client is not feeling well.
5. **Break down the task into clear steps based upon what the client can do.** This helps clients accomplish the portions of the task of which she or he is able.
6. **Take the time to learn how the client does things.** Your client has had a great deal of experience in adapting to the effects of his or her impairment. You can often learn many good techniques this way.
7. **When you are assisting the client, plan the task with the person.** If possible, plan the tasks in a way that establishes a routine.
8. **Recognize that your client will have good days and bad days.** Adapt your approach to your client's level of ability and interest.
9. **When possible, make use of labour-saving techniques.** For example, place a sheet of waxed paper under mixing bowls to catch spills. Place newspapers under the vacuum when you change the bag. If your client permits, try using a cooking spray to make pots and pans easier to clean. Minimizing cleanup may encourage your client to do things he or she enjoys.
10. **Relax and encourage your client to do the same.** Any task is easier when you can relax and even laugh a little.
11. **Work with the client.** You are partners in getting the tasks done.

12. **The client's diagnosis is not as important as his or her functional ability.** Worry less about the medical diagnosis. Focus on the client's ability and where he or she needs help.

13. **Remember that a condition is not necessarily an illness.** There is a difference between having a physical impairment and having an illness (such as the flu). Your client will not appreciate being referred to as ill or sick if, in fact, he or she has a disability that is not caused by an illness.

14. **Not all tasks are an opportunity for rehabilitation.** Respect your client's wishes for how—and how often—he or she practises tasks to develop a skill.

15. **Use available adaptive aids to make a task easier.** Many clients have identified aids that assist them. Use these as the client wishes. If your client has a need for a particular adaptive aid, speak with your supervisor.

16. **Recognize that the client's condition may mean that the client is more isolated.** In some cases, a client's condition may make it impossible for him or her to get out, or to take part in social interaction. Whenever possible, take the time to chat with your client, if that is her preference. Do remember that not everyone sees isolation in the same way; you might feel that someone does not have enough opportunity to interact, while that person feels that he or she has more than enough.

17. **Recognize that the client may see the condition very differently than you do.** A client may feel that a particular condition is the result of something he or she has done "wrong" in the past. In some communities, particular conditions may be seen as a sign of shame. Respect the client's view and try to see the situation the client does. This does not mean that you must agree with the client, but that you are trying to understand how significant the situation is to her.

COMMON CONDITIONS

This section covers many common diseases and other conditions. Each section briefly describes the process of the condition, any known causes, and any hints specific to the condition that may make providing support easier.

Please be aware that a client with a particular condition will have had considerable advice from doctors, therapists, and other persons knowledgeable about the condition. Many clients have done considerable research and are extremely knowledgeable. As well, each client will experience the condition differently. Remember that your client is the expert in how he or she is affected.

The information provided in this chapter is accurate at the time of publishing. Be aware that developments in the understanding and treatment of conditions occur regularly. It is important for you to remain up to date with information on conditions. Local condition-specific associations can be excellent sources of information as can your local public health unit. As well, many reputable organizations have established websites to provide information on specific conditions.

This chapter organizes conditions by the body system that is primarily affected. However, few conditions affect a single body system, leaving others unaffected. For example, a stroke (cerebral vascular accident) affects the nervous system; it does so usually because of a circulatory system problem (a clot or a hemorrhage). As well, a stroke may produce paralysis of one side of the body, resulting in gait changes and musculoskeletal problems. The experience of the stroke may also cause the person to feel overwhelmed. As Case Examples 20-2 and 20-3 illustrated, it's important to see the person—not just the condition.

Conditions Affecting Vision

In Chapter 10, we discussed common age-related changes to vision. In this section, we'll discuss other vision conditions.

Cataracts

A cataract describes a clouding of the lens of the eye. The clouding may involve the entire lens, or just a part of it. Figure 20-1 shows a normal eye and one with a cataract clouding the lens. The amount of a person's vision that is impaired will depend upon the size of the clouding and what part of the lens is clouded. If the area is small, vision may not be greatly affected and the person may not have to have the cataract removed. Cataracts are very common. They can be caused by a number of things: medications, injury, and some diseases. They are also more common with age, although they can occur at any age. Infants can be born with cataracts (called congenital cataracts). Cataracts are not contagious, although they may develop in both eyes at the same time.

The only effective treatment for cataracts is removal of the affected lens. This is a very common surgery. The Canadian National Institute for the Blind (CNIB) estimates that 1.5 million cataract operations are performed each year in North America. Most of these surgeries don't require the person to stay in hospital overnight. Complications can happen but are not common. The CNIB states that more than 95 percent of those who have the surgery see an improvement in their vision.

FIGURE 20-1
An eye with a normal lens and one with a cataract

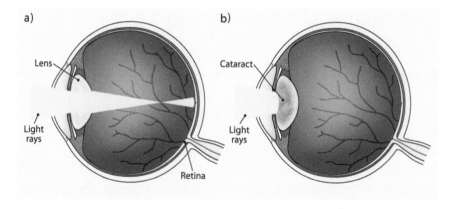

Age-Related Macular Degeneration (AMD)

Age-related macular degeneration (AMD) is the leading cause of vision loss in people over age 50 (CNIB, 2006). The CNIB estimates that more than 2 million Canadians have the disease. There are two forms of AMD: wet and dry. Wet AMD makes up about 10 percent of the cases; dry AMD 90 percent. Both types affect the macula, the part of the back of the eye that handles central vision—the things we look directly at.

Wet AMD is caused when small blood vessels break and bleed into the macula, blocking vision. It progresses rapidly; a person can lose all central vision within weeks or months if it is not treated. Dry AMD progresses slowly and may not be noticed at all until identified in an eye exam. Photo 20-1 shows an image with normal central vision and the same image as seen by a person with advanced AMD.

Women, Caucasians, and people with blue eyes are more likely to develop AMD. Smoking, obesity, and exposure to sunlight also increase risk. Treatments are available for the condition, but there is no cure at present. Early detection may limit vision loss; persons over 50 should have their eyes examined annually.

Glaucoma

Glaucoma is caused by increased pressure in the eye. It affects 1 in 100 Canadians and is a leading cause of blindness (CNIB, 2006). The pressure likely damages the optic nerve, resulting in the loss of peripheral (side) vision. It can occur in people of any age, but is more common in people over age 40. People who have had an eye injury or eye disease are also at greater risk.

There are two types: open-angle glaucoma and closed-angle glaucoma.

Open-angle glaucoma is the most common type. Patients don't usually notice any symptoms until it is very advanced. Closed-angle glaucoma is less common. The symptoms of acute closed-angle glaucoma may occur suddenly. Symptoms include a sudden dull, aching pain over one eye, a change in vision, or seeing blurring and halos around lights. Acute closed-angle glaucoma is a medical emergency. A client with these symptoms should be seen by a doctor immediately.

There are no symptoms of glaucoma other than vision loss. Unfortunately, once vision loss has occurred, it cannot be restored. Eye examinations usually include a test for glaucoma. Treatment is usually eye drops, but in some severe cases, other medications or an iridotomy (a surgical technique that makes a tiny opening in the iris to relieve pressure) may be used.

Diabetic Retinopathy

This is an eye condition that can occur in persons with diabetes. In this condition, there are changes to the blood vessels that feed the retina. Eventually, the vessels can become blocked, cutting off the blood supply to part of the retina. When this happens, two things occur: the part of the retina that was nourished by those vessels dies and new blood vessels develop to take the place of the damaged ones. The new vessels are fragile and often bleed into the eye, blocking vision. Early diagnosis and treatment can slow or delay vision loss. Good management of blood glucose levels can also help.

Photo 20-1
Normal central vision and central vision in AMD
Source: Courtesy of National Eye Institute, National Institutes of Health

Supporting the Person with Vision Loss

Throughout the text there are guidelines for assisting a person with vision loss to communicate, to eat, and do other routine tasks. The following guidelines supplement those listed elsewhere in the text:

1. **Identify what the person can and cannot see.** For example, can the person see things when looking directly at them? Only when looking away? Use this information to place food and other items the person needs within the line of sight.
2. **Describe what the person can't see, if the person wants you to do so.** Make certain that you learn what level of detail your client prefers. Describing things in too much or too little detail may frustrate him or her.
3. **Remove hazards the person cannot see.** Always check with the person first if you are moving something that has been in one spot for some time.
4. **Find out what helps the person to see better, if possible, and make use of what you learn.** Does better light help? Positioning the light in another spot? Using a magnifier?

Cancer

Cancer is the term used to describe the abnormal and out-of-control growth of cells. A mass of these abnormal cells is called a *tumour*. We call a cancerous tumour a *malignant tumour*. Malignant tumours not only grow in size (as a result of the cell growth), but they can invade and damage healthy tissue. When a tumour spreads to other parts of the body, we say that it has *metastasized*.

The Canadian Health Network identifies cancer as the leading cause of premature death in Canada. It states that 44 percent of men and 38 percent of women will be diagnosed with some form of cancer in their lifetime, but with current treatment more than half of those diagnosed with cancer survive.

There are more than 100 types of cancer. Most affect specific parts of the body. Some risk factors contribute more to one type of cancer than to another. For example, exposure to the sun increases one's risk of skin cancer, smoking increases the risk of lung cancer, and chewing tobacco increases the risk of mouth cancer. It's estimated that 5 to 10 percent of cancers are the result of inherited traits.

Health Canada estimates that 153 100 new cases of cancer and 70 400 deaths from cancer occurred in Canada in 2006.

In Canada, lung cancer is the leading cause of cancer death for both women and men. However, breast cancer is the cancer most often diagnosed cancer in women; prostate cancer is the most often diagnosed in men (Health Canada, 2007).

We often think of cancer as an adult disease and, indeed, it is much more common in adults. However, the Public Health Agency of Canada states that 1300 children/teens are diagnosed with cancer each year. Furthermore, cancer is the second leading cause of death among people aged 5–19. (Accidents are the most common cause of death in this age group.) The most common cancers are leukemias (cancers of blood-forming cells), lymphomas (cancers of lymphatic tissues), and tumours of the central nervous system. Together, these account for approximately 60 percent of all child/youth cancers (Public Health Agency of Canada, 2007).

The Canadian Cancer Society estimates that 60–70 percent of cancers could be prevented if people adopted healthier lifestyles. Three behaviours are seen as significantly increasing a person's risk of cancer: smoking; a high-fat, low-fibre diet; and exposure to the sun. Table 20-1 describes what Health Canada suggests that you do to reduce your risk.

TABLE 20-1	Reducing Your Risk

While you can't change inherited traits, there is much that you can do to reduce your risk of developing cancer. Health Canada suggests the following:

- Eat better – reduce fats and follow Canada's Food Guide
- Be more active
- Protect yourself from the sun
- Don't smoke
- Avoid second-hand smoke
- Tell your doctor when your health changes
- Screen for cancer
- Handle hazardous materials carefully

Today, most cancers can be treated. Although treatment may not cure the cancer, it may lead to a longer and better quality life for the person with the disease.

Early detection plays an important role in cancer treatment. In general, the earlier a cancer is detected and treated, the greater the person's chances of surviving the disease.

Table 20-2 describes the steps the Canadian Cancer Society suggests you take to help detect skin cancer.

TABLE 20-2	The Canadian Cancer Society's Skin Cancer Detection Checklist

- Learn what to look for and check your skin regularly, as most skin cancers can be treated if they're caught early enough.

- If you notice changes or are confused about what you should be looking for, ask your doctor for help.

- Make sure that you or someone else checks "hard-to-get-at" places such as your back, back of your neck and ears and backs of your legs.

- What you should watch for:

  - any change in a birthmark or a mole that changes shape, colour, size or surface

  - any new growth on your skin – pale, pearly nodules that may grow larger and crust, or red, scaly, sharply defined patches

  - any sore that doesn't heal

  - any patch of skin that bleeds, oozes, swells, itches or becomes red and bumpy

STOP AND REFLECT   20-1

At the turn of the last century, untanned skin was considered chic.

Perhaps we should adopt that notion today!

Supporting the Person with Cancer

Because of the variety of cancers, it's important to keep in mind that each will have its own treatment plan. What is appropriate for one person is not necessarily appropriate for another.

You must also keep in mind that the person's level of ability may change in response to the effects of treatment as well as to changes in the person's condition. Chemotherapy and radiation therapy (two common forms of cancer treatment) can have significant side effects that will alter the person's ability. Some treatments (such as chemotherapy) may make the person more susceptible to infections. You must be careful to prevent transmitting infections to your client.

Be prepared to make the most of the client's "good" days. This may mean changing your schedule of tasks to do something that the client enjoys, even though the task would usually be done on another day.

Having cancer can be a frightening experience. Many people equate cancer with death, even if the particular type of cancer is treatable with a good chance for recovery. Your client may feel frightened or be angry. He or she may want to talk about the fears and other feelings. It is important to listen and to offer support. Your client may turn to you for advice. If this happens, offer your support for the decision the client makes, but do not offer advice as to what to do. Encourage your client to discuss these feelings with the doctor, health professional, or family. Let your supervisor know if your client regularly asks you for advice. Your supervisor may be able to offer resources to the client.

Cancer treatments can cause physical changes that can be distressing to the client. Chemotherapy can cause hair loss. Radiation can alter appearance. Surgery can dramatically alter appearance. Your client may need special support and encouragement to cope with these changes in body image. Hairpieces, scarves, or other coverings may be used to mask hair loss. Cosmetics may be used to mask skin discolouration. Your client may use a prosthesis. Be aware that physical appearance is important to your client—assist him or her to look attractive.

Some clients will not acknowledge the diagnosis. Others will deny that they have the disease. Always respect your client's wishes. Do not force the client to discuss the disease if he or she does not want to.

Some clients find that food tastes different or unappealing. Sometimes, previously "favourite" foods may even make the person feel nauseous. A person may only want small meals or snacks. This may happen because of the cancer or as a result of the treatment. Be prepared to prepare different meals or snacks, doing your best to make them nutritious. The Canadian Cancer Society suggests that the following may also help:

- Eating smaller amounts every 1–2 hours.
- Keeping foods high in protein and calories handy so that they are ready to eat when the client is hungry.
- Eating favourite foods at any time of the day, whether or not they are "usually" eaten at that time.
- Eating the biggest meal when the client feels most hungry.
- Drinking fluids between meals instead of with meals to avoid filling up too quickly.
- Using beverages high in calories and protein such as milkshakes and commercial nutrition supplements between meals. You may find chilled or room-temperature beverages are easier for the client to drink.
- Exercising lightly, if the client is able, such as taking a walk before meals to increase appetite.

The Canadian Cancer Society's website (www.cancer.ca) provides some recipes that may be useful.

Pain control is often an important component of support. Although not all people with cancer experience pain, many do. Your client may use medications to control pain. He or she may also use nonmedicinal methods such as relaxation, distraction, or mental imagery to control pain. Some clients may benefit from massage.

Most professionals now believe that most if not all cancer pain can be controlled, that a person should not have to experience pain. If your client is experiencing pain, encourage him or her to discuss this with a doctor. It may be helpful for the person to keep a log of the time, frequency, and severity of the pain, as well as what seems to lessen or aggravate it. This can be useful when adapting a person's routine or for the person to use in a discussion with a doctor.

CASE EXAMPLE 20-4

Mrs. Voornam is a 75-year-old resident of a retirement home. She was diagnosed with breast cancer six months ago. She has had a mastectomy (a removal of the breast) and is currently receiving chemotherapy.

Kara is one of Mrs. Voornam's support workers. She knows that Mrs. Voornam's immune system is weakened by the chemotherapy. She is particularly cautious to practise good infection control to avoid any transmission of germs that could harm Mrs. Voornam.

Mrs. Voornam often experiences some nausea after chemotherapy, and her mouth becomes dry. Kara knows that sucking on ice chips moistens Mrs. Voornam's mouth without making her become more nauseous. She makes sure that Mrs. Voornam has a good supply of ice chips. With Mrs. Voornam's approval, Kara has started freezing orange juice into cubes for Mrs. Voornam to try.

Mrs. Voornam's hair has thinned as a result of the treatment. As a result, she prefers to wear a wig when going out. Kara helps her don the wig and style it.

Hypertension

Blood pressure is the measure of the pressure of blood against the walls of your blood vessels as it circulates through the body. High blood pressure is called hypertension. The Heart and Stroke Foundation estimates that 20 percent of Canadians have hypertension and of this 20 percent, about 40 percent do not know that they have the condition (HSF, 2007). Generally, a blood pressure reading of over 140/90 is considered high; however, a reading of 130/90 is considered high if the person is also diabetic. Over time, hypertension causes scarring of the artery walls, allowing plaque to build up, making it easier for clots to block blood flow. It is dangerous. It is the most common cause of stroke. Left untreated, it can also result in heart problems, and kidney problems.

Hypertension has been called the silent killer because there are often no obvious symptoms. The only certain way to tell if a person has high blood pressure is to have a blood pressure reading taken by a person trained to do so. Blood pressure should be checked annually if normal, more frequently if it's high. People with risk factors or other health concerns should follow the advice of their doctor or health professional.

There are several risk factors for hypertension. Some factors, such as obesity, drinking, smoking, and physical inactivity can be changed: a person can lower the risk by changing habits. Other risk factors, such as age, sex and family history, cannot be modified. For example, women are at greater risk of hypertension when pregnant and after menopause. Some women are also at greater risk when taking oral contraceptives.

Supporting the Person with Hypertension

Support may take many forms. For example, you may be asked to:

- Check food labels for fat and/or sodium content
- Use low/no fat cooking techniques
- Prepare "healthy" meals or follow a specific diet
- Encourage or assist in physical activity (such as walking with the client, etc.)
- Remind the client to take medications

Heart Disease

Heart disease is a term that describes a group of cardiovascular conditions. The leading cause of heart disease is *atherosclerosis* (also known as *arteriosclerosis*).

Atherosclerosis

Atherosclerosis describes the condition in which arteries harden and narrow. It is caused by the buildup of plaque on the inside walls of the arteries. As plaque builds up, it narrows the inside of the artery and, in time, may restrict blood flow. It can affect the arteries of the brain, heart, kidneys, and the arms and legs. The narrowing of the vessels can also make the heart work harder and, over time, weaken the heart. Try the exercise listed in Stop and Reflect 20-2 to get an idea of the effect of the narrowing of the vessels.

STOP AND REFLECT 20-2

You can get an idea of how much harder your heart has to work to pump blood through narrowed blood vessels by trying this experiment.

Make a loose fist with your hand. Leave an opening about the size of a dime, as shown in Figure 1. Place your lips against the opening and blow.

Now, make a tight fist with your fingers curled so that they touch your palm. Try again to blow through the opening.

You likely found it much harder to blow through the closed fist. You probably had to blow very hard to get any air through at all.

FIGURE 1

Effects of Heart Disease

Be aware that the person with a heart condition may not always look ill or disabled. A person with heart disease can be anxious about his or her condition. The person may fear being left alone in case he or she has a heart attack and there is no one there to help. A person who has survived a heart attack may feel particularly vulnerable. You may need to reassure the person that you are there.

It's important to identify your client's limits with regard to the type and duration of any activity. Realize that the person may tire quickly. Encourage the client to do what is comfortable and to follow the plan set by his or her health professional. Help the client to pace his or her activities.

Heart disease can result in a heart attack (also called a *cardiac arrest* or a *myocardial infarction*) or in chronic problems that can limit a person's activities. However, there are many other conditions in this group. We'll discuss some of the more common ones in this section.

Peripheral Arterial Disease

Some people with heart disease also experience a condition where blood flow to their neck, arms and legs is reduced due to atherosclerosis and arteriosclerosis. This condition is called *peripheral arterial disease (PAD)*. It's also known as *peripheral vascular disease*. It is most common in those over 65 who smoke or have diabetes, hypertension, or high cholesterol.

Though some people with this condition experience pain, many do not. People with PAD are at increased risk of developing infections and skin ulcers. In extreme cases, the loss of blood flow can cause the tissue to die or become gangrenous, requiring amputation.

Supporting the Client with PAD

A client with PAD may be very sensitive to touch. If so, handle the affected limb very carefully to avoid bumping, rubbing, or causing an abrasion. Watch for clothing or shoes that are too tight; the client may not be aware that something is restricting the limb. If the client has ulcers or wounds, wear disposable gloves, use clean technique, and follow the support plan when caring for the limb. Poor circulation will make any infection harder to heal.

Photo 20-2
A person with Peripheral Arterial Disease. Note the shiny taut texture of the skin.
Source: Dr. P. Marazzi/ Photo Researchers, Inc.

Congestive Heart Failure

Congestive heart failure (CHF) results when the heart does not pump as strongly as it should. As a result, the body does not get the amount of blood and oxygen that it requires. CHF can cause fluid to build up in parts of the body (called edema). CHF can be caused by many things: heart muscle damage (such as occurs with a heart attack); long-term hypertension; heart valve disease; heart muscle disease; or, as the result of coronary artery disease, long-standing reduced blood flow to the heart.

People with CHF usually experience swollen legs and ankles, but there may be fluid buildup in other parts of the body, such as the abdomen or lungs. They may be short of breath even when at rest. Some people with CHF find it hard to lie down and prefer a semi-sitting position. The shortness of breath often worsens with activity. The person may also feel tired or may tire easily.

Most people with CHF are on medications to reduce the fluid build up and to strengthen the heart. Some of these medications cause vitamin or mineral loss—you might be asked to prepare special meals or remind your client to take supplements. The client may also be on a low-salt or no added salt diet. Some clients will use special stockings called compression hose to help control leg swelling.

You may be asked to put these on your client's legs. If so, be certain to fit them properly, with no bunching or binding. If you are in doubt, ask the client, family member, or your supervisor for guidance. Do bear in mind that compression hose are not the same as support hose. Compression hose give much firmer support. Photo 20-3 shows one type of compression hose.

Photo 20-3
Compression hose can be hard to distinguish from regular hose.
Source: JOBST a brand of BSN Medical

Coronary Artery Disease (CAD)

The buildup of plaque on the interior of the coronary arteries (the arteries providing blood to the heart muscle) causes these vessels to narrow. When this happens, the person develops coronary artery disease. Coronary artery disease is the most common form of heart disease (Heart and Stroke Foundation, 2007). It can lead to congestive heart failure, angina, and heart attack.

Angina

The proper health care term for angina is *angina pectoris*, which means heart pain. Angina can be a symptom of a heart problem, or it can exist alone. It usually—but not always—results from a blockage in the coronary arteries. There are three types of angina: stable, unstable, and syndrome X. Stable angina generally occurs as a result of activity. It usually stops when activity ceases or the person takes prescribed medication. Unstable angina does not have a predictable pattern and may occur even if the person is resting. Unstable angina does not always respond to medication.

Syndrome X angina does not result from coronary artery disease. It is more common in women and if it occurs, it is often with physical activity. People with syndrome X do not have arterial blockage and are not at greater risk of a heart attack. One cause may be a tightening of very tiny blood vessels in the heart. These vessels are so small that this temporary tightening does not put the person at risk of heart attack, but are strong enough to cause pain (Texas Heart Institute, 2007). Another possible cause is inflammation of these very tiny vessels (Espliguero and Kaski, *Canadian Medical Association Journal*, 174 (13): 1833. (2006)).

The person experiencing the pain may still respond with alarm to the pain, however. Medications are often prescribed to treat the pain.

Heart Attack

A heart attack is a sudden condition that can result in death if not treated immediately. The Heart and Stroke Foundation of Canada estimates that 23 000 Canadians die of a heart attack each year, and that half of these people die before they reach hospital.

Keep in mind that a person with a heart condition is at increased risk of a heart attack. It's important to know the warning signs of a heart attack so that you may provide help. The Heart and Stroke Foundation identifies the following symptoms.

Pain
- sudden chest discomfort or pain that does not go away with rest
- pain that may be in the chest, neck, jaw, shoulder, arms or back
- pain that may feel like burning, squeezing, heaviness, tightness or pressure
- in women, pain may be more vague
- chest pain or discomfort that is brought on with exertion and goes away with rest

Shortness of breath
- difficulty breathing

Nausea
- indigestion
- vomiting

Sweating
- cool, clammy skin

Fear
- anxiety
- denial

If your client has these symptoms, be prepared to calmly take charge of the situation. The Heart and Stroke Foundation suggests that you do the following, as appropriate:

- CALL 9-1-1 or your local emergency number immediately
- Ask the client to stop all activity and sit or lie down, in whatever position is most comfortable.
- Assist the client to take nitroglycerin or other medication prescribed for the situation, if the client has it.
- Have the client rest comfortably and wait for emergency medical services (e.g., ambulance) to arrive.
- Remain calm.

Supporting the Person Who Has Had a Heart Attack

A heart attack can result in changes that are not immediately life threatening but that can significantly limit the activity of the person. Sometimes, a person who has had a heart attack does not fully recover and must adjust to limitations imposed by his or her condition. Often, this means making lifestyle changes (such as stopping smoking or eating a low-fat diet), as well as reducing activity and stress to reduce strain on the heart. Some people take part in *cardiac rehabilitation*, an exercise and fitness program designed specifically for people who have had a heart attack. A person in a cardiac rehabilitation program will have a specific diet and exercise plan to follow.

Sometimes, the person who has had a heart attack becomes fearful of exertion or of being left alone, that he or she might have another heart attack when no one is there to get help. The following five items may help you support your client:

- **Listen to your client and offer support that does not make the fear worse.** Don't minimize the fear, but do help the person put it into perspective. As well, don't overreact and cause the client to become more frightened.
- **Learn about what the client can do and what the signs of overexertion are, and help the client to attain a safe activity level.**
- **Identify any emergency response equipment or procedures the client can use and make certain that the client can access them.** Put emergency response call buttons within easy reach, and make certain the client knows how to use them and what will happen when they do.
- **Ensure that any emergency medication is within the client's reach.**
- **Encourage the client to discuss concerns with his or her health professional.**

Other Heart Conditions

There are a number of other heart conditions that are less common. A detailed discussion is beyond the scope of this book, but a brief description of two is included in this section.

Cardiomyopathy   A condition in which the heart muscle walls are weakened. There are a number of types. Many different things can cause cardiomyopathy: alcohol or drug misuse, a virus, or an inherited condition, among others. The person's specific experience will determine what support is required.

Rheumatic Heart Disease   About 60 percent of people who have acute rheumatic fever develop some form of heart disease. Though this fever can damage any part of the heart, it's often the valves that are damaged. Damaged valves may be narrowed or may not close properly. The heart then does not pump as efficiently as a normal heart.

Stroke

It is very likely that you will work with a client who has had a stroke. According to the Heart and Stroke Foundation of Canada, stroke is the leading cause of adult neurological disability in Canada. The Heart and Stroke Foundation of Canada estimates that more than 50 000 strokes occur in Canada each year.

A stroke (also called a cerebral vascular accident or CVA) is caused by an interruption of blood flow to the brain. This interruption causes death to the nerve cells nourished by the affected vessel. It is considered to be a cardiovascular problem because the impairment is caused by damage or disease of the blood vessels.

The risk of stroke increases with age, certain ethnic backgrounds (First Nations, African, or South Asian), and if a close relative has had a stroke before age 65. High blood pressure, coronary artery disease, smoking, obesity, and lack of physical activity are among other risk factors. A previous stroke also puts a person at greater risk for another. As a result, it's important to know the warning signs of stroke, as identified by the Heart and Stroke Foundation of Canada. Table 20-3 describes these.

TABLE 20-3	The Warning Signs of Stroke
Sign	**Description**
Weakness	sudden weakness, numbness, and tingling in the face, arm, or leg
Trouble speaking	sudden temporary loss of speech or trouble understanding speech
Vision problems	sudden loss of vision, particularly in one eye, or double vision
Headache	sudden, severe, and unusual headache
Dizziness	sudden unsteadiness or sudden falls, especially if you have any other warning signs

The Causes of a Stroke

There are two main causes of stroke: a blood clot in a blood vessel in the brain, or a hemorrhage (a burst or leaking blood vessel in the brain). Two cardiovascular conditions contribute to many strokes: arteriosclerosis and atherosclerosis. Arteriosclerosis is a loss of thickness and loss of elasticity in vessel walls that narrows the vessel. Atherosclerosis is the buildup of plaque and other deposits on the inside of the blood vessel. Either condition can make it easy for matter to block the flow of blood in a vessel, causing the cells the vessel nourishes to die. Figure 20-2 shows a blockage due to atherosclerosis.

The Heart and Stroke Foundation estimates that 60 percent of all people who have had a stroke experience some ongoing disability. The effect a stroke has on a client will vary by the location and size of the stroke. Some strokes affect an area so small that the client may not

FIGURE 20-2
Blockage due to buildup of plaque on artery walls

even know that it has occurred. Others can cause significant changes in the person's ability or even death. Stroke is the fourth leading cause of death in Canada (Heart and Stroke Foundation, 2007).

The brain is made up of the *brain stem, the cerebellum, and the cerebrum* (Figure 20-3). The cerebrum is further divided into left and right hemispheres. A stroke may affect any of these structures.

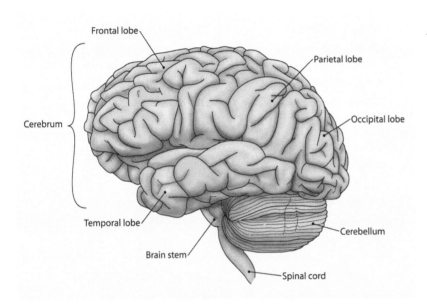

FIGURE 20-3
Areas of the brain

The Brain Stem The brain stem is at the bottom of the brain and connects the brain to the spinal column. It controls functions essential for life such as breathing, heartbeats, swallowing, balance, and movement. A stroke in the brain stem is often fatal.

The Cerebellum This area coordinates fine movements, the ability to walk, to reach out and grab objects, as well as contributing to balance and speech. A stroke in this part of the brain might cause tremors, slurred speech, loss of coordination, clumsiness, or other problems moving.

The Cerebrum This part of the brain is divided into right and left hemispheres. Each hemisphere has four "zones" called lobes. Each lobe has specific functions. For example, a stroke in the temporal lobe of the left hemisphere will often result in a specific language disorder called *Wernicke's aphasia*. A stroke usually affects the structures in either the left or right hemisphere of the client's brain. Because the right hemisphere controls the body's left side and the left hemisphere controls the body's right side, physical effects are usually seen on the side of the body *opposite* the damaged hemisphere.

Many functions are controlled by a specific part of one hemisphere. For example, the ability to use language is usually found in the left side of the brain only. Table 20-4 lists the hemisphere of some common functions.

The location of the stroke may also affect the client's pattern of behaviour. The client with damage to the left hemisphere may become very cautious. The client with damage to the right hemisphere may become impulsive.

Many persons who have had a stroke experience some level of sadness or depression. Others may find that they cry easily, experience strong emotions in response to everyday events, or experience rapid mood swings (such as being elated one moment and despondent the next). Researchers differ on the degree to which these emotional

TABLE 20-4	Hemisphere Controlling Some Common Functions	
Lobe	Left Hemisphere Damage in this Lobe can Cause	Right Hemisphere Damage in this Lobe can Cause
Temporal Lobe	Language problems Memory problems (usually temporary)	Memory problems (usually temporary)
Frontal Lobe	Partial or total paralysis of the right side of the body (hemiplegia) Difficulty controlling skilled movements, such as the ability to button a blouse, even though the body may be capable of making those movements	Partial or total paralysis of the left side of the body (hemiplegia)
Parietal Lobe	Loss of sensation on the right side of the body	Loss of sensation on the left side of the body Diminished or no awareness of the left side of the body or of the left side of the person's vision; called lateral neglect or left-sided neglect Spatial-perceptual problems, such as an inability to identify objects, to distinguish an object from the background on which it sits, to judge distance, or to judge shapes Inability to understand what is heard or felt
Occipital Lobe	Loss of sight on right side	Loss of sight on left side

states are the result of a stroke or are caused by the number of changes that the person has experienced as a result of the stroke. No matter the cause, it is important to be empathetic. Your client is not able to control the flow of emotions and needs your support.

Phases of Stroke Recovery

There are two general phases of stroke recovery. The first happens in the weeks and months after the stroke and can be fairly rapid. The second phase continues throughout the person's life. Although recovery in the second phase is usually much slower than in the first, recovery does continue to happen. For example, while 37–79 percent of persons who have had a stroke are incontinent (unable to control bowel or bladder function) in the first year after the stroke, only about 30 percent remain so after the first year (Canadian Stroke Network, 2007). You should never assume that a client will not recover ability.

There are two aspects to recovery. The first aspect is to deal with the changes (including perceptual problems) posed by the stroke. The second aspect is to make the psychological and social adjustment to the disability that the impairment creates. It's generally accepted that the psychological and social adjustments are more difficult for most clients.

Supporting the Person Who Has Had a Stroke

How you assist the client will depend upon the impairment the client has. It's very important to learn what disability the client experiences and what assistance is helpful to the client. Make sure that you follow the general approaches listed earlier in this chapter.

Here are some techniques useful in assisting the client who has had a stroke.

1. **The client may take a great deal of time to do tasks.** This is particularly true of clients who are attempting a new or complex task. Make sure you allow time for what the client is to do.
2. **Be aware that a client who is somewhat impulsive as the result of a stroke may appear very self-assured even if he or she is not.** Get to know what your client's behaviour signifies.
3. **If the client has hemiplegia (partial or total paralysis of one side of the body), assist the client to dress the affected side first.** For example, assist the client to put the affected arm in a sleeve first.
4. **Remember that language or perceptual problems are not dementia.** The client will not necessarily have problems understanding, problem solving, or sequencing tasks. Do not assume that the client is confused.
5. **A person with lateral neglect will not see items to the left or even the left side of things.** For example, your client may complain that his or her dinner plate is cleared when in fact only the right side of a plate is clean. Try turning the plate so that the remaining food is on the right. Similarly, placing often-used items to the right of the client will help him or her to find them.
6. **If your client has a language problem, learn how to adapt your technique so as to be able to communicate effectively.** Often, the client will share with you the techniques he or she has found useful. You may also find some useful hints in the guidelines for working with clients with aphasia discussed in Chapter 10.
7. **Help your client may make use of specific aids or use specific techniques to address issues.** For example, a client may use clothing that closes with Velcro or have shoes that use elastic laces. He or she may use a special plate, cup, or spoon, or need to avoid certain foods. He or she may have a toileting schedule that is designed to reduce or eliminate bouts of incontinence. The client's home may have been rearranged to allow the client to easily get to the bathroom or kitchen.

Your provincial Heart and Stroke Foundation has a great deal of information about stroke and stroke recovery.

Transient Ischemic Attack (TIA)

A transient ischemic attack (TIA) happens when there is a temporary blockage in the blood flow to a part of the brain. It produces changes much like a stroke, but these changes disappear completely within twenty-four hours.

Several things can cause TIAs. The main cause is atherosclerosis (discussed later in this chapter). TIAs can also be caused by:

- spasms in the arteries of the brain
- abnormalities in the shape of the blood vessels
- certain blood disorders that can cause inflammation of the arteries in the brain
- abnormal blood pressure changes
- uncontrolled bleeding (hemorrhage) in the brain caused by structural problems with the blood vessels in the brain, such as an aneurysm.

A TIA puts a person at significant and immediate risk for another TIA or a stroke. It is extremely important for the person with these symptoms to seek immediate medical attention. The signs of a TIA are the same as those for a stroke. If your client has any of the symptoms, contact emergency services and your supervisor.

Arthritis

It's been said that if you live long enough, you'll likely develop some form of arthritis—a condition that causes inflammation of the joints or other tissues. The Public Health Agency of Canada estimates that 4 million Canadians over 15 have arthritis—16 percent of this population (PHAC, 2000). The term arthritis actually includes over 100 different conditions. Some are hereditary, but most are not.

Arthritis is more common among older adults, but some forms occur in children. Arthritis usually does not affect how long a person lives, but it can have a significant effect upon the person's quality of life. A person's ability to do things and her or his body image may be significantly affected.

Table 20-5 lists some of the more common forms of arthritis, their effect, and common treatment.

Some degree of joint inflammation and pain are a part of all forms of arthritis. Figure 20-4 compares a normal joint to a joint affected by arthritis.

FIGURE 20-4
Normal and arthritic joints

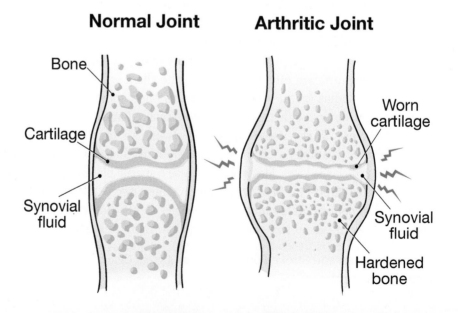

TABLE 20-5	Common Forms of Arthritis	
Type	**Description**	**Common Treatment**
Osteoarthritis	The most common form of arthritis, osteoarthritis affects 2.7 million Canadians. It's often called wear and tear arthritis because it is characterized by cartilage that is damaged or worn away, but it is not caused by normal movement. Risk factors include injury, joint damage, excess weight, and heredity. It usually occurs in weight-bearing joints like the hips or knees, but can appear elsewhere.

It is more common in older people, although people of almost any age can develop the condition. | Moderate activity usually helps this type of arthritis, as can the application of heat and cold.

Proper positioning will reduce stress on joints.

Many people benefit from the use of labour-saving devices like luggage carts and trolleys that can minimize the stress on affected joints.

Medication is often used to control pain. |
| Fibromyalgia | This is actually considered a syndrome, as the condition can present with a wide variety of symptoms. People with the syndrome experience widespread pain on both sides of the body. It may be difficult for the person to sleep, yet fatigue beyond that which could be accounted for by lack of sleep is also a symptom.

Weakness, difficulty concentrating, and poor memory are also symptoms. | Exercise and physical therapy are beneficial.

Pacing tasks, adapting to a slower pace, and balancing rest and activity are often of greatest benefit.

Medication is often used to enable the client to sleep more soundly. Pain medication is not usually beneficial. |
| Lupus | Lupus refers to three types of conditions, of which systemic lupus erythematosus is the most severe and most common. Lupus is an autoimmune disease. In this disease, the body's immune system malfunctions and begins to attack the person's normal, healthy tissue.

Many types of tissue can be attacked and become inflamed: the heart, lungs, joints, muscles, blood vessels, and the nervous system.

Anyone of any age can develop lupus, but it is most common in women of childbearing age.

Many people with lupus experience "flare-ups," in which the effects of the condition are pronounced, mixed with periods of few or no symptoms. Exposure to the sun, excessive stress, and fatigue can all be triggers for these flare-ups. | Alteration of lifestyle can eliminate or reduce triggers.

Medication can be useful in combatting many symptoms of the condition. |
| Rheumatoid Arthritis (RA) | This causes inflammation in the lining of the joints and, possibly, other internal organs. | Moderate exercise is often beneficial, but the optimal level of activity must be carefully determined. Low impact activities are best. |

TABLE 20-5	Common Forms of Arthritis *(continued)*	
Type	**Description**	**Common Treatment**
	RA can affect people of any age, although it most often appears between the ages of 25 and 50 years. In children, the condition is now called childhood arthritis. Fatigue is often a result of RA. RA can have significant effects on the person's function.	Pacing tasks, avoiding repetitive movements, and using assistive devices, like canes and utensils with built-up handles, are all beneficial. Medication is useful in many cases.
Ankylosing Spondylitis	This condition is arthritis involving the spine. It causes pain and stiffness in the back and bent posture. This is caused by the inflammation of the spinal joints (vertebrae). In severe cases, the vertebrae can eventually fuse together leading to severely limited mobility. If tendons and ligaments are also inflamed, the person may experience pain and tenderness in the ribs, shoulder blades, hips, thighs, shins, and heels and along the bony points of the spine. Some people experience iritis—inflammation of the iris of the eye. It's much more common in men and usually first appears between aged 15 and 40, although it can appear at any age.	Moderate exercise (including range of motion and strengthening activities) is often recommended. Contact sports and those that pose a risk of falling are not recommended, as people with AS are at greater risk of spinal fracture. Many people find that applying heat (e.g., taking a hot shower or using a heating pad) provides benefit. A number of medications are prescribed. Some control pain, while others alter the body's immune system to reduce inflammation. Many of these medications have significant side effects and must be carefully monitored.
Gout	Gout occurs when there is too much uric acid in the body. This can occur for two reasons: when the body makes too much uric acid or cannot get rid of enough of it. Crystals of uric acid often build up in the joint, causing pain and inflammation. These crystals can also appear in soft tissues and form tophi—yellowish deposits. These often appear in the feet, hands or elbows. Crystals can also appear in the kidneys and urinary tract. Gout usually affects the big toe but it can also involve the entire foot, ankle, and knee, as well as the hand, wrist and elbow. Once described as *the disease of royalty*, as shellfish and organ meats aggravate it. Gout affects 1 in 30 Canadians and is at least 4 times more common among men than women.	There is no cure, but the focus of treatment is aimed at minimizing joint damage and pain. Diet and medications are the two most common treatments for Gout. Avoiding shellfish, organ meats (liver, etc.) as well as spinach, peas, lentils and beans. Caffeinated drinks and alcohol should also be avoided, as should chocolate. Heat and cold treatments may be useful. Exercise is usually not recommended until the inflammation and pain have diminished.

Source: The Arthritis Society of Canada, 2007

Supporting the Person Who Has Arthritis

Arthritis encompasses many conditions, many of which have *exacerbations*—periods of acute (and often painful) symptoms and periods of no or little pain. For this reason, it's important to take into account the client's level of ability each time you work with him or her. It's also important to learn what helps the person avoid exacerbations and what aids recovery. If your client has had arthritis for some time, it's likely that she or he knows what helps and what doesn't. Here are some general guidelines that may be appropriate for your client:

- **Help the client to pace himself or herself, and to rest when required.** On some days, your client may prefer that you do some or all of a task so as to avoid pain or fatigue.
- **If treatment includes a specific diet, do your best to follow it.** Check ingredient labels for "hidden" ingredients that are to be avoided. For example, peas and lentils may be in soups; spinach may be included in mixed salad greens.
- **Assist with the application of heat or cold, if permitted by your agency.** Check with your supervisor if you are uncertain.
- **Provide medication reminders, if asked to do so.** Check with your supervisor if you are not certain that this is within your role.
- **Assist with exercise when it is appropriate for the client.**
- **Help your client to enjoy good days.** If your client is interested and your role permits you to do so, make use of good days by taking a walk or doing another activity the client enjoys—in moderation.

CASE EXAMPLE 20-5

Mr. Gerard is 58 years old. He has had rheumatoid arthritis most of his adult life. As a result, he has lost some function in his arms, hips, knees, and hands.

Mr. Gerard's condition fluctuates. He often has long periods of time without significant pain. At these times, he is able to do almost all routine activities without problem. At other times, he experiences an exacerbation and can do very little for himself without pain.

Julie, his support worker, knows that Mr. Gerard's condition can change from day to day. She is prepared to vary her tasks to best meet his level of ability.

What tasks might Julie be asked to do when Mr. Gerard has an exacerbation?

Osteoporosis

The term osteoporosis literally means "porous bones." Osteoporosis causes bones to become brittle and weak. Although it can affect anyone, it is most common in women who have gone through menopause. Twenty-five percent of women and about 13 percent of men over age 50 have osteoporosis. The Osteoporosis Society of Canada estimates that 1.4 million Canadians have the condition.

In extreme cases, simple acts such as sneezing or rolling over in bed can break bones. Seventy percent of hip fractures are the result of osteoporosis (Osteoporosis Society of Canada, 2007).

The condition occurs when bones lose calcium. This can happen because of insufficient calcium intake, or because of aging. Virtually all the cells in the body require calcium to function. If the supply of calcium from food or supplements is not enough to meet the need, the body will take calcium from the bones to nourish cells. As well, as a person ages, the body gradually becomes less able to absorb calcium efficiently and becomes less efficient at creating bone. Vitamin D3 has been found to enhance the body's ability to absorb calcium. The Osteoporosis Society of Canada recommends that **Canadians aged 19 to 50, including pregnant or lactating women, receive 400 international units (IUs)** of Vitamin D3 per day. **Adults over 50 should receive 800 IUs.** One of the most plentiful sources of D3 in our diet is milk. However, a glass of milk provides only about 100 IUs of Vitamin D3; a person over 50 would have to drink eight glasses each day to meet the requirements. As well, many people were not raised to drink milk. For this reason, many people take a vitamin supplement to meet the daily requirement.

A person's peak bone density is thought to occur at about 20 years of age. If a person had low bone density as a young adult, he or she is more likely to develop osteoporosis as an older adult. Bone loss is often so slow and gradual that a diagnosis is often not made until the person has fractured a bone.

No single factor causes osteoporosis. Many things can put a person at risk. Spotlight 20-1 identifies risk factors for osteoporosis.

SPOTLIGHT 20-10 ARE YOU AT RISK?

Are you at risk to develop osteoporosis? The Osteoporosis Society of Canada has identified the following risk factors:

Major risk factors

Age 65 or older

Vertebral compression fracture

Fracture with minimal trauma after age 40

Family history of osteoporotic fracture (especially if your mother had a hip fracture)

Long-term (more than three months) use of glucocorticoid therapy such as prednisone

Medical conditions (such as celiac disease, Crohn's disease) that inhibit absorption of nutrients

Primary hyperparathyroidism

Tendency to fall

Osteopenia apparent on X-ray

Hypogonadism (low testosterone in men, loss of menstrual periods in younger women)

Early menopause (before age 45)

Minor risk factors

Rheumatoid arthritis

Hyperthyroidism

Prolonged use of anticonvulsants

Prolonged heparin use

Body weight less than 57 kg (125 lbs.)

If your present weight is more than 10 percent below your weight at age 25

Low calcium intake

Excess caffeine (consistently more than four cups a day of coffee, tea, cola)

Excess alcohol (consistently more than two drinks a day)

Smoker

Research has shown that physical exercise, particularly weight-bearing and resistance exercise, are extremely useful in reducing the impact of osteoporosis. Weight-bearing (or load-bearing) activity actually builds bone mass. It also improves balance and coordination, which reduces the risk of falls.

The amount and frequency of exercise will depend upon the person and his or her specific circumstances.

Supporting the Person Who Has Osteoporosis

Encourage calcium and Vitamin D3 intake. Bear in mind that some clients do not (or cannot) drink milk, so other sources must be found. If your client does drink milk, consider using it instead of water in recipes, if appropriate and the client approves.

Assist and encourage the client to exercise. Be certain to follow the pattern and pace set out for the client. Do not push the person to pain or fatigue.

Take on the heavier or more demanding portions of a task, as the client will allow. If possible, do the lifting and bending that may pose a risk.

With the client's permission, assess and remove safety hazards that might cause the person to slip or fall. If within your tasks, keep walks and porches clear and free of ice in the winter (even if the client only goes outside to get the mail).

Post-Polio Syndrome

Post-polio syndrome is a condition that can occur in people who have had the poliomyelitis virus. It results in a further weakening of the muscles initially injured by the virus. Post-polio syndrome can occur as many as 40 years after the original infection. Polio Canada estimates that approximately 50 percent of the people who had the virus will develop post-polio syndrome.

It's important to note that post-polio syndrome is not a virus itself. It is not contagious. Although the exact mechanism is not known, it likely results from two factors: nerve cell stress and age. In polio, nerve cells are damaged or destroyed. Usually some cells remained unaffected, or less affected, and still able to function. These cells eventually adapt to help the person regain partial use of the muscles. Over time, these stressed cells apparently become tired and cease to function as they once did. As well, we all lose nerve cells as we age. For most people, this loss does not result in significant changes in function, as there are more than enough nerve cells to do the job. However, a person who has had polio has lost a great number of nerve cells, so the age-related loss is much more noticeable (March of Dimes, 2001).

The symptoms of post-polio syndrome are

- Unaccustomed fatigue, requiring rest in the middle of the day, or earlier
- New joint and muscle pain
- Muscle weakness and/or loss of muscle use, even in muscles that were not affected by the polio
- Respiratory problems and/or swallowing difficulties
- An intolerance for cold that causes muscle weakness, and sometimes a burning pain and/or discoloration of limbs

The person who experiences these symptoms may also experience distress at the thought of losing function that he or she worked so hard to get and keep after the polio.

CASE EXAMPLE 20-6

Mrs. Bibb is a 68-year-old woman who had polio as a teen. As a result, her left leg is weaker than the right, and she has lost some fine motor control in both arms. With extensive rehabilitation, she was able to walk with a leg brace and two canes. She completed college and worked as a store manager while raising a family. She was most determined to remain independent.

As Mrs. Bibb grew older, she began to notice greater weakness in her left leg and in both arms. She began to tire much more easily and to experience pain in her upper arms. At first, Mrs. Bibb and her family thought *that these changes were the result of "getting older," but she became distressed, because it seemed almost as if the polio had returned. However, her doctor confirmed that the changes were due to post-polio syndrome.*

Once again, Mrs. Bibb has had to adjust to impairment. She has had to accept assistance from support workers. Carmita, her support worker, is careful to respect Mrs. Bibb's independence. She plans work with Mrs. Bibb so that Mrs. Bibb may save her energy for the tasks most important for her.

Supporting the Person Who Has Post-Polio Syndrome

The person who experiences post-polio syndrome often benefits from pacing his or her activities to provide periods of rest as required and changing positions used to work, sleep, or eat. Keeping warm is essential, as cold seems to affect the person's ability to function. Some people benefit from water exercise routines and massage. Many times, adaptive aids can be of benefit.

It's important to bear in mind that this syndrome is not the result of a person's inability to cope with impairments. Assist the person to plan tasks to balance activity. Be prepared to take on parts of a task that cause the person pain. Help the person stay warm and recognize that he or she may be cold even if others are not.

Most people with this syndrome will be able to define the tasks or parts of a task that they would like you to do. Work with your client to determine the best approach.

Multiple Sclerosis

Multiple sclerosis (MS) is a central nervous system disease that occurs when the myelin sheath (the protective coating that surrounds the nerve fibre) becomes inflamed and scarred. The term actually means "many scars." Nerve impulses do not get to where they are supposed to go, or they produce a response that is different from what the person intended. The myelin sheath is much like the insulation on an electrical cord. If the insulation breaks, the wire shorts out and doesn't work.

Exactly what causes MS is not known. However, it is now thought to be an autoimmune disease in which the person's body attacks its own myelin. This attack results in inflammation and scarring of the myelin.

The MS Society of Canada estimates that between 55 000 and 75 000 Canadians have multiple sclerosis. MS affects approximately twice as many women as men, mostly people between the ages of 20 and 40, although children as young as two can be affected. A rare, severe form can also affect younger persons. It occurs more frequently in countries furthest from the equator. Canada has one of the highest rates of MS in the world (MS Society of Canada, 2007).

There are three main types of MS. The *clinically isolated syndrome* causes a single attack of the disease. MS lesions are diagnosed, but the symptoms do not return. *Relapsing-remitting MS* (RRMS) is the most common form, accounting for 75 percent of all diagnoses. In this form, there are exacerbations (periods of functional loss) and remissions (recovery). *Benign MS* is a subtype of RRMS and usually occurs in 10–15 percent of cases. In benign MS, the person has only minimal symptoms 10–15 years after the initial episode. Many people with benign MS develop RRMS over time.

Progressive MS has two forms: *primary-progressive MS* (PPMS) and *secondary-progressive MS* (SPMS). In PPMS, the condition worsens without any real recovery or period of remission. In SPMS, an initial phase or relapsing-remitting MS becomes progressive.

There is no cure for MS. A number of therapies can be used to treat specific symptoms the person experiences. With current treatment, most people with MS have a normal life span.

MS can cause many things: loss of balance, impaired speech, extreme fatigue, double vision, and paralysis. The most common symptom of MS is fatigue. This fatigue is different than the fatigue that comes from lack of rest or overexertion. It is more intense and lasts longer. It's thought that the body requires more energy to transmit messages when the myelin sheath has been damaged. About 10 percent of people with MS will experience some problems with memory. Approximately 15 percent will experience pain as a result of the disease.

People with MS experience periods in which their symptoms are severe. These are called exacerbations. Some things, such as having a child, can increase the risk of an exacerbation. However, many people have long periods of time when they have few or no symptoms.

Supporting the Person Who Has Multiple Sclerosis

In addition to the general approaches, keep the following in mind.

1. **A person with MS may be very impaired one day and fine the next.** Some exacerbations appear and disappear quite suddenly. Be prepared to accept rapid variations in your client's level of ability.
2. **Vision problems, although usually temporary, can be quite severe.** These include double vision, an involuntary jerking of the eyes that makes it impossible for the person to focus, or even total loss of vision for a period of time. Be aware that some clients may be very frightened by the changes even if they have experienced them before. Provide support and assistance.
3. **Fatigue can be overwhelming and not easily addressed by a nap.** You may have to provide additional support if your client is extremely fatigued.
4. **Be aware of the effect heat can have on the client and help the client to stay cool.** Heat can make it particularly difficult for a person with MS to function. Some clients have air conditioning; others use fans. A cool bath or shower or cool drinks may also help.

Parkinson's Disease

Parkinson's disease is a progressive neurological disorder that affects the person's ability to initiate movement. It results from the death of cells in a part of the brain called the *substantia nigra*. These cells produce dopamine, a chemical that assists nerves to communicate. It most often affects people over 60 years of age but can occur in younger people. According to the Michael J. Fox Foundation, Parkinson's disease affects 1 in 100 people over 60.

There are many ways that Parkinson's affects people. Some notice only minor changes. A tremor is one of the early signs of Parkinson's disease. In later stages, it can significantly affect a person's ability to move as well as to speak. The person may experience rigidity and move slowly. Not all people with a tremor have Parkinson's: there are other causes, including essential tremors and medication-induced tremors.

Some research has suggested that depression is more likely to occur in a person with Parkinson's disease. Parkinson's can produce cognitive changes that may be very mild to severe.

Many people with Parkinson's disease develop a rigid facial expression that does not easily change. This is called "masking" and can cause other people to wrongly believe that the person does not understand what is going on around them.

At present, there is no known cause or cure. The effects of the disease can be controlled to some extent by medication. However, medication cannot stop the progression of the disease. Recently, surgical techniques have been used to relieve symptoms.

Supporting the Person Who Has Parkinson's Disease

There are many techniques that can assist the person with Parkinson's disease. Keep in mind that your client will be the best source of information as to which techniques work best.

1. **Attempt only one task at a time.** Attempting to pick up a pen with one hand while dialling a telephone number with the other will cause the hand that is dialling to stop working. This means that most tasks will take more time. Be patient.
2. **Pay particular attention to slight changes in the floor surface as your client walks.** Doorjambs, stoops, and even slight differences in the level of the sidewalk can cause a person with Parkinson's to trip and fall.
3. **Activity is essential for present and future health.** Because of the difficulty initiating activity, many people become less active. Help your client to start activities (most clients will have a preferred way of doing this) and encourage him or her to keep active.
4. **Be prepared to do difficult tasks without fuss.** For example, your client may not be able to butter toast. Be prepared to "fill in" for her or him if the inability is too frustrating.
5. **Help the client to reduce or avoid stress.** Stress worsens every Parkinson's symptom.
6. **Use the methods set out for the client to help her or him initiate movement.** Some clients use a 1-2-3-move pattern to initiate movement; others do not. Forcing a client to move (such as by physically moving the person's feet) will usually increase rigidity and may cause the client to fall.
7. **Appreciate that medication may take some time to take effect.** If necessary, plan tasks to take advantage of periods of greater mobility.

CASE EXAMPLE 20-7

Mr. Romanov is 68 years old. He has had Parkinson's disease for more than ten years. Medication has controlled most of Mr. Romanov's symptoms; however, he does have difficulty starting to move (freezing). As well, his facial expression has become "mask-like" and his tremors are more noticeable.

Gerald assists Mr. Romanov with bathing and other personal care. He also accompanies him shopping. Despite Mr. Romanov's mobility problems, both he and Gerald realize how important it is for Mr. Romanov to

remain active. They plan out the activities beforehand to ensure that they are not rushed or doing too many things at once.

Gerald has noticed that people often speak to him instead of Mr. Romanov. It seems as though others assume that, because of his facial expression, Mr. Romanov is not able to answer. When this happens, Gerald turns to Mr. Romanov for the answer. In this way, he encourages the other person to speak directly to Mr. Romanov.

Huntington's Disease

Huntington's disease (HD) is a progressive neurological disease that eventually affects all the person's abilities, both physical and cognitive. An older name for this disease was *Huntington's chorea*. The term *chorea* means dance, and it referred to the uncontrolled movements that people with HD develop. One in every 10 000 Canadians will develop HD (Huntington Society of Canada).

HD causes a loss of *neurons* in the part of the brain called the basal ganglia. The basal ganglia controls motor and intellectual function, so when these neurons are lost, function is significantly affected. The disease is caused by a single gene and is passed down from one generation to the next. The child of a person with HD has a 50 percent chance of developing the disease. A test is available that will determine whether a child of a person with HD carries the gene, but it is not given unless the person agrees to pre- and post-test counselling.

HD usually appears in middle age, although one rare form appears in school-age people. It can appear as late as age 70. The duration of HD ranges from 10–20 years. In general, the earlier the disease appears, the quicker it progresses. There are no medications or treatments that can stop the progression of the disease. Some medications are used to treat the physical and cognitive effects of the disease.

Supporting the Person Who Has Huntington's Disease

1. **Help the person participate in everyday communication.** Although HD affects both physical and cognitive function, it is impossible to know how much the person understands. A person may well understand the communication but be unable to easily speak and participate. Help the person by restating what he or she has said so that he or she knows you have understood.
2. **Help the person to maintain adequate nutrition.** People with HD can burn more than 5000 calories per day. Remember that the person may have trouble chewing and swallowing. Cut foods into small pieces to reduce the amount of chewing required. Sometimes, puréed food is easier to eat. Thin or thicken liquids for easier swallowing.
3. **Learn about and make use of the adaptations the client and family have made to make the environment safer.** For example, some people with HD sleep on a mattress placed on the floor. This helps to minimize the risk of injury if the person's movements propel him or her out of bed. Others have removed obstacles or bric-a-brac to lessen the possibility of injury. Make sure that you do not place items in areas that could pose a hazard to the person.
4. **Do your best to keep a calm environment.** The effects of HD worsen when the person is anxious.

Muscular Dystrophy

The name **muscular dystrophy (MD)** actually refers to a group of conditions. Each condition is caused by a defect in a specific gene. Most people think that MD is a children's disease, but different forms of the disease can affect people of any age. In general, MD causes muscle tissue to degenerate and be replaced by fatty and connective tissue. There is no loss of intellectual function in the person with MD.

There are many types, but among the most well known are Duchenne MD, a form that affects mostly boys (Duchenne in girls is extremely rare). It's usually diagnosed when a boy is three to five years old. Friedreich's Ataxia also affects boys, usually before puberty. It usually progresses slowly. Limb girdle muscular dystrophy (LGMD) actually describes a group of disorders affecting the voluntary muscles, mainly around the pelvic (hip) and shoulder regions. Most diseases in this group occur before age 40, but some occur later. Many have been traced to a specific gene.

The age of onset, the muscles affected, and the rate at which the disease progresses vary from form to form. Most forms are inherited; others appear in people who do not have a family history of the disease.

Supporting the Person Who Has Muscular Dystrophy

Because of the number of forms of MD, as well as the variations in the way each form can progress, it's vitally important to learn what works for the client. Some clients may require only minimal assistance, while others may require extensive support. As with most other conditions, your client will know very well what works best for him or her. Discuss methods and techniques with your client.

Cerebral Palsy

Cerebral palsy (CP) is the term used to describe a group of disorders that result from an anomaly or an injury to the brain as it develops. Although many infants are born with CP, the condition may occur after birth and up to three years of age. The condition is not progressive; it will not get worse.

A person may experience a wide range of problems with physical sensation and motor skills. Some people with CP experience a great deal of muscle rigidity. This is called spasticity. Some people may experience learning disabilities or developmental problems. Many people with cerebral palsy have difficulty producing speech.

Supporting the Person with Cerebral Palsy

1. **Do not assume that your client has difficulty understanding simply because he or she has difficulty speaking.** A speech problem is a motor skill problem, not a cognitive one. Treat the person as the adult he or she is.
2. **Learn from your client.** Many clients with CP can give specific instructions as to how you should assist.

CASE EXAMPLE 20-8

Jenny Redbird is a 24-year-old woman with CP. She has significant problems with walking and speaking. Despite these impairments, she has completed a degree in mathematics and works for a research company.

Like anyone her age, Jenny enjoys going out. She is fond of bluegrass music and tries to see new plays as they come to town. In order to do this, Jenny has set up a network of support. Mylee, her attendant, assists her with dressing and getting ready for work each weekday morning. Two other support workers, Edralin and Cassie, assist Jenny mornings and nights on weekends.

Jenny enjoys a friendship with all three attendants. She has selected all three not only for their skills but also their personalities. She and Cassie attend plays. Mylee and Jenny head for music clubs periodically. Jenny has introduced all three women to her other friends. In this way, she finds the need for support less intrusive.

Spinal Cord Injury

Spinal cord injuries occur when the spinal cord is damaged or severed, usually as a result of injury to vertebrae. When the vertebrae are damaged, parts of the bone may irritate, sever, puncture, or compress the spinal cord. When this happens, the nerves in the spinal cord are damaged and they no longer carry nerve impulses as they did before.

Sometimes, damage is complete (i.e., all the nerves in the spinal column at a specific point are damaged). When the damage to the spinal cord is complete, no impulses can travel from the brain to beyond the point of injury. Any muscle groups controlled by nerves that are damaged will not function, and the person will not have any sensation in the affected areas. If there is partial damage, some, but not all, movement and sensation may be affected.

Paraplegia describes the injury in which a person has use of the upper part of the body but not the lower part. *Quadriplegia* is the term used to describe the condition in which a person has lost use of the upper part of the body as well as the lower. Some, but not all people with paraplegia or quadriplegia also lose sensation in the affected limbs, however.

The Canadian Paraplegic Association estimates that 900 Canadians sustain a spinal cord injury each year (CPA, 2007). Motor vehicle accidents account for 41 percent, falls for 16.5 percent, sports (including diving) for 12 percent, and other causes (including industrial accidents) make up the remaining cases. It is a condition that usually affects young people aged 18 to 35.

Supporting the Person Who Has a Spinal Cord Injury

Most clients with a spinal cord injury will need help with specific physical tasks. Aside from the impairment, the person may be quite physically fit and able (Photo 20-4)—perhaps more so than you! Most clients will discuss with you the tasks they need done and how they would like you to do them. This can involve learning special techniques.

Depending upon the extent of the disability, the client may ask you to assist with skin care and positioning. Skin breakdown is a serious problem for anyone who cannot easily move about. If your client does not have sensation, he or she may rely upon you to observe for skin problems.

Many people with spinal cord injuries require assistance with bowel and bladder care. If so, you should receive specific instructions about the type of help you are to provide. Often, the client will provide the information. If not, or if you have concerns about what you are asked to do, review the situation with your supervisor.

Photo 20-4
Most people with a spinal cord injury live full lives.

Chronic Obstructive Pulmonary Disease (COPD)

Chronic obstructive pulmonary disease (COPD) is the name given to a group of irreversible lung (pulmonary) diseases that are characterized by decreased inspiratory and expiratory capacity. The two most common diseases are emphysema and chronic bronchitis. Both diseases cause the airways in the lungs to become obstructed. In chronic bronchitis, the airways become partially blocked with mucus. Emphysema results in an enlargement of the air sacs in the lungs that causes the airways to collapse. COPD causes shortness of breath and, as the body has to work harder to get oxygen, can have negative effects on the cardiovascular system as well. Approximately 714 000 Canadians have been diagnosed with COPD (Lung Association, 2007).

COPD occurs as the result of damage to the lungs over a long period of time. It happens slowly and is often not noticed until the effects have become disabling. Although more than 90 percent of COPD cases are caused by smoking, exposure to chemical fumes, second-hand smoke, organic dust, or mining dust can also cause the condition, as can a history of childhood lung infections (Lung Association, 2007). A very rare form of emphysema is linked to an inherited lack of a specific protein.

While COPD cannot be cured, it can be controlled to some extent. Medications can help open airways. Techniques can help the person breathe more effectively and help clear the lungs of mucus. Even proper sitting and standing can help the person cope with the effects of the condition.

Though the best treatment for a smoker with COPD is to stop smoking, this is an extremely personal decision and is one that the client must make on his or her own. You should not encourage smoking, but an attempt to "police" the client's smoking will likely not work and may destroy the client–worker relationship. If you are concerned about a client's smoking, discuss the issue with your supervisor.

Supporting the Person Who Has COPD

1. **As with many conditions, pacing is important.** Shortness of breath can be severe and occur very suddenly. Many persons with moderate COPD may not be able to walk 10 m without stopping to rest.
2. **Encourage the person to sit while performing activities.** Sitting takes less energy than standing.
3. **Adapt tasks so that the client avoids bending or lifting.**
4. **Plan tasks so that you can help with the more physically demanding components.**
5. **If your client allows, help him or her to organize belongings so that what is needed is within easy reach.** This is particularly important if the client will be using the items when you are not there.
6. **If you are permitted to do so, assist the client with breathing exercises as required.** Be certain you know how to correctly help, as improper techniques may not help the client and may actually put the person at risk. Ask your supervisor or the client for direction.

Tuberculosis

Tuberculosis (TB) is a disease caused by bacteria that usually affects the lungs. A person can contract TB only through exposure to a person who has *active* or *infectious* TB. It usually takes prolonged exposure to TB to put a person at risk, unless the person has a weak immune system.

It's important to be aware that exposure to TB does not mean that the person will develop the active disease, even if a Mantoux test (a screening test for TB) is positive.

TB is not common in Canada, but its incidence is increasing. The Lung Association estimates that 70 percent of the cases in Canada actually began outside the country. TB is considered to be more common in long-term care facilities. This is partly because many people with weakened immune systems live in close proximity to one another. Many infections can spread more easily in these situations. For this reason, most health care workers are regularly tested for exposure to TB.

Only 10 percent of the people exposed to active TB will develop the active form. The remaining 90 percent will not develop the active form of the disease, do not become ill, and cannot infect others. Active TB can be treated by a course of medications given over a long period of time. Some people are hospitalized for treatment, while others can be treated at home. People exposed to TB, but who do not have the active form, usually take preventative medication for six months to one year. This substantially reduces their chances of developing active TB.

Recently, forms of TB have been identified that are resistant to common treatments. These are called *drug-resistant strains* and are very difficult to treat.

Pneumonia

Pneumonia is an inflammation or infection of the lungs. There are two types of pneumonia: bronchial and lobar. Bronchial pneumonia occurs in spots on both lungs; lobar affects a section (a lobe) of a lung.

Pneumonia causes the lungs' air sacs to fill with fluid. This prevents oxygen from reaching the blood. There are more than 30 causes of pneumonia, but a virus causes more than half of the cases. Pneumonia can also be caused by bacteria, the inhalation of a substance (called aspiration pneumonia), by organisms such as mycoplasma (an agent with both viral and bacterial properties), rickettsia, tuberculosis, or an obstruction like a tumour. Many of these conditions are serious and can be fatal if left untreated.

Medication is effective against bacterial and some other forms of pneumonia. However, there are few medications to treat viral pneumonia. It may take weeks or even months to recover form a bout of pneumonia. It can be fatal to people with other medical conditions or who are otherwise frail.

Asthma

We often think of asthma as a children's disease. According to the Canadian Lung Association, asthma is the leading chronic respiratory disease among children (CLA, 2003). Asthma can occur at any age however.

People with asthma have difficulty breathing. Their airways may become inflamed and swollen, or the muscles may go into spasms, causing the airway to constrict (Figure 20-5).

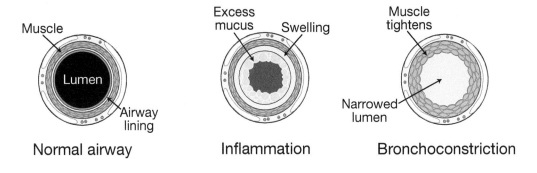

FIGURE 20-5
Normal, inflamed, and constricted airways

There are two main reasons for an asthmatic episode: triggers and causes. Triggers cause the airways to go into spasm. Common triggers include smoke (particularly cigarette smoke), cold air, dust, strong fumes, inhaled irritants, stress, and exercise. Causes produce inflammation and swelling. Common causes include inhaled allergens (e.g., pollen, mould, pet dander, dust mites) and respiratory viral infections.

Reducing exposure to allergens can be of tremendous help in reducing asthmatic episodes. Anti-inflammatory medication is often prescribed. Despite careful management and environmental control, an episode may occur. The onset of asthma symptoms is often sudden and severe. However, most people with asthma manage their symptoms without panic. In many cases, prescribed medication quickly addresses the symptoms. It is important for you to learn how the client with asthma responds to the onset of symptoms and to calmly support the client in taking necessary actions.

Diabetes

Diabetes is a disease that results from the pancreas's inability to produce enough insulin or to properly use insulin that is produced. A person with diabetes cannot metabolize food properly and may be at risk for cardiovascular and kidney problems. Diabetes also causes vision problems due to changes in the blood vessels in the retina of the eye.

There are three types of diabetes: type 1, type 2, and gestational. Type 1 diabetes occurs when the body does not produce any insulin or does not produce enough insulin. This type accounts for about 10 percent of the cases. Most children who develop diabetes have type 1. Type 2 diabetes is sometimes called *late-onset diabetes*, as it tends to occur in people over 45 years of age. It can be the result of insufficient insulin or from the body's inability to use the insulin that the pancreas does make. Gestational diabetes is a form of the disease that develops when a woman is pregnant. It usually disappears after the pregnancy is over, but may result in an increased risk of both mother and child developing diabetes at a later date.

Diabetes cannot be cured. The condition requires close monitoring of blood sugar levels, food intake, and activity. Medication may have to be taken orally or by injection each day. Even when treated, diabetes can have devastating effects on a person's circulatory system. As a result, even a small wound may pose serious risk to the person. It may not heal or gangrene may set in. Diabetics also are at an increased risk of kidney and vision problems.

Diabetes can have a dramatic affect on the person's life. Even such simple things as joining a friend at a coffee shop for a snack may require planning. Daily blood tests may be required. Some people are able to control their condition by careful management of their diet. Others must take daily doses of insulin to control blood sugar levels. Insulin must be injected to be effective, and most people who take insulin learn to self-inject. Others train a family member to assist. Some people must take two or more injections per day.

People with diabetes must also guard against two conditions related to the amount of sugar in the blood: *hyperglycemia* (high blood sugar) and *hypoglycemia* (low blood sugar). Hypoglycemia can result in a condition known as *insulin shock*. Hyperglycemia can result in a *diabetic coma*. Both conditions are serious and can result in death if not treated. Table 20-6 summarizes the causes and symptoms of each condition. Note that some of the symptoms are identical.

Supporting the Person Who Has Diabetes

Each person has his or her own regime for managing diabetes. It's important to know your client's regime and what you can do to help him or her maintain it. This may include preparing special meals or helping the client to find acceptable alternates to favourite foods. If part of the client's diabetes management plan involves losing weight, you might be asked to assist your client to prepare low-calorie meals or to take part in an exercise program. You might be asked to help the client test urine. You will not usually be expected to administer insulin. Speak with your supervisor if your client or another caregiver asks you to administer any medication.

Some people with diabetes may experience a decreased blood supply to the legs and feet. This may result in infections or poor wound and cut healing. Also, in some cases, the nerve cells become damaged and the person with diabetes may not feel temperature changes, touch, or pain. Serious conditions may occur, including gangrene (death of body tissue).

TABLE 20-6	Hypoglycemia and Hyperglycemia		
Condition	Causes	Symptoms	Possible Remedy
Hypoglycemia (low levels of glucose in the blood)	Too much insulin Omitting a meal Eating too little food Increased exercise Vomiting	Weakness Headache Low blood pressure Dizziness Rapid pulse Perspiration Trembling Hunger Cold, clammy skin Confusion Convulsions Unconsciousness	Orange juice Hard candy
Hyperglycemia (greater than normal levels of glucose in the blood)	Insufficient insulin Eating too much Too little exercise Stress Undiagnosed or untreated diabetes Infection	Weakness Headache Low blood pressure Rapid and weak pulse Drowsiness Thirst Flushed face Frequent urination Slow, laboured breathing Dry skin Nausea or vomiting Coma	Insulin

When you provide support to a client with diabetes, make certain to note the condition of the client's feet. Report to your supervisor any observations of shoes that are too tight or feet that are discoloured or swollen even if the client does not report any pain. The client may not sense discomfort because of nerve damage.

Human Immunodeficiency Virus

Human immunodeficiency virus (HIV) is the virus that causes AIDS (**acquired immune deficiency syndrome**). HIV attacks the body's immune system, making the person susceptible to many infections and diseases. These are called *opportunistic infections and diseases*. When a person develops these conditions, he or she is considered to have AIDS. Over time, these infections and diseases result in the person's death. There is no cure for HIV or AIDS, although the opportunistic conditions can usually be treated or prevented to some degree.

HIV cannot be spread by social contact. Hugging, holding hands, and touching do not spread the disease. Insect bites cannot transmit the virus. HIV can be spread by the exchange of body fluids: semen, vaginal secretions, breast milk, and blood. A person can contract HIV by having unprotected sex with an infected person, by using needles that have been used by an infected person (and not sterilized), by having a transfusion of infected blood or blood products, or by a puncture of the skin or mucous membrane by an infected object (such as a needlestick).

Supporting the Person Who Has HIV

1. **Keep in mind that you may pose a risk to your client.** The person who has HIV is susceptible to many infections. Colds, viruses, and other infections that you can easily fight off could be quite serious for your client. Use standard precautions to protect both of you.
2. **Keep the disease in perspective.** HIV is a serious disease that can be transmitted. However, proper precautions can ensure that the virus is not transmitted. Do not focus so much on your client's condition that you cease to see her or him as a person.

Hepatitis

Hepatitis refers to a group of diseases that affect the liver. There are actually six types, but three of them—Hepatitis A, Hepatitis B, and Hepatitis C—account for more than 90 percent of the cases (Health Canada, 2007). The causes and effects of each are different.

Hepatitis A

Health Canada reports that Hepatitis A cases occur in 2.9 out of every 100 000 Canadians. Eating raw, undercooked, or contaminated food or drinking contaminated water are the primary ways Hepatitis A is transmitted. Though it can be transmitted via contact with infected blood or through sexual relations, this is not common. Symptoms include jaundice (yellowing of the skin), appetite loss, stomach pain, and fatigue. There is no treatment for Hepatitis A, but most people recover in four to six weeks. People who have had the disease or have been vaccinated against it are immune from contracting it.

Hepatitis B

Hepatitis B is the most prevalent strain of the virus. Health Canada estimates that less than 1 percent of the population has had the virus. It is transmitted by contact with infected blood, blood products, and semen. Use of contaminated personal care items such as toothbrushes and razors, as well as unclean equipment used to pierce or tattoo, pose a risk, as do needlestick injuries. Hepatitis B can also be passed from mother to baby at birth.

There are acute and chronic forms of Hepatitis B. About 90 percent of people infected with the acute form recover. However, 15–40 percent of those with the chronic form go on to develop liver damage and disease. Babies infected at birth have a greater risk of developing a chronic form of Hepatitis B later in life.

Symptoms are similar to those of Hepatitis A, with the addition of joint pain and a general feeling of sickness. However, Health Canada estimates that up to 30 percent of people with Hepatitis B do not have symptoms. Treatment is aimed at helping the body's own defences overcome the virus.

Hepatitis C

Hepatitis C was first described in 1989. Health Canada estimates that between 210 000 and 275 000 Canadians are currently infected. Approximately 70–80 percent of those infected have the disease for the rest of their lives.

Symptoms are the same as for the other forms of Hepatitis, but it's estimated that only 20–30 percent of people infected with Hepatitis C actually show symptoms. It is primarily transmitted through contact with contaminated blood or blood products, although an infected mother can pass it on to a baby during birth. Persons who received organ transplants, blood, or blood products before 1989 are also at greater risk and have likely been tested.

Kidney Disease

The term kidney disease actually describes a group of conditions that can cause kidney damage and loss of function. Most kidney diseases damage the organ's ability to filter toxins from the blood.

The leading causes of kidney disease are diabetes and hypertension. However, there are also many other causes. Some are inherited; others are more likely as a person grows older. Some types are caused by medications. The cause of some kidney disease is not unknown.

Kidney disease is often progressive; it will get worse over time, particularly if not treated or if underlying causes are not treated. There is no cure for chronic kidney disease, although some underlying causes can be resolved. In the early stages, treatment is focused on removing or reversing an underlying cause or by reducing the effects upon the person's kidneys. Management in early stages usually includes medications and a specific diet. In later stages dialysis or transplant may be required.

Supporting the Person with Kidney Disease

In addition to the general guidelines in this chapter, the following may help you to assist the person with kidney disease:

1. **Assist the client to follow the diet set out.** A special diet is almost always required. This diet usually restricts protein and potassium to certain levels, but each diet is customized to the specific person. Fluid intake is usually restricted.
2. **Support the client in taking part in activities, as she or he is able.** Moderate exercise is beneficial to the client.
3. **Encourage the client to talk with family or a health care professional if certain symptoms are present.** These include unusual itching, cold intolerance, leg cramps, weakness, nausea, shortness of breath, or chest pain. These are some of the symptoms that the person's condition may be changing. There may be other important signs, depending on the person's specific situation.

ACUTE CONDITIONS

Not all conditions are chronic and serious. Many conditions are relatively minor and will often disappear in a short period of time with treatment. Some will disappear without treatment. Many of the conditions in this group are described as illnesses, but some are symptoms of an illness. For example, diarrhea is a symptom of many conditions, not a condition itself.

This section describes some of the more common acute conditions. In most cases, your client, supervisor, or other designated person will provide specific instructions to follow if your client has one of these conditions. Information in this section provides general information only.

Because of your role, you may be the first person to notice a condition. For example, you might be the first person to notice a rash on a client's back. Notify your supervisor if your client develops any of these conditions.

Skin Conditions

Eczema Eczema describes several conditions that usually produce dry and itchy skin. Some types are found most often on certain parts of the body. One form, atopic dermatitis, is seen most often in babies and young children. Varicose eczema usually occurs in older adults and people with varicose veins. Treatment usually includes a skin moisturizer; sometimes diet changes and stress reduction are also recommended.

Contact Dermatitis Contact dermatitis (sometimes called contact allergy) is an allergic reaction to something that is touching or was touching the skin. It usually starts at the site of contact, but can spread. Many things, including skin care products, some metals, and some medications can cause it. In most cases, treatment includes removing contact with the substance. If the possible cause is a medication, the client must discuss the issue as soon as possible with his or her doctor.

Shingles Shingles is the common term for herpes zoster. People who have had chicken pox can develop this condition, as the virus that causes chicken pox remains dormant in the body. If the person's resistance drops, the virus can reactivate and cause shingles. The first symptom is a sense of skin burning or pain. Within a few days, a rash forms and blisters appear. They usually appear on the trunk and most often on one side of the body.

Shingles is contagious, but less so than chicken pox. It is passed from person to person by contact with the rash, not by coughing. Blisters appear on parts of the body that are usually covered by clothing, making contact harder. However, shingles can

Photo 20-5
Picture of shingles on torso
Source: Copyright 2008 C.M.S.P. – Custom Medical Stock Photo, All Rights Reserved

pose a risk to pregnant women who have not had chicken pox, babies, and those with compromised immune systems or who are ill.

The condition usually clears up on its own; medication is prescribed to control symptoms. You should wear disposable gloves when coming into contact with the rash, blisters, or fluid from the blisters.

Viruses and Bacterial Infections

Urinary Tract Infections Urinary tract infections (UTIs) are infections that occur frequently. Approximately 500 000 women seek treatment for UTIs each year (Ontario Ministry of Health, 2007). UTIs are usually bothersome and painful, but are often not serious unless the infection spreads to the kidneys. Kidney infections can be serious and lead to disabling conditions.

Though not everyone with a UTI has symptoms, the following are among the more common ones:

- Burning sensation when urinating
- Feeling urge to urinate more often
- Feeling the urge to urinate but not being able to do so
- Leaking urine
- Bloody, cloudy, or bad-smelling urine
- Pain in the lower abdomen

You may also notice that your client avoids drinking liquids or delays voiding. If so, ask the client if she experiencing any of these symptoms and suggest that she seek the advice of a doctor. Avoiding liquids can make a UTI worse and may cause the client to become dehydrated, causing other health problems.

The following symptoms may be a sign that an infection has spread. A person with these symptoms should seek medical attention as soon as possible.

- Blood or pus in the urine
- Fever, chills, or vomiting
- If the person has diabetes or chronic illness, a history of kidney infection or disease
- Pain on urination during pregnancy
- Severe back pain

MRSA MRSA stands for methicillin-resistant staphylococcus aureus, a bacterial infection that is resistant to the methicillin. Staphylococcus aureus (also called Staph A) is common. It's found on the skin of healthy adults. If it gets into the body, it can cause infection that may be mild or severe. MRSA usually infects people whose immune systems are weakened. People who develop it usually do so when they are in hospital. Most healthy people are not at great risk of contracting MRSA. Support workers should use handwashing and standard precautions to avoid contracting or spreading the infection (Canadian Centre for Occupational Health & Safety, 2007).

VRE VRE stands for Vancomycin-Resistant Enterococci. Like MRSA, this is a bacterial infection that has become resistant to a common treatment. Though enterococci can cause serious infections, VRE is not any more serious than other enterococci infections. Most healthy people are not at risk of contracting VRE, unless they have been treated frequently with Vancomycin. A healthy person with VRE does not usually require treatment, although those with an infection do. Handwashing is the best precaution anyone can take to prevent the spread of VRE (British Columbia Centre for Disease Control, 2007).

Flu Flu is the common term for *influenza*, viruses that causes fever, cough, sore throat, runny nose, head and muscle aches, and fatigue. Most healthy people recover from the flu, but older adults and those with chronic conditions or weak immune systems may develop pneumonia or other serious complications. Many provinces now provide a flu vaccine (the "flu shot") to their residents. These annual vaccinations usually protect the person against the three strains of the virus that are expected to be most common that particular year. The expected strains do change from year to year, so last year's vaccination may not protect a person against the virus. Good handwashing, proper infection control, and disposal of used tissues can all help to limit risk to an unvaccinated person.

Encourage the client who has symptoms of the flu to contact his or her doctor. Advise your supervisor if your client develops flu or flu-like symptoms.

Common Symptoms

Fever describes a body temperature higher than normal (39°C or 98.6°F). It is usually a sign that the body is fighting an infection. Viruses and bacteria do not easily survive in higher temperatures, so the body raises its temperature to become less "friendly" to the infection. A person with a fever may complain of feeling chilled. Report a fever to your supervisor. Treatment is aimed at removing the cause (e.g., infection) if possible and to control symptoms. You may be asked to give your client liquids to drink or, if the fever is high, to apply cold compresses. A fever that lasts for more than three days, is accompanied by a stiff neck or chest congestion or redness or swelling, or occurs in a person with a serious medical condition can be serious and should be treated by a doctor.

Nausea is a sick feeling in the stomach. Vomiting is the forced expulsion of stomach contents up the esophagus. Nausea and vomiting can be caused by many, many conditions. Most are not serious, but some causes, such as heart attack, head injury, stroke, are very serious and must be treated. Nausea and vomiting can cause dehydration, either because fluids do not stay in the body or because the person avoids drinking to avoid nausea and vomiting. Dehydration can be particularly serious in older adults or persons with other health concerns. It should be reported to your supervisor.

Diarrhea occurs when the intestines push stool through the bowel before all the fluid in the stool is absorbed. It also happens when bowel inflammation allows fluid to seep into the stool. It is one of the most common symptoms and has literally hundreds of causes. In most cases, there are other symptoms; the cluster of symptoms will point to a particular diagnosis and treatment. Diarrhea usually is not serious, although some cases are severe and require immediate treatment. For example, diarrhea accompanied by dehydration or vomiting should be investigated immediately.

Constipation usually refers to hard stool that the person finds difficult to pass. Some people with constipation also experience bloating or abdominal discomfort. It does not necessarily mean not having a daily bowel movement. If stool is soft and easy to pass, the person is usually not constipated, even if the person does not have a bowel movement each day. Many things can cause constipation and in most cases it is not serious. However, some forms can lead to fecal impaction.

Fecal impaction occurs when a mass of dry, hard stool collects in the rectum and is so hard that it cannot be passed. In some cases, watery stool from higher in the bowel may leak around the impaction. Treatment includes removal of the impaction and treatment of the cause. Removal (or disimpaction) must usually be done by a regulated health professional who is skilled in the technique. In very rare cases, you may be trained to perform the technique. Disimpaction can be dangerous if done improperly.

WHAT TO DO WHEN YOU ENCOUNTER A NEW CONDITION

This chapter provides you with an overview of many conditions. It's very likely that you'll have a client who has a condition not discussed here. When that happens, you'll need to get accurate and reliable information on the condition and support approaches. The following guidelines will get you started:

- Ask your client, his or her family and caregivers. Most clients and those who assist them are very knowledgeable about their conditions and how to best be assisted.
- Seek out the local support groups or associations for the particular condition. They can be a great source of general information. Always make certain that you check out what you've learned with your client, however, as some information may not apply to the client's situation.
- Check out websites that discuss the condition. A word of caution here: make certain that the websites you access provide reliable information. Many associations have websites (a number are included at the end of this text) and are generally quite reliable. Other sites may be set up by people advocating a particular treatment or use unverified information. They may suggest harmful or useless approaches. Be certain that you are comfortable with the information you see. If in doubt, check with your client, supervisor, or with the association connected to the condition.

Questions for Review

1. Describe functional change. How does it relate to the concept of disability?

2. What are the six common types of changes?

3. You have a new client who needs physical assistance due to arthritis. What eight questions should you ask yourself in order to learn how to best assist the client?

4. What approaches should be used no matter what assistance you are providing?

5. What is the most common cause of vision loss in people over age 50?

6. What are the symptoms of glaucoma?

7. What are the two major causes of heart disease?

8. What is hypertension? What are the risk factors for hypertension?

9. What are the two main types (categories) of stroke?

10. What cardiovascular conditions contribute to an increased risk of stroke?

11. What functions are commonly controlled by the left hemisphere of the brain? The right hemisphere?

12. What is a TIA? Why is it important for a person to seek treatment if he or she has had a TIA?

13. What are the warning signs of a heart attack?

14. What should you do if your client has the signs of a heart attack?

15. What is gout? What foods should a person with gout avoid?

16. What is lupus?

17. What is the most common symptom of multiple sclerosis?

18. What techniques may assist the client with Parkinson's disease?

19. What techniques may assist the client with COPD?

20. List three major ways diabetes can affect a person.

21. What two things should you keep in mind when you are supporting the client with HIV or AIDS?

22. What is Hepatitis C? Is it curable?

23. What is a UTI? What are four of the symptoms?

24. What symptoms of a UTI mean that the person should see a doctor as soon as possible?

25. When should a person with a fever seek immediate medical attention?

26. Where can you go to find information on a specific condition?

27. What do you need to verify when you are getting information from a website?

Chapter 21

Infant and Child Care

Learning Objectives

Through reading this chapter, you'll be able to

1. List the six common situations in which the support worker may provide support to infants and children.
2. Describe the role of the support worker in providing support to the family with infants and children.
3. Outline a child's stages of development from birth to age one.
4. Demonstrate care of the well infant.
5. Describe the characteristics of support provided to new mothers.
6. Describe the signs of illness in infants.
7. Identify selected conditions that may require children to have support needs.
8. Discuss the characteristics of support provided to children with developmental or physical disabilities.

Chapter at a Glance

- Common Situations
- Establishing a Relationship with Parents
- Infant and Child Development
- Infant Care
- Infants and Children with Special Needs
- Postpartum Depression

Terms You'll Use

Autism Spectrum Disorder A group of disorders that affect verbal and non-verbal communication and social interaction caused by abnormalities in brain structure or function.

Circumcision The surgical removal of the foreskin of the penis.

Cleft Lip A congenital fissure or opening in the upper lip.

Cleft Palate A congenital fissure in the roof of the mouth, resulting from incomplete fusion of the palate during embryonic development.

Club Foot A congenital condition that may result in the following: an infant's foot (especially the heel) being smaller than normal, pointing downward, the front of the foot rotating toward the other foot, or the entire foot turning in. In extreme cases, the bottom of the foot can point up.

Congenital Hip Dysplasia A condition resulting in partial or total hip dislocation.

Down Syndrome A condition caused by an unusual arrangement of chromosomes, most often due to the presence of an additional copy of chromosome 21 in each cell.

Engorgement A painful overfilling of the breasts.

Fetal Alcohol Effect (FAE) A disorder that can occur when a woman drinks alcohol during pregnancy; milder than FAS.

Fetal Alcohol Syndrome (FAS) A disorder that can occur when a woman drinks alcohol during pregnancy; more serious than FAE.

Fragile X Syndrome A genetic disorder caused by a weakness or break in a portion of a child's X chromosome.

Hydrocephalus A condition related to an increase of intracranial fluid in the brain that causes increased head size and pressure in the brain.

Jaundice A condition that causes yellowing of the skin.

Milestone The time at which particular events, skills, or behaviours are generally expected to occur.

Multiple Births The birth of more than one baby during one pregnancy.

Parent A person who has the primary responsibility of caring for a child.

Phenylketonuria A disease caused by the absence of a liver enzyme.

Postpartum Depression A depression that can occur in women who have recently had a baby.

Spina Bifida A congenital condition caused by a defect in the way the spinal column has formed.

COMMON SITUATIONS

The support provided to a family usually falls into one of these six categories. Keep in mind that some support may address more than one type of need.

1. **Support to the new parent or parents of multiple births.** You may be asked to provide support to new parents of multiple births, which refers to the birth of twins, triplets, or quadruplets. This type of support usually focuses on helping with infant care, with any other children in the home, as well as with the new mother as she recovers from childbirth.

2. **Support to the premature infant and to parents of a premature infant.** You may be asked to assist with care for the infant or to undertake household tasks so that the parents may care for the child. Many premature babies have medical conditions that are treated by a professional member of the support team. You may be asked to assist with care appropriate for a support worker to perform.

3. **Support to an infant or child with a physical or developmental disability.** You may be asked to assist with care for the infant or to undertake household tasks so that the parents may care for the child. Many infants or children with disabilities have conditions that are treated by a professional member of the support team. You may be asked to assist with care appropriate for a support worker to perform.

4. **Support for the parent with physical disabilities.** You may be asked to assist a parent who cannot perform all parenting activities as the result of a physical disability. You may be asked to perform specific infant and child care tasks, to assist the parent to perform tasks (such as bathing an infant) that he or she cannot do alone, or be asked to perform specific household tasks so that the parent can devote time to child care.

5. **Support for the parent who lacks parenting skills or experience.** You may be asked to assist a parent who does not have parenting skills. The parent may be a spouse who has to assume parenting because the primary caregiver is ill or away. The parent could also be a young person who has no experience or self-confidence.

In these situations, you may spend a great deal of time teaching the parent to care for the infant or child, as well as coaching the parent as he or she practises skills.

6. **Support for the parent who has difficulty coping with the demands of parenting.** You may be asked to assist a parent who has difficulty coping for many reasons. The parent may have multiple sources of stress: a mental health condition, a substance abuse problem, or a history of abuse. In these situations, you may provide emotional support, coach the parent as he or she practises skills, as well as complete household tasks so that the parent does not become overwhelmed.

ESTABLISHING A RELATIONSHIP WITH PARENTS

In this section, we'll use the term **parent** to refer to any person who has the primary responsibility of caring for the child. This may include grandparents, aunts, uncles, and mothers and fathers. Also, families come in many types, such as single parent, nuclear (a mother and father with children), and extended (a nuclear family with grandparents or other relatives in the same home), among many others.

The role of a parent is a special one. It implies a special love, closeness, and caring between the child and the parent. Consider the situation in Stop and Reflect 21-1.

STOP AND REFLECT ((21-1))

If you are a parent, recall a time that your child had a minor injury (such as a cut, scrape, or bruise).

_____
_____

_____

How did you feel when your child asked or reached out to you for comfort?

_____

_____

How do you think you would feel if your child had reached out to someone else for comfort?

_____

_____

Many times, the parent you are assisting has mixed feelings about your help. The parent may feel that he or she is a "bad" parent because of a need for assistance. The parent may be concerned that the child will begin to rely upon you instead of him or her. Occasionally, a parent will feel that you are there to judge him or her in some way.

You must do your utmost to put the parent at ease. If possible, you should have the opportunity to go over the support plan before your first visit. This allows you to get an accurate description of the purpose of your support, as well as the specific tasks you may be asked to perform.

As you make your first few visits, you will need to take time to get to know the parent and others involved in the child's care. It's particularly important to establish how you can work together to best meet the child's needs. Keep in mind that you are not there to comment on how the family is organized. You must respect the ways in which family members relate to one another, even if it is not the way that you would prefer.

INFANT AND CHILD DEVELOPMENT

The period between birth and age three is one of extensive growth and development. At birth, the nervous system is relatively mature and directs most of the newborn's activity. The newborn displays many reflexes that attest to the maturity of the nervous system. Table 21-1 describes some of the more common ones.

TABLE 21-1	Common Reflexes in the Newborn
Reflex	**Happens When...**
Moro	The crib is jarred, and the infant startles by drawing its legs up and folding its arms on its chest.
Rooting	The infant's cheek is touched, and the infant moves its head toward the source looking for food.
Sucking	The infant's lips are touched, and he or she begins to suck.
Tonic Neck	The infant is sleeping, the head is turned to one side and one arm is raised over its head as if the infant is "fencing."
Grasp	The infant's hands are touched, and the fingers grasp your fingers.
Blink	The bridge of the infant's nose is touched, and he or she blinks.

The newborn can also hear, taste, smell, see, and fixate on objects. At full term, all of the body's systems are working but are immature. Keep these things in mind as you care for a newborn.

1. Full expansion of the lungs does not take place for a few days after birth in an infant carried to full term. A premature infant's lungs may be very immature.
2. Infants cannot easily regulate or conserve their body heat. Therefore, room temperature should be kept at 20°C to 22°C, as infants lose heat very quickly.
3. The immaturity of the infant's musculoskeletal system means that movements are random and uncoordinated. However, an infant should never be limp.
4. It is common for an infant's eyes to be crossed at birth, as the eye muscles are immature. This should correct itself as the infant grows.
5. The infant's urinary system is not fully developed. Therefore, it is not unusual for the infant to have several wet diapers each day.
6. The infant's immune system is immature at birth. Take steps to prevent any infectious contacts.
7. At birth, small pimples (called *milia*) are evident on nose and chin; these will disappear in the first few weeks.
8. The infant's skin peels within the first few weeks.
9. Stools are initially black-green and tarry. They change within the first week to bright yellow, soft, and pasty for breast-fed infants. Bottle-fed infants' stools are yellowish brown and are usually firmer than those of breast-fed infants. It is normal for a newborn to strain when having a bowel movement.
10. Hiccups occur often. Burping infants and offering warm water helps to calm them.

Conditions That Require Special Care

There are other conditions that may require special care:

1. Circumcision (the surgical removal of the foreskin of the penis) may be performed prior to discharge from hospital. If so, there may be special instructions for bathing and monitoring urine output.
2. Infant jaundice (yellowing of the skin) itself isn't a disease. In most cases infant jaundice occurs as a baby's liver isn't mature enough to metabolize the molecule bilirubin. If you notice any yellowing of the infant's skin or eyes, report the observation to your supervisor.

Developmental Milestones

Researchers have developed milestones—the times at which particular skills or behaviours are generally expected to develop. It's important to remember that milestones are guidelines, not absolute deadlines. Each child will be somewhat different, attaining some milestones ahead of schedule and others somewhat later. These minor variations are not usually a cause for concern. However, a consistent delay in developing abilities is something to discuss with your supervisor. Table 21-2 describes some common milestones from birth to one year.

Caregiving Tips

Research suggests that the more you interact with the infant, the more complete the infant's development will be. Keep these guidelines in mind to make the most of the time with the child.

1. **It's important to spend time with the infant.** This stimulates many senses and encourages awareness.
2. **Learn and follow the infant's schedule.** Most infants will fall into a routine after a period of time. Don't be alarmed if the routine differs from infant to infant.

TABLE 21-2	Milestones from Birth to One Year		
Age	Physical Development	Cognitive Development	Social Development
Birth to 4 months	lifts head and chest when lying on stomach follows a moving object or person with eyes grasps rattle or finger wiggles and kicks rolls over (stomach to back) sits up with support plays with fingers, hands, toes	explores objects with mouth can discriminate between people, places, shapes, and colours turns head toward bright colours and lights responds to a shaking rattle or bell	cries (with tears) to communicate pain, fear, hunger, discomfort, fatigue, or loneliness stops crying when lifted or touched babbles and coos loves to be touched and held close responds to voices returns a smile responds to "peek-a-boo" and other simple games

▶▶|

Table 21-2	Milestones from Birth to One Year *(continued)*		
Age	Physical Development	Cognitive Development	Social Development
4 to 8 months	<ul><li>develops a pattern for feeding, sleeping</li><li>rolls from back to stomach and stomach to back</li><li>sits alone without support</li><li>holds head erect</li><li>raises up into crawling position; may rock back and forth, but not move forward</li><li>uses finger and thumb to pick up objects</li><li>transfers objects from one hand to the other</li><li>first teeth begin to appear</li><li>drools, mouths, and chews on objects</li><li>drinks from a cup with help</li><li>reaches for cup or spoon</li><li>closes mouth firmly or turns head when not hungry</li></ul>	<ul><li>develops ability to think</li><li>learns through smelling, tasting, touching, seeing, hearing</li><li>can focus eyes on and reach for small objects</li><li>plays at length with one or two items</li><li>uses voice to indicate pleasure or displeasure</li><li>can assign simple words to people and objects (e.g., "dada" or "mama")</li><li>recognizes and seeks familiar voices</li><li>looks for ball rolled out of sight</li><li>seeks toys hidden out of sight (e.g., under a blanket, basket, or container)</li><li>recognizes names of family members</li></ul>	<ul><li>cries in different tones or pattern to indicate hunger, fear, loneliness, and other needs</li><li>responds to own name</li><li>responds differently to strangers and family members</li><li>imitates sounds, actions, and facial expressions of others</li><li>squeals, laughs, babbles, or smiles in response to others</li><li>smiles at own reflection in mirror</li><li>raises arms to be held</li><li>shows mild to severe anxiety at separation from parent</li></ul>
8 to 12 months	<ul><li>needs 2–3 meals per day</li><li>enjoys drinking from a cup</li><li>begins to eat finger foods</li><li>enjoys opening and closing doors</li><li>crawls well</li><li>pulls self to a standing position</li><li>stands alone holding onto furniture for support</li><li>walks holding onto furniture or with help</li><li>prefers one hand over the other</li></ul>	<ul><li>says first words</li><li>interested in picture books</li><li>pays attention to conversations</li><li>claps hands, waves bye if prompted</li><li>likes to place objects inside one another</li><li>uses 3–4 word speech</li><li>responds to own name</li><li>likes to watch self in mirror</li></ul>	<ul><li>imitates adult actions such as drinking from a cup, talking on phone</li><li>expresses fear or anxiety toward strangers ("makes strange")</li><li>wants caregiver or parent to be in constant sight</li><li>may become attached to a favourite toy or blanket</li><li>offers toys or objects to others but expects them to be given right back</li></ul>

3. **Respond to the infant's cries.** The cry is the only way the infant can communicate his or her needs. Responding also makes the infant feel secure ("my needs will be met").

4. **Hold and cuddle the infant when feeding him or her.** Physical contact is very important to a child's development. Holding the infant means that you are not propping a bottle up with a pillow—an action that can lead to choking and later, tooth decay.

5. **Make use of the pre-crawling period (birth to five months or so) to childproof everything.** Safely store *all* household chemicals and cooking supplies. Be aware that ingesting even a "safe" substance (such as vinegar) can be harmful to an infant. Install safety latches on cabinets and place covers on electrical outlets. Pad sharp corners of tables or shelves or remove them from the area in which the child plays. Remove fragile, breakable items from lower shelves and low tabletops.

6. **Provide good stimulation.** Provide bright colours and a variety of objects to look at and handle. These need not be expensive toys. Clean, bright socks or washcloths, small plastic containers, plastic measuring cups, a kettle, spoon, or spatula will often do. Big pictures cut from packaging can also amuse. Simple music (played on a radio or stereo) provides auditory stimulation.

7. **As the child grows, offer variety in tastes, temperature, texture, and aroma.** Infants are often very sensitive to tastes. Even foods that do not seem spicy to you may be too spicy to the infant, so experiment with caution.

8. **Talk and read to the infant.** This helps the infant to learn language.

9. **Play games like peek-a-boo and pat-a-cake.** This encourages intellectual and motor skill development as well as promotes social interaction.

10. **Provide a safe area for the infant to crawl about.**

INFANT CARE

This section includes procedures for many types of infant care. There may be a number of safe variations for each procedure, and some procedures will have to be adapted to take into account the specific setting. If you are assisting a parent, make sure not to discourage him or her from performing tasks. Do your utmost to follow the style of care provided by the parent—if it is safe.

Bathing the Newborn

Bathing is a wonderful opportunity to spend time with the infant. Parents will usually pick the best time of the day to bathe their infant based upon the needs of the infant and others in the household.

Preparing the Environment

1. Make sure that the room is warm and that all windows are closed to prevent drafts.
2. Remove any jewellery to prevent scratching the infant's skin.
3. Bathe the infant before a feeding. Bathing stimulates the infant to feed better. Bathing before a feeding can also prevent vomiting or bowel movements during the bath.

Procedure 21-1
Bathing the Newborn

EQUIPMENT

basin or infant tub

towel and washcloth

baby soap

diaper

alcohol swab
(optional) or cotton
swab with rubbing
alcohol

petroleum jelly

brush or comb

clean clothing

blanket

1. Wash your hands.
2. Fill the basin or tub with lukewarm water. Always test the water with your wrist. Never add warm or hot water while the infant is in the basin or tub.
3. Undress the infant and immediately wrap in towel to prevent chilling. Support the infant under your nondominant arm and close to your body in a football fashion. Figure 21-1a illustrates this position.

FIGURE 21-1A
*Proper support
for an infant*

4. Use a clean washcloth without soap to wash eyes, face, and ears.
   a. Gently wipe each eye from inner corner to outer corner. Use a separate corner of the washcloth for each eye. This prevents spread of bacteria from one eye to the other.
   b. Wash off particles at entrance to the nose. Do not use cotton-tipped swabs, as they may push mucus further into the nose or cause damage to the nasal lining.
   c. Do not use cotton-tipped swabs to clean the ear canal as they may push wax further into the canal and damage it. Wax will work itself out naturally. Be very careful in handling a premature infant's ears as they are very soft.
5. While holding the infant's head over the tub, use a washcloth and soap to wash the hair. Hair can be washed daily or twice a week. Wash the hair quickly as the infant rapidly loses heat through the head. Massage the scalp gently in a circular fashion. Avoiding the soft spot is not necessary, but be sure to use gentle motions. Be careful not to get soap into the infant's eyes.
6. Lather and rinse thoroughly. It is important to get all of the soap out to prevent irritation from soap residue.
7. Dry the hair thoroughly with the towel.
8. Unwrap the infant and place him or her into the tub, supporting the upper torso and head at all times with your arm. Figure 21-1b illustrates the positions. (Do not immerse the infant totally into the tub until the umbilical cord has fallen off.)
9. Using your dominant hand, wash the infant with a soaped hand or washcloth starting at the neck and working down. Pay special attention to the creases.

FIGURE 21-1B
Supporting the infant in the tub

10. Turn the infant over with the head to the side and wash his or her back.
11. Rinse well.
12. Wash genitalia as follows:
    a. Female genitalia: Wash from front to back to prevent spreading anal bacteria into the urinary system and the vagina. The female infant may have a scant amount of bloody vaginal discharge, which is normal due to the hormones received from her mother.
    b. Male genitalia: Do not retract the foreskin of the uncircumcised penis as it is attached firmly to the head of the penis. The foreskin will retract naturally at about five years old. Wash the penis and scrotum gently, paying special attention to keeping the creases clean.
13. Dry the infant thoroughly with the towel with special attention to the creases.

Caring for the Umbilical Cord Stump

Some physicians recommend that the umbilical cord stump be wiped with rubbing alcohol to aid in drying. This will help it fall off within a week or so after birth. If this is the case, wipe after each bath and diaper change. Be sure to wipe the base of the cord itself, not the infant's skin. Umbilical cord stumps can become infected. If the cord area becomes red, has an odour or discharge, is swelling, or develops a pimply red rash, notify the parents and advise them to contact the infant's doctor.

Signs of Illness in an Infant

Infants do become ill despite the best of care. Illness in infants can be serious if not treated promptly. Table 21-3 lists signs of illness for which you should observe. Bear in mind that any change in the infant's normal routine may be important and should be carefully monitored.

TABLE 21-3	Signs of Illness in Infants
Sign	**Description**
Fever/Body Temperature	Any fever in a baby younger than six months old Fever over 38°C in a child older than six months Fever below 38°C lasting more than two days Fever accompanied by a rash Body temperature below 36.5°C
Dehydration	Pale, dry skin Sunken eyes Dry lips and tongue Infrequent urination (less than 6 wet heavy diapers a day) Urine that is dark in colour Fewer bowel movements than usual in the last 24 hours Diarrhea (frequent, watery bowel movements) Vomiting
Breathing	Having a hard time breathing Gasping or grunting Breathing faster than usual or long pauses (more than 10 seconds) in breathing Persistent coughing or wheezing Lips and fingertips have a blue tinge
Feeding	Not wanting to suck or feed Rapid sucking for several feedings Falls asleep on the breast or bottle without drinking and does not wake up for next feeding
Behaviour	Very fussy Fidgety—won't settle down Weak cry Extreme sleepiness, lethargy Unresponsiveness
Other	Blood in the stool Yellow or green discharge from eyes Yellow tint to the skin (jaundice) over the whole body Persistent diaper rash with blisters or pimples

Dressing the Infant

After drying the infant well, dress him or her in clean clothing. Clothing should be weather appropriate and unrestrictive. Be aware that an overdressed infant can overheat quickly and that an underdressed infant can lose heat quickly. A good guideline is to dress the infant in the same amount of clothing as an adult.

For the first week after birth, it is sometimes recommended to wrap the infant snugly in a blanket. This gives the infant a secure feeling and makes it easy to position the infant on his or her side or back. Avoid placing the infant on his or her stomach until the infant's physician advises it is safe. An infant under one year of age should never be placed on his or her stomach to sleep.

Doing the Infant's Laundry

Because infants have sensitive skin, you must take special care with their laundry. The following guidelines will help you keep clothing looking nice and avoid irritating the infant's skin:

1. Wash diapers separately from other baby clothing. Use Procedure 21-2 to launder cloth diapers if used.
2. Wash clothing in a mild detergent. Avoid scented products or those with added bleach. Avoid using "natural" animal-fat-based soaps as they may affect the clothing's flame-retardant properties.
3. Avoid using scented fabric softener. Perfumes in both liquid and dryer-sheet softeners can irritate an infant's skin.
4. Soak stained items in cold water. Do not use hot water as it may cause the stain to set. Stubborn stains can be soaked in a solution of detergent and water before washing. If possible, soak the stain until it disappears. Never dry stained items in the dryer as the heat will cause the stain to set.
5. Avoid using starch when ironing clothing. The chemicals and the stiffness can irritate the infant's skin.

Procedure 21-2
Laundering Cloth Diapers

1. Fill the diaper pail with warm water.
2. Add 125 mL (1/2 cup) of borax.
3. Rinse dirty diapers by holding the diaper in the toilet bowl while flushing the toilet to remove soil.
4. Place rinsed diapers in the diaper pail; the borax solution will help remove stains.
5. Run diapers through a wash cycle. Use detergent, hot water, and bleach according to the recommendations for the client's machine.
6. Run diapers through a second wash cycle. Do not add detergent. Use water and add white vinegar to the final rinse. (The vinegar gets rid of soap residue and whitens diapers.) As an alternative, you may add baking soda to the final rinse to help soften the fabric. Do not use both vinegar and baking soda in the same rinse.
7. Dry diapers in the dryer without any softener.
8. Fold and place in proper location.

EQUIPMENT

diaper pail with a cover

borax

baking soda

bleach

white vinegar

Feeding the Infant

Usually after the bath, the infant is ready to eat. If the infant is breast fed, assist the mother into breast-feeding position. If bottle-fed, prepare a bottle for the infant.

Assisting the Mother with Breast Feedings

Breast feeding is a wonderful experience for mother and infant. Most mothers receive help from postpartum nurses in the hospital prior to discharge but will still require support and encouragement when they return home. A mother's milk is not present until approximately the third day after birth. At that time, the milk is usually present, and the infant can receive adequate nutrition. The infant is receiving adequate nutrition from the mother when the infant:

1. appears comfortable at the breast
2. latches on easily
3. is satisfied after feeding
4. is sleeping well (four to five hours)
5. has six to eight wet diapers per day
6. has one or more stools per day,
7. is gaining weight

A breast-feeding mother must maintain a nutritious diet. In most cases, an additional intake of 500 calories a day over the mother's normal intake is required. A nursing mother should avoid gassy foods that are passed to the infant, such as cabbage, beans, or broccoli. She should also avoid all medication and alcohol; these will be passed to the infant.

Breast feeding is done on demand usually every two to three hours. Frequent breast feeding prevents **engorgement**, a painful overfilling of the breasts.

Procedure 21-3
Assisting the Mother with Breast Feedings

1. Wash hands prior to assisting the mother.
2. Help her into a comfortable position. No one position is necessarily better than another as long as the mother is comfortable. Some mothers find a nursing pillow useful. It is most important that the mother is comfortable and relaxed during feeding to promote the let-down reflex and allow a good flow of milk.
3. Bring the infant to the mother's breast to avoid strain on the mother's back.
4. Advise the mother to brush the infant's cheek with the nipple. This causes the infant to turn toward the nipple (the rooting reflex).
5. Advise the mother to guide the infant's mouth toward the nipple so that the infant can latch onto the whole nipple and areola. If the infant sucks only on the nipple, the nipple becomes cracked and sore. Figure 21-2 illustrates the proper and incorrect positions.
6. As the infant nurses, watch to ensure that the infant's nose is not covered by the mother's breast.
7. The infant should feed from both breasts at each feeding. Burp the infant after finished feeding from the first breast. An infant receives most of each breast's milk within five minutes, but 10 to 30 minutes of sucking stimulates the breast to produce more milk. As well, alternating the breasts (starting one feeding with the right breast, the next with the left) allows for equal replenishing of breast milk.
8. To remove the infant from the breast, advise the mother to insert her finger into the infant's mouth to break the suction.

FIGURE 21-2
*Infant latching
onto nipple*

Preparing Formula

If a mother decides to bottle feed, a commercially prepared formula is often recommended by the physician. Formula may come in many forms from ready-to-use in cans to powder that must be mixed.

Formulas that must be mixed have simple instructions on the can. These instructions must be followed exactly. The formula must be used within the time limit set in the instructions. Stale prepared formula loses nutritional value and can become contaminated. It must be discarded to prevent infection in the infant.

Most mothers prefer to heat formula, but it is fine to feed the infant formula at room temperature. Avoid heating the bottle in the microwave, as this form of heating can destroy nutrients. If you heat formula, use a pan of water into which you place the formula in a heatproof container. Do not heat plastic bottles in a pan, as they will melt. Pour the warmed formula into a bottle, placing a nipple and bottle ring on top.

Always test the formula on your wrist before feeding the infant to make sure it is not too hot. This is also an opportunity to check that the nipple hole is the correct size. If it is, the formula should come out in drops but not flow steadily. An infant can tire easily if the hole is too small or receive too much formula and choke if it is too big.

Bottle-fed infants usually feed every three to four hours. Each feeding should take 15 to 20 minutes.

Procedure 21-4
Bottle Feeding

1. Assist the mother to find a comfortable position. If you are feeding the infant, hold the infant in your nondominant arm. Make sure that the infant's head is higher than the torso.
2. Tilt the bottle so that the nipple fills with formula.
3. Place the nipple in the infant's mouth. You will know you have the right position when you can feel the infant sucking on the nipple.
4. Burp the infant after each 15 to 30 mL (one-half to one ounce) of formula is taken. You can burp the baby over your shoulder or over your lap as shown in Figures 21-3 and 21-4.
5. Continue to feed until the infant takes no more formula. Do not allow formula to pool in the baby's mouth, as it can cause choking.

6. Discard unused formula after each feeding.
7. Document the amount of formula the infant drank.
8. Change the infant if required.
9. Place the infant on his or her side to promote digestion.

All bottles and nipples should be sterilized before their first use. After that, a thorough cleaning in hot soapy water or in the dishwasher is usually sufficient. However, there may be situations where repeated sterilization is necessary. These situations include when the client uses well water or when the infant's doctor has recommended sterilization.

FIGURE 21-3
Burping the infant on the shoulder

FIGURE 21-4
Burping the infant on the lap

Procedure 21-5
Sterilizing Bottles and Nipples

EQUIPMENT

bottles	water
nipples	tongs
rings	clean dish towel
caps and lids	
saucepot large enough to hold bottles laid on their sides	

1. Fill pot two-thirds full with clean water. Bring to rolling boil.
2. Submerge bottles, rings, nipples, lids, and caps in boiling water.
3. Boil for five minutes.
4. Remove items with tongs.
5. Place on a clean towel to dry.

Diapering the Infant

Parents may choose to use cloth or disposable diapers. They may also choose a diaper service to deliver and pick up cloth diapers. The choice of which type to use is a personal decision and is often based upon cost, comfort, convenience, and environmental factors. You should not attempt to convince parents to use a type you prefer.

The infant should be changed several times a day, prior to feedings, after feedings, and at any other time necessary. Infants frequently wet and soil diapers. As the infant gets older, diaper wetting and soiling will become less frequent.

Procedure 21-6
Diapering the Infant

1. Wash your hands.
2. Lay the infant on the change table. Always have one hand on the infant when on the change table to prevent falls.
3. Undo the diaper (unpin or open Velcro® if cloth diaper, pull adhesive tab on disposable diaper). Close pins and make sure they are well out of infant's reach.
4. Pull the front of the diaper down between the infant's legs.
5. Wipe the infant from front to back with a clean area on the inner front of the diaper.
6. Roll the front of the diaper so that the inner portion is inside.
7. Pull the back of the diaper so that it is away from the side of the infant.
8. Lift up the infant's buttocks by holding the infant's legs and lifting up.
9. Wipe off soil with a cloth.
10. Remove the soiled diaper from under the infant.
11. Lower the infant's buttocks to the table.
12. Wrap the diaper and set it aside out of the infant's reach.
13. Lift the infant's legs as in step 8. Using baby wipes or a wet washcloth, cleanse the genital area. Always wipe from front to back. If the infant is very soiled or has a rash, use a mild soap with the washcloth. Wet wipes do not need additional soap. Rinse well and pat dry.
14. Apply cream if used.
15. Lift up the infant's legs as per step 8. Place a fresh diaper under the infant's buttocks. Disposable diapers and fitted cloth diapers have a front and back. Disposable diapers have tape tabs on the back. Fitted cloth diapers are usually larger in the back. Make sure that you position the diaper properly.
16. Lower the infant's legs and bring the front of the diaper up between the legs.
17. Fasten the diaper securely. If pins are used, insert them from the front to the back.
18. Make sure that the diaper is snug around the hips and abdomen. If the umbilical cord stump is present, fold the diaper edge so that it is below the stump to prevent irritation.
19. Place the baby in a safe place.
20. Dispose of diaper according to type. Wrap disposable diapers up tightly and dispose of promptly. Flush cloth diaper in toilet to remove excess soil and place in diaper pail.
21. Wash your hands.
22. Report any unusual bowel movement or rash to parent and, if appropriate, your supervisor.

EQUIPMENT

diaper (if cloth, fold as per parent's instructions)

wet washcloths or wipes

petroleum jelly, diaper cream, or other ointment as used by parents

INFANTS AND CHILDREN WITH SPECIAL NEEDS

There are many conditions that cause an infant to have special needs. Some result in effects on physical development, others on cognitive development. Some conditions affect both physical and cognitive development.

Providing Support to the Child with Special Needs

In many cases, the child's family will have gained extensive knowledge of their child's condition and will be quite involved in their child's support. In some cases, you may be assisting a family just learning to cope with a condition. The family is an integral part of the support team: you must work together to support the child. It's likely that you will follow a specific support plan developed for the child. It's also possible that you will be asked to perform household tasks so that a parent can devote more time to working with the child. You must be prepared to adapt your role and to be flexible in order to be effective.

In this section, we'll discuss some of the more common conditions. Table 21-4 on page 463 describes other conditions you might encounter.

Autism/Autism Spectrum Disorders

In general use, the term *autism* describes both the specific Autistic Disorder and is also often used to refer to all Autism Spectrum Disorders (ASD). The most accurate term is Autism Spectrum Disorder, which describes a group of developmental disorders that cause disability in verbal and non-verbal communication and social interaction. These disorders are caused by abnormalities in brain structure or function. Researchers have identified five types. The three most common types are Autistic Disorder (also called autism, classic autism, and AD); PDD-NOS (Pervasive Developmental Disorder – Not Otherwise Specified); and Asperger's Disorder (also called AS, Asperger's Syndrome, and Asperger Syndrome). The remaining two (Childhood Disintegrative Disorder and Rett's Disorder) are extremely rare.

Researchers don't know exactly what causes ASD. Current research has linked ASD to genetic, metabolic and possibly environmental cases. ASDs are not caused by bad parenting.

ASDs are called *spectrum disorders* because the symptoms of the disorder are unique to the person. These disorders can usually be identified by age 2, but this may vary.

The number and particular kinds of symptoms may vary and symptoms may range from mild to severe. Ability to function, to interact with others may differ significantly from person to person. As with all conditions, it's important to identify what your client's abilities and needs are, and not to make assumptions based upon general information.

Approximately two-thirds of children with ASD have below-average intelligence. A child may possess extraordinary ability in a specific task (such as mathematics), even though he or she might not possess average intelligence overall. Most children with ASD have difficulty forming and maintaining social relationships. They avoid interaction with others and usually play alone. Many of them have an altered response to sensory stimulation (sights, sounds, tastes, and touch). They may be overly sensitive to sensory stimulation or appear to ignore all stimulation. Many children with ASD have a focused or narrow attention span and exhibit repetitive behaviour.

There is no cure for ASDs. Treatment is usually centred on encouraging social interaction and addressing specific problem behaviours. Some children with ASD undergo intensive one-to-one therapy. Therapy started when the child is very young can help to minimize symptoms. You may be asked to assist in specific play therapy or to work with the child to help change how he or she responds to sounds or sights.

Children with ASD do not "grow out" of the condition. Some adults with ASD are able to live and work independently. Others require support with everyday activities.

Cerebral Palsy

We discussed cerebral palsy (CP) in Chapter 20. If you choose to provide support to children, it's quite likely that you will be assigned to assist a child with special needs at some time in your career. CP affects one child in every 1000 births. CP is caused by an anomaly in or injury to the brain before, during, or shortly after birth. People with CP usually have difficulty with muscle control (having muscle tone that is too tight or too loose). Sensory problems, developmental problems, learning disabilities, and speech problems may also occur.

Down Syndrome

Down syndrome is a condition caused by an unusual arrangement of chromosomes, most often due to the presence of an additional copy of chromosome 21 in each cell. It affects one of every 800–1000 births (Saskatchewan Down Syndrome Society, 2006).

Children with Down syndrome often have distinctive physical features. Some of the more common features include small nose, wide-set eyes, an upward slant to the eyes, small hands and feet, short stature, and low muscle tone. Most children with Down syndrome have mild to moderate mental retardation and often have heart and respiratory problems as well as reduced resistance to disease. They are at increased risk for developing Alzheimer disease or leukemia as adults. The symptoms can differ widely from person to person. Always take the time to identify exactly what your client's abilities and needs are.

Fetal Alcohol Effect and Fetal Alcohol Syndrome

Fetal alcohol effect (FAE) and Fetal alcohol syndrome (FAS) are two disorders that can result from a woman drinking alcohol when pregnant. FAE is a milder and much more common form of the two disorders. Both FAE and FAS can produce physical and psychological impairments. Many people with FAE or FAS will require support all their lives. It is estimated that one in 750 children born has FAE or FAS.

Children with either disorder can have difficulty learning. Many have difficulty paying attention to tasks or are easily distracted. The ability to problem-solve and to learn from previous mistakes is often impaired as well. Some children act impulsively or are extremely stubborn. FAE or FAS may also be linked to learning and attention disorders.

Children with FAE or FAS can benefit from therapy aimed at helping them learn life skills and practise problem solving. Children with FAE or FAS often benefit from a consistent routine free of overstimulation and distraction.

Fragile X Syndrome

Fragile X syndrome is a genetic disorder caused by a weakness or a break in a portion of a child's X-chromosome. It is an inherited condition and is thought to be the leading cause of inherited learning disabilities and mental retardation.

Children with Fragile X syndrome often have distinctive facial characteristics, such as a long narrow face, prominent jaw, flat feet, or prominent ears. Psychological problems, including learning disabilities, autism-like symptoms, anxiety, or a dislike of being held or touched, can also appear. Speech and language problems are almost always present.

Children with Fragile X syndrome are often helped by speech and language therapy. You may be asked to help with any exercises the therapist prescribes. Children with Fragile X Syndrome are often helped by a consistent routine that limits distraction and overstimulation.

Spina Bifida

Spina bifida is a congenital condition caused by a defect in the way the spinal column has formed. This defect can leave a gap in the spinal column and cause the spinal cord to protrude out from the spinal column. Most often, the condition involves vertebrae at or below waist level.

There are three main types of spina bifida: spina bifida occulta, spina bifida cystica, and cranium bifida. The most common is spina bifida occulta (occulta means hidden). Some studies suggest that 5–10 percent of the population has this condition. The vast majority of people with this condition have no symptoms. In fact, they may not even know that they have the condition until an X-ray for other reasons brings the condition to light.

A small number of people with spina bifida occulta do experience physical problems, such as loss of sensation in the legs, bowel problems, and incontinence. Sometimes, the condition is noticed when the child has a growth spurt. Surgery can reduce or eliminate the symptoms. Figure 21-5 illustrates the spine of a person with spina bifida occulta.

Spina bifida cystica occurs when the gap in the spinal column is so large that a sac forms in the column. In many cases, this sac contains nerves and part of the spinal cord. When it does, there is usually loss of sensation and paralysis below the damaged vertebrae. Incontinence and bowel problems are almost always present. However, the exact impairment will depend upon the location of the sac as well as the nerves affected. In a few cases, the sac contains fluid only and does not cause significant impairment. Figures 21-6 and 21-7 illustrate the two types of spina bifida cystica.

Cranium bifida occurs when the bones of the skull fail to develop properly. This can cause brain damage and, in severe cases, death.

Photo 21-1
Computer-aided communication system

Communication Aids for Children

Many children with communication impairments use communication aids. These aids range from word boards and simple physical adaptations to sophisticated computer systems that generate speech (Photo 21-1). Some clients use voice-recognition software to "type" by speaking into a microphone attached to a computer. You may need training to help your client use communication aids.

FIGURE 21-5
Spina bifida occulta

FIGURE 21-6
Spina bifida cystica (myelomeningocele or meningomyelocele)

FIGURE 21-7
Spina bifida cystica (meningocele)

TABLE 21-4	Other Conditions That Can Affect Development	
Condition	**Cause**	**Effect**
Hydrocephalus	Increase of intracranial fluid in the brain, causing an increased head size and pressure changes in the brain	It can result in cognitive delays. Hydrocephalus can be treated and impairment diminished.
Cleft Lip	A fissure or opening in the upper lip	It affects speech and appearance. It can be corrected surgically.
Cleft Palate	A more serious condition in which there is a passageway between the nasopharnyx and the nose	This condition complicates feeding and leads to infections. It can be corrected surgically.
Club Foot	A malformation of the bones in which one foot is twisted inward or outward	It affects gait. It can be corrected surgically.
Congenital Hip Dysplasia	Partial or total hip dislocation	It affects gait and posture. Some forms can be corrected surgically; others may only be partially corrected.
Phenylketonuria	A disease caused by the absence of a liver (hepatic) enzyme	If not treated, it can result in cognitive delays.

POSTPARTUM DEPRESSION

It is normal for a new mother to experience emotional feelings after the delivery of her child. A woman's hormones shift very rapidly after delivery. This can cause mood swings.

Two conditions, postpartum blues and postpartum depression, are more serious forms of these mood swings. These conditions can produce depression or feelings of sadness in women who have recently delivered a baby.

Postpartum Blues

Researchers estimate that more than 75 percent of all new mothers experience postpartum blues. This condition usually occurs within the first ten days after delivery and is related to the rapid drop of estrogen and progesterone levels in the woman's body. A mother with postpartum blues may feel irritable, tired, and down. She may cry for no apparent reason.

Postpartum blues can last for two to three weeks. In most women, it will disappear over time. Reassure the new mother that this condition is quite normal and will pass with time. Work with the new mother to divide tasks so that she can rest or get out of the house for a bit.

Postpartum Depression

Postpartum depression is a serious depression in women who have recently had babies. It affects about 10 percent of new mothers and is more serious than postpartum blues. It results from a combination of biological and psychological factors. Sometimes, postpartum depression occurs in a woman who has experienced depression prior to or during her pregnancy.

Many symptoms of postpartum depression can also be those of extreme fatigue. You should report to your supervisor any observation of the following:

1. A lack of enjoyment in life
2. Disinterest in others
3. Loss of normal give-and-take in relationships
4. Feelings of inadequacy and inability to cope
5. Loss of mental concentration
6. Disturbed sleep
7. Constant fatigue and feelings of ill health

As a support worker, you may be asked to assist the mother by taking on a number of routine activities so that she can rest. Actively listening, encouraging, and supporting the new mother may also provide some support. In some cases, the mother may require medication.

A more serious form of postpartum depression is that of postpartum psychosis. This condition affects less than one mother in 1000. A mother with postpartum psychosis is not in touch with reality and could harm or neglect her infant. Some mothers with this condition contemplate suicide. You must immediately report to your supervisor any observations of potential harm or neglect as well as any expressed thoughts of suicide. If the mother attempts to harm her infant or herself, you must contact emergency services immediately.

Questions for Review

1. What are the six types of situations in which you may be asked to assist a family with children?

2. What are six common reflexes in the newborn?

3. What milestones would you expect a child to attain by eight months of age?

4. What are five signs of illness in an infant?

5. Define postpartum blues. How does this condition differ from postpartum depression?

6. What are seven signs of postpartum depression? How can you assist the mother who has postpartum depression?

Questions for Discussion

1. Why is it important to establish a good relationship with the parents? What concerns might the parents have about receiving support?

2. You have been assigned to Mrs. Renard, a new mother of premature triplets. Two of the triplets are home. The third is still in hospital. Mrs. Renard spends time at the hospital every day, in part so that she can breast feed the infant. You are assigned to a six-hour shift. The first three hours are spent with the infants at home while Mrs. Renard is at the hospital. Mrs. Renard is at home for the second three hours.

   What sorts of tasks would you expect to do? Why?

3. Your client, a new mother, has been crying a great deal for the past month and a half. She seems very tired. When you ask how she is, she tells you that she never realized that being a parent would be so difficult. What should you do?

Chapter 22

Mental Health

Learning Objectives

Through reading this chapter, you'll be able to

1. Define mental health and mental health condition.
2. Discuss the role of the support worker in assisting clients with mental health conditions.
3. Outline the following five major mental health conditions that may affect adults: depression, schizophrenia, bipolar disorder, anxiety, and substance abuse.
4. Discuss the signs, symptoms, and common causes of depression.
5. Describe common signs and symptoms of bipolar disorder, schizophrenia, and anxiety.
6. Describe ten ways you can support the person with a mental health condition.
7. Describe a crisis plan and list the common components.

Chapter at a Glance

- What Is Mental Health?
- Mental Health across the Life Span
- Mental Health Conditions
- Common Mental Health Conditions

Terms You'll Use

Anxiety Disorders A group of conditions in which anxiety becomes extremely disabling over a long period of time.

Bipolar Disorder A condition in which a person has alternating periods of hyperactivity and depression; also called manic depression.

Continuum A range.

Crisis Plan a document that includes information to help address any worsening symptoms to avoid further deterioration and list the client's wishes for support or care if the client becomes unable to express these wishes because of a mental health crisis.

Depression A range of conditions from a feeling of sadness to a clinical syndrome.

Mental Health The ability to deal with the conditions of life effectively.

Mental Health Conditions Conditions that affect a person's self-concept, behaviour, thoughts, or feelings to such an extent that they interfere with the person's ability to deal with situations effectively.

Multiple Loss The loss of more than one thing at a time.

Omnipotent The state of being above all harm.

Paranoia A range of conditions in which a person believes that he or she is being persecuted or threatened.

Risk Factors Factors that put a person's mental health at risk.

Schizophrenia A chronic mental health condition that affects a person's ability to take part in everyday activities. The condition may cause delusions, hallucinations, and disordered thinking.

Substance Abuse The misuse of medications, illicit drugs, or alcohol.

WHAT IS MENTAL HEALTH?

In understanding mental health, it's helpful to review the definition of health in general. As we discussed in Chapter 14, health can be defined as optimum physical, social, and emotional well-being, not just the absence of disease.

Thus, **mental health** refers to having a sense of well-being—having the ability to deal with the conditions of life effectively. Having good mental health can be said to mean that the person is able to adjust to changes in his or her life and is able to make some changes that will maintain or improve his or her quality of life. Being in good mental health is not the same as simply not having a mental illness, in much the same way that being physically healthy is not the same as not being sick.

Researchers have proposed six characteristics of mental health. These are presented in Table 22-1.

TABLE 22-1	Characteristics of Mental Health
Self-acceptance—to have a positive, yet realistic, appreciation of yourself	
To have positive relationships—to make and keep friends, get along with people in a social situation, avoid relationships that are harmful to yourself or others	
To be able to make decisions for yourself—without feeling obligated to conform to the expectations of other people	
To feel that you are basically in control of your own life—to have confidence that you can cope with setbacks or get through hard times	
To have a purpose in life—to have goals, a sense of direction, and a sense that life is worth living	
To have a sense of ongoing development—to be open to new ideas and new skills	

Source: National Advisory Council on Aging, Mental Health and Aging, *Paper #10 in the Writings on Gerontology series, March, 1991.*

Mental health is not an "either/or" situation. It is defined by how well we are able to function and how satisfied we are with how we function. Health is thus measured in degrees, not by whether or not a factor is fully met. Figure 22-1 illustrates the **continuum**, or range, of mental health.

Most of us have at least one of the four factors that are less than ideal, yet we see ourselves as mentally healthy. For example, we all have some anxieties and challenges

FIGURE 22-1
*The continuum
of mental health*

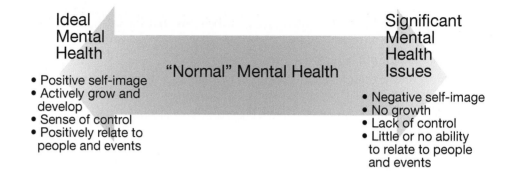

or feel sad or stressed sometimes, yet we are still able to relate to others, as well as do what we need and want to do. It's quite normal to have changes in mood or energy level from day to day. It's also normal to feel stressed or down for a brief period of time or to be angry or frustrated over something.

MENTAL HEALTH ACROSS THE LIFE SPAN

People of any age can experience mental health conditions. Some conditions are more common at certain ages. In general, however, older adults do face more problems, losses, and challenges than do people of other ages. Many of these conditions, losses, and challenges can put older adults at greater risk of developing a mental health condition.

Risk Factors

Several social factors that can put a person's mental health at risk have been identified and are called **risk factors**. These include the following:

- **A recent loss of spouse or close family member.** The loss of a spouse is considered to be one of the greatest, if not the greatest, loss one might experience. However, the loss of a close family member, or even an exceptionally close friend, may also be extremely significant. These losses often bring with them other changes: financial, social, and lifestyle.
- **Being socially isolated.** Social contacts may decline as people get older. About 30 percent of seniors report spending most of their time alone (Stone & Fletcher, 1986). Friends and family members die, making family size smaller, which means that there are fewer family supports or opportunities for contact. Social contacts can also diminish if a person has a condition that limits his or her ability to get about, particularly in a Canadian winter. Living alone puts a person at greater risk for isolation.
- **Having a physical disability or poor health.** Chronic conditions, including physical impairments, have been linked to depression, anxiety, and substance abuse.
- **Low income.** Having limited finances can limit a person's social activity. Unexpected costs—for home repairs, for example—can mean significant stress for a person on a limited budget.
- **Sensory defects.** Vision and hearing problems have been linked to anxiety and even paranoid behaviours. Significant sensory loss may increase social isolation by making it difficult to talk with others or get out to events.
- **Stressful life events.** Losses and changes in roles, finances, and health are often stressful. Even "positive" events, such as a new job or a move to a new location, can cause stress.

CASE EXAMPLE 22-1

Mr. and Mrs. Chang, both 78, lived together in the home they had owned since coming to Canada from Hong Kong in 1982. They managed well on their old age security and Mr. Chang's private pension. Mrs. Chang has had arthritis for a number of years, but had been able to manage with Mr. Chang's help. Mrs. Chang also relied on Mr. Chang to interpret for her as she speaks very little English.

When Mr. Chang died suddenly, Mrs. Chang was not comfortable living on her own and, without her husband's pension, could not really afford to keep up their home. She felt that she had to sell her home and move into an apartment. The only suitable apartment Mrs. Chang could find was in a neighbourhood several blocks from her old home. She now rarely goes out, as the neighbourhood is not familiar and she knows no one there. Her limited English makes the transition even more difficult, and there are few people who speak Cantonese.

What losses has Mrs. Chang experienced? How might she react to these losses?

In this case, her husband's death has caused Mrs. Chang to experience a number of other losses. She lost not only her spouse, but also her home and some of her financial security—all in a very short period of time. This is a common event among older people and is often called multiple loss.

MENTAL HEALTH CONDITIONS

Mental health conditions (also called mental problems, mental illnesses, or psychiatric disorders) are conditions that affect a person's self-concept, behaviour, thoughts, or feelings to such an extent that they interfere with the person's ability to do what he or she wants or needs to do. For example, a person may have extreme feelings of sadness or worthlessness that make it very difficult or impossible for the person to function.

The term *mental health condition* can be described as a situation in which a person's ability to adapt is affected or limited in some way that affects the person's well-being. Generally, mental health conditions affect the person over a period of time, not just once or once in a while.

Most of us have experienced a problem coping with something. Perhaps you can recall a situation when you simply had too much going on and that last thing was just one thing too many. You might have burst into tears. Perhaps you lost your temper.

Whatever happened, you were probably able to get through it and found the next day better. Does this mean you have a mental health condition? Probably not.

Mental health conditions can be caused by any one of four factors: social causes (such as isolation), biological causes (such as the lack of a specific chemical in the brain), psychological factors (such as extreme stress or emotional trauma), and genetic factors. Sometimes, more than one factor is involved.

Warning Signs of Mental Health Conditions

Mental health conditions often change a person's behaviour. Table 22-2 lists some behaviours that can be warning signs of a mental health condition. It's important to remember that these signs can be a symptom of many conditions, not just mental health conditions. As well, these signs are usually changes in the client's normal

TABLE 22-2	Signs of a Mental Health Condition

Warning Signs of a Mental Health Condition in Adults

confused thinking	prolonged sadness or irritability
feelings of extreme highs and lows	excessive fears, worries, or anxieties
social withdrawal	dramatic changes in eating or sleeping habits
strong feelings of anger	
growing inability to cope with daily problems and activities	delusions or hallucinations
	suicidal thoughts
denial of obvious problems	numerous unexplained physical ailments
substance abuse	

Warning Signs of a Mental Health Condition in Younger Children

changes in school performance	frequent temper tantrums
excessive worry or anxiety	hyperactivity
persistent nightmares	persistent disobedience or aggression

Warning Signs of a Mental Health Condition in Older Children and Pre-Adolescents

substance abuse	excessive complaints of physical ailments
change in sleeping and/or eating habits	
defiance of authority, truancy, theft, and/or vandalism	prolonged negative mood, often accompanied by poor appetite or thoughts of death
intense fear of weight gain	
inability to cope with problems and daily activities	frequent outbursts of anger

Source: National Mental Health Association.

behaviour. Speak with your supervisor if you notice that any of these signs are present for a prolonged period of time.

Responding to Warning Signs

1. **Be sensitive to changes in behaviour, particularly if you have not noticed the behaviour before, such as a client who suddenly seems more anxious than usual.** Look for cause and effect: does a particular event or situation seem to cause the behaviour?
2. **Tell your supervisor about the behaviour.** Be careful to describe it, not to evaluate it. Instead of saying, "Mrs. G. was really paranoid when we were shopping," say, "Mrs. G. accused me of wanting to leave her alone in the store."
3. **Identify with your supervisor the steps to take if the person is in danger of hurting himself, herself, or another person.**

COMMON MENTAL HEALTH CONDITIONS

In this chapter, we'll discuss five common mental health conditions: depression, schizophrenia, bipolar disorder, anxiety, and substance abuse. As you read the following information, be aware that each condition may affect one person differently than it does another. The information presented here provides some general information. You must be careful to follow the support plan developed for your client.

Depression

STOP AND REFLECT ((22-1))

Take a minute and think back to a time in the past when you experienced feelings of sadness. Perhaps you described it as depression at the time, perhaps not. Keeping that experience in mind, consider the following questions.

At the time, were you aware of having other feelings? If so, what were they?

_____

_____

_____

How did you express those feelings to others? What did you do or say?

_____

_____

_____

At the time, were you aware of the cause of these feelings?

_____

_____

_____

What helped you to get over these feelings? (others, time, thinking about it differently, etc.)

_____

_____

_____

Keep these things in mind as you read on.

Most of us have used the term *depression*, whether about others or ourselves. We've had a bad afternoon, day, or week. We're frustrated at events or overwhelmed by them. We might feel helpless or hopeless. For most of us, this is a temporary state; after a bit, the feelings lift and we go on. The situation you described above probably did not last a long time although it might have seemed to.

Depression is used to describe a wide range of conditions, from a casual feeling (such as "I was so depressed about that assignment") to what is called a clinical syndrome or depressive episode—a diagnosis that a doctor or psychiatrist might make. Most of this section is concerned with depression as a state of feeling.

Depression as a State of Feeling

This is probably the most common use of the term depression. The feelings are not so strong as to keep us from doing most of our usual activities, although we might not have the usual interest or energy. Usually, these feelings are a reaction to something that has happened to us. These causes can range from things that are fairly minor—a cold that has dragged on a long time, for example—to things that are much more significant, such as the loss of a loved one.

As well, we are generally aware of these causes. Think back to your situation. Were you aware of the cause(s) of your feelings at the time? Chances are that you were, although you might not have always connected your reactions to the event. For example, you might have found it strange that you didn't have your usual interest in something, only later realizing that the lack of interest was related to the sadness.

Depression as a Clinical Syndrome

Depression as a clinical syndrome is less common. In this situation, the feelings of sadness are often quite extreme—the person may feel unable to do anything at all. She or he may lose interest in most activities or not have the energy to act. This type of depression usually lasts much longer than the feeling-state type—sometimes months or years. The person may not be able to identify any reason or cause for the condition. A physician or psychiatrist must diagnose this type of depression. It is a serious condition but can be treated by a combination of medication and counselling.

When you are working with a client who has been diagnosed as having this type of depression, it is very important to learn what approaches are best to use with the client and to follow those approaches carefully.

Signs and Symptoms of Depression

One of the most difficult problems in identifying any type of depression is that the list of signs and symptoms of depression includes things that are opposites. For example, both weight gain and weigh loss can be a symptom, as can an inability to sleep or an inability to remain awake. Sometimes, the symptoms don't seem to be consistent with our idea of what depression is. For example, we don't normally associate frustration with depression, yet it is often present in people who are depressed. Finally, many of these symptoms are also symptoms of other conditions.

Go back to your situation. Did you experience other feelings? What were they? You probably weren't only sad but had a number of other feelings as well. These might have included anger, guilt, frustration, or anxiety. You may have shown these feelings in a variety of ways. Perhaps you cried a lot. You might have withdrawn from others or found yourself unable to relax. Perhaps you lost all interest in food; maybe you ate much more than usual.

Beyond that, depression is a condition we define by how severe a symptom or set of symptoms is, not just whether or not it's present. We don't have a list of symptoms that we can simply check off to identify the condition like we could if the person had, for example, chicken pox. The symptoms listed in Table 22-3 can be signs of depression.

Can you see the difficulty? All of us have experienced some of these symptoms, yet very few of us would consider ourselves to be depressed in any sense of the word. Some of these symptoms are opposites of others; some are also symptoms of a great many other conditions. All of this makes depression difficult to identify.

TABLE 22-3	Possible Signs of Depression
weight loss	weight gain
lethargy—too tired to move	hyperactivity—can't settle down
feelings of worthlessness/hopelessness	blames self for things, angry, frustrated
lack of emotions—flat effect	crying easily
sadness	loss of interest in others
headaches	constipation
dizziness	rapid heart beat

Depression and the Older Person

Older people, like people of any age, can become depressed. Like people of other ages, older people can experience the short-term, feeling-state kind of depression as well as the clinical syndrome. As above, we'll focus on the feeling-state type for now. As many as 20 percent of older adults experience depression, according to the study *Seeking Solutions: Canadian Community Action on Seniors and Alcohol Issues.*

Social Attitudes and Depression

Despite the fact that depression is one of the most common mental health conditions among older people, attitudes about the condition can make it harder to identify. Many older people feel that a "mental illness" is an embarrassment and are very reluctant to discuss it. As well, people who work with older people sometimes overlook or misinterpret possible symptoms of depression. This can happen because the worker might do the following:

1. Accept the signs and symptoms as things that can't be changed because they come with growing old.
2. Feel that the person's losses aren't really that significant or that the person could "shake these feelings off" if he or she really wanted to.
3. Confuse the symptoms of depression with those of cognitive impairment (dementia). At first glance, many symptoms of depression do seem to be much like the symptoms of cognitive impairment. However, they are not, as Table 22-4 shows.

Supporting the Person with Depression

Many clients who are depressed will have a support plan that identifies specific responses to the client's needs. Be sure to follow the client's support plan. The following are general guidelines only.

1. **Accept the client where she or he is.** If you make the client feel that he or she must behave in a specific way to gain your acceptance, you won't likely be able to establish rapport.
2. **Avoid giving simplistic advice**—such as "Why don't you get some exercise? It will help you." While it is true that exercise can help moderate a person's mood, the decreased activity is part of the cycle of depression. An older person who is

TABLE 22-4	Dementia and Depression
Dementia	**Depression**
Client tries to hide cognitive losses, or seems unaware.	Client complains of memory loss or other cognitive losses and is upset over them.
Symptoms progress slowly.	Symptoms progress fairly quickly.
Client tries to answer, but may give vague answers or answers that aren't quite right.	"Don't know" types of answers are common.
Client tries hard to perform tasks well and is frustrated when unable to do them.	Client makes little effort to perform, and seems not to care.
The client's emotions seem to change easily—one minute upset, the next OK.	The client's mood is consistently sad.
Attention and concentration may be impaired.	Attention and concentration are usually present.

depressed may intellectually know what needs to be done or how to do it, but often does not know how to carry it along.

3. **Keep the client at the centre of the activity.** The client who helps plan things will have more desire to follow the plan.

4. **Be prepared to accept "objective" inconsistencies.** Look for the meaning behind the behaviour and base your interaction on that. A person may tell you that your visit "doesn't matter," yet you know that he or she looks for you to come. Respond to what is meant, not always what is said.

5 **Recognize your client's need for control.** Situations often rob clients of the ability to make decisions or exert control. The perception of loss of control can, in some clients, be sufficient to withdraw.

6. **Display your faith in the client's ability to act effectively in the situation to the degree possible.** This includes the offering of structured choices (where neither option is incorrect) if necessary.

7. **Present challenges that are appropriate.** A rule of thumb is to begin with the most complex task that the person is assured of completing. Positive experiences encourage positive approaches.

8. **Some challenges begin with simple interaction.** Display your interest by showing pleasure in the relationship with the client.

9. **Support self-esteem by direct reinforcement of the person.** Comment on current attributes and activities. If there are none obvious, comment upon those past and still possible.

10. **Encourage physical activity whenever possible.** There are demonstrated relationships between physical activity and outlook.

11. **Use the strength of the interpersonal relationship to help compensate for needs.** Your faith may be transferred through you to another person or activity. (I believe in you; you believe in X; I believe in X.)

Suicide

Suicide is more common among older people and people who have recently experienced significant physical disability. The Mood Disorders Association of Ontario states that suicide is five times more likely in individuals over 60 than in younger groups. They note that:

- Suicide is more likely to occur in those living alone.
- Bereavement is highly associated with suicide. Death of a spouse, other family member, or friend is more common in later life than in other age groups.
- Loss of mobility, functionality, and independence are all related to higher suicide rates.

We also know that older people who attempt suicide are more likely to be successful in taking their life.

Finally, we know that older people who talk about suicide or make comments like "I may as well do myself in," should always be taken seriously. Never assume that a person who says things like this is just trying to get attention or to scare you.

Supporting the Person Who Appears Suicidal

As a support worker, you may be the first—or only—person to notice that a person appears to be suicidal. Your proper response to these observations is essential if the client is to receive proper care. Always report these situations to your supervisor immediately. The following are some additional guidelines. Listen carefully and with concern, but don't try to argue or tell the client that he or she "couldn't mean that."

1. Ask person directly if he or she is contemplating suicide.
2. Tell the person what specific behaviours worry you.
3. Listen to the person's response in a supportive, non-judgmental way.
4. Attempt to identify the stressor.
5. Ask the person if he or she has a specific plan. If so, remove the means. Tell the person you are doing this for her or his safety.
6. If the person does not want to talk to you, ask if there is someone else he or she would be willing to talk to.
7. Ask person to postpone the decision.
8. Let the person know that these feelings don't mean that she or he is a "bad person" and the person doesn't need to be ashamed.
9. Let the person know that his or her life is important to you and to others.
10. Seek help from your supervisor, trusted family members, friends, distress line, physician.
11. Do not leave the person alone.

Schizophrenia

Schizophrenia is a chronic mental health condition that often has significant effects on a person's ability to take part in everyday activities. Schizophrenia is thought to be caused by biological factors, although it appears that a person can inherit a likelihood of developing the condition.

Schizophrenia can cause the person to have delusions (false ideas or beliefs), hallucinations (hearing, seeing, feeling, smelling, or even tasting things that do not really exist), and disordered thinking (rambling, disconnected, or incoherent speech). The person can also lose motivation, interest, and any ability to express emotion. These experiences can be frightening to both the person and those around him or her. They can cause the person to withdraw from social contact.

Schizophrenia usually appears in people aged 20 to 30. Men often show symptoms at an earlier age than do women. There are four major types of schizophrenia. These are:

- **Catatonic schizophrenia:** A severe form in which the person is withdrawn and mute.
- **Disorganized schizophrenia:** A form that results in incoherent speech and behaviour but does not usually cause the person to experience delusions.
- **Paranoid schizophrenia:** A form that causes the person to feel persecuted or suspicious or to have delusions of grandeur (such as being very powerful or rich).
- **Residual schizophrenia:** A form that causes the person to have no interest in life or motivation to act. Delusions or hallucinations are usually not present or have ceased.

Medication is the most common treatment for schizophrenia, although counselling may help the person to cope with everyday life. Many medications are available to treat schizophrenia. Most treatments cannot fully control the symptoms and many medications have significant side effects. Only about 20 percent of the people diagnosed with schizophrenia recover.

Supporting the Person with Schizophrenia

Most clients with schizophrenia will have a support plan that identifies specific responses to the client's needs. Be sure to follow the client's support plan. The following are general guidelines only:

1. **Help the person to stick with his or her medication regimen.** Regularly and conscientiously taking medication can control many symptoms.
2. **Follow a consistent routine for all activities.** This can reduce anxiety and promote a sense of control.
3. **Have patience.** Do not become anxious or frustrated; this will only heighten the client's anxiety.
4. **Actively listen to the client and support his or her efforts to cope.**
5. **Keep things simple.** Do one task at a time. Use short sentences. Make it easy for the client to follow what you are saying. Do not abruptly change topics.
6. **Do not argue with a person about whether or not a delusion is real.** The delusion is real to the person experiencing it. Comfort the person if the delusion is frightening to him or her.

Bipolar Disorder

Bipolar disorder is known also as manic depression and occurs when people experience periods of hyperactivity (called mania) that alternate with periods of depression. There are many variations of this disorder but virtually all cause the person to alternate (or cycle) between mania and depression. How frequently these cycles occur depends upon the variation. Some people experience eight to ten cycles in a lifetime; others rapidly move from mania to depression several times a day.

The symptoms of depression in bipolar disorders are almost identical to those of a clinical depression, although they are less likely to be as severe. Manic phases often follow immediately after a period of depression. A manic phase is sometimes seen as recovery as the person has renewed interest in activity, in life, and is often quite social. The person soon becomes irritable and may not sleep much at all. Some people in the manic phase feel that they are **omnipotent**—above all harm. The person may talk rapidly, may hallucinate, or have rambling, incoherent speech. People with bipolar disorder have a greater risk of suicide.

Bipolar disorder is thought to be the result of a chemical imbalance in the brain. Medication often offers effective treatment. Some studies suggest that maintaining a consistent sleep routine can reduce the number of cycles the person experiences.

Supporting the Person with Bipolar Disorder

Most clients with bipolar disorder will have a support plan that identifies specific responses to the client's needs. Be sure to follow the client's support plan. The following are general guidelines only.

1. **Help the person to stick with his or her medication regimen.** Regularly and conscientiously taking medication can control many symptoms.
2. **Follow a consistent routine for all activities, particularly sleep.**
3. **Actively listen to the client and support his or her efforts to cope.**

Paranoia

Like the term depression, we often use the words paranoia and paranoid in many ways. We may say that someone who thinks someone is talking about him or her is paranoid. We may also think that someone who fears that "someone" will hurt him or her is paranoid.

The term **paranoia** is used to describe many conditions—from those mentioned above to the psychiatric condition *paraphrenia*, a condition in which the person has delusions (false beliefs) and is constantly feeling persecuted.

Paraphrenia is relatively rare among older adults. When this condition exists, it is often something diagnosed earlier in the person's life. This condition may affect people with another form of mental illness or dementia.

More common is what we might call "paranoid behaviour." For example, we might say that someone who accuses people of taking things is paranoid. Like paraphrenia, this type of behaviour often happens when a person has another condition, such as dementia or delirium (acute confusion). It's important to remember that, although paranoid behaviours can be a sign of another condition, they do not mean the person has a delirium or dementia.

Sometimes, the paranoid behaviour is related to other things. Research has shown us that people with hearing loss may seem "paranoid." For example, they may think that people are talking about them. People with vision problems may also seem paranoid. They may fear someone whose face they cannot clearly see, for example. These changes more likely are due to the difficulties the person has in seeing and hearing well, not to a mental health condition. Unfamiliar places or people and unexpected events may cause a person to become suspicious or paranoid.

Supporting the Person with Paranoia

Most clients with paranoia will have a support plan that identifies specific responses to the client's needs. Be sure to follow the client's support plan. The following are general guidelines only:

1. **Don't argue with the person.** It seldom works and may make the person very angry at you.

2. **Focus on areas where the person is not paranoid.** Some people may feel very positive about their sister, but be very (unrealistically) suspicious about their brother. Trying not to dwell on the negative situation may help.

3. **Remember that this behaviour may be related to sensory loss.** Help clients to remember to put on their glasses or use their hearing aid if they have one. Use techniques to enhance vision and hearing.

4. **Explain noises or sights that have been misinterpreted.** For example, "That noise was a car backfiring." Or, "The rapping sound was me opening this package."

5. **If the behaviour is related to a lost item, help look for misplaced articles but don't scold the person for losing things.** If something is frequently lost and can easily be replaced (e.g., a favourite mug), you might suggest that the family get an extra one. If need be, learn where favourite hiding places are.

6. **Don't forget that even the most suspicious person may actually be a victim.** Advise your supervisor of any situation that seems based on fact.

7. **If possible, use distractions such as music, going for a walk, etc.**

8. **Keep a consistent routine.** This may reduce uncertainty and reassure some persons.

Anxiety and Anxiety Disorders

Anxiety as a Normal Emotion

Everyone feels anxious at one time or another. (Think back to the night before you wrote your first test.) An older person may feel anxious about becoming ill or dependent upon other people. A person who has recently had a car accident may feel very anxious about driving again. For most of us, anxiety allows us to generate energy, focus our efforts, and move into action.

Anxiety as a Disabling Condition

Sometimes, anxiety keeps us from taking any action at all. This may be due to an extreme reaction to a situation, such as being so anxious about speaking in front of a large group that a person cannot talk at all. This type of anxiety can also come from drug or alcohol abuse or as a side effect of some medications. Sometimes, anxiety increases for a period of time when the person stops taking certain medications, such as Valium. This type of anxiety is not usually considered a mental illness, although a person may benefit from treatment. It is common in older adults. Studies estimate that between 10 and 20 percent of older adults living in the community have symptoms severe enough to require treatment.

Anxiety disorders are a group of conditions in which anxiety becomes extremely disabling over a long period of time. There is usually no identifiable reason for the anxiety. People with anxiety disorders may experience panic attacks with significant physical symptoms (such as shortness of breath, dizziness, a racing heart beat, or chest pain). The person may become unable to do everyday activities, such as going to the mailbox or grocery shopping. Anxiety disorders are the result of biological and psychological causes. They most often appear in persons who are between 20 and 30 years of age.

Anxiety disorders can be treated with medication and a specific type of counselling. It helps the person to change the way he or she sees the anxiety and includes specific ways that the person can reduce the anxiety.

Supporting the Person with Anxiety or an Anxiety Disorder

Most clients with anxiety or anxiety disorders will have a support plan that identifies specific responses to the client's needs. Be sure to follow the client's support plan. The following are general guidelines only:

1. **If the person has a specific technique used to address the anxiety, remind or help the person to use it.**
2. **Help the person to relax.** If the person is in a public place, try to move to a quieter spot.
3. **Do not tell the person that he or she should not be anxious.** Remember that the person knows this but is still having difficulty. Be calm and reassuring.

Substance Abuse and Misuse

Substance abuse refers to the intentional misuse of medications, illicit drugs, or alcohol. Substance misuse is the unintentional misuse of medications. People of any age, sex, or income level can have a substance abuse or misuse problem.

Recent research has identified that alcohol abuse is not uncommon among older adults. Alcohol abuse among older persons is grouped into two types: early onset (when alcohol has been a problem since early or middle adulthood) and late onset (alcohol problems that arise in response to stressors in late life). Social isolation, multiple losses, and lack of coping mechanisms all contribute to late-onset alcohol abuse. In some cases, other factors may influence the person's alcohol consumption.

Alcohol Abuse

Symptoms of alcohol abuse include many symptoms common to other conditions: frequent falls, tremors, memory problems, difficulty focusing one's attention, and confusion. This can lead others involved with the person to overlook a potential condition. You should advise your supervisor if you note any of these symptoms. As these symptoms can indicate many conditions, you should report your observations, not make a conclusion about a person's alcohol use.

Supporting the Person with an Alcohol Problem

If your client has an identified support plan, be sure to follow it. The following are general guidelines only:

1. **Reduce social isolation.** Many studies have linked social isolation with alcohol abuse. Spending time with the client and helping him or her to renew or maintain social contacts may provide valuable connections with others and reduce isolation.
2. **Assist the client to find ways to overcome challenges of later life.** Assisting a client to manage her or his household or to shop or even to prepare a meal may reinforce the client's sense of control and ability to cope and reduce the need to escape.
3. **Assist the client to find creative positive ways of coping with stressors.** A walk, a creative activity, even a telephone contact may provide a more positive alternative to alcohol consumption.
4. **You cannot force a client to change his or her behaviour.** You should never attempt to coerce or force a client to alter his or her alcohol consumption. Speak with your supervisor if you have concerns about your client's alcohol consumption.

Medication Misuse and Abuse

Medication abuse or misuse among older adults may be higher than for any other age group. This is likely due in part to the number of medications prescribed to older adults, as well as to misunderstandings about how a medication is to be taken.

Sometimes, a person unknowingly takes too many medications because he or she has received prescriptions from more than one doctor (for example, a family doctor and a specialist). In this instance, neither doctor may know that the other has prescribed medications for the person.

The symptoms of medication misuse vary depending upon the medications used and the amounts taken. You should be alert for any change in your client's condition that appears to be the result of medication. Report any changes to your supervisor.

Supporting the Person Who Has or May Have a Medication Use Problem

If your client has an identified support plan, be sure to follow it. Do not advise the client on the proper use of medications: this is a task for the client's pharmacist or physician.

1. **Discuss with your supervisor any medication problem you observe.** For example, vision problems may make it difficult for a client to see if he or she has taken the right medication at the right time. A client who is forgetful may not remember that he or she has already taken medication and repeat the dose.
2. **Be alert to the signs of medication misuse if requested.** As signs vary with the specific medication, you may have to discuss the possible signs with your supervisor or other person responsible for the client's medication.

Crisis Plans

Some clients have a crisis plan as part of their support plan. The crisis plan includes information that can help address any worsening symptoms to avoid further deterioration and list the client's wishes for support or care if the client becomes unable to express these wishes because of a mental health crisis.

Crisis plans can take many forms, but they most often include the following five parts:

- Part one includes methods and activities that help the client to stay healthy on a daily basis. This information may also be found in the client's support plan.
- Part two includes a list of triggers: events, or circumstances that may trigger, or bring on, a crisis. This may include things such as busy environments, noisy environments, or questions about specific topics.
- Part three includes early warning signs that that may signal the client's need for help. These things may include changes in appearance, behaviour, or communication patterns.
- Part four includes a description of symptoms that occur when the client's ability to cope is breaking down or getting worse. As in part three, this may include changes in appearance, behaviour, or communication patterns.
- Part five sets out the plan to follow if others must make decisions for the person. This usually involves contacting one or more members of the client's family, friends or support team.

Crisis plans are developed for each person. They list specific things that work for that person. In your role, you may be able to observe things that are useful to include in the crisis plan. Discuss your observations with the care team. Don't assume that something that works for one client will work for another.

You may be called upon to use the information in the crisis plan to support the client. Be certain to clarify any questions you may have about the plan and what specific interventions mean.

Questions for Review

1. Describe the continuum of mental health.

2. What six factors can put older adults at risk of developing a mental health condition?

3. Are the warning signs of a mental health condition the same in children as in adults? If not, how are they different?

4. What should you do if you observe any of the warning signs?

5. What are the two types of depression? How are they different?

6. What are some common signs of depression?

7. Why is depression often overlooked in older adults? State at least two reasons.

8. Depression and dementia have similar symptoms. How might you tell the difference between the two?

9. What can you do to assist a client who is depressed?

10. Is suicide a problem among older adults? Why or why not?

11. What can you do to respond to someone who appears suicidal?

12. What five things can you do to assist a client diagnosed with schizophrenia?

13. What is bipolar disorder? By what other name is it sometimes called?

14. What is a crisis plan? What are the common parts of a crisis plan?

Questions for Discussion

1. How might you support the person who has a degree of paranoia?

2. Can anxiety actually help you to function? When is anxiety helpful? When can anxiety make it harder for you to function?

3. Your client is a single woman. You are aware that she has abused alcohol in the past and that reducing the possibility for abuse is part of her service plan. What can you do to assist your client to reduce alcohol abuse?

4. You work in a long-term care facility. You are out to dinner with friends when you see one of your residents out to dinner with his family. You stop to say hello and you notice that he is drinking a beer. Residents in your facility cannot have alcohol unless a doctor allows it. You don't know if this resident has permission. What do you think that you should do? Why? Does the resident have the right to drink alcohol when he or she is out of the facility?

Chapter 23

Cognition and Cognitive Impairment

Learning Objectives

Through reading this chapter, you'll be able to

1. Describe cognition and how it changes as we age.
2. Describe the Seven A's of cognitive impairment.
3. Outline the three major causes of cognitive impairment.
4. Identify common reversible and irreversible causes of cognitive impairment.
5. Discuss the difference between frontotemporal dementia and Alzheimer Disease.
6. Describe how the symptoms of Alzheimer Disease differ when the person has the type associated with Down syndrome.
7. Describe the six fundamental principles of providing support to a client with a cognitive impairment.
8. Explain common approaches to communicating with a client with cognitive impairment.
9. Describe interpretative communication and list its seven principles.
10. Discuss common approaches to assisting a client to perform tasks.
11. Identify challenging behaviours and describe the problem-solving approach to addressing these behaviours.

Chapter at a Glance

- What Is Cognition?
- Cognitive Impairment
- What Is Confusion?
- Delirium
- What Is Dementia?
- Caring for the Person with Dementia
- Supporting a Client with the Performance of Tasks
- Challenging Behaviours
- Acquired Brain Injury

Terms You'll Use

Acquired Brain Injury Brain injury that occurs as the result of trauma, anoxia, hemorrhage, seizure, or toxins.

Cognition The ability to process information; it includes six cognitive processes.

Cognitive Impairment A situation that disrupts the way the brain works to think, use language, remember, and coordinate movements.

Cognitive Processes The six factors that contribute to cognition: perceiving, recognizing, interpreting, and organizing information; judging; and reasoning.

Delirium A reversible cognitive impairment often related to extremely high fever, medications, or infections.

Dementia A term used to describe a set of symptoms that occur in some types of cognitive impairment.

Early-Onset Dementia Dementia that occurs in younger people.

Heterotopic Ossification Abnormal bone growth in joints after a brain injury.

Irreversible Not curable or capable of being restored to a previous state.

Progressive Worsens over time.

Reversible Curable or capable of being restored to a previous state.

Traumatic Brain Injury Brain injury caused by traumatic events such as motor vehicle accidents, gunshot wounds, or falls. This is sometimes called acquired brain injury.

WHAT IS COGNITION?

There are many definitions of cognition. For the purposes of this text, we'll define **cognition** as including a number of processes, as illustrated by Figure 23-1. Cognition includes thinking, or **cognitive processes**: perceiving, recognizing, interpreting, and organizing information, judging, and reasoning. It also controls memory and motor functions, helping a person to decide how to move, as well as how to sequence the movements into purposeful action. In other words, cognition controls all we do.

The brain is the control centre of the body. It is a complex organ, and researchers are just beginning to understand how it works. Much is yet to be discovered. We do know that different areas of the brain are responsible for different cognitive processes. Some functions are held in a relatively well-defined area of the brain. Others appear to be spread out over larger areas. Figure 23-1 illustrates the functions controlled by specific areas of the brain.

Cognitive processes change over time. Adults process information differently than do infants or children. Most researchers agree that older adults process information differently than younger adults. Despite these differences, most people do

FIGURE 23-1
Functions controlled by specific areas of the brain

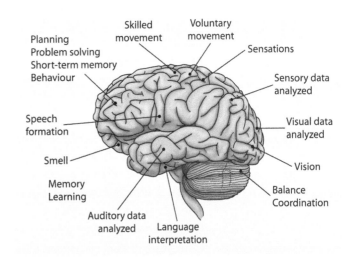

not experience a significant decline in cognitive function over their lifetimes. Researchers have identified that in most people, cognitive function remains intact at least until the person is in his or her 80s (Duke University, Longitudinal Study of Aging).

COGNITIVE IMPAIRMENT

Cognitive impairment is the term used to describe the symptoms of conditions that disrupt the way the brain works to think, remember, use language, and coordinate movements. Cognitive impairment is often called dementia, particularly when it occurs in older adults

As part of an educational program on dementia, Ontario has developed a set of seven descriptions of the changes in intellectual function. This is part of a program—called U-First!—provided by the Ontario Community Support Association. The "Seven A's" provide a framework to describe these changes and are listed in Table 23-1. We'll look at each in greater detail in this section.

TABLE 23-1	The Seven A's of Dementia

1. **Amnesia**: loss of memory
2. **Aphasia**: loss of language
3. **Agnosia**: loss of recognition
4. **Apraxia**: loss of purposeful movement
5. **Anosognosia**: no knowledge of illness/disease
6. **Altered Perception**: loss of perceptual acuity
7. **Apathy**: loss of initiation

Amnesia

Amnesia is a loss of memory. Although we talk about memory as though it is one thing, there are actually five different types of memory: sensory memory, short-term memory, long-term memory, habitual memory, and unconscious learning. We'll look at each type of memory in this section.

Sensory memory describes the ongoing screening of all sensory information: visual, auditory, tactile, taste, and scent information. It also includes proprioception, how the entire body, or a single body part, is positioned at any given moment (Brooks, Provincial Fitness Unit, Alberta, 2007).

We're usually unaware that we're receiving and screening all this information; we often don't realize that we're responding to it. We're usually aware only of new or unusual information. For example, did you ever reach into a drawer to take out a sweater and feel a texture you didn't expect to feel? Likely you began to pay attention to this new and unexpected texture. In other words, the tactile information moved from your unconscious into your conscious.

Short-Term Memory (STM)

Short-term memory is the most significant aspect of memory. If it does not function properly, the person will not be able to remember well, or even at all. It also affects learning.

Short-term memory's purpose is to keep information in conscious memory until the person decides what to do with it. As Figure 23-2 illustrates, it's a bit like a loading dock. Information in short-term memory must be moved within a short period of time. Memory that moves into long-term memory is retained. Memory that is not is forgotten.

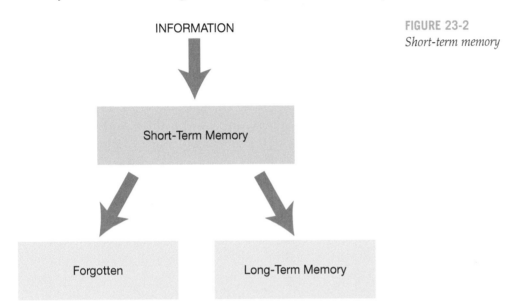

INFORMATION

Short-Term Memory

Forgotten

Long-Term Memory

FIGURE 23-2
Short-term memory

If memory cannot be placed into this storage, or cannot be held long enough to be moved to long-term storage, the person cannot learn, as Case Example 23-1 illustrates.

CASE EXAMPLE 23-1

Adjit has been diagnosed with probable Alzheimer Disease. He lives at home with his wife. One of his usual chores at home has been to put away the dishes once they were washed.

Adjit and his wife used to do dishes by hand, but his wife recently had a dishwasher installed. Now, Adjit cannot remember where the dishes are, even though his wife shows him every day. He keeps looking for the dish drainer in the sink and asks why his wife hasn't washed the dishes. His wife has become frustrated, as she sometimes thinks that he is simply being "stubborn." He is not. Adjit's short-term memory is damaged; he cannot store this information or decide what to do with it (place in long-term memory or forget it).

Long-term memory has unlimited capacity. It is divided into two areas:

- declarative (all the information you learned or experienced over time)
- procedural (all the tasks you've learned how to do)

Both declarative and procedural memory are put down in layers; the first thing you have ever experienced or learned is at the bottom, and as you proceed through life, you pile your memories on top of each other so that the last thing you have learned is at the top.

In a progressive dementia, memory is lost in reverse (i.e., the last thing learned is the first thing lost). It's a bit like knitting a sweater and then unravelling it row by row; starting with the row you knitted last. People with memory loss cannot remember what happened this morning, last week, or last year, but they still have intact memory for information that happened a long time ago.

As a result, a person with dementia does not live in the past; she or he lives in the moment but has access only to information in the past. We can usually access the information from this morning, yesterday, last week, or last year. The person with dementia may be able to access only information from 30 or 40 years ago.

Habitual Memory

Well-learned tasks move out of our conscious awareness so that we can do them automatically without thinking. For example, habitual memory is what we use when we are taking a shower or bath. We don't consciously think about the actions involved, we simply do them. There is some evidence that this habitual memory is stored in a different place than other memories.

People with a cognitive impairment dementia may have difficulty responding to a simple request like "tie your shoes," yet may be seen doing it later when the lace has become untied. This is because the act of tying shoes is stored in habitual memory. The ability to understand the instruction is not. The person is able to do the task, but not to understand what was meant when she was asked to do it. You can probably see why this is so frustrating for caregivers—including you: when asked, the person cannot perform the task; later, the person does it without a flaw, in response to a particular stimulus.

CASE EXAMPLE 23-2

Mrs. Molodani has been diagnosed with vascular dementia. She has moved to her daughter's home, as she cannot safely live alone. You are assisting her. It is cool; Mrs. Molodani is shivering. You suggest that she put on her sweater, but she only looks blankly at you. When you hand her the sweater, she puts it on.

This happens because the sequence is stored in habitual memory and does not require conscious thought. Mrs. Molodani responded to the stimulus—your offer of the sweater, and her habitual memory handled the rest.

Unconscious Learning

Even though a person with memory loss can no longer consciously learn, he or she can still learn unconsciously by doing the same things in the same way, day after day. These repetitive actions create a "memory trail." This is why routines are very important.

As the term implies, this learning happens without the person realizing that it is happening. Unconscious learning can be durable. For example, a person continues to return to her "old room," even though she has moved to a new one on the same unit. As you saw in Case Example 23-1, Adjit kept looking for the clean dishes in the dish drainer in the sink where they always had been.

Aphasia

Language includes both speech and comprehension. However, the speech and comprehension are actually located in different areas of the brain.

Different conditions can affect speech or comprehension in different ways. For example, the speech of a person with frontal lobe dementia is often the first aspect of language affected. Alzheimer Disease, however usually first affects language comprehension.

Language is fundamental to a person's ability to relate. If the ability to use language is diminished, the person may withdraw. For example, a person with difficulty comprehending may have difficulty talking with others, as she has difficulty sorting out what is being said. The person may try to create his or her own interpretation of the conversation that he or she believes to be absolutely true. The person will likely become increasingly dependent on nonverbal cues to help him or her make sense of the world around.

Language difficulties can affect both understanding and expression. You may have heard the terms *receptive aphasia* and *expressive aphasia* to describe these issues. The person may have one or both. If the person has difficulty understanding (receiving) what is said, he or she may not reply correctly or do what was asked. If the difficulty lies in expression, the person may not be able to state what she or he wants or needs.

This results in communication difficulties and misunderstandings between family/staff and the person. For example, a caregiver may assume that the person's communication skills are intact because the person is able to express specific needs, discomfort, or frustration. When that very same person cannot understand what is being asked of him or her, the caregiver may think that the person is intentionally trying to be difficult.

Second Languages

You may have had a client who could speak a second language at one point, but no longer can. A second language is often lost earlier than a primary language. Languages learned later in life may be held in an area different than the one in which the person's primary language is held. Remember that even if a person can speak the words of a primary language, she or he may not be able to understand or communicate needs.

When a client develops the symptoms we call cognitive impairment or dementia, the last-in-first-out rule applies:

- What is learned last is usually lost first.
- What is remembered last is usually forgotten first.

Agnosia

Agnosia causes people to lose the ability to recognize people, objects, and sounds. The person loses recognition of people, usually in the order that they last came into his or her life. For example, a person's grandchildren (the group most recently known) are the first forgotten. As we discussed earlier, as the disease progresses the person gradually has access only to information from the remote past.

This can cause a number of difficulties. For example, if a person can only access information from 30 years ago, then the person thinks of herself or himself as 30 years younger. Who is the 75-year-old spouse if the person is only 40? Who are these adult children who are the same age as the person? Who is that person in the mirror if he or she has lost access to the memory of getting older and recalls herself or himself with a much younger face?

Mirrors can be very disturbing to the person experiencing agnosia. We usually have mirrors in bathrooms and bedrooms—our most personal spaces. The person perceives a stranger watching very personal activities: undressing, bathing, and toileting. If a caregiver is also present, then the mirror shows two strange people in the room.

STOP AND REFLECT ((23-1))

Imagine that you are at home. A person you don't know at all—you're certain you have never seen before—comes into the room and starts to talk to you. You can't understand all she says, but you follow her to your bedroom. She then starts to unbutton your shirt.

What is your first reaction?

_____

_____

_____

Why do you think you react this way?

_____

_____

_____

You then notice that there is an old person and another person watching you. This old person is the same sex as you are, but you are certain you have never seen the person before.

What is your reaction now?

_____

_____

_____

Why do you think you react this way?

_____

_____

_____

Did you say you'd be frightened or angry? Perhaps you said you'd resist or even try to get away. If so, you have some idea of what it may be like for the person with agnosia. In her 1993 book *Living in the Labyrinth: A Personal Journey Through the Maze of Alzheimer's,* Diana Friel McGowin describes a time when she, not yet diagnosed, meets a very friendly man in the hall of her office. Ms. McGowin does not know him, and is very apprehensive. Even though they speak for some time, she does not recognize him until he tells her who he is—her nephew who has come for an interview with Ms. McGowin's employer. She has known him all his life, yet did not recognize him, even with the cues present in their conversation.

Agnosia also causes the person to lose recognition of objects and their purpose. This can become a safety issue. It is not uncommon for someone to use an object in the wrong way. For example a person may mistake a disposable razor for a toothbrush. Or, she or he may no longer recognize a toothbrush as a toothbrush and react with anger when a caregiver tries to put this foreign object in her or his mouth.

Finally, the person loses recognition of sounds. A previously familiar sound, such as a cat meowing, could become a baby crying or something unknown that upsets the person.

CASE EXAMPLE 23-3

Ruth Tartan is 65, diagnosed with frontal lobe dementia. Ruth came to Canada from England in the 1960s, when she married. She had lived in England all her life prior to coming to Canada. She now lives with her son and his family.

Ruth's family notices that she becomes very upset whenever the teakettle whistles. She cries and crosses her arms over top of her head. They are very confused about this behaviour and worry that it upsets her. Ruth cannot tell them what the problem is.

A family friend is able to provide some information. "That sound is just like the air raid siren we used to hear in Britain," she says. "I wonder if Ruth thinks that the kettle sound is the air raid siren?" Ruth cannot understand enough to say whether or not this is the case, but her behaviour stops when the family begins using a kettle that does not whistle in the same tone.

Apraxia

A person with dementia loses the ability to plan, sequence, and execute the steps of particular tasks. Every task has an order, and even the simplest of tasks has a number of steps.

STOP AND REFLECT

Do you remember when you first learned to drive? Was it easy to figure out what came first and what sequence the other tasks were supposed to be in?

Chances are that it took you a bit of time to get everything in the correct order. You may have felt frustrated or overwhelmed at times.

As with other components, the last thing learned is the first to be lost. In early stages, the person may begin to have difficulty managing the remote control or the microwave oven. Next the person loses the skills learned as a young adult—driving the car, cooking, hobbies, etc. Eventually, the person will have difficulty with tasks learned as a child (i.e., dressing, bathing, and toileting).

Some situations can be hard to understand. For example, learning to read is a skill learned early in life. It may be retained even though other seemingly simpler skills have been lost. This can cause caregivers to feel that the person "knows what she is doing," when in fact she does not. Similarly, a caregiver may assume that a person who reads can use written clues. This may not be the case; it is important to determine if the person can understand what those words mean.

It's also possible that a person is physically capable of performing a task, such as getting dressed, but cognitively the person cannot organize and sequence the tasks required to do so. A caregiver may think that the person is refusing to do a task when the person may actually not know how to start or organize it.

Tasks that are too difficult, unfamiliar, or have multiple steps and demands may exceed a person's abilities and result in frustration and inappropriate behaviours. Recall the time when you learned to drive. There probably were times that you became frustrated or even wanted to cry or just give up. The difference between you and the person with cognitive impairment is in the degree of skill required; you can manage a much more complex task than the person with dementia is able to manage.

Apraxia also makes it difficult to attend to tasks and shift from one task to another. This means the person will have difficulty with complex tasks and may become upset when confronted with numerous stimuli, instructions, competing noises, or other distractions. Again, this is much like the difficulty we have when many things come at us at once, or when we need to really concentrate on how we are doing something.

STOP AND REFLECT 23-3

Imagine that you are in the car, going shopping. You have other people in the car. They are talking and the radio is on. When you get to the store, the only parking space available is really small—just large enough for you to get into, but no room to spare. You'll really have to concentrate in order to park without hitting another car. What do you do?

_____

_____

_____

_____

_____ ∎

Chances are that you asked the others to be quiet and you turned down the radio. If you did one or both of these things, you've done them to reduce the distraction, to help you focus on what you need to do. The distraction is the same thing that happens to the person with cognitive impairment; only our "threshold"—the point at which the distraction is too much to deal with—is much higher than it is for the person with the impairment. As well, the person with cognitive impairment may not be able to tell you that the distraction is too much—you may only see it in the person's behaviour.

Anosognosia

Anosognosia means that the person doesn't know that she or he doesn't know. This is also called impaired insight. Impaired insight is often the reason why a person refuses help; the person doesn't know he or she needs help.

Insight is one of the functions called "executive functions" or "higher-level functions of the brain." These functions are:

- insight and judgment
- controlling impulses
- appreciating the consequences of behaviour (e.g., safety, how it makes other people "feel")

- problem solving and planning
- knowing when to "quit" a task
- shifting from one task to another
- attention/concentration

Executive functions are necessary for appropriate, socially responsible, self-directed behaviour. They appear to be stored in the frontal lobe of the brain.

Perhaps you've been in a situation in which someone tells you that she or he is going to do something. You have done a similar thing and know that it is not very likely to work out. You explain this, but the person does not believe you; the person's perception says something different. Or, perhaps you've heard someone say that a person "didn't know enough to be afraid." In a sense, these situations are similar to anosognosia—the people "don't know what they don't know." The difference is one of degree—this happens to us in rare circumstances. It happens to the person with cognitive impairment *every day*.

The person with anosognosia feels that he or she is still doing things the same as always. For example, your client may get up and get ready for work, because the person's memory is of a time 30 years ago, when going to work was the daily routine. When you try to redirect the activities, the person may become angry. Bear in mind that the person is not in denial or intentionally being difficult. He or she is simply acting upon what his or her brain says is the truth.

Anosognosia can make some behaviour difficult to understand. Although some intellectual abilities may remain relatively well preserved, the person with frontal lobe impairment has difficulty understanding consequences of behaviour—appreciating how the behaviour makes other people feel. This does not mean that the person doesn't care. Rather, it's an indication of the person's inability to understand how what he or she has done affects the other person.

For the same reason, anosognosia can also pose safety risks. For example, a person may attempt to drive a car when one is not able. Another person may see help with cooking as an aggressive or controlling. Based on what the person's brain is telling him or her ("I'm able to do this"), these behaviours make sense.

Altered Perception

Some people with dementia experience hallucinations—seeing something that isn't there. However, most often the person is experiencing an illusion—*misperceiving* what is there.

Altered perception is more of a problem in the late afternoon and evening. During those times, the person is losing the ability to perceive images correctly and is losing colour. You've probably experienced this yourself—things look different at twilight; colours are less vivid and some seem to "stand out" more than others. Again, we process these changes and realize the effect on what we're seeing. The person with cognitive impairment is usually unable to do this.

This loss is compounded by normal, age-related changes in vision and hearing. These changes make it more difficult to see or hear clearly, adding to the likelihood that something will be misperceived.

For example, a garbage bag at the end of the driveway may be perceived as a person in a black coat sitting at the road. Similarly, a coat rack or coat tree in the corner may be seen as people.

Another major loss is depth perception, our ability to see in three dimensions. This affects the person's ability to judge how far or close something is, or how high, deep, long or wide something is.

STOP AND REFLECT ((23-4))

Consider the following common issues:

If you are without depth perception, and the doors and walls are the same colour, where is the door?

If the carpeting on the floors and stairs is the same, where do the stairs start?

If there is water in the bathtub, are you willingly going to step into the tub if you think there is no bottom?

If the television screen looks like everything else in the room, two-dimensional, then does it not make perfect sense that everyone on TV is in the room?

CASE EXAMPLE 23-4

Vera Small has Alzheimer Disease. She has always watched certain shows on television. Lately, she has become focused on the speaker in the Canadian Tire commercials. The commercial shows his head, neck, and shoulders only as he speaks. Mrs. Small believes he is visiting her and becomes very upset when he disappears. Her daughter tries to tell her that he is not "real," it's a commercial, but Mrs. Small says her daughter is "crazy," that the man was just here, in the room.

Loss of depth perception greatly affects the ability to navigate freely through the environment. It can change the way the person walks and sits. The following are a few examples:

- Dark carpets or tiles may look like holes in the floor. The person may fear stepping onto them, being certain she or he will fall into the hole.
- In sitting, the person will cautiously put a hand on the edge of the seat, brush the edge of the seat with a leg, and then sit on the edge or even arm of the chair. You will tell the person to move to the middle but he or she is not sure where the middle is or how far down, or how far over to go.
- The person may be unable to relate to distance in space and therefore bump into objects or people.

These perceptual changes, combined with the person's difficulty in processing information, can cause the person to focus only on what's directly ahead. In a sense, the person develops tunnel vision—not because of any change to the eyes, but because the brain can't take in all the extra information from peripheral vision.

Apathy

Over time, individuals with progressive cognitive impairment develop a form of apathy; they lose the ability to initiate conversation or initiate involvement in activities. Apathy occurs when damage is done to or there are interruptions in the connections to parts of the frontal lobes.

Often, it isn't that the person doesn't want to initiate or take part; the person simply doesn't know how. In this type of apathy, the person will try to participate if someone engages her or him. For example:

- A person may sit in front of a meal and may not touch it until someone gets him or her started. Once verbal cues or hand-over-hand technique is used, the person may finish the meal independently.
- When asked, a person may say "No" to offers of going to the chapel to sing, but staff have noticed that if brought to the chapel, the person sings and smiles.
- A person spends most of the day in silence, head down, chin on chest; but if approached and called by name, the person will lift his or her head to make eye contact and smile.

This isn't the same type of apathy that occurs with depression. A person who is depressed will not participate even when someone tries to interact. Such a person feels too low to motivate himself or herself to interact socially.

Causes of Cognitive Impairment

Like dementia, cognitive impairment is not a disease, but a group of symptoms that may be the result of many different conditions. There are more than 100 conditions that can produce cognitive impairment. These conditions can be broken into two general categories: reversible and irreversible conditions. Reversible conditions can be partially or fully cured by treatment. Examples of reversible conditions include delirium and overmedication.

Other conditions produce irreversible impairment, which cannot be cured. These include many traumas, vascular dementia, and senile dementia of the Alzheimer type. These conditions affect the structure of the brain, damaging and destroying brain cells. Many conditions that produce irreversible impairment are also progressive—they become worse over time. Table 23-2 lists the common categories and conditions of cognitive impairment.

TABLE 23-2	Common Conditions Causing Cognitive Impairment	
Irreversible and Progressive	**Irreversible and Nonprogressive**	**Reversible**
Alzheimer Disease (senile dementia of the Alzheimer type)	Trauma	Infection
	Hemorrhage	Drug Toxicity
Vascular Dementia		Vitamin Deficiency
Creutzfeldt-Jakob's Disease		Tumour
		Depression
Huntington's Disease		Normal Pressure Hydrocephalus
Parkinson's Disease		Thyroid Disease
Alcohol-Related Dementia		Metabolic Disorders
AIDS-Related Dementia		Subdural Hematoma (a bruise under the skull)
Frontal-Lobe Dementia		

It's important to remember that a person can have both an irreversible cognitive impairment (like Alzheimer Disease) and a reversible, or curable, cognitive impairment (from an illness or overmedication, for example). Treating the reversible impairment may reduce the symptoms of the disease and help the person to function better. Some reversible conditions can cause permanent damage if they are not treated soon enough. You should never overlook symptoms of a possible reversible impairment. Report any changes to your supervisor. Later in this chapter, we'll discuss what to look for and what information is useful when you report.

WHAT IS CONFUSION?

STOP AND REFLECT ((23-5))

Have you ever said that someone was confused? What made you say that about the person?

_____

_____

_____ ■

Look at your answer. Did you say that the person was confused because of something she or he did—such as answering a question inappropriately or losing something?

Confusion is not cognitive impairment. Sometimes hearing loss, stress, or lack of attention can result in a behaviour that seems wrong. A person with cognitive impairment is often confused, but a person who appears confused doesn't always have a cognitive impairment.

DELIRIUM

Delirium is caused when some agent (a medication, substance, infection, or other medical condition) temporarily affects a person's ability to follow and make sense of what is going on around him or her. Delirium is a medical emergency that must be immediately treated. A person with delirium may have poor concentration, be easily distracted, be disoriented to time and place, or have visions or hallucinations. The person may seem as though he or she is in a dream state, even though he or she is awake. People of any age can develop delirium, but it is the symptom of a condition that requires treatment.

The treatment for delirium depends on the cause. Some types, such as those provoked by medication or general anaesthetics, will usually disappear once the medication is stopped. Delirium resulting from infection will cease when the infection is resolved.

You should immediately report any sudden decline in your client's ability to understand or perceive what is around him or her. Cognitive changes that occur suddenly are often due to a treatable cause. It's important to advise your supervisor or other designated person so that the client can be assessed and treated. Even after treatment has been provided, it may be some time before the person regains function. It is important to closely supervise the person to minimize the risk of harm.

WHAT IS DEMENTIA?

As we discussed earlier, *dementia* is a term that is often used to describe the symptoms that accompany many types of cognitive impairment when they occur in older adults. Some rare forms of dementia can occur in people as young as age 30. When it occurs in a younger person, the condition is called early-onset dementia. People may speak of dementia as only occurring when the person has an irreversible condition. This is not entirely accurate: Though dementia does describe the symptoms that accompany irreversible conditions such as Alzheimer Disease, it also refers to symptoms that come from overmedication, poor diet, and sensory loss, among other conditions.

Irreversible Dementias

There are many different types of irreversible dementias. Figure 23-3 shows the percentage of each cause, based upon data from the Canadian Collaborative Cohort of Related Dementias (ACCORD) study. In this section, we'll discuss the most common causes: Alzheimer Disease, vascular dementia, Lewy body, and frontotemporal dementia. We'll also discuss the specific type of Alzheimer Disease that occurs in people who also have Down syndrome.

Alzheimer Canada estimates that more than 400,000 Canadians have some type of irreversible dementia. The risk of dementia increases with age. About 8 percent of the population over 65 has some form of dementia, and this rises to 35 percent of people over 85 (Canadian Study on Health and Aging, 1994). Despite the fact that it is more common in people over 85, dementia is not a normal part of aging.

Remember that the terms acquired brain injury or traumatic brain injury are used to describe cognitive impairment in a person of any age when the impairment is caused by a trauma. The impairment caused by trauma differs from that caused by non-traumatic causes. We'll look at these conditions in a separate section of this chapter.

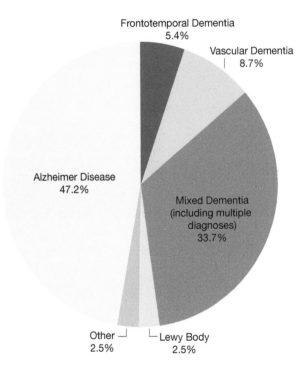

FIGURE 23-3

Causes of irreversible progressive dementia (ACCORD Study)

Source: A Canadian cohort study of cognitive impairment and related dementias (ACCORD): study methods and baseline results. Feldman H, et al. Neuroepidemiology. 2003;22(5):265-74

Alzheimer Disease

Alzheimer Disease is the most common cause of dementia in older people. Women are more likely to be affected; two-thirds of those with Alzheimer Disease are women (Alzheimer Canada, 2007). The disease is named after Dr. Alois Alzheimer, a German doctor who first described the disease in 1906. Dr. Alzheimer noticed changes in the brain tissue of a woman who had died of an unusual mental illness. Upon an autopsy, he found abnormal clumps (now called senile plaques) and tangled bundles of fibres (now called neurofibrillary tangles) in the brain. These plaques and tangles are considered to be the hallmarks or characteristics of Alzheimer Disease.

Scientists also have found other changes in the brains of people with Alzheimer Disease. There is a loss of nerve cells in areas of the brain that are vital to memory and other mental abilities. There also are lower levels of the chemicals in the brain that carry complex messages back and forth between the billions of nerve cells. Alzheimer Disease may disrupt normal thinking and memory by blocking these messages between nerve cells.

We don't know for certain what causes Alzheimer Disease. We do know that some things increase a person's risk of developing it. The major risk factors are age and family history. Another possible risk factor is a serious head injury. Researchers are also examining the possibility that metals (such as aluminum, zinc, and lead) may cause the disease.

Genetic Predisposition

Researchers have identified some cases where there is a genetic predisposition to developing a dementia. For example, the disease has been traced though families and it has been found that on these relatively rare cases, a specific gene seems to trigger the disease.

We also know that persons who have Down syndrome will, almost certainly, develop a form of Alzheimer Disease. People who develop this form often have different symptoms than a person with Alzheimer Disease who does not have Down syndrome. We'll look at this condition and others in the next section.

It's important to remember that most cases of Alzheimer Disease are probably not caused by any single factor. It is more likely to be the result of several factors that act differently in each person. For example, genetic factors alone may not be enough to cause the disease. Other risk factors may combine with a person's genetic makeup to increase his or her chance of developing the disease.

General Symptoms

Usually, irreversible dementias begin slowly. The only symptom at first may be mild forgetfulness. The person may lose keys or misplace his or her wallet. Because forgetfulness is something that happens to us all at some time, the person or those around him or her may not notice this symptom.

Later, memory loss becomes more obvious. The person may have trouble remembering recent events, where familiar things are located (such as the post office or the grocery store), or even the names of familiar people or things. The person may have difficulty solving simple problems. At this stage, driving a car is difficult and dangerous although the person may not realize it.

As the disease goes on, the symptoms become serious enough to cause concern. For example, the person with dementia may not remember how to do simple, everyday tasks, such brushing teeth or combing hair. The person can no longer think clearly and may begin to have problems speaking, understanding, reading, or writing.

In the later stages, the person with dementia may become anxious or aggressive or wander away from home. It is at this later stage that families often begin to consider admitting the person to a long-term care facility. Despite this, the Canadian Study on Health and Aging estimates that 50 percent of all people with dementia live in the community. Most of these people live with family members, often with a husband or wife.

Diagnosis

We don't have a test that will tell us for sure whether a person has Alzheimer Disease or other irreversible dementias. Examining brain tissue for tangles and plaques is the only way to make a firm diagnosis of the disease. However, doctors use a number of things to help to diagnose probable Alzheimer Disease. They often look for other causes for the dementia—like overmedication, sensory problems, or illnesses. They also often run a series of medical tests. Doctors at specialized centres can correctly diagnose "probable Alzheimer Disease" 80 to 90 percent of the time.

Duration of the Condition

The course the disease takes and how fast changes occur vary from person to person, as well as from one type of dementia to another. Some people may live as little as five years after the diagnosis, while others may live with it for as many as 20 years. Some people may lose abilities very quickly; others may see a decline over a much longer period of time.

You may hear colleagues talk about the stages of Alzheimer Disease. This term refers to a general description of the changes in abilities that occur. There are many descriptions of the stages, but the descriptions recognized by the Alzheimer Society of Canada are the most widely accepted, as described in Table 23-3. However, you may hear of the Global Deterioration Scale, also called the Reisberg Scale. It is a seven-stage scale and it is described in Table 23-4.

Bear in mind that the stages are a guideline only. Each person is an individual. Also, the disease will affect each person differently. For example, a person may show symptoms of the early stage in some areas and the middle stage in others.

Treatment

At present, there is no treatment that can cure or stop the progression of Alzheimer Disease or most other irreversible dementias. However, some new medications seem to help the person to think more clearly.

Also, some medications may help control symptoms of Alzheimer Disease, such as sleeplessness, agitation, wandering, anxiety, and depression. Treating these symptoms often makes the person more comfortable and makes it easier for caregivers to provide care. Medications may not help in all cases, however, and may make the symptoms worse for some people.

It is important to be aware that symptoms may also be the result of other causes, and that they may respond to treatment. Sometimes, the treatment is simple. For example, a person who has Alzheimer Disease and who also wears glasses will generally be more responsive if he or she is wearing the glasses. The person will be able to see better. This means that it's more likely that information will reach the person's brain more clearly, which, in turn, can help him or her to function.

Dementia in Persons with Down Syndrome

Most, but not all people who have Down syndrome also develop a progressive, irreversible dementia, if they live long enough. The disease usually first appears when the person is in his or her 40s or 50s, much younger than the average for a person

TABLE 23-3	Stages of Alzheimer Disease		
Abilities Affected	**Early Stage**	**Typical Symptoms Middle Stage**	**Late Stage**
Mental Abilities	mild forgetfulness; difficulty learning new things and following conversations; difficulty concentrating; limited attention span; problems with orientation, such as getting lost or not following directions; communication difficulties such as finding the right word	continued memory problems; forgetfulness about personal history; inability to recognize friends and family; disorientation about time and place	loss of ability to remember, communicate or function; inability to process information; severe speaking difficulties; severe disorientation about time, place, and people
Moods and Emotions	mood shifts; depression	personality change; confusion; anxiety/apprehension; suspiciousness; mood shifts; anger; sadness/depression; hostility	possible withdrawal
Behaviours	passiveness; withdrawal from usual activities; restlessness	declining ability to concentrate, restlessness (pacing, wandering); repetition; delusions; aggression; uninhibited behaviour; passiveness	nonverbal methods of communicating (eye contact, crying, groaning)
Physical Abilities	mild coordination problems	assistance required for daily tasks (e.g., dressing, bathing, using the toilet); disrupted sleep patterns; appetite fluctuations; language difficulties; visual-spatial problems	sleeps longer and more often; becomes immobile (bed-ridden); loses ability to speak; loses control of bladder and bowels; has difficulty eating and/or swallowing; unable to dress or bathe; may lose weight

Source: ©Alzheimer Society of Canada, 1997–2007. Revised October 2005.

Table 23-4	Global Deterioration Scale

Stage 1: No cognitive decline

- Experiences no problems in daily living.

Stage 2: Very mild cognitive decline

- Forgets names and locations of objects.
- May have trouble finding words.

Stage 3: Mild cognitive decline

- Has difficulty travelling to new locations.
- Has difficulty handling problems at work.

Stage 4: Moderate cognitive decline

- Has difficulty with complex tasks (finances, shopping, planning dinner for guests).

Stage 5: Moderately severe cognitive decline

- Needs help to choose clothing.
- Needs prompting to bathe.

Stage 6: Severe cognitive decline

- Needs help putting on clothing.
- Requires assistance bathing; may have a fear of bathing.
- Has decreased ability to use the toilet or is incontinent.

Stage 7: Very severe cognitive decline

- Vocabulary becomes limited, eventually declining to single words.
- Loses ability to walk and sit.
- Becomes unable to smile.

Source: Modified from Global Deterioration Scale, Reisberg, 1982.
Reisberg, B., Ferris, S.H., de Leon, M.J., and Crook, T., American Journal of Psychiatry, 139:1136-1139, 1982.

without Down syndrome (Alzheimer Society of British Columbia, 2008). Alzheimer Disease is the most common, but others are also possible.

Many of the symptoms are similar to those in Alzheimer Disease; however, some are different or occur at a different time. Most differences occur in the early stages of Alzheimer Disease (Down's Syndrome Association of the UK, 2004). Table 23-5 illustrates some of these differences.

Vascular Dementia

Vascular dementia occurs when strokes impair a person's cognitive function. It is important to remember that though most strokes do not cause dementia, some do. As well, having had a stroke that does not result in vascular dementia still puts the person at greater risk of developing vascular dementia.

TABLE 23-5	Changes Associated with Dementia in a Person Who has Down's syndrome

- Subtle changes in behaviour that are often only seen by a person who knows the person with Down's very well
- Inability to do tasks, often expressed as a refusal or seen as stubbornness
- Rapid speech, repetitive comments, restlessness
- Hallucinations
- Seizures occurring earlier than in other forms of AD

Source: Adapted from Down's Syndrome Association of the UK and Stanton and Coetzee, Down's syndrome and dementia, *in* Advances in Psychiatric Treatment (2004) 10: 50-58

Sometimes, the dementia is the result of a single stroke. Other times, it is the result of a number of strokes. When more than one stroke has caused the dementia, it may be called *multi-infarct dementia*. In Canada, vascular dementia is the second greatest cause of dementia (The Canadian Study of Health and Aging, 2000). Its incidence increases with age, and it affects more men than women. Vascular dementia and Alzheimer Disease can occur in the same person.

People with vascular dementia often have a "stair step" progression to the disease: a sudden loss of function that stabilizes, then drops and stabilizes again. It's also likely that the person will have mood and behavioural changes. In some cases, the person may have delusions or other psychiatric symptoms. A person with vascular dementia is more likely to also have severe depression than a person who has Alzheimer Disease.

Lewy Body Dementia

Photo 23-1
Lewy bodies in brain matter
Source: *Photo courtesy of Kondi Wong, Armed Forces Institute of Pathology*

Lewy body dementia is a progressive disease and is named because the disease is identified by abnormal structures in brain cells called Lewy bodies. Lewy bodies are abnormal collections of proteins. Photo 23-1 shows Lewy bodies in brain matter.

The disease is more common in men than women. Researchers have not identified a definite cause of Lewy body dementia, but some researchers are exploring a possible link between the condition and Parkinson's and Alzheimer diseases, as Lewy bodies contain a protein associated with these two diseases. Other researchers are exploring a genetic link.

A person with Lewy body dementia may experience symptoms similar to those of both Parkinson's and Alzheimer diseases. The person usually experiences progressive loss of language, reasoning and other higher mental functions. He or she may also experience depression and anxiety. Problems with short-term memory are common, as are progressive losses of memory, but these losses often occur later than they would in a person with Alzheimer Disease. The person may have visual hallucinations that may be very vivid. The person may also experience muscle rigidity, tremors, stooped posture or slow, shuffling movements—symptoms similar to those of Parkinson's disease.

Creutzfeldt-Jakob Disease

Creutzfeldt-Jakob Disease (CJD) is a rare form of progressive dementia. It is caused by infectious agents called prions (misfolded proteins). These prions attack the brain,

Lewy body

destroying cells and leaving microscopic holes in the brain. Photo 23-2 shows the holes created by CJD in brain matter.

CJD is always fatal. It progresses rapidly. In 70 percent of cases, the person with CJD dies within six months onset of the disease.

There are two forms, variant and classical. Variant CJD is a new disease in humans. It is linked to eating beef products from cattle infected with BSE (commonly known as Mad Cow Disease). The Public Health Agency of Canada states that there has been only one case of variant CJD in Canada, and that case occurred in a person who had lived in the United Kingdom for a long time. No cases have been linked to eating Canadian beef (Public Health Agency of Canada, 2007).

Classical CJD is a human prion disease. It is not linked to eating beef and is seen rarely in populations around the world. About 30 cases are diagnosed in Canada each year, most in people 45–75 years of age (Public Health Agency of Canada). There is some concern that CJD may be transmitted through blood, organs, or other body products, but the Public Health Agency of Canada states that this is extremely rare; only one case in Canada has been identified.

Early symptoms may include memory lapses, mood swings similar to depression, lack of interest, and social withdrawal. The person may become unsteady on her or his feet. Later symptoms may include blurred vision, sudden jerking movements, and rigidity in the limbs. The person may experience slurred speech and have difficulty swallowing. Eventually, movement and speech are lost.

Brain shrinkage and deterioration occurs rapidly

Brain section showing spongiform pathology characteristic of Creutzfeldt-Jakob

✷A.D.A.M.

Photo 23-2
The dark spots in the brain matter (inset, upper right) show the holes created by CJD.
Source: © 2008
A.D.A.M., Inc.

Frontotemporal Dementia (FTD)

Unlike Alzheimer Disease, which generally affects most areas of the brain, frontotemporal dementia is a progressive dementia that affects specific areas of the brain—the frontal and temporal lobes. Frontotemporal dementia includes a number of variations: Pick's disease, frontal lobe dementia, and primary progressive aphasia, among others.

The age of onset of FTD is also earlier; in most cases, occurring in the mid-50s. Incidence increases with age only to about age 62, then incidence declines (Association for Frontotemporal Dementias, 2007). In 25–50 percent of the cases, there is a family history of the condition (Vancouver Coastal Heath Research Institute, 2006).

How FTD progresses depends upon the type. In some cases, brain cells in the frontal or temporal lobes can shrink or die. In other cases, the brain cells in these areas get larger, containing round, silver "Pick's bodies." In both situations, the changes affect the person's functioning.

People with FTD demonstrate changes in behaviour and understanding that result from changes in the "executive functions" of the brain. They can show lack of concern for social norms or other people or lack of insight into their own behaviours. They often retain the cardinal features of memory, keeping track of day-to-day events and orientation to space and time. Sometimes the language loss is very specific (for example, being unable to name a specific item).

In the early stages, this pattern of loss can make a person with FTD simply seem uncaring and abrasive, or appear to have a mental health problem, not a problem with cognition. It is not uncommon for an individual to first be diagnosed with mental illness (for example, bipolar disorder, schizophrenia, or depression) before learning about their FTD diagnosis. This is especially common in people who develop the behavioural symptoms first.

Table 23-6 identifies the general changes often occurring in a person with FTD.

Table 23-6	General Changes Occurring in a Person with FTD

Behavioral Symptoms

A progressive deterioration in the person's ability to control or adjust his/her behavior appropriately in different social contexts is the hallmark of all of these behavior changes.

- *Hyperoral* behaviors include overeating, dietary compulsions, in which the person restricts himself to eating only specific foods (such as a certain flavor of Lifesaver, or eating food only from one fast food restaurant), or attempts to consume inedible objects. Patients may consume excessive amounts of liquids, alcohol and cigarettes.

- *Stereotyped and/or Repetitive* behaviors can include re-reading the same book multiple times, hand rubbing and clapping, humming one tune repeatedly, or walking to the same location day after day.

- *Personal hygiene* habits deteriorate early in the disease progression, as the person fails to perform everyday tasks of bathing, grooming, and appropriate dressing.

- *Hyperactive* behavior is exhibited by some patients, and can include agitation, pacing, wandering, outbursts of frustration, and aggression.

- *Hypersexual* behavior can range from a preoccupation with sexual jokes to compulsive masturbation.

- *Impulsive acts* can include shoplifting, impulsive buying, and grabbing food off of another person's plate.

Language Symptoms

There are some FTD subtypes (semantic dementia and progressive non-fluent aphasia) that have specific language deficits as their cardinal feature. Listed below are the general symptoms of language deterioration that can accompany any FTD diagnosis.

- *Aphasia* (reduced output of speech)

- *Dysarthria* (increased difficulty producing speech due to weakness or incoordination – speech sounds are weak, imprecise and uncoordinated)

- *Agrammatica* refers to an increasing difficulty in remembering or understanding the rules of grammar that help us get meaning from a sentence.

- *Decrease in Reading and Writing Comprehension* occurs as the patient experiences problems with word meaning and recognition.

- *Echolalia* refers to a repetition of a word or phrase said by another person.

- *Perseveration* is the repetition of a word or phrase said by the patient himself.

- *Mutism* eventually develops in many FTD patients during advanced stages of the disease. Though at this stage the person has lost all ability to speak, he or she may still be able to retain some understanding of what is spoken to them.

Cognitive Symptoms

FTD patients typically suffer increasing impairment in "executive functions," listed below.

- *Distractibility and impersistence* mean the person has increasing difficulty staying on task mentally.

- *Mental rigidity and inflexibility* develop as the person may insist on having his or her own way, or have increasing difficulty adapting to new or changing circumstances.

Table 23-6	General Changes Occurring in a Person with FTD *(continued)*

■ *Planning and problem solving* impairments develop as the ability for abstract reasoning decreases. Examples of this would include difficulty planning and coordinating the cooking of a meal, or making a shopping list and performing necessary errands.

■ *Poor financial judgment* can produce additional, troubling situations for families.

Emotional Symptoms

■ *Apathy* or indifference toward events and the surrounding environment can be marked by reduced initiative, and lack of motivation.

■ *Lack of insight* into the person's own behavior develops early. The patient typically does not recognize the changes in his or her own behaviors, nor do they exhibit awareness or concern for the effect these behaviors have on the people around them, including loved ones.

■ *Emotional blunting* develops early in the course of the disorder, and is manifested as a loss of emotional warmth, empathy, and sympathy, and development of what appears to be indifference toward other people, including loved ones.

■ *Mood changes* can be abrupt and frequent.

Neurological Symptoms

■ *Movement dysfunction* symptoms may be some of the first to develop, and are similar to those seen in Parkinson disease, although they do not mean that the person has Parkinson disease. These include: decreased facial expression, bradykinesia (slowness of movements), rigidity (resistance to imposed movement), and postural instability. A very small number have difficulty with eye movements, dystonia (abnormal muscle postures), or alien hand syndrome (in which the person does not recognize his hand as being part of his own body).

■ *Muscle dysfunction.* People with FTD experience many of the muscular problems seen in ALS: weakness, muscle atrophy, and myoclonus (muscle jerks).

Psychiatric Symptoms

Some people with FTD may experience psychiatric symptoms, including depression, mania, persecutory delusions (thinking people are "out to get them") and visual or auditory hallucinations.

Source: Association for Frontotemporal Dementias, April 2007

Other Dementias

Other dementias may be the result of poor circulation in the brain, heavy metal poisoning, or metabolic conditions.

CARING FOR THE PERSON WITH DEMENTIA

Fundamental Principles of Support

There are six fundamental principles you must keep in mind when working with a client with dementia. Relate the first four principles to what you would do in response to Stop and Reflect 23-6.

STOP AND REFLECT ((23-6))

Consider the following situation. You are home alone on a stormy night. No one else is expected to be at home. It is 2:30 a.m. when you hear pounding on the front door. You go to answer the door. You try to switch on the outside light, but it does not turn on. In the brief glare of a flash of lightning, you see a person in a dark, hooded sweater. You do not recognize the person.

How do you feel? What are you thinking? Will you open the door?

_____

_____

_____

_____

You ask the person at the door to tell you who he or she is. When the person speaks, you realize it is one of your friends who lives nearby.

How do you feel now? Have your feelings changed from the ones you had before you knew who the person was? Would you open the door?

_____

_____

_____

Did your past experiences affect how you responded in this situation? Perhaps your home has been burglarized, or this situation has happened to you before. Either way, your experience would be affected by your past experiences.

1. **Every action has a purpose to the person performing the action.** Even the most aimless activity is purposeful to the person who is performing it. For example, studies have shown that clients who wander do so for a number of reasons: to get exercise, to relieve boredom, or to be with others. Whether or not you understand the client's purpose does not matter.
2. **Every action has meaning for the person doing it.** No activity is meaningless.
3. **The world, as the person perceives it, is as real to him or her as our world is to us.** For example, a client may refuse to enter an elevator because he or she sees the elevator as a small, dark hole, and the client fears that he or she will fall. Do your best to see what the client might see. This will help you to understand the behaviour. Never argue with a client about what he or she perceives.
4. **The person may lose words, but never loses feelings.** The ability to experience emotions remains with the client long after he or she loses the ability to verbally communicate. Use nonverbal forms of communication to help get your message across.
5. **You are the person who must adapt and change.** The client with dementia has little, if any, ability to adapt his or her behaviour. You must adapt your approach to the client's needs.
6. **Your approach to the client will determine whether or not communication is successful.**

Problem Solving

It's often helpful to answer the following questions when you're faced with a situation that's hard to understand. These questions are adapted from the U-First! Strategy and are summarized in Table 23-7. You'll note that these questions are very similar to those you ask yourself when you notice any change in a person.

TABLE 23-7	Questions to ask when behaviour is hard to understand

1. What do I notice? What are the changes?
2. What risk does it pose?
3. What is the person trying to tell me?
4. What could be the cause(s)?
5. What is my response?
6. What happens when I respond this way?
7. What needs to be shared with others?

Source: Ontario Community Support Association, 2006

Question 1—What Do I Notice? What Are the Changes? Answering this question will help you put what you see in behavioural terms: appearance, behaviour, and communication. As we discussed in Chapter 10, it's important to describe in specific terms, not to make a generalization, judge it, or make an assumption. If you're tempted to say, "Gee, she's frightened," ask yourself what makes you say that. Look for the reason for your assessment—it's likely in what the person did or how she or he did it.

Question 2—What Risk Does It Pose? This is an important question. Sometimes behaviour is simply different; it doesn't put the person or others at risk. It may even be comforting to the person. If the behaviour falls into this category, leave it alone. It (literally) isn't hurting anyone. Do share your observation with others, though, so that you can all use the same approach with the client.

Question 3—What Is the Person Trying to Tell Me? Communication with the person with dementia is one of the most important parts of caring for the person (Photo 23-3). It can also be one of the most challenging. The person may not be able to find the right words or many words at all. This can be painful, frustrating, and embarrassing for the person and for the caregiver.

Communication

As we discussed in Chapter 7, nonverbal components of communication (body language) can often be more significant than the words used. In communication with clients with dementia, body language may be the most significant component of communication. This is because the person gradually loses the ability to understand concepts and words. The person may also be less able to tell that someone is trying to get his or her attention and may have difficulty following a conversation.

You should focus on four things when communicating with a person with dementia: the setting, your approach, the message, and the client's response. Remember that the person will pay attention to your body language no matter what you are saying. Make sure that you know how you look and act as you speak with the client. The following tips can make communication easier.

Photo 23-3
Good communication requires patience and creativity when there are barriers to overcome.
Source: CHATS

The Setting

1. **Talk to the person in a place free from distractions.** Move away from background noise (such as an open window, air conditioner, television, or a crowded room).
2. **Do not position yourself between the person and a window.** The glare from the window will make it impossible for the person to see your face. This can frighten the person.

Your Approach

1. **Approach the person from the front.** Many people with dementia ignore their peripheral (side) vision.
2. **Approach the person slowly.** Walking quickly up to a person may startle or frighten him or her.
3. **Do not invade the person's personal space.** Doing so will make the person uncomfortable and hamper his or her ability to understand your message.
4. **Identify yourself at the beginning of your conversation.** Allow time for the person to acknowledge you. If possible, gain eye contact before proceeding.
5. **Use a calm and gentle approach.** Don't demand that a person do something. Make sure that your body language does not convey that you are upset or in a hurry.
6. **Make sure that you are at eye level.** Crouch, sit, or kneel in front of the person if necessary.
7. **Try using touch to help convey your message, if acceptable to the client.** Be aware that touch may not be helpful to communication with every person.
8. **Make sure your body language is in tune with your words.** Remember that the person will take his or her cue from your body language.
9. **Don't patronize or talk down to the client.** The person will sense your tone and respond negatively.

The Message

1. **Use short sentences with simple words.** Long sentences or words with many syllables will make it harder for the person to follow your message.
2. **Speak slowly.** Consciously slow down your rate of speech.
3. **Keep your tone gentle and normal.** Avoid shouting or speaking forcefully. (This is easier to do when you are speaking slowly.)
4. **Make time for social pleasantries before beginning a task or asking for information.** Most people with dementia retain social skills well into the later stages of the condition. Allowing the person to use these familiar skills can help to put the person at ease and make the remaining communication easier.
5. **Use concrete terms and words you know are familiar to the client.** If possible, use words the client uses.
6. **Allow the person time to understand what you've said before continuing.** It is very frustrating for the person to have too little time to understand. As a result, the person may cease trying to communicate at all.
7. **Give the person time to answer a question before going on to another.** This encourages the person to participate in the conversation.
8. **Ask simple questions that have a "yes" or "no" answer.**
9. **Don't order the person to do something.** The person is still an adult and should be asked and encouraged, not ordered.

10. **Don't argue with the person about his or her statements.** If something is incorrect, gently state the correct information. In some cases, it may be better to distract the person by changing the subject. Whatever you do, try to avoid embarrassing the client. For example, if a client says that another person's purse is hers, you might gently respond that, although the purse looks like the client's, it actually belongs to another person.

11. **Use notes if the person can read and follow them.** Some people can follow only printed notes. If you use a note, make sure that it is clear. List any steps the person is to take in the order the person is to do them.

12. **Be flexible.** If the client has difficulty understanding a word or phrase, try a different one that means the same as the first.

13. **Be patient.** Communication takes time.

14. **Remember that an ill or tired person will not hear as well.** Take this into account as you decide how much you will attempt to get across at one time.

The Client's Response

1. **Be sensitive to the person's body language and the tone of his or her words.** This is often the first indication you will have of how well your message is getting through.

2. **Acknowledge and respect the person's feelings.**

3. **Actively and carefully listen to what the person is trying to say.** This will do two things. First, it will enhance the likelihood that you will understand. Second, your body language will also let the person know that you are interested in his or her thoughts.

4. **Be aware that the person may only be able to speak in concrete terms.** In particular, the ability to make comparisons may be lost. The person who says to you, "I was hit by a Mack truck" likely means that the person feels like he or she was hit, not that the event actually happened.

5. **Focus on a word or phrase that makes sense or seems to be key to the client's message.** Often, once you have a key word or phrase, you can make guesses and ask questions to get the whole message.

6. **Ask family and friends about possible meanings of words or phrases you don't understand.**

Communication Techniques

There are many techniques used to communicate with a person with dementia. Two of the more common are interpretative communication and reorientation. Properly used, each type can help you to better understand your client.

Interpretative Communication You may have heard of validation therapy or other interpretative approaches to communicating with clients who have dementia. Although the specifics of these approaches differ, they generally share the following principles:

1. **All communication has meaning.** It is up to you to attempt to learn the meaning of the communication.

2. **A person loses the ability to use comparisons such as "I feel like...," using instead the phrase itself.** For example, a person may say, "I've been hit by a truck,"

when he or she means that it feels like he or she has been hit by a truck. Respond to the implied message instead of the actual words.

3. **A person may ask for people, places, or things that have provided comfort or good feelings, even though those things are no longer available.** For example, a person may repeatedly ask to go home, even if he or she is at home. He or she no longer recognizes home now as a source of comfort. The person looks for that "other" home where he or she was comfortable. Respond by asking about the person's home to get an idea of what he or she needs to have.

4. **Use exploring words to learn more about what the person wants.** Your goal is to learn what the person is wanting. For example, if a client wants to go home, you might ask questions like the following: Who is at home? What sorts of things did you do at home? What things do you need to do there now?

5. **Use reminiscence to explore the person's statements.** For example, if a client says that he or she needs to get home to take care of the children, you might try talking about what life was like when the person was at home with his or her children. This may give you an idea of what the client is missing.

6. **Look for ways that the client can meet needs in the present.** For example, the client who needs to get home to care for the children may be missing the caregiving role she or he once had. Knowing this, you may be able to find some way that she or he can be a caregiver now. You might tell the client how much you appreciate her or his hugs, or that you know that the person looks out for you.

7. **Validate the person's feelings and needs.** The person's feelings and needs for someone or something are valid and reasonable to him or her. Respect them. Don't minimize the situation or say that the person shouldn't feel that way.

STOP AND REFLECT 23-7

A resident repeatedly wanders the halls of the facility. She asks people if they have seen her husband. When a staff member tells her that he has passed away, she says, "I know, but that doesn't mean that I don't need him."

CASE EXAMPLE 23-5

Mrs. Lavigne is a resident of a long-term care facility. She has vascular dementia. Support workers have noticed that she calls every female who helps her "Claire." At first, staff members assume that she is confused. One day, a support worker asks Mrs. Lavigne's family about the name. She learns that "Claire" is the *first name of the niece who cared for Mrs. Lavigne before she moved into the facility. Thus, "Claire" is the name Mrs. Lavigne uses to refer to any woman who helps her.*

How might you use the principles of interpretative communication to respond to Mrs. Lavigne?

Reorientation Reorientation refers to providing clients with useful information about the environment. It works best when the information provided is meaningful to the client and can be used with interpretative approaches. The following guidelines will help you to appropriately use reorienting technique:

1. **Make certain that the information is useful to the client.** For example, knowing the day of the week may not matter to a client unless something special happens on

that day. Useless information makes it difficult for the client to remember more important items.

2. **Don't provide too much information.** Too much information can confuse the client and make it hard to retain the information he or she needs.

3. **Provide information that comforts the client.** For example, if a client asks when lunch will be served, it's most appropriate to tell, even if he or she forgets and asks again, as long as the answer is satisfying.

4. **Don't quiz the person on reality "facts."** This can be embarrassing and frustrating and often has no real purpose. For example, insisting a client tell you the name of a visitor (e.g., "Who's here to see you? Don't you know who this is?") can be very upsetting to the person if he or she cannot remember. It is far better to supply the information by saying something like: "I see that your daughter Susan is here. You must be really glad to see her."

5. **Make orienting materials such as clocks and calendars handy if the client uses them.** Some clients are comforted by the presence of these items.

CASE EXAMPLE 23-6

Mrs. Jankowski was a supervisor in a large office. She was responsible for supervising 20 telephone operators and ensuring that they were doing their jobs and that no problems arose.

Mrs. Jankowski is now 86 and has developed dementia. She lives with her daughter and attends a day program. As the daughter must leave early for work, you are *assigned to assist Mrs. Jankowski to get up, have breakfast, and get dressed. Today Mrs. Jankowski meets you at the door partially dressed. She says, "I'm sorry, I can't have a visitor today. I'm late for work. You'll have to come some other time."*

How might you use an interpretative approach to communicate with Mrs. Jankowski?

Communicating with Others When the Client Is Present

There will be times when you and your client are with other people. Make sure that you include the client in any conversation to the extent that he or she can participate. Even if the client cannot take active part in the conversation, attempt to include the person by making sure he or she is physically a part of the group (Photo 23-4). These tips can help you keep the person included:

Photo 23-4
Support the client to do his or her best. Here, a worker encourages discussion.
Source: CHATS

1. **Don't ask questions that rely on a good memory.** This relies upon an ability that is not strong. This can be frustrating and embarrassing for the client.

2. **Don't talk to others about the person in front of the person.** Respect the person's presence. If there is information about the client that you must convey to another, do so when the person is out of the room.

3. **Don't ignore the person.** The person will notice the lack of inclusion. If possible, ask the person questions that you know he or she can answer to help keep the person part of the conversation.

SUPPORTING A CLIENT WITH THE PERFORMANCE OF TASKS

As a support worker, you often will be required to assist a client with routine tasks of living. The eight questions we described in Chapter 20 can be a good starting point for determining what the client can do and when the client will need help. Table 23-8 recaps these eight questions.

TABLE 23-8	Assessing a Client's Ability to Perform Tasks

- WHAT tasks does the client see as important to do?
- WHAT does the client enjoy doing?
- WHAT is the client able to do?
- HOW does the client do those things?
- WHEN is it easiest for the client to perform the task?
- WHICH parts of a task is the client unable to do?
- WHY is the client unable to do those parts?
- HOW does the client want you to assist?

In addition to the eight questions, there are several steps you can take to make the process easier for you both:

1. **Focus on familiar skills or tasks.** Familiar is easier and can boost the person's self-esteem.
2. **Break the task down into simple steps.** Small simple tasks are much easier to do.
3. **Give choices whenever you can.** We all like to have control over the things we do.
4. **Allow plenty of time for tasks to be done.** All cognitive processes will take longer. If the client feels pressured to respond quickly, anxiety may further hamper ability.
5. **Allow time to rest when needed.** The client will not be able to function well when tired or overstimulated.
6. **Follow the client's cues.** Learn what parts of the task are frustrating or impossible. Plan on completing these steps before the client becomes frustrated.
7. **Sincerely praise any success.** Genuine praise lifts anyone's spirits. Make sure that your praise is appropriate for an adult.

CHALLENGING BEHAVIOURS

Often, people with dementia develop some behaviours that are hard for us to understand. These behaviours include wandering, becoming angry, becoming frightened, refusing to take a bath, or even refusing to go into a room. The behaviours seem to happen without warning and may last a few minutes or a long time. These are called challenging behaviours. You may hear other people refer to these behaviours as problem behaviours or difficult behaviours. They should not be seen as problems or difficulties; they simply are behaviours caregivers must strive to understand. They pose a challenge to caregivers who must unravel the meaning of the behaviour, the cause of the behaviour, as well as determine what, if anything, can alter the behaviour. The last four problem-solving questions listed in Table 23-7 (page 505) are useful here: *What could be the cause(s)? What is my response? What happens when I respond this way? What needs to be shared with others?*

Understanding the A-B-Cs of Behaviours

One helpful way of looking at actions is to use the A-B-C (Action, Because, and Communication) approach. This approach is based upon the belief that no action or behaviour just happens. Each is a product of some reason or stimulus. Additionally, each action is affected by others' responses to the behaviour.

This approach asks the caregiver to look at each challenging behaviour in terms of what causes (or seems to cause) the behaviour and what the caregiver's response communicates to the client.

Table 23-9 describes the Action, Because, and Communication approach. Through this method, the caregiver may be able to figure out what triggers the behaviour. The caregiver may also be able to determine what may be changed in order to reduce the incidence of the behaviour. Let's take a look at each of the steps.

TABLE 23-9	The A-B-Cs of Behaviour

Action

- What you see the person doing
- May include signals before the behaviour
- Generally, the action is the event to which we react

Because

- The reason or "why"
- The thing that triggers or cues the behaviour
- Often not readily seen

Communication

- How we respond to the behaviour
- How we signal that we have "understood"
- Communication can be used to encourage or discourage the behaviour

The Action

This is the action or behaviour that you see, such as wandering, yelling, or striking out at another person. Some actions are preceded by other actions called warning signs or signals. For example, a client who is about to strike out may narrow his or her eyes. Determining warning signs can help you to prevent an undesired behaviour from happening.

The Because

The because is the reason for the behaviour. Because they trigger the behaviour and occur before the behaviour happens, we often overlook these things. The because is important. If you can determine what triggers an undesirable behaviour, you may be able to remove the trigger and stop the behaviour from happening.

There are four main sources of triggers. Examining each as a potential source of the action may help you to define the likely reason.

1. **Emotional and physical health.** A person who is ill, in pain, tired, already frightened or upset may react unpredictably. Sometimes, the trigger is a biological need. For example, a person who wanders may have to use the washroom. Similarly, emotional needs can trigger behaviours. A person who needs the comfort of others may refuse to leave an area where other people are present.
2. **Environment.** Sometimes, the environment is too busy, too noisy, or even too hot or cold. Environmental distractions can overstimulate the person, causing the person to react unpredictably. A loss of personal space can cause a person to strike out at another. A confusing environment can heighten a person's disorientation and trigger anxiety or fear. For example, a resident of a long-term care facility who cannot tell which room is his or hers may end up in other residents' rooms, causing upset to all concerned. Placing a distinctive wreath on the resident's door may help the resident to find the right room more easily.
3. **Tasks or demands.** A task that is too complex or that needs to be done too quickly may overwhelm the person and trigger anger or anxiety. Similarly, too much to do at any one time may overwhelm the person.
4. **Communication.** Difficulty in understanding communication or in making oneself understood can trigger anxiety or aggression.

CASE EXAMPLE 23-7

A facility noticed that cognitively impaired residents regularly refused to enter a particular elevator in the home. This elevator was in a wing that had been recently renovated. The problem was not noticed until after the renovation. Staff members decided to observe resident behaviour to see if they could find out what the problem was. They soon realized that a black rubber strip placed at the entrance to the elevator was apparently frightening the residents. It appeared as though residents felt that the black strip was a hole into which they might fall. Replacing the strip with a brighter coloured one solved the problem.

Once you've determined the possible triggers, you can attempt to eliminate or change them so that they do not provoke the behaviour. Preventing the behaviour will likely save the client a great deal of distress as well as make your job easier.

The Communication

It's extremely important to share what you have learned with others who assist the client. First, this improves the quality and the consistency of the support provided, making it easier for you and the client. Second, you may have identified an approach that works, or works many times. This may (and likely is) a problem that others have had. Sharing this information will help them to better do what they do.

Never assume that something is obvious, just because you've figured it out. Share what you know and what you know works with others. Make certain that the useful information is communicated to your supervisor and included in the client's support plan.

You will not be able to prevent every challenging behaviour. There will be situations when you will have to respond to an unexpected and challenging situation. How you respond to a challenging behaviour is important because it can either reduce the behaviour or make it worse. This section discusses some common behaviours and possible responses.

Wandering

Wandering can often be linked to a specific event, such as the need to use the bathroom, the desire to see others, or to get exercise. Remember that the activity has meaning for the person. Try to identify the reason the person is wandering. If you cannot determine this, or if the wandering seems to be in response to a need for exercise or stimulation, the best approach may be to provide a safe area in which he or she can wander. If you must stop a wandering client, try to distract him or her or gently guide the person in the desired direction. A restraint should not be used to control wandering, as it can cause the client to become very angry and aggressive.

CASE EXAMPLE 23-8

Eddah Ampar often wanders throughout the halls of the long-term care facility where she lives. The support workers who care for her have determined that Mrs. Ampar's wandering is related to a need for exercise and a need to see other people.

Occasionally, support workers have to stop Mrs. Ampar in order to bring her to the dining room or to help her get ready for bed. The support workers have found that trying to stop Mrs. Ampar makes her upset and can cause her to yell at the staff.

The support workers spoke with their supervisor. The supervisor arranged a meeting so that the issue could be discussed and some possible approaches identified. As a result of that meeting, the support workers have begun to walk with Mrs. Ampar for a bit as they gently guide her in the direction they desire her to go. When the workers approach Mrs. Ampar is this manner, she rarely becomes upset. In fact, she seems to enjoy the workers' company as they walk.

Anger or Aggression

Anger and aggression are usually signs that the person is frightened and feels the need to defend or protect himself or herself. These behaviours can be linked to many causes. The environment can be too stimulating, the environment may be unfamiliar, or there may be many unfamiliar people or sounds in a familiar setting. Losing sight of a familiar person or object can cause the person to feel suddenly alone and insecure. Sudden movements or startling noises (such as a yell or scream) may put the person on guard. Even the difficulty of adapting to varying levels of light (such as when the person leaves a brightly lit hallway to enter a dark room) may upset the person, as he or she cannot see well enough to become comfortable with the surroundings.

Physical causes can also trigger anger or aggression. Fatigue or sleep deprivation can cause the person to become angry when bothered (much as it might cause you to become irritable). Physical discomfort (such as that caused by pain or even constipation) can trigger anger. Other potential triggers include the side effects of medications, hallucinations, or sensory loss.

Anger or aggression can be triggered for psychological reasons as well. The person may be reacting to the pressure of too many demands at once. The person may be frustrated in response to a lack of ability or upset over a change in routine. As well, many people with a dementia can easily adopt the emotions of others (for example, becoming angry if there is another angry person in the area). Inappropriate communication, such as being scolded, confronted, or treated in an offensive manner, can cause the person to become angry or aggressive.

The best response to angry or aggressive behaviour is to eliminate the trigger. Attempt to determine the reason for the anger or aggression. Can you eliminate or reduce it? Sometimes, you can minimize an angry or aggressive outburst if you can "catch" it as it begins. Many times, a person's body language will warn of anger before it happens. Get to know these signs. As well, avoid surprising a client. Surprise often turns to fear when the person cannot easily understand what is going on.

If you must respond to a client who is angry or aggressive, use these guidelines:

1. **Use a quiet approach.** Be gentle and calm. Do not yell or be forceful.
2. **Do not ridicule or attempt to "laugh off" the situation.** Your actions will tell the person that you are making fun of him or her.
3. **Make sure that the person's surroundings are calm and quiet.** Turn off radios or televisions. Ask others nearby to leave the area if possible.
4. **Don't overwhelm the person with too many commands, too many words, or speech that is too rapid.** This simply heightens the person's sense of a loss of control and may heighten the anger.
5. **Listen to the person's words and body language.** He or she may say or do something that indicates the source of the anger. As well, the act of calmly listening and attempting to understand may calm the person.
6. **Don't challenge the person.** Attempting to reason with the person or to force the person to do something may provoke more anger or even physical violence.
7. **Distract the person if possible.** You can sometimes reduce the anger by causing the person to focus on something else.
8. **Give the person private space when necessary.** Leave the room if possible. Ask others to do the same. Give the person a few minutes to calm down before returning.
9. **Avoid restraining the person.** The use of a restraint will almost certainly be seen as a sign of aggression. It usually heightens the person's anger. Try leaving the person alone in a room instead.

CASE EXAMPLE 23-9

Mr. Krall has Alzheimer Disease. He is in the middle stages of the disease. He lives at home while he awaits admission to a long-term care facility. He receives support service five days per week. Mr. Krall can very quickly become angry if he is startled or if someone near him is moving very quickly. In particular, he will become angry if someone tries to quickly make him do something. He will strike out at a support worker who insists he do something.

Support workers have learned that they can best assist Mr. Krall by gently asking him to participate. If he refuses, the support worker does not press the issue. She leaves him alone for a few moments. When she returns, Mr. Krall is often no longer angry. This information is now included in Mr. Krall's support plan, so any new worker knows how to approach this situation.

10. **Use touch carefully.** To an angry person, touch can be perceived as a sign of aggression.
11. **Do not argue with the person.** Instead, gently repeat information.
12. **Never approach anger with anger.**

Catastrophic Reactions

A catastrophic reaction is an overreaction to a situation. The person is not able to control these reactions, which are often unpredictable, although the reaction may occasionally be preceded by flushing, restlessness, or a refusal to receive care.

When you respond to the client, you must be aware that the behaviour is not wilful. Attempt to reduce the resident's feelings of anxiety and panic by providing comfort and support.

You may be able to prevent some catastrophic reactions by maintaining familiar routines and a quiet environment. Interpersonal approaches can also help. Always approach the person from the front, and remain in his or her field of vision. Introduce new persons and situations carefully and slowly. Avoid attempting to force the person to do things beyond his or her capacity.

Delusions, Paranoia, and Hallucinations

Remember that delusions, paranoia, or hallucinations are the person's reality. Telling a person that what he sees, hears, or believes is wrong will not help. Focus your efforts on preventing frightening episodes by ensuring that the person feels safe and secure. Try to create a calm and nonthreatening environment. You should also attempt to identify any physical causes of hallucinatory behaviour (such as fever, dehydration, or poor nutrition).

If a person is experiencing delusions, paranoia, or hallucinations, try the following:

1. **Do not argue or try to rationalize with the person.** This will only upset the person.
2. **Reassure or distract the person if he or she feels threatened.** Some hallucinations may not be threatening to the person.
3. **Ensure that the person is not misinterpreting the situation.** It may help to explain that what the person sees as a dead body is actually a pile of laundry on the floor. If the person cannot accept your explanation, do not argue.
4. **If the person is not in distress or causing others distress, ignore the behaviour.**
5. **Problems in hearing or vision may contribute to hallucinations and paranoia.** Monitor the person for physical causes of the behaviour and report as necessary.

ACQUIRED BRAIN INJURY

Acquired brain injury, or traumatic brain injury, refers to brain injuries that occur as a result of any one of the following five factors:

- **Trauma:** This includes injuries caused by motor vehicle accidents; by being hit with a pole, brick, or bat; by sustaining a fall; as well as gunshot wounds.
- **Anoxia:** This is an injury caused by the lack of oxygen in the brain (such as that caused by carbon monoxide poisoning, a cardiac arrest, or an airway obstruction).

- **Vascular:** These are injuries caused by a hemorrhage, the result of surgery, or a vascular malformation. Some definitions also include strokes in this category. Others exclude all strokes except those caused by a hemorrhage.
- **Seizure:** This is an injury caused by seizures.
- **Toxins:** This is an injury caused by substance abuse, ingestion of lead, or inhaling volatile agents (such as glue or gasoline).

Acquired brain injuries do not include conditions that are inherited, that are present at birth, or that are progressive. Acquired brain injuries are not caused by dementias.

The majority of acquired brain injuries are the result of motor vehicle accidents. More men than women are affected by this type. Most accident-related brain injury occurs in people between the ages of 16 and 24 years of age. Falls account for a significant number of brain injuries. In fact, falls are among the leading causes of acquired brain injuries among older adults.

The Effect of Brain Injuries

The effect of a brain injury will depend upon the size and location of the injury, as well as whether or not the person has experienced any secondary problems such as infection, problems that arise from the brain's reaction to the injury (such as changes in the affected blood vessels, swelling, bruising), or increased pressure in the brain. Cells damaged by the primary injury can release chemicals and other products that cause additional damage. In many cases, the secondary effects can be more damaging than the initial injury.

Keep in mind that the person's ability to recover may change from day to day or even hour to hour. What could be done easily at one time may be impossible just hours later. Identifying when, where, and with whom the person is most able is important to understanding when a particular task is appropriate and when it is too difficult.

Loss of memory is one of the most common effects. The person may find it difficult to remember common and familiar information, such as people's names. New information, such as remembering details of a phone message or an appointment, may be difficult. The person may become lost in familiar territory or forget where he or she left things.

CASE EXAMPLE 23-10

Carlos Martino is a 34-year-old who sustained a head injury in a car accident two years ago. Until the accident, he was a senior sales representative for a utility company. Although Carlos had few physical injuries from the accident, his brain injury impaired his ability to coordinate his activities. He finds it difficult to drive.

A year ago, Carlos's employer offered him a job that did not require him to drive. However, Carlos has memory problems that are minor on one day and very significant on the next. As a result, he was not able to do the tasks required. He received a disability pension and "retired."

Carlos has found his inability to work frustrating. He has always kept busy. Now, sometimes even the simplest things are impossible for him to do. He does enjoy working in a volunteer position with a local agency. He is able to go to the agency on his "good" days.

Carlos uses support services to help him organize himself, to get ready for his volunteer work, and to help him manage his banking and bill paying. His support workers adapt to the dramatic changes in Carlos's ability from day to day. They also recognize that Carlos is an intelligent person who has significant impairments in some abilities.

Brain injury can also affect the person's ability to plan, initiate, or properly organize activities. Simple, once-familiar tasks, such as getting a glass of milk, may become very frustrating. Problem-solving abilities may also be impaired. A person may make quick and poor judgments or not react at all to a situation. Common social skills may also be lost, making it difficult and embarrassing for the person to take part in social activities.

There also may be losses in the ability to focus one's attention, to respond quickly to a situation, to sequence physical movements, as well as to control impulses. Hearing, vision, and perception may become altered either as a result of the primary injury or a secondary injury.

The person also may experience loss of the ability to actually control movement. In some cases, the person may develop abnormal bone growth in certain joints (such as the hips, shoulders, knees, and elbows). This bone growth is called heterotopic ossification and is a secondary effect of the brain injury.

Supporting a Person with a Brain Injury

Supporting a person with a brain injury is a complex and daunting task. Most people who sustain a moderate or severe injury will have to make adaptations and adjustments throughout their lives. Even people who have made significant recovery will have to cope with problems related to the injury.

Each person's situation will be different. People with the same type of injury will often require different coping and support strategies. It is extremely important that a support plan be developed with the person and that the plan be followed by all persons supporting the person.

You may find that some strategies used to support a person with a brain injury are similar to those used for other conditions, such as stroke or dementia. Do not assume from this that the person's brain injury is the same as the other condition. It is not.

In many cases, the person will have family support. Note that the family will also be making adjustments as they learn to get along with the changes the injury has brought about. Like your client, the family may show a mixture of joy (that the person has survived) and grief (that the person has changed). Support the client and family members as they deal with these emotions.

Questions for Review

1. What six processes make up cognition?

2. What are the seven A's of cognitive impairment?

3. What are the two main categories of cognitive impairments?

4. Do all irreversible cognitive impairments continue to get worse with time? If not, which conditions are nonprogressive?

5. Is confusion the same as cognitive impairment? Why or why not?

6. What do we call dementia that occurs in a younger person?

7. What is the most common cause of irreversible dementia?

8. How does vascular dementia differ from Alzheimer Disease?

9. What seven principles are fundamental to the support of the person with dementia?

10. What questions should you ask when you are trying to problem-solve new or puzzling behaviour?

11. What are five principles of interpretative communication?

12. Are all hallucinations distressing to a person? Why or why not?

13. What causes an acquired brain injury?

14. You are assigned to a client who has an acquired brain injury. What should you keep in mind as you work with this client?

Questions for Discussion

1. You are assigned to a client with dementia to complete his or her care. How might you assess the client's ability to do the tasks involved? How might you support the client to perform the tasks of which he or she is capable?

2. You are to take your client for a walk. When you get into the hallway, the client looks from side to side, backs up, and refuses to enter the doorway. Use the A-B-C approach to identify what might be the cause of the situation and report on your response. Discuss your approach with your colleagues.

3. Today, you are preparing Mr. Urich for a bath. When you approach him with the towels, he begins to scream at you. He raises his fist to strike out. What do you do?

4. You have been assigned to assist a client with Alzheimer Disease. What can you do to make communication with the client easier?

Chapter 24

Abuse

Learning Objectives

Through reading this chapter, you'll be able to

1. Define abuse.
2. Discuss the role of the support worker.
3. List the four major forms of abuse.
4. Explain the cycle of abuse.
5. Describe the possible indicators of infant or child abuse, spousal abuse, and elder abuse.
6. Outline the steps a support worker should take if abuse is suspected.

Chapter at a Glance

- Abuse
- The Effect of Abuse
- The Role of the Support Worker
- Forms of Abuse
- The Cycle of Abuse
- Child Abuse
- Spousal Abuse
- Elder Abuse
- What to Do

Terms You'll Use

Abuse Harm to a victim caused by anyone upon whom the victim relies for basic needs or support.

Cycle of Abuse A term used to describe the three phases of abuse: abuse, remorse, and anger escalation.

Failure to Thrive A condition that occurs when abuse causes a child to fail to grow and develop.

Infantilize The treatment of an adult like a child.

Neglect The intentional or unintentional failure to provide the essentials of life.

ABUSE

When I hear the term abuse I think of the following things:

_____
_____
_____
_____

The emotions I associate with the term abuse are:

_____
_____
_____

If I am faced with a situation that I think might be abusive, my first reaction is (or would be) to:

_____
_____
_____

If I had to identify factors that might be linked to abuse, I would list the following:

_____
_____
_____

What came to your mind when you thought of the term abuse? Many people first think of physical violence. However, the definition is much broader than just physical abuse. **Abuse** can be defined as any harm to the victim caused by anyone upon whom the victim relies for basic needs or support. Abuse occurs in relationships where the victim is under the control or influence of the offender. The definition of abuse generally does not include self-neglect or victimization by an unknown assailant.

Some types of abuse are easier to define than others. Physical and financial abuse are sometimes much easier to identify than are other types of abuse. Sometimes people (even professionals trained to work with situations of abuse) can disagree on whether a specific situation is abusive. Sometimes, the person others see as a victim does not agree that abuse has taken place. All these issues can make it difficult to determine what, if anything, should be done.

Abuse can occur across the life span. Children and spouses as well as older adults can be abused. People of any financial status may be abused. Sometimes, more than one type of abuse occurs within the same family.

Abuse is an issue that often provokes strong feelings. Review your answer to Stop and Reflect 24-1 about the emotions you associate with abuse. Did you have feelings of anger? Perhaps you felt sadness or even embarrassment for a victim. People in abusive relationships often are embarrassed to admit that it is happening or are ashamed of their behaviour. Some victims may feel that they have done something to provoke the abuse—that the abuse is somehow their fault. Some (both abusers and victims) may be afraid of what may happen if the abuse is reported or discovered.

THE EFFECT OF ABUSE

In addition to the effects directly related to the abusive actions, the experience of being abused may affect the person's emotional, social, physical, and sexual development and well-being. The effect abuse has on a person is most often determined by four factors: the nature and severity of the abuse, the abuser's relationship to the victim, the type(s) of threat or coercion used, and the quality of the intervention made by others to stop the abuse.

THE ROLE OF THE SUPPORT WORKER

If you were faced with a situation you felt might be abusive, what would your first reaction be? You might have said "to stop the abuse," or "to help the person leave the situation," or even "to make the abuser stop." You might have very strong feelings about your need to help. While you have a role to play in helping the victim of abuse, you are not responsible to deal directly with the abuse (or suspected abuse) unless the victim is in a life-threatening situation in your presence.

As a support worker, your responsibilities are threefold. First, you are responsible for accurately reporting any observations or suspicions of abuse to your supervisor immediately so that your supervisor may take the appropriate action. Second, you are responsible for providing emotional support to the client. Third, if you are assigned to a client who has been abused, you are responsible to follow the support plan established to support the client. The last section of this chapter discusses how you might fulfill these responsibilities.

FORMS OF ABUSE

There are five major forms of abuse: psychological, physical, sexual, financial, and neglect. All forms of abuse involve one person exercising power over another. A person might not experience all types of abuse, but most abuse also causes psychological harm.

Psychological Abuse

Psychological abuse is sometimes called verbal abuse. Because it attacks a person's needs to feel safe, secure, and to belong, psychological abuse can be very damaging to the person. Someone who abuses another in this manner may humiliate the person (such as intentionally embarrassing the person in front of others) or insult the person by calling the person "stupid," "a moron," or "an idiot." Some people infantilize an adult by treating him or her like a child.

Another form of psychological abuse includes not speaking to the person, ignoring the person, or behaving as though the person wasn't there. It also includes isolating the person by not allowing him or her to take part in conversations and activities or by not allowing the person to have visitors. A third form consists of saying things to frighten or threaten the person.

Physical Abuse

Physical abuse occurs when a person experiences actual physical harm. The harm can take many forms: slapping, pushing, kicking, pinching, hitting, or beating. It can also take the form of intentionally rough treatment, such as pulling hair, allowing someone to drop when being helped from a bed to a chair, and using bath water that is far too hot or cold. Chemically or physically restraining a person is also a form of physical abuse.

Sexual Abuse

This form of abuse includes inappropriate sexual comments or jokes, intimidation of the person by jealous comments or actions, and unwanted or uncomfortable touching or kissing. Sexual assault (assault, forced intercourse, harassment, or use of the person as a subject of pornography without the person's knowledge and consent) is also a form of sexual abuse.

Financial Abuse

Financial abuse includes the misuse or theft of a person's money or possessions. It includes forcing a person to sell property, stealing his or her money or personal possessions, forging a person's signature on pension cheques to obtain money, as well as using a legitimately obtained power of attorney to improperly use the client's resources or dispose of the client's property.

CASE EXAMPLE 24-1

Mrs. Fiona McGillvray had always lived in the same province. Because of increasing health problems, she recently moved to a different province to live with her son, his wife, and three teenaged daughters. Mrs. McGillvray's family was unprepared to help her meet her care needs. They were not able to arrange for the time to take her to many medical appointments. They also did not know how to help her find friends and social activities in her new home.

As Mrs. McGillvray's condition worsened, tension grew. Mrs. McGillvray was asked to eat in her room, not with the rest of the family. When her calls to friends at "home" increased the telephone bill, the calls were limited to no more than five minutes once each week.

What factors indicate that there may be abuse occurring against Mrs. McGillvray?

Neglect

Neglect is defined as the intentional or unintentional failure to provide the person with the essentials of life. This can include abandoning (even for short periods of time) a person who cannot safely be left at home or denying a dependent person food, liquid, medication, or access to health services (such as not taking the person to the doctor or not allowing health professionals to visit). Neglect can also occur when the person is left in an unclean or unsafe environment or when a person is not allowed to have the stimulation of social contacts, entertainment, or exercise.

Sometimes, neglect results from the caregiver not performing the duties required to appropriately care for a person. The person might be careless, forget, or not learn the proper methods of caring for specific needs (such as how to properly apply a dressing).

When an infant, child, or frail older adult is involved, neglect can be particularly serious due to the victim's size and the extent to which the victim depends upon the person. Neglect can easily be fatal in infants or very dependent older people (for example, if the caregiver does not even feed the person). Neglect also includes the denial of necessary affection.

THE CYCLE OF ABUSE

Once an abusive incident happens, it usually happens again and again unless something is done to stop it. This is called the cycle of abuse. It has three phases: the incident phase, the guilt or remorse phase, and the anger escalation phase. Figure 24-1 illustrates these phases.

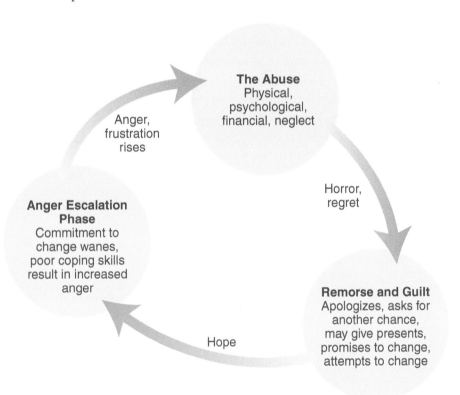

FIGURE 24-1
Cycle of abuse

The Incident Phase

This is the phase when the abusive incident or incidents occur. Keep in mind that the abuse takes place even if the person who has been abused does not know that it has happened. In cases of financial abuse or neglect, the person who has been abused may not be aware at all.

The Guilt or Remorse Phase

This is the phase when the abuser reacts to the event. Many abusers will react with guilt or remorse. The person may vow not to abuse again and may make this promise to the victim. It's important to be aware that the abuser may have genuine guilt or remorse. The abuser may truly believe that he or she will be able to break the cycle. However, it is unlikely that the cycle will be broken unless help is sought.

The client may truly believe that the abuser will change based upon his or her change in behaviour. This may allow the person to deny a problem for an extended period of time.

The Anger Escalation Phase

This is the phase when the abuser's commitment to changing wanes and poor coping skills give way to another incident of abuse. Without assistance, this phase culminates in another abusive incident, starting the cycle anew.

CHILD ABUSE

Most information on child abuse is divided into two types: physical abuse and sexual abuse. Researchers estimate that about 10 percent of all children experience physical abuse by a parent or caretaker. It's estimated that about one in five male children and one in four female children will experience unwanted sexual acts.

We sometimes have an image of a child abuser as a stranger. This is not usually the case. Most abusers are people known to the child. Only a small percentage are strangers. Researchers suggest that the abuser may have once been a victim and that the likelihood of abuse may increase with stress or economic or internal pressures.

Many provinces have special regulations for the reporting of child abuse or suspected child abuse. In some provinces, you may be legally required to report observations or suspicions directly to the provincial Children's Aid Society. You must learn the reporting requirements for your province.

Indicators of Child Abuse

Remember that the presence of certain behaviours does not necessarily mean that abuse is occurring. There may be other reasons for these behaviours. Report your observations to your supervisor immediately if you notice any of these indicators. Remember, your province may require you to report suspected child abuse to a local or provincial authority.

Psychological Abuse

The following behaviours may be associated with psychological abuse.

The adult abuser may use the child as a scapegoat, blaming the child for things that are beyond the child's control. The adult may tell the child that he or she is bad or tell other people (in the child's presence) that the child is bad. The adult may reject the child, withhold affection, or isolate the child from other children or all other people. The adult may use power to coerce the child to do something, such as bribing, manipulating, or intimidating.

The child may have a variety of responses. He or she may appear depressed, withdrawn, aggressive, or display extreme attention-seeking behaviours. The child may attempt too hard to please others, be overly compliant, or extremely well mannered.

Children may also have physical problems, such as an inability to control their bowel or bladder. The child may also have frequent psychosomatic complaints (complaints of physical problems for which a physical cause cannot be found).

Physical Abuse

In addition to bruises, cuts, burns, and other physical injuries, there may be other indicators of physical abuse. It is extremely important to keep in mind that many of these indicators may be the result of other factors, not abuse.

The adult may have little or no knowledge of child development and may express difficulty coping with the child or show little or no affection toward the child. The adult may indicate that the child is injury prone. The adult may also lie about the child's injuries, give inconsistent explanations about injuries, or even delay seeking treatment.

The child may have several injuries at various stages of healing. He or she may "forget" how injuries happened or have explanations inconsistent with the injuries. The child may be wary of adults or cringe if touched unexpectedly. Some children may display extreme behaviours, such as extreme aggression, withdrawal, overt compliance, or excessive eagerness to please others.

Failure to Thrive

In extreme cases, the abuse may cause the child to fail to grow and develop. This condition is called **failure to thrive**. This is an extremely dangerous form of child abuse that can be life threatening.

The adult may reject the child or ignore the child's attempts to be affectionate. The adult may indicate that the child was and is unwanted or label the child difficult to care for.

The child may appear lethargic, to move very little, or to be disinterested in the surroundings. It is not uncommon for these children to display little anxiety or cry very little, if at all. The child may appear pale and extremely thin with an extremely low body-fat ratio. Some children will stop growing altogether. Most of these children will not have met developmental milestones normal for children their age.

SPOUSAL ABUSE

CASE EXAMPLE 24-2

Carrie Worth is a 32-year-old woman with three children all under five years of age. She is recovering from a severe fracture of her left leg. She fractured her leg when her husband threw her down the basement stairs. When hospital emergency room staff asked her about the incident, she told them, "He had a right to be angry. I burned the mashed potatoes and dinner was late." Hospital staff encouraged her to enter a shelter, but she refused. She returned home with her husband.

Why do you think Carrie returned home? How would you feel if you were working with her? Could you act on your feelings?

Both men and women can be victims of spousal abuse, although women are most often the victims. It's estimated that almost 50 percent of women have experienced some form of abuse. Unlike children, we see adults as able to make decisions and take action. It may be difficult to understand why the victim does not simply leave an abusive relationship. You must become aware that there may be many factors that make it difficult for the victim to leave.

The abuser may intimidate and isolate the victim, gradually stripping the victim of all outside contacts and supports. The victim may believe that he or she is incapable of leaving the relationship.

Abusers may exert control over the victim through the victim's children, by using the children to convey messages, by threatening to take the children away, or by attempting to make the victim feel guilty about all the "upset" the victim has caused. The abuser may also threaten to withdraw economic support, prevent the victim from getting a job, or prohibit the victim access to family funds.

Indicators of Spousal Abuse

Psychological Abuse

It's very likely that indicators of psychological abuse will accompany indicators of physical or financial abuse. Isolation, lack of social contacts, loss of contact with family, as well as a reliance upon the abuser for the necessities of life may all be present. The victim may feel helpless or state that the abuse was deserved.

Physical Abuse

Indicators of physical abuse include old and new injuries. In many cases, recent injuries are more severe than earlier injuries. The victim may deny the injuries or have explanations for their cause that do not make sense. He or she may cover injuries with clothing or makeup.

ELDER ABUSE

Although both men and women can be victims of elder abuse, a typical victim is likely to be over 75 and female. She is likely to be widowed or single. While the victim may have progressive physical or mental impairments, most are competent. Most victims are socially isolated and increasingly dependent upon the abuser to meet their needs. The victim may take on the role of a child.

Many victims of elder abuse deny the abuse and, even if they don't, they are reluctant to report the abuse. Some may feel that discussing abuse brings shame to them or to their family. They may worry about the abuser and fear that the family will be broken up if the abuse is reported. They may fear that they will lose contact with the person, even if that contact is abusive. The person may fear finding another place to live or having to move to a long-term care facility. Some older adults may not recognize the abuse as abuse or may feel that the abuse is deserved. The person may also fear more abuse if the abuser is reported.

The abuser is usually middle-aged, and often is the child of the victim. The abuser is frequently experiencing stress (such as financial, medical, marital, substance abuse, or unemployment). The abuser may feel that increasing demands of the caretaking role deplete family resources and often resents the need to care for the parent. The abuser may also feel dependent upon the victim for emotional or financial support.

Potential Indicators of Elder Abuse

Caregiver Characteristics

The following caregiver behaviours may indicate an abusive (or potentially abusive) situation. As with all indicators, you must not make the assumption that the presence of one or more means that abuse is present. Discuss any observations with your supervisor.

A caregiver may respond defensively when asked about the health of the older adult. The caregiver may make excuses or be hostile, suspicious, or evasive about explanations. The caregiver may not want the older adult to be interviewed alone.

The caregiver may appear excessively concerned or unconcerned about the older person. He or she may "blame" the elder for conditions, like forgetfulness or incontinence, yet refuse to permit hospitalization or diagnostic tests.

The caregiver may show signs of stress, often as the result of needlessly taking on all the older adult's care without help. He or she may have been a caregiver for an extended period of time and may appear tired. The caregiver may have been forced (or felt forced) to take on the caregiving situation and, as a result, may resent having to provide care.

Victim Characteristics

The older adult may show signs of neglect (unclean, thin, or dehydrated) or physical abuse. He or she may have medical needs that have not been addressed.

The older adult may withdraw from contact with others or be anxious or fearful of communication. He or she may be unwilling to discuss the relationship with the caregiver or any problems in caregiving. The older adult may be demanding or hostile and may be verbally abusive.

Some older adults may express fear of having "no place to go" or fear that they will have to leave their home if abuse is discovered. There may be evidence that a competent person has lost control over his or her financial affairs.

Indicators of Elder Abuse

The indicators of elder abuse are virtually identical to those of spousal abuse.

Psychological Abuse

It's very likely that indicators of psychological abuse will accompany indicators of physical or financial abuse. Isolation, lack of social contacts, loss of contact with family, as well as a reliance upon the abuser for the necessities of life may all be present. The victim may feel helpless or state that the abuse was deserved.

Physical Abuse

Indicators of physical abuse include old and new injuries. In many cases, recent injuries are more severe than earlier injuries. The victim may deny the injuries or have explanations for their cause that do not make sense. He or she may cover injuries with clothing or makeup.

Neglect and Failure to Thrive

An adult who suffers neglect will show many of the same symptoms of a neglected infant or child. The adult may shun communication, show no interest in others, or even seem to fear contact. There may be evidence of poor personal care and lack of medical attention.

WHAT TO DO

It is extremely important to be aware of the scope of your role in reporting observations and supporting the client. Your agency will have specific guidelines for providing support in these cases. The nine guidelines below provide some general guidance as to assistance you can provide.

1. **Report suspicions of abuse to your supervisor.** Do not assume that someone else will do it.
2. **If asked, assist the abuser in obtaining help.** Contact your supervisor to determine the specific steps you should take when assisting the abuser.
3. **Find out what resources for victims of abuse exist in your area.** Make sure that you have telephone numbers available if a client should ask for them.
4. **Observe for indicators and report your observations to your supervisor immediately.**
5. **Listen to the client.** Do not judge the client or insist that he or she do something.
6. **Offer information if the client wants it.**
7. **Support the client in taking action, but do not insist that the client do so.** Recognize that a competent abused person has a right to maintain his or her lifestyle—you cannot force the client to make changes he or she does not want.
8. **Do not assume that one person's method of addressing an abusive situation will apply to all others.** What has worked for someone else—or even for you—may not be right for the person. Do not insist that a person take a particular approach.
9. **Maintain your relationship with the client, even if other types of assistance are refused.** The client still needs your support. If you withdraw support, the client may find it very difficult if he or she does decide to seek help at a later date.

Questions for Review

1. What are the five general types of abuse? What are the signs of each type?

2. Describe the cycle of abuse.

3. What factors can make it difficult for a person to admit that he or she has been abused?

4. Identify indicators of abuse in infants and children.

5. Why is neglect so dangerous? What three types of people are most at risk of neglect?

6. What are indicators of spousal abuse?

7. What are the indicators of elder abuse?

Questions for Discussion

1. Is the existence of abuse always easy to define? What factors can make it difficult for the people involved to agree that abuse exists?

2. Imagine that a client tells you that his family is abusing him. He says that his daughter is making him sign over his Canada Pension cheque. He tells you that he doesn't know what she does with the money, and when he asks his daughter, she yells at him. What are your feelings? What should you do? Why?

3. Review this case study. As a support worker, what steps would you take?

You are assigned to assist Sandy Rendor to care for her newborn twin girls. She also has a two-year-old daughter and a four-year-old son. The twins were born prematurely and spent some time in hospital. One was in critical condition for some time. They are both now home but are still frail. Both babies require monitoring to ensure that they do not stop breathing. Sandy's husband, Dale, travels a great deal, so the primary responsibility for care rests with Sandy.

Today, as you are assisting Sandy with the laundry, the four-year-old comes into the room holding one of the twins' breathing monitors. It is supposed to be on the baby as she is napping. The four-year-old says: "Baby's sleeping, mom—this could wake her up." You know that he has heard the alarm sound.

Sandy yells at the four-year-old, grabbing the monitor from him. She grabs his arm and tells him he's a bad boy and to never do that again. You are surprised at the level of her anger as she is normally a loving parent.

Chapter 25

Palliative Care

Learning Objectives

Through reading this chapter, you'll be able to

1. Describe the range of attitudes Canadians have toward death.
2. Define palliation and palliative care.
3. Discuss the role of the support worker providing palliative care.
4. Outline the impact of life-threatening illness on the client, the client's family, and the support worker.
5. Explain the client's rights with regard to treatment and resuscitation.
6. Demonstrate specific techniques (within the scope of support work) to promote comfort and help alleviate pain.
7. Describe signs of apparent death and care of the body after death.
8. Define grief and discuss aspects of grief work.

Chapter at a Glance

- Attitudes Toward Dying and Death
- Culture, Life-Threatening Illness, Dying, and Bereavement
- Palliative Care (or Palliation)
- The Role of the Support Worker in Palliative Care
- The Impact of Life-Threatening Illness
- Living Wills and Do-Not-Resuscitate Orders
- Promoting Comfort and Reducing Pain
- When Death Is Near
- At the Time of Death
- Care of the Body After Death
- Grief and Grief Work

Terms You'll Use

Anticipatory Grief The sense of loss, grieving, and preparing to move on that can occur before an expected loss happens.

Do-Not-Resuscitate Orders A document that states a person is not to receive life-sustaining measures.

Grief Work Tasks associated with moving through the phases of grieving.

Hospice A form of support and care for people who are terminally ill.

Life-Threatening Illness An illness that is likely to cause death.

Living Will A document that gives specific instructions as to the care and treatment a person wants; also called an advance directive.

Palliative Care Active and compassionate care with the purpose to provide comfort and control pain, not to cure.

ATTITUDES TOWARD DYING AND DEATH

The experience of dying and death is intensely personal. No two people—even two siblings who experience the death of a parent—will see the experience in the same way. Our responses are the result of our personalities, culture, coping mechanisms, experiences with previous deaths, as well as the social supports we have to assist us.

Nonetheless, Canada is seen as a death-ignoring society. By this we mean that, although we all are aware that people die, as a society we do not see death as a natural consequence of living. Researchers attribute this to two things: that we have moved death from the person's home to the institution, and that we have developed technology to treat many conditions, leading to a belief that death can be avoided in many cases. Let's look at each of these more closely.

Where People Die

At the turn of the last century, most deaths occurred at home. People did not go to the hospital to die. Care was provided in the person's home, often by family members who learned how to give the necessary care. This gave people the opportunity to see death as a natural occurrence as well as to be able to assist in making a person comfortable.

Gradually, people began to go to institutions such as hospitals or long-term care facilities near the end of their lives. In part, this was due to advances in treatment that were available only in hospitals. Additionally, Canadians were increasingly becoming two-career families, leaving no one at home to care for a dying person.

Today, we estimate that about 70 percent of people die in a hospital or long-term care facility. This has made death less familiar to people and, therefore, somewhat frightening.

Treatment Advances

Many treatment advances have occurred in the last century. As a result, many conditions once thought incurable can now be cured. This has altered how we see illness and death, making it easier to believe that almost everything can be cured. It is called the medicalization of death, and it has had the effect of making dying and death seem to be something beyond the scope of families, requiring it to be managed only by professionals.

The Hospice Movement

The hospice movement is dedicated to the compassionate care of people who are dying. Canada's hospice movement is based on the St. Christopher's Hospice of London, England, that was founded by Cicely Saunders in 1967. A hospice is a residence where terminally ill people can receive support and care. There are only a few hospice residences. In Canada, the hospice movement provides support to many people who choose to die in their homes.

The hospice movement has been instrumental in changing Canadian attitudes about dying and death. Because of this movement, people are once again seeing death as a natural part of life. People who are terminally ill are now more likely to remain at home. Families are becoming more involved in the support of the dying person. As a result, support workers are frequently involved in supporting both the client and his or her family.

STOP AND REFLECT ((25-1))

How do you see death?

_____

_____

_____

From whom did you learn about death?

_____

_____

_____

To what extent are your views about death influenced by your culture?

_____

_____

_____

_____

To what extent are your views about death influenced by your personal experience?

_____

_____

_____

_____

Your Own Attitudes

Support workers providing palliative care must carefully examine their beliefs and attitudes about death prior to working with clients requiring this care. It is extremely important that the worker ensures that personal attitudes, fears, or anxieties do not interfere with the ability to care for the client.

CULTURE, LIFE-THREATENING ILLNESS, DYING, AND BEREAVEMENT

Canada is a multicultural country. Death is a significant event in most cultures, but there are many ways in which death is viewed. This challenges us to both question and adapt our approaches to better meet the needs of people who view dying and death differently.

CASE EXAMPLE 25-1

An older Asian woman feels that her cancer is punishment for not having cared for her mother when her mother was ill many years ago. She feels that she is not deserving of care and asks her support workers to leave because of this.

What are some of the different views you have heard about life-threatening illness and dying? Why do you think the differences in views exist?

As you'll recall from our discussion in Chapter 7, each person is the product of a unique personal culture. A person's views on life-threatening illness, dying, death, and bereavement may be heavily influenced by religion, previous experiences, as well as ethnic practices (Figure 25-1).

Ethnic rituals Personal
experiences Religious beliefs
Notions of what is a "good death"
The right age Role of
Expectations traditional
of family or folk
members treatment
Spiritual Role of
needs medical
treatment

FIGURE 25-1
Perceptions of life-threatening illness, dying, and death are influenced by many things

It is not helpful to assume that people will act a certain way or hold certain beliefs just because they are members of a particular ethnic group. You must learn how your client sees the situation, what he or she feels is appropriate treatment, and how the client sees your role. Equally important is how the client sees the role of the family, as well as the type and extent of emotional and spiritual support the client desires.

Even people who have not observed religious or ethnic practices throughout their lives may turn to these practices and rituals when faced with a life-threatening situation.

As a support worker, your role is to support the client and the client's family, however new or different the practices they choose to observe might be.

PALLIATIVE CARE (OR PALLIATION)

There are many definitions of palliative care (also called palliation). For our purposes, we will define palliative care as active and compassionate care whose purpose is to provide comfort and control pain so that the person may live life fully until he or she dies. It is not to cure or to prolong life.

Palliative care implies four things: that death is a natural process, that the person is entitled to measures that support comfort and reduce pain and other symptoms, that the person has the right to maintain his or her lifestyle as he or she chooses until death, and that the person has the right to die with dignity. Many hospice services have formalized their thoughts about the rights of the dying person. Exhibit 25-1 contains a sample "Bill of Rights."

EXHIBIT 25-1
A dying person's bill of rights

THE DYING PERSON'S BILL OF RIGHTS

1.   I have the right to be treated as a living human being until I die.

2.   I have the right to maintain a sense of hopefulness, however changing its focus may be.

3.   I have the right to be cared for by those who can maintain a sense of hopefulness, however changing this might be.

4.   I have the right to express my feelings and emotions about my approaching death, in my own way.

5.   I have the right to participate in decisions concerning my case.

6.   I have the right to expect continuing medical and nursing attention even though "cure" goals must be changed to "comfort" goals.

7.   I have the right not to die alone.

8.   I have the right to be free from pain.

9.   I have the right to have my questions answered honestly.

10.   I have the right not to be deceived.

11.   I have the right to have help from and for family in accepting my death.

12.   I have the right to die in peace and dignity.

13.   I have the right to retain my individuality and not be judged for my decisions, which may be contrary to the beliefs of others.

14.   I have the right to discuss and enlarge my religious and/or spiritual experiences, regardless of what they may mean to others.

15.   I have the right to expect that the sanctity of the human body will be respected after death.

16.   I have the right to be cared for by caring, sensitive, knowledgeable people who will attempt to understand my needs and will be able to gain some satisfaction in helping me face my death.

THE ROLE OF THE SUPPORT WORKER IN PALLIATIVE CARE

As a support worker, you will likely be asked to support both the client and his or her family. You will likely assist clients with personal care as well as provide social and emotional support. You may provide respite services (such as assisting the client so that another caregiver can get needed rest or recreation). You may help with household tasks so that a family member is free to provide the client's personal care.

In most cases, you will be part of a team comprising the client, the client's family, friends and other supports, other caregivers, and the client's doctor. You will work closely with the other team members to ensure that the client receives the support he or she desires. It is particularly important that you share information with all other team members.

CASE EXAMPLE 25-2

Erica Huber is a support worker with Hometown Support Services. She is assigned to provide palliative care to Mr. Stokes, a client. Erica is a part of a team that is made up of Mr. Stokes, his wife and daughter, a visiting nurse, and two hospice volunteers.

When she was first assigned to Mr. Stokes, Erica spent a bit of time getting to know him. Erica learned Mr. Stokes's preferences as well as his expectations of her. She was also able to get a sense of how Mr. Stokes's condition affects him.

Erica knows Mr. Stokes will often share information with her that he would like to be passed on to other team members. She makes sure to carefully listen to him as well as to pass on significant information to other team members.

How does palliative support differ from other types of support work?

THE IMPACT OF LIFE-THREATENING ILLNESS

The Client

Although each person and situation is different, most people experience a range of emotions when faced with a life-threatening illness, an illness that is likely to cause death. Denial, anger, bargaining, and acceptance are the emotions that have historically been associated with dying, but we now know that the person may experience many other emotions as well. A client may also experience despair, fear, uncertainty, or hope. Sometimes, a client experiences many strong emotions or experiences a single emotion for a period of time. He or she may also alternate between emotions (for example, between despair and hope).

The client may also question his or her faith or purpose in life. She or he may search for meaning in past activities or need to know that he or she will leave a legacy for others.

The client faces many changes in his or her life as a result of the illness. The client may not have the energy to maintain social relationships or take part in activities he or she once enjoyed. Sometimes, friends drift away, perhaps because they are uncomfortable with the client's illness or because the client can no longer take part in the activities they once shared. A client whose illness has forced him or her to leave work may have to deal with financial uncertainty, as well as the concern that family members may not have the resources necessary to live comfortably.

People with a life-threatening illness have the same range of needs as anyone. However, their priorities may be very different. Exhibit 25-2 illustrates a list of needs identified by people with life-threatening illness. As you read this list, make note of how many needs relate to everyday activities. As a support worker, it's likely that you will have a great opportunity to assist a client to attain what is important to him or her.

EXHIBIT 25-2

*The needs of
the dying person*

NEEDS OF THE DYING PERSON

Psychological Needs

To be heard
To be with people I wish
To know that the person's life has made a difference
To be a part of their community
To be loved
To be touched
To make peace

❖

Spiritual Needs

To participate in the rituals that are a part of one's beliefs
To have spiritual beliefs recognized and respected
To have access to religious symbols (Bibles, rosaries, statues, etc.)
To have visits with a member of the clergy, if desired

❖

Physical Needs

To be free from pain, as much as is possible
To have needs for food, water, and body function met
To be as comfortable as possible
To be touched as desired

Most Importantly, the Person Needs to Live Until They Die

The Family

Like clients, each family member will react differently to the diagnosis of a life-threatening illness. It is not uncommon for family members' reactions to be different than the client's. For example, a client may be accepting of a diagnosis although the family members are not. Like clients, family members may experience many feelings and may alternate among them.

For many families, the time after a diagnosis is made is one of many changes. The client may have many new needs. There may be a number of other caregivers involved in the client's support. Familiar patterns of activity (ways of doing things) change, and there is usually a period of uncertainty as family members get used to new roles and activity. Sometimes, the family becomes very protective of the client and must balance their need to keep the client "safe" with respect for the client's need to make decisions and take risks.

Everyone may need time to come to terms with the diagnosis and its meaning. Family members may find it hard to balance the client's need for support with their own needs for support. The family may also have to deal with **anticipatory grief**— the sense of loss, grieving, and preparing to move on that occurs before an expected loss happens. Anticipatory grief can cause the family members to distance themselves from the client.

As a support worker, you will likely be involved in supporting the family. Family members may need to discuss the way the client's illness affects them and how they must adapt to those changes. Be assured that each client (and family) will come to his or her own unique way of responding. No single way is the "right" or "best" one. You must be nonjudgmental as you listen and provide support.

The Support Worker

> ### CASE EXAMPLE 25-3
>
> *Jenna Mace assisted Mr. Moreau and his family as Mr. Moreau was dying of cancer. As one of two support workers assigned to Mr. Moreau, Jenna came to know him well. As she was often the worker assigned to overnight shifts, Jenna and Mr. Moreau spent a great deal of time talking. Mr. Moreau shared his family photographs with her and told her many stories of growing up in a farming community.*
>
> *After a period of remission, Mr. Moreau's condition suddenly and dramatically worsened. Within one week, he was dead. Jenna found that she experienced shock and grief at the sudden loss of the client she had come to know so well.*
>
> **Put yourself in Jenna's place. How would you feel?**

You must not overlook the effect that supporting a terminally ill client has on you. Even though you are not a family member, you will get to know the client very well. You will establish a relationship with the client that will require you to share a bit of yourself even as you maintain professional boundaries. It's very likely that you will feel a sense of anxiety at the impending loss of the relationship.

Make certain that you have a support system that can assist you as you assist your client. You may want to speak with your supervisor to see if you can discuss issues in palliative care with other workers who provide this type of support.

LIVING WILLS AND DO-NOT-RESUSCITATE ORDERS

A client receiving palliative care has likely made a decision to cease extensive treatment aimed at attaining a cure. Some clients have made this decision informally with their loved ones. In these cases, all caregivers understand the client's wishes and act accordingly even though there is no written document that outlines them.

Some clients, particularly those who are in long-term care facilities or hospitals, may choose a more formal way of stating their desires. Two common ways are by naming a person to make decisions for them when necessary and by completing a do-not-resuscitate order.

Most provinces have legislation that allows a person to name another to act on the person's behalf if the person becomes unable to do so. Usually, the person naming another person to act for them completes a legal document that names that person and sets out the scope of the decisions that person could make. The person who acts on another person's behalf in this manner is often called a *substitute decision-maker*, although some provinces may use other terms. The substitute decision-maker is expected to consider any wishes the person has made when making decisions on their behalf.

A **living will** (or advance directive) is a document that sets out a person's wishes for care should the person not be able to make those decisions. These documents may be useful to the substitute decision-maker, but may not be legally binding.

A **do-not-resuscitate order** is a document that states that a person is not to receive heroic measures to sustain his or her life. A do-not-resuscitate order is concerned only with life-sustaining measures, while a living will may address other forms of treatment.

When these documents are written to conform to legal requirements and are in place, their contents must be respected. Your agency will have specific guidelines for following the instructions in a living will or do-not-resuscitate order. Make sure that you know your agency's procedures.

As a rule, you should not witness any living will or do-not-resuscitate order. It may seem to others that you could have influenced the client to write or sign the document. If you are asked to witness, you might suggest that one of the client's friends or neighbours be asked instead.

PROMOTING COMFORT AND REDUCING PAIN

Comfort takes many forms. It can be physical, as in freedom from pain. It can be emotional, as in being in the company of someone who genuinely cares. With all that the client is experiencing, comfort may be difficult to attain.

Many clients with a life-threatening illness will experience physical pain. In some cases, the pain is mild or moderate and is not always present. In other cases, pain may be severe and constant.

Many clients may receive medication for pain. If so, there should be a person who is responsible for monitoring the medication. Usually, you will not be expected to take responsibility for a client's medication. However, there may be a number of other things that you can do to promote comfort and reduce pain.

Promoting Comfort

A Positive Self-Image

Having a life-threatening illness can be very destructive to a client's self-image. First, the effects of the illness or treatment may alter a client's appearance. For example, there may be visible scarring from surgery or hair loss from chemotherapy. Some medications may cause the person to develop reddened or flaky skin. Second, the client's ability to maintain personal hygiene may be compromised by the illness, the treatment, or both.

You can promote a positive self-image by helping the client to bathe, dress, and groom in whatever way makes him or her comfortable. Many clients may not have the stamina for a daily bath. However, most will appreciate daily sponge baths, clean clothing, and having their hair neatly styled.

Communication

Do you remember the last time you really communicated with someone? Can you recall the satisfaction you got from knowing that the other person was "on the same wavelength"? The ability to establish rapport, actively listen, and relate to another person can provide great comfort.

Through the practice of good communication skills, you can make sure that your client feels that someone who is genuinely interested has listened to him or her. You can also ensure that your client has the opportunity to spend time alone with friends.

Basic Nutrition and Personal Care

STOP AND REFLECT ((25-2))

Recall a time when you were ill with the flu or a cold. Focus for a moment on the physical discomfort associated with the illness.

How did you feel?

_____
_____
_____
_____

What made you feel better?

_____
_____
_____
_____

Chances are that you felt out of sorts when you were ill. An ill client, particularly one who spends a great deal of time in bed, may share many of those feelings. Scratchy, wrinkled sheets can irritate fragile skin. A client may also experience a variety of physical irritants: his or her mouth may become dry, the tongue may become coated, or dried secretions may collect in the corners of the mouth. Poor swallowing may allow particles of food to stick to the client's teeth.

Techniques to Support Client Comfort

There are many techniques you can use to promote client comfort. Table 25-1 identifies some useful techniques.

Pain Control

Although medications are often the most effective means of controlling pain, there are other techniques for controlling pain. In particular, four techniques may be of benefit to clients: massage, relaxation techniques, visualization, and music.

Massage

A back rub or hand or foot massage may provide great comfort to the client. Even clients who decline most touch may appreciate a massage if offered. Do not force a client to accept a massage, however.

TABLE 25-1	Techniques to Support Client Comfort

Area of Concern	Comfort Measure
Confusion, possibly due to drugs or pain	Reassure the client, be patient, provide orientation information, but don't force the client to accept the information.
Constipation, possibly due to inactivity, weakness, or dehydration	Help the client maintain an upright position for bowel movements, if possible. Increase mobility, if possible. Increase fluid intake.
Difficulty swallowing	Moisten dry foods. Substitute more easily swallowed foods for those that are difficult. Chop or puree foods.
Dry, irritated, or sore mouth Dry or coated tongue	Assist the client to brush teeth or provide mouth care. Encourage client to rinse mouth frequently. Encourage client to suck on ice chips, frozen juice cubes, or popsicles. Avoid acidic drinks or fruits if mouth has sores. Use lip gloss or petroleum jelly to keep lips moist. Ensure tongue is brushed or cleaned.
Lack of interest in eating, possibly due to fear of vomiting, drugs, chemotherapy, dry mouth, diarrhea, or constipation	Respond to the factor causing the lack of interest.
Nausea or vomiting	Provide smaller meals. Encourage starchy foods: crackers, pasta, rice, potatoes. Offer clear fluids. Avoid spicy, greasy, or overly sweet foods. Offer cold foods (cold foods do not have as much of an aroma and may not trigger nausea).

Relaxation Techniques

These techniques cause the person to focus on body rhythms and away from pain. Table 25-2 outlines a simple relaxation technique.

Visualization

Imagining oneself in a pleasant place or reliving a pleasant experience can provide respite from pain.

TABLE 25-2	A Simple Relaxation Technique

1. Find a quiet spot where you are not likely to be distracted.

2. Get into a position that is comfortable. This can be sitting, reclining, or lying down. Use a pillow to provide support if required.

3. Close your eyes if you wish.

4. Breathe in deeply. As you do, tense your muscles.

5. Keep your muscles tense for a few seconds as you hold your breath.

6. Exhale and relax your muscles.

7. Repeat the process for 5–10 minutes.

Music

Music can lift spirits and distract a person, minimizing the sensation of pain. Any type of music or sound that relaxes the client is appropriate, whether it is new age, rap, or jazz.

The suggestions in this section are general ideas. Many clients have developed their own measures. It's important to learn effective comfort and pain control approaches from your client, his or her family, as well as other caregivers.

It is helpful to learn about the quality of the pain that the client feels. Knowing some basic information about the type, frequency, and severity of the pain, as well as what makes the pain worse or better, can help you to comfort your client. Often, this information is recorded in the client's support plan. If not, talk to your supervisor about obtaining this information. Report to your supervisor your observations about when pain begins, how long it lasts, what makes it better or worse, as well as how severe it is.

WHEN DEATH IS NEAR

It is likely that you will be asked to assist at a time when your client is near death. There may be a number of physical signs that death is near. It is important to remember that the dying person is often conscious to the very end.

Concepts

1. **Senses are dulled and finally fail to respond.** However, do not assume that the person cannot hear. This sense may remain after all others diminish.
2. **The person's pulse and respirations gradually change.** Sometimes, there is a marked change from laboured breathing to a peaceful rhythm.
3. **Urine output diminishes.** If output ceases, death is likely within 48–72 hours.
4. **The sensation of pain likely is diminished and the person may seem more "content."**
5. **Sensation and ability to move diminish first in the client's legs, then in the arms.**

6. **Body surfaces cool as peripheral circulation diminishes.** The client's skin will often feel cold and clammy to the touch.
7. **Despite being cool to the touch, most dying persons do not feel cold.** In fact, any restlessness is often caused by the sensation of heat.

Techniques

The following techniques may be helpful. Always take your cues from the client. A technique that calms a client is useful, no matter where the idea came from.

1. Offer lighter-weight clothing to help minimize the sensation of heat. You may have to explain to the family that although the client feels cold to the touch, his or her internal temperature is quite warm.
2. Providing for fresh-air circulation helps to reduce the sensation of heat as well as to diminish any odours.
3. Some people are more comfortable when sheets are not tucked in. Sometimes, leaving the client's feet exposed can help to reduce the sensation of heat.
4. Reposition the person frequently to prevent sore spots.
5. The room should not be darkened unless it appears to comfort the client.
6. Encourage family to be seated near the client's head and to touch the client (if this has been acceptable in the past). The nearness and physical contact helps to compensate for diminished sensory perception and to promote a sense of connection.

AT THE TIME OF DEATH

At the time of death, the client's respirations and pulse will cease. Unless asked to do otherwise, allow the family time with the client.

The client's support plan should offer detailed information as to the actions to be taken at the time of death. It is extremely important to make sure all tasks are defined beforehand so that there is no confusion.

It's often helpful if the support worker makes any calls or handles any tasks identified in the support plan that a family member does not want to do. This allows the family to focus on their grieving.

CARE OF THE BODY AFTER DEATH

It is usually acceptable to straighten the sheets and cover the client's body to ensure modesty. Client preferences as well as agency policy will determine what, if any, additional care is provided to the client's body. Make sure you know your agency's policy beforehand.

GRIEF AND GRIEF WORK

The pain of grief is as much a part of life as the joy of love.
It is, perhaps, the price we pay for love, the cost of commitment.

Parkes

It is normal to feel loss when a client dies. The process of grieving allows us to deal with the loss, to work through the changes the loss has brought about, to begin to adapt to the new reality, and, finally, to begin to create a new life for ourselves. **Grief work** is defined as the tasks that are associated with moving through these phases.

As a support worker who has supported a client who has died, your grief work is twofold. You must support the client's family and loved ones in their grief, as well as work through the stages of your own.

Each person's grief is unique. It results from the unique relationship between the person and the client. However, there is a general pattern to the process of grieving. Knowing that one's reactions are "normal" may be a comfort to some people. The three phases most people experience are numbness, confronting, and redefining.

It is important to remember that people do not move through these phases in an orderly fashion. For example, a person may still experience periods of denial long after the death. It is not uncommon for a person to "automatically" telephone the deceased person on a birthday or anniversary, only realizing the error when the person does not answer.

Phase One—Numbness

The first phase is one of shock and denial. The person may say something like "I can't believe that he is gone." The person may appear shocked or overwhelmed. Sometimes, the person seems to behave almost as if nothing happened. Attention and concentration are usually diminished, and the person may find it incredibly difficult to do routine things like eating or dressing. The person may have no appetite and find it difficult to sleep.

At the same time, there is often a great deal of activity in the home. Family, friends, and neighbours may visit. Arrangements may have to be made. There are many details to attend. These tasks can provide a purpose—in effect, a ready-made list of things to do. In turn, this allows the person some time to adjust to the loss.

The task of this phase is to move from the initial shock to acceptance of the death. As a support worker, you can help the person by listening without challenging, by making sure that support is available, and by making sure that the necessities of life are provided. Perhaps you have taken part in the ritual of bringing food to the family of the deceased person. This helps to provide the grieving person with nourishment, as well as provide a way for others to help.

Phase Two—Confronting the Loss and Pain

As the activity in the home subsides and the shock wears off, the person can begin to focus on the pain of the loss. This can be a time of uncertainty, a time in which the person questions his or her ability to "go on." It may also be a time of desiring to maintain contact with the deceased person's memory by doing things like going to the restaurant the deceased person really liked.

The task of this phase is to work through the uncertainty and yearning. This also involves rediscovering one's strengths as a way of preparing to go on. As the survivors may not be receiving support services, it may not be possible for you to assist them through this phase. If you are present, your task is to help the person balance the grieving with periods of time devoted to maintaining the person's health and well-being. This is often called "taking a break from grieving," as it allows the person to regain energy necessary to deal with this phase. It's often helpful to assist the person to focus on the strengths he or she does have that can be of help.

Phase Three—Redefining and Reconnecting

The third phase of grief deals with the survivor's gradual focus on life without the deceased person. It is in this phase that the person begins to believe that he or she will have a life and begins to focus on making plans, forming new relationships, and reconnecting with old relationships.

The task involved in this phase is to reinvest energies into new goals, activities, and relationships. A support worker involved with the survivor during this phase should assist the person to believe in his or her strengths and abilities. The support worker should also offer encouragement to reconnect with old friends as well as take steps to make new ones.

The Support Worker's Grief

It's not unusual for you to experience aspects of these three phases as well although they will not be as intense as they are for a loved one. It's not uncommon to feel shock as well as a loss of purpose in the period right after the death. You must be sensitive to your needs and ensure that you have proper support. If your agency provides palliative care to many clients, it may offer support groups or other help for workers who have experienced a client's death.

Questions for Review

1. What factors have shaped our attitudes toward death?

2. What is the hospice movement? How has it changed Canadian attitudes toward death?

3. You are assigned to assist a person who is dying. What might you expect your role to be?

4. Do people with a life-threatening illness have the same needs as other people? Why or why not?

5. How can a life-threatening illness affect the family of the client?

6. What are living wills and do-not-resuscitate orders called in your province? What are your responsibilities with regard to these documents?

7. Medication is the only thing that can reduce pain. Do you agree? Why or why not?

8. What are four signs that death is near?

9. What can you do to promote client comfort at the time near death?

10. What are the phases of grief work? What are the tasks (grief work) of each phase?

Questions for Discussion

1. What is a good death? Is your definition the same as that of your colleagues?

2. Are there times when it is better for a person to go to a hospital to die? Under what circumstances might this be a good choice?

3. *You have been assigned to assist Mrs. Ross, a 58-year-old woman who has breast cancer that has metastasized. Her doctor has advised her that further treatment would not be effective. Mrs. Ross tells you that she has made peace with the prognosis and has put her affairs in order.*

   Mrs. Ross has two children who are at university 2000 km away. Her husband's job requires him to travel and he is often away. Mrs. Ross is an independent woman who does not want to disrupt her family members' lives. An architect, she has always been active in professional associations and has socialized with a small group of friends. Since her diagnosis, however, she has become less and less active. She tells you that part of the reason for this is that she has little energy for socializing. She also says that she feels that she is "not a pretty sight" and is uncomfortable with going out. Mrs. Ross's hair did not grow back well after chemotherapy and is patchy. As well, she is uncomfortable with her breast prosthesis and prefers not to wear it. She seems to miss the social interaction and often seems lonely and sad.

   Explain how her behaviour relates to the process and stages of dying.

   What are your thoughts and feelings? Explain how they relate to your beliefs about illness, health care, and death.

   Describe the approaches that you should take to help Mrs. Ross.

Chapter 26

Assisting with Medications

Learning Objectives

Through reading this chapter, you'll be able to

1. Describe the four factors that determine how you may assist a client with medications.
2. Discuss to what extent a support worker can assist with medications in your province, as defined by both legislation and agency practice.
3. Define what items are considered drugs and the conditions under which you may assist a client to take medications.
4. Outline the four general ways in which you may assist a client to take medication and describe any special precautions you must take when using each.
5. Specify the information you must have in order to safely administer medication to a client.
6. Describe the role of medication monitoring and discuss its importance.
7. List the seven "rights" of medication administration.
8. Explain the difference between over-the-counter and prescription medications and between generic and brand-name medications.
9. Identify and describe common medication terminology and the information found on a prescription medication label.
10. Accurately measure liquid medications.
11. Demonstrate the proper administration of oral and topical medications and eye, ear, and nose drops.
12. Outline the steps to take if a problem arises.
13. Describe the Canadian Pharmaceutical Association's A.C.T.I.O.N. Plan for addressing possible medication problems.

Chapter at a Glance

- Can a Support Worker Administer Medications?
- What Is a Drug?
- Generic and Brand-Name Medications
- Roles of Other Professionals
- Assisting a Client with Taking Medication
- The Seven "Rights" of Medication Administration
- Administering Medications
- Medication Monitoring
- Factors That May Affect a Person's Compliance
- If Problems Arise

Terms You'll Use

Blister Pack A card containing single doses of one or more medications prescribed for a person.

Buccal Tablet A dose of medication that is dissolved in the mouth and absorbs through the mucous membrane of the mouth.

Dossette A container that holds individual doses of medication.

Drug An agent that alters the body's mechanisms.

Generic Name The name of the active ingredient in a medication.

Herbal Medications Substances that contain naturally occurring chemicals.

Narcotics Medications that dull the senses to provide pain relief and may be addictive.

Over-the-Counter Medications Medications that can be purchased and used without a prescription.

Prescription Medications Medications that are prescribed by a doctor for the treatment of specific conditions.

Sublingual Tablet A dose of medication that is dissolved under the tongue and absorbs through the mucous membrane of the mouth.

Syringe A hollow tube that can be filled with a medication for administration.

CAN A SUPPORT WORKER ADMINISTER MEDICATIONS?

The answer to this question depends upon four factors:

- the province in which you work
- the policy of your employer
- possibly the decision of a regulated health professional who supervises your care to a particular client
- your ability to safely carry out the correct procedure

Provincial Legislation and Regulation

Each province has legislation that regulates specific health procedures. How provinces do this varies; some have legislation that sets out controlled acts; others include this information in a number of profession-specific acts (such as a *Nursing Act*, etc.). In most provinces/territories, some aspect of medication administration is regulated. Each province and territory differs in what is regulated. Table 26-1 summarizes each province's applicable legislation.

As a support worker in Canada, you are an unregulated caregiver. There is no legislation describing your scope of practice; nor are you as a support worker mentioned in legislation regulating health professionals. However, because these acts describe activities that only members of designated professional groups may do, they indirectly define some limits to your practice.

TABLE 26-1	Home Support Workers and Medication Administration: A Cross-Canada Overview	
Province	Role	Delegation and Responsibility
British Columbia	■ Unclear	■ Registered Nurses Association of British Columbia (RNABC) Nursing Practice Guidelines (August 2002), Section 8 (Administering of Medications): Nurses may delegate the task of administering medications to home support workers in accordance with RNABC policy and agency policies and procedures. ■ Delegating nurse continues to assume responsibility for the overall assessment, determination of client's status, care planning, interventions and care evaluation related to the administering of medication (Registered Nurses Association of British Columbia, 2002). ■ RNABC's policy statement Delegating Tasks to Unregulated Care Providers (November 2000): Responsibility for nursing practice cannot be delegated. The decision to delegate is that of the client's registered nurse, and the accountability for safe delegation is shared between the agency, the home support worker and the registered nurse (Registered Nurses Association of British Columbia, 2000).
Alberta	■ HSWs often involved in medication administering ■ Many of their functions delegated by the nurses (Mansell, 2003)	■ Alberta Association of Registered Nurses (AARN) issued a position statement, AARN Position Statement on the Utilization of Auxiliary Health Care Workers in the Delivery of Health Care (1993, re-endorsed 1998): Designated tasks and activities may be delegated to auxiliary health care workers under specific conditions. ■ Registered nurse remains accountable and responsible for the overall nursing care delivered and is responsible for determining the appropriate delegation of tasks and activities. ■ The employers of the HSW have joint responsibility in ensuring the competency of the HSW (Alberta Association of Registered Nurses, 1993). ■ Guidelines of Delegation and Supervision of Patient and Client Care (AARN, June 2002);

▶▶|

TABLE 26-1	Home Support Workers and Medication Administration: A Cross-Canada Overview *(continued)*	
Province	**Role**	**Delegation and Responsibility**
		provides guidelines outlining the overall supports within the health system that are needed to enable safe supervision and delegation of care, key steps for safe delegation and supervision of client and client care, and measures that registered nurses should take when they are unable to provide safe supervision and delegation of care (Alberta Association of Registered Nurses, 2002).
Saskatchewan	▪ HSWs remind clients to take medications but they do not actually administer them (Sullivan, 2003)	▪ Saskatchewan Registered Nurses' Association (SRNA) released a document, Guidelines for Mediation Administration (Apr 2000): RNs are accountable when they teach, delegate, or supervise home support workers. Nurses may teach medication administering, which is defined as the actual physical act of administering the medication to the client, and documentation of the time and date it was administered. ▪ While a nurse may teach medication administering to home support workers, he/she still maintains the responsibility of assessing health care needs, developing a care plan, evaluating the client's health status, and evaluating the ongoing effectiveness of the medication (Registered Psychiatric Nurses Association of Saskatchewan et al., 2000). ▪ Nursing in Collaborative Environments (jointly prepared by the Registered Psychiatric Nurses Association of Saskatchewan, the Saskatchewan Association of Licensed Practical Nurses, and the SRNA, 2000): The assignment of a nursing task or procedure to an unregulated health care provider must be appropriate (appropriate assignment means that the Registered Psychiatric Nurse (RPN), Licensed Practical Nurse (LPN), or Registered Nurse (RN) must consider the client's status and requirements for care, the competence of the unregulated health care provider, and the practice environment. The RPN, LPN or RN who is assigning a task or procedure to an unregulated health care provider is responsible for ensuring appropriate support is provided).

⏭

TABLE 26-1	Home Support Workers and Medication Administration: A Cross-Canada Overview *(continued)*	
Province	**Role**	**Delegation and Responsibility**
Manitoba	■ "Home care attendants" may only remind clients to take their medications, cannot administer medications, and may help clients with blister packs (Matthes, 2003)	■ Manitoban nurses may delegate medication-related tasks to home support workers who are designated as "home care attendants" (Matthes, 2003; Matthes, personal communication). ■ The College of Registered Nurses of Manitoba (CRNM), the Manitoba Association of Licensed Practical Nurses, (MALPN), and the Registered Psychiatric Nurses Association of Manitoba (RPNAM) jointly prepared a discussion paper entitled Decision Making: A Framework for Delegation released January 1999. The document discusses the overlap between the scopes of practice of the three regulated nursing professions in that province. It also states that in clients' specific situations, and according to agency policy, an unregulated home support worker may be trained by a Registered Nurse (RN), Licensed Practical Nurse (LPN), or Registered Psychiatric Nurse administering to home support workers by the nurse in this document (College of Registered Nurses of Manitoba, Manitoba Association of Licensed Practical Nurses, & Registered Psychiatric Nurses Association of Manitoba, 1999).
Ontario	■ HSWs have no involvement with medications, though they may ask the client if they have taken their medications (Kirstein, 2003)	■ Guidelines for Working with Unregulated Care Providers (College of Nurse of Ontario (CNO), 2000): Paid care providers, including personal support workers, generally assist with or provide personal care, and may deliver some basic elements of nursing care, including assisting with medications (College of Nurses of Ontario, 2000). ■ The CNO's Standards of Nursing Practice includes a section called Delegation of Dispensing. However, this section is not relevant to the role of the unregulated home support worker regarding medication administering for isolated seniors in the community. The document pertains to the transfer of function of prescribing and distributing drugs, normally performed by physicians, pharmacists, and dentists, to the nurse (College of Nurses of Ontario, 1996).

▶▶

TABLE 26-1	Home Support Workers and Medication Administration: A Cross-Canada Overview *(continued)*	
Province	Role	Delegation and Responsibility
Quebec	■ HSWs can remind clients to take medications but cannot administer them (Lapointe, 2003)	■ Règlement sur les Actes Visés a l'Article 36 de la Loi sur les Infirmières et les Infirmiers qui Peuvent Etre Posés par des Classes de personnes Autres que des Infirmieres ou des Infirmiers (The Ordres infirmières et infirmiers du Québec): Position of delegation on nursing takes to unregulated home support workers remains unclear.
New Brunswick		■ Not required to have involvement in medication management, may remind client to take medication or bring the medications to the client (Lepine, 2003). ■ Under certain conditions, or in some circumstances, support workers are authorized to perform delegated functions relating to medication administering (Lepine, 2003; Lepine, personal communication). ■ Delegating Nursing Tasks and Procedures (Nurses Association of New Brunswick, May 1996): Nurses are ultimately responsible for the quality of nursing services provided to the client; nurses may delegate appropriate activities to other categories of health care workers (regulated and unregulated), family, and friends.
Nova Scotia	■ Can only remind clients to take medication and cannot administer medication (MacDonald, 2003)	■ Regulation of Personal Care Workers (College of Registered Nurses of Nova Scotia, 2002): The College does not support the ad hoc and inconsistent approach to the training and employment standards of home support workers (personal care workers) and believes that provincial standards for entry requirements and training programs for home support workers and other ancillary health workers must be established under the authority of the government though the Departments of Health and Education. RNs who supervise home support workers are accountable for assigning tasks that are within the personal care worker's level of competence. The Statement makes no specific reference to delegation of medication-related tasks to personal care workers (College of Registered Nurses of Nova Scotia, 2002).

TABLE 26-1	Home Support Workers and Medication Administration: A Cross-Canada Overview *(continued)*	
Province	**Role**	**Delegation and Responsibility**
		▪ Report and Recommendation of the Committee on Unlicensed Assistive Personnel (CRNNS, Nov. 1998, reprinted 2002), developed as a response to the many concerns heard from nurses about their experiences in supervising and delegating to Unlicensed Assistive Personnel (UAPs). The purpose of the document was to provide registered nurses with a framework to assist them in supervising and delegating to UAPs in any care setting and regardless of model of care used. It states that a home support worker employed by an agency shall not perform the following activities: medication administering, nursing procedures, and any tasks for which they have not been trained.
Prince Edward Island	▪ Can't administer medication; may give the container to the client at the client's request (only if the client is not cognitively impaired) (Stewart, 2003)	▪ Support workers may also apply ointments in some cases (although a family member is preferred) and may remind clients to take medications (Stewart, 2003; Stewart, personal communications).
Newfoundland & Labrador	▪ May be delegated the task of administering medication to clients (Dooley, 2003)	▪ Delegation of Nursing Tasks to Support Workers in Community Settings (Association of Registered Nursed of Newfoundland and Labrador, 2002): All tasks that home support workers are requested to perform, which are outside their scope of practice, require delegation by an appropriate health care professional. ▪ Delegation is a shared responsibility between the nurse, support worker, employer, and the client (when appropriate). When nursing tasks are delegated, the nurse still maintains responsibility for assessment, planning, implementing, and evaluating care (Association of Registered Nurses of Newfoundland and Labrador, 2002). ▪ Assisting the client to take medication is part of the basic requirements of home support worker practice; thus, nurses do not need to delegate this task. Medication administering is outside the support worker's approved scope of practice and must be delegated.

▶▶|

TABLE 26-1	Home Support Workers and Medication Administration: A Cross-Canada Overview *(continued)*	
Province	**Role**	**Delegation and Responsibility**
Northwest		HSW can remind the client to take medication and may ensure the client takes medications in bubble pack and/or dossettes (Chetwynd, 2003).
Yukon Territory		May remind clients to take medication but cannot administer them (Sullivan-Curtis, 2003).
Nunavut		No role in medication administering or management (Barns, 2003).

Source: Reproduced with permission from Screening and Managing Medication Problems in Isolated, Independent-living Seniors, *Final Report – Phase I, Ottawa, ON: Canadian Pharmacists Association © 2004*

In addition, some provinces have legislation that restricts acts in certain settings. For example, Ontario's long-term care facility legislation restricts medication administration to regulated nursing personnel, even though the administration of oral and topical medications in other settings is not a controlled act.

The lack of consistency among provinces may reflect the differences in how each province organizes its health care. However, it does promote a lack of understanding of the support worker's role. The Canadian Pharmacists Association has recommended that the role of support workers be clearly defined, preferably at the national level (CPA, Screening and Managing Medication Problems in Isolated, Independent-Living Seniors, 2004).

Employer Policy

Employers have the right to determine what their support workers will do, within the bounds of legislation. It's not unusual for an employer to prohibit workers from performing certain acts, simply because the acts are not appropriate to the job the worker is to do, or because the task is prohibited by an agreement the agency has with a funder. For example, an outreach worker may not be permitted to make meals or to accompany a client to shop, by terms of an agreement that the employer has with the agency who funds the services.

Decision by a Health Professional Authorized to Perform the Act

In most provinces, a health professional authorized to perform a controlled act can ask an unregulated provider to perform some of those acts, if certain conditions apply. In these cases, the health professional delegating the task is responsible to make certain that the worker performing the act is doing it correctly and as instructed. Many professional colleges have provided guidelines for their members to follow when determining whether an act may be delegated.

Support Worker Ability

Finally, the support worker's ability determines whether he or she is able to perform any permissible act. *Bear in mind that no act is appropriate or safe if you are not trained to perform it.*

STOP AND REFLECT ((26-1))

What is the role of support workers in your province? How is this role shaped by provincial legislation? How is this role shaped by agency policy?

_____

_____

_____

_____

_____

Talk with two or three agencies. What are their policies on medication administration? How are these policies similar? How are they different?

_____

_____

_____

_____

_____

Photo 26-1
Medications
Source: © David
Young-Wolff/Photo Edit;
Shutterstock; Photo by
Mario Tama/Getty Images

WHAT IS A DRUG?

When we hear the term *drug,* we often think of prescription medications, but there are many more items that are actually drugs. For the purposes of this text, we'll define a **drug** as an agent that alters the body's mechanism (Photo 26-1). This definition includes:

- prescription medications
- over-the-counter (nonprescription) medications
- vitamins and minerals
- herbal medications
- alcohol
- tobacco

Prescription Medications

Prescription medications are those that must be prescribed by a doctor (or, in some cases, a dentist or other specific health professional). Prescription medications are approved by Health Canada. Many medications are approved for the treatment of specific ailments or conditions and cannot be prescribed for other conditions.

Controlled medications and narcotics are two special types of prescription medications. These medications are seen as having the potential for dependency or abuse if their use is not carefully controlled.

Controlled medications include many antidepressants. Prescriptions for these medications can be refilled, but it is expected that the doctor will keep very close supervision of the person taking the medication. Narcotics are medications that dull the senses to provide pain relief and that have great potential for addiction. Narcotic prescriptions cannot be refilled. The doctor must write a new prescription each time the prescription runs out.

Over-the-Counter Medications

Over-the-counter medications are those that can be purchased and used without a prescription. Many remedies, pain medications, and ointments are available over the counter. In some cases, the over-the-counter medication is a low-dose version of a prescription medication. Over-the-counter medications usually have a product code that begins with the letters DIN. Over-the-counter medications include medications that a person can buy to treat a minor condition or minor symptoms of a condition.

Be aware that over-the-counter medications can be harmful if taken improperly. Taking too much medication, taking it with other medications, or combining it with alcohol or certain foods can all cause serious side effects.

Vitamins and Minerals

Vitamins and minerals are regulated by Health Canada. Although they are sold as over-the-counter medications, some vitamins and minerals can be harmful in large quantities or when combined with other medications. In some cases, the effect of large doses of a vitamin or mineral is simply not known.

Herbal Medications

Herbal medications are those that contain naturally occurring chemicals and can be just as potent as prescription medications. In fact, the chemicals found in some herbal medications are the same as those found in prescription medications. For example, the chemical found in the herb foxglove is the same as that found in the heart medication digitalis (a medication that slows and strengthens heart rate). Because herbal medications are regulated as food supplements, the quality and potency may vary widely from one manufacturer to another.

Alcohol

Alcohol is classified as a drug although it is regulated differently than are other drugs. Alcohol can alter or heighten the effects of other medication. Alcohol is also seen as potentially addictive and has a potential for abuse. Excessive consumption of alcohol can cause alcohol poisoning or death.

Tobacco

Among many other chemicals, tobacco contains nicotine, an addictive agent that stimulates the central nervous system. Nicotine also can have adverse affects on the cardiovascular system. In Canada, tobacco is regulated under separate legislation.

GENERIC AND BRAND-NAME MEDICATIONS

Every medication has a generic name, the name of the active ingredient in the medication. When a medication is first brought to market, it is protected by a patent issued to the manufacturer who discovered the medication. The manufacturer gives the medication a brand name that is trademarked, meaning that only that manufacturer can use that brand name to describe the medication.

The trademark does not expire, but the drug patent only lasts for a period of time and cannot usually be renewed. After the drug patent expires, other manufacturers can duplicate the medication. For example, a common pain reliever is ASA, or acetylsalicylic acid. The name Aspirin is the brand name that the manufacturer, Bayer, has patented for its brand of ASA. After the patent expires, many manufacturers can make the same medication, but only the manufacturer that holds the trademark may use that brand name.

A medication whose patent has expired may be sold by the original manufacturer as well as a number of other manufacturers. Those other manufacturers give their own name to their version of the medication. For example, the generic medication furosemide is sold under four different brand names.

A generic medication must have the same active ingredient as the brand-name version. However, the inert ingredients (the things that make a pill easier to swallow or that coat a pill) may be different. Some people may be sensitive to an inert ingredient and thus respond differently to different versions of the same generic medication.

A client's doctor may allow a pharmacist to substitute a generic version for a brand-name version. Because the name of the medication may be different, you must be cautious that any medication you are asked to administer is, in fact, the medication in the container.

ROLES OF OTHER PROFESSIONALS

Chances are, you have taken a medication prescribed by your doctor. At least three people are involved in the proper use of a medication:

- the doctor who prescribes the proper medication
- the pharmacist who fills the prescription accurately
- the person who takes the medication properly

If the client requires assistance with medication, there will be other support workers involved depending upon the type of assistance needed. Often, a family member and a nurse are involved. As a support worker, you may be asked to assist a client. Remember that every person involved has an equally important role in ensuring that the medication is properly taken.

As described earlier in this chapter, each agency has its own policies and procedures for assisting a client to take medication. As well, each province regulates certain types of medication administration (such as injections). It is extremely important that you learn and follow your agency's policies and procedures for assisting a client to take medications. You should also understand any provincial regulations that apply to these activities.

SPOTLIGHT 26-1 A SIMPLE ACT?

At first glance, handing a person a pill or applying a medicated cream may seem like a simple act. It is not. Though the physical act is simple, the risk that it carries can be significant. Medication improperly taken can harm or kill a person. It's much like driving—the act of turning the steering wheel is simple; the risk driving can incur can be significant.

Administering a medication requires that you know—and take responsibility for—several things: that you are authorized to give the medication; what you are to give; when it is to be given; how it is to be given; what to look for or to look out for; and what to do if the client refuses or something goes wrong. You need to know who to contact if there are problems and what information that person will need to have.

A simple act? Not at all.

ASSISTING A CLIENT WITH TAKING MEDICATION

When we speak of assisting with taking medications, we are speaking of administering or assisting a client with administering medication. Administration means the act of taking a medication. When we take medication, we are considered to be self-administering the medication.

Your ability to assist a client with medication will be determined by three things:

- the type of medication and the way it is administered
- the setting (such as a client's home, a long-term care facility, or a rest home)
- the specific assistance you provide

Each province has legislation that restricts who may administer some types of medication. For example, in most cases, many provinces require that specific registered health professionals administer injected medications. Many provinces require that a registered nurse administer medications in a long-term care facility. Beyond the restrictions posed by legislation, your agency's policy will also determine how you can assist a client to take medication. You always must be careful to follow your agency's policies. Be aware that agencies will vary in how they allow a worker to assist a client. If you work for more than one agency, you may find that one allows you to assist in ways that are prohibited by the other.

Types of Assistance

There are four general types of assistance. You may assist a client by:

- reminding him or her to take the medication when the client is physically able to do so;
- providing some help with physical tasks, such as helping the client to open a bottle or blister pack when the client asks you to do so;

- handing the clients the contents of a dossette or individual-dose blister pack at the proper time; or
- opening the prescription or over-the-counter medication bottle, pouring out the proper amount of medication, and giving the medication to the client.

Each level of assistance requires you to ensure that the action you are taking is correct. For example, if your role is to remind the client to take a medication, you must do so at the proper time. The more involved you are in assisting your client, the more responsibility you will bear in making sure the act is done accurately (Photo 26-2).

Photo 26-2
*Assisting the client
with medication*

What You Need to Know to Assist the Client

There is specific information you must know in order to safely assist a client to take his or her medications. You must know the following:

1. Any pertinent information about the client, such as allergies or health concerns that may be affected by the medication
2. What other medications the client is taking, when they are taken, and if any of these medications may affect the action of the medication you are asked to give the client
3. Foods or beverages that may affect the action of the medication or cause side effects
4. The reason the client is taking the medication
5. The effects that should be expected (such as reduced joint pain) and action to take if the expected results do not appear
6. What side effects may arise and what to do if they do arise
7. The time the medication is to be administered, the correct dosage, and the method to be used to administer the medication (for example, orally or by ear or nose drops)
8. What to do if the client refuses the medication or skips a dose
9. The name of the person to contact if any problems arise
10. The records to be kept and the procedure to be used for recording

If you are uncertain as to whether a medication can be safely given, contact the designated person or your supervisor as your agency requires. Do not give the medication unless you are certain that it is safe to do so.

CASE EXAMPLE 26-1

Yasmin provides support for Mr. Patel. One of her tasks is to remind and observe Mr. Patel take medication. He usually takes the pills form the dossette his daughter fills for him. Today, Mr. Patel opens the dossette and looks at his pills. "These are not the right pills," he tells Yasmin. "My morning pills are white, and these are orange." Yasmin looks into the dossette and notes two orange pills. She is also aware that the last time she observed Mr. Patel take his medication, the pills were white.

What Yasmin Does

Yasmin knows that Mr. Patel's daughter is the person who manages most of his medication needs. She asks Mr. Patel if he would like to call his daughter. He does. His daughter reminds him that his doctor has changed his medication. The white pills have been discontinued. The orange pills are the correct pills. Mr. Patel takes his medication.

Yasmin notes the incident in the activity log.

If you were Yasmin, what would you do in this situation?

THE SEVEN "RIGHTS" OF MEDICATION ADMINISTRATION

In addition to all the information you must know in order to assist the client, you must know and follow the seven "rights": the right person, the right medication for the right purpose, the right dose, the right time, the right method, and the right documentation. Each of these "rights" is explained in this section. Small errors in medication can have significant effects on the client. Keep your mind on your work. If it is difficult to concentrate due to noise or commotion, move to a quiet area if possible.

The Right Person

In a client's home, this is usually obvious. However, if you are in a group home or assisted living situation, make sure that you have the proper client. Ask the client his or her name. If the client's chart has a photo, compare it to the client.

The Right Medication

Most medications will be stored in one of three types of containers: the prescription bottle, a dossette, or a blister pack.

How you check for the right medication depends upon the container from which you will remove the medication.

If removing the medication from its prescription bottle:

1. **Check the prescription label.** Figure 26-1 illustrates a typical medication label. Ensure that the medication is prescribed for the person and that the date on which it was dispensed is within the last six months. If the medication is older, verify its use with the appropriate person.
2. **Check that the medication name and strength listed on the bottle are the same as the medication name and strength listed in the support plan.**
3. **Check that the pills in the bottle are all the same.** If not, contact the appropriate person before giving the medication.

FIGURE 26-1

A prescription medication label

Photo 26-3
Various dossettes

Photo 26-4
*Single-dose
blister pack*
Source: Shutterstock

Photo 26-5
*Multiple-dose
blister pack*
*Source: Manrex Pill
Pak Card*

4. **Check the pills to ensure that they are not split, chalky, wet, or discoloured.** If any of these conditions exist, contact your supervisor.

Some clients may use a dossette (Photo 26-3). If removing medications stored in a dossette:

1. **If possible, review the contents of the dossette with the person responsible for filling it.** Know which medications should be given during your visit.
2. **Store the dossette properly until use.** Make sure that the dossette is not left where its contents can be tampered with by others in the setting or by the client. Do not leave the dossette in direct sunlight (for example, on a window sill).
3. **If you have any concerns about the contents of the dossette, contact the appropriate person before administering the medication.**

Blister packs (sometimes called unit dose) are used in both facility and community settings. There are two general types: those that store a single medication and those that store all medications taken at a specific time.

The first type stores a single medication for a period of time, usually one month. Each blister contains a single dose. In this system, there will be a card for each medication prescribed to the client. Photo 26-4 illustrates this type of blister pack.

The second type contains in each blister all medications that a person takes at a particular time. In this type, there may be a single pill (unit dose) or multiple (multi-dose) pills in each blister. The client will usually have a blister pack card for each 7 or 28 days. Photo 26-5 illustrates this type of blister pack.

The Right Purpose

Medications are prescribed for a specific purpose. It can be dangerous to use a medication for a purpose other than that for which it was prescribed. The medication may not treat the condition, allowing it to worsen. It may react with other medications that the person is taking or have unwanted side effects. Even over-the-counter medications can be dangerous if taken for the wrong purpose.

Discuss your observations with your supervisor if you suspect that your client is taking a medication that was not prescribed for the condition your client is trying to address.

The Right Dose

Any medication can be dangerous if taken in the wrong amount. Too little may not effectively treat the condition, putting the person at risk. Too much may cause harm or even death. Follow these steps to ensure you are providing the client with the correct dose.

1. **Read and reread the order written in the support plan.**
2. **Confirm any changes in the usual dose** (e.g., two tablets instead of one, or a different strength of medication).
3. **Compare the information on the prescription bottle with the strength listed on the support plan.**
4. **Know the meaning of abbreviations for medications.** Table 26-2 lists common abbreviations.

TABLE 26-2	Sample Prescription Abbreviations

This table lists some sample abbreviations. **Before you use any abbreviation, make sure that you find out if your agency approves of it.** The use of an incorrect or misunderstood abbreviation can pose a significant danger to a client.

Abbreviation	Meaning
a.c.	before meals or food
ad lib.	at pleasure
amp.	ampoule
b.i.d.	twice daily
caps.	capsule
fl., fld.	fluid
fort.	strong
gtt.	drops
h.s.	at bedtime
i.c.	between meals
liq.	liquid
NPO	nothing by mouth
p.c.	after meals or food
per os.	by mouth
p.r.n.	when or as required, whenever necessary
q.i.d.	four times daily
qh, q1h	every hour
q2h	every two hours
q.s.	a sufficient quantity
stat.	at once
t.i.d., t.d.	three times daily
t.i.d.a.c.	three times daily before meals
ung.	ointment

5. **Make sure that you measure liquids accurately and that you use the correct number of pills.** When measuring liquids, make sure that you are using the proper system of measurement (imperial or metric). Do not use household spoons to measure, as they vary widely in size.
6. **Make sure that the person takes all of the medication.**

The Right Time

Medication is taken at specific times for many reasons. Sometimes a medication must be taken before meals, or before or after another medication. Medication taken more than once in a day must usually be taken to ensure a consistent level of the medication in the body. Follow these guidelines to provide the right medication at the right time:

1. **Double-check the time of administration on the support plan.**
2. **Know the meaning of common terminology related to frequency.** Table 26-2 lists common short forms for timing.
3. **Make sure that the client's meals are timed so that the client takes the medication on an empty stomach, with meals, or after eating, as required.**
4. **Make sure that medications ordered for the same time can be safely given together.** If not, make sure that you know which medication must be given first and how much time must elapse between administering the medications.
5. **If going out with a client, make sure that any medication to be taken while out is checked before departure and brought with the client.**

The Right Method

Medications must be administered in specific ways to be effective. For example, some medications must be taken with milk or other coating liquid to be effective. Others cannot be taken on an empty stomach, or with certain types of liquids, such as grapefruit juice. As well, some tablets must be placed under the tongue.

1. **Make sure you know how to administer the medication.**
2. **Make sure that you are familiar with any special measuring devices prior to using them.**
3. **Carefully follow any instructions for preparation.** Be aware that some pills can be crushed and mixed with jelly or applesauce to make them easier to swallow, but others cannot. If you don't know whether a client's pills can be crushed or mixed, contact the appropriate person. *Never* crush or split pills or open capsules unless you have been instructed to do so.
4. **Do not handle medications with your bare hands.** Pour liquids directly into the measuring device. If the device has been washed, ensure that it is dry before using. Water left in the device may reduce the amount of medication.
5. **Pour the required number of pills into the inverted top of the pill container and then into the client's hand.** If using a dossette, check the contents of the appropriate vial, then pour directly into the client's hand.

Photo 26-6
Worker documenting medication

The Right Documentation

Accurate recording of the medication given is essential. It is critically important that other caregivers know what medication was given, when and how it was given, as well as any observations about the procedure. The following guidelines will help ensure that your documentation provides accurate and clear information (Photo 26-6):

1. **Document the medication given, the amount given, the time given, and any other pertinent observations you make.** If you have been asked to make specific observations (for example, a change in condition), make certain that you do so.
2. **Use the appropriate form.** For example, you may be asked to record information on a medication administration form as well as in a progress note.
3. **Follow all rules for documentation.** It is extremely important that your note clearly state all required information.
4. **Make certain that you immediately report any concerns to the appropriate person.** Concerns should be reported to the appropriate person, not simply documented in the client's record. Discuss with your supervisor the specific procedure you are to use to report concerns about medications.

MEDICATION MONITORING

According to the Canadian Pharmacists Association, almost one-third of older adults receiving home care have a medication-related problem. Among these problems, most are related to medication *administration* (CPA, 2004).

Many things may interfere with a client's ability to take a medication as prescribed. The client may not understand the need for the medication, may find the medication regime too complex, or may feel that the side effects outweigh the benefit of the medication. The client may not be able to see well enough to select the correct pills, or may be unable to open the bottle, blister pack, or dossette. A client with dementia may not be able to remember, understand, or initiate the process to properly take prescribed medications.

As a support worker, you have a valuable role to play in the monitoring of a client's medication regime. Because you may spend more time with the client than any other caregiver, you are in a unique position to observe any difficulties or concerns the client may have. You may also be the first caregiver to note the presence of a side effect or when a medication has not had the desired effect.

You may also have the opportunity to discuss the client's concerns with him or her. These observations may then be passed on to your supervisor or to another designated person for follow-up.

FACTORS THAT MAY AFFECT A PERSON'S COMPLIANCE

Have you ever been prescribed a medication but did not take it? Perhaps you missed doses or accidentally took the medication at the wrong time or in the wrong amount. Perhaps you had a reaction or experienced unpleasant side effects. You might not have finished the medication as directed or never even filled the prescription.

There are many things that can cause a person to not take a medication properly, or perhaps to not take the medication at all. We often call the person who doesn't take medication as prescribed noncompliant, but the reason he or she is not following the prescription may have nothing to do with a desire to avoid the medication. The reason may be related to physical, cultural, communication, misinformation, past or current experiences, complexity of the plan, cognitive ability, or financial factors. Though these factors can affect a person of any age, they may more likely occur in older persons. This section examines the more common factors.

As a support worker, your role is to observe for these situations and accurately report them to the appropriate person. Many of these factors can co-exist (e.g., a client may have difficulty seeing and not be comfortable with the language). It is not appropriate for a support worker to give advice on medications or suggest that a person modify dosages, etc.

Sensory and Physical Factors

Older adults may have conditions that make it difficult for them to see the medication, read or hear instructions, or open the medication vials. Vision problems may make different pills seem identical or make it impossible to read the prescription label.

A person with impaired hearing may not have clearly understood the instructions or may not have heard the reason for using the medication in the first place.

Additionally, the person may not understand the response to any question he or she asked.

Arthritis or other conditions may make it painful or even impossible for the person to open a prescription vial or even flip up the top of a dossette.

Language Factors

Language factors can arise from two situations. They can arise when a person's preferred language is not the language in which the medication instructions are provided. For example, a client whose preferred language is Polish may find it very difficult indeed to follow medication instructions in English, whether verbal or written.

Language can also be a factor when a person's ability to read in the preferred language is limited or when terminology is new or unfamiliar. For example, a person may be quite able to converse in English, but not able to easily read it. Another person may have functional reading but have difficulty understanding the terminology used, as it is unfamiliar.

CASE EXAMPLE 26-2

Mr. Pelliter has high blood pressure. He is prescribed a medication. He does not take the medication regularly. When the support worker asks why he is not taking the medication, he tells her that the pills are only for when he is "nervous"—the doctor told him that they are for hypertension. Mr. Pelliter believes that hypertension is anxiety—high tension—not high blood pressure. The support worker advises her supervisor, who contacts Mr. Pelliter's case manager. When the case manager explains the terms to him, he begins to take his medication properly.

Cultural Factors

Cultural factors can mean many things. Perhaps a person's ethnic upbringing may not have included liquids recommended for taking the medication. One of the most common examples of this is milk. Many ethnic communities do not include milk in their diets. If a person who does not drink milk is to take medication with milk, he or she may well not take the medication, or take it incorrectly.

Culture can also include religious or ethnic prohibitions about medications. Some religions advise members to avoid all medications, or certain medications or medical procedures. Some communities simply do not condone the use of prescriptions.

Additionally, a person's individual upbringing may influence his or her compliance with a prescription. Some people have been raised to avoid medications. This has nothing to do with ethnicity or religion, but is rooted in the way the person was raised.

Misinformation

People receive information about medications from many sources: the pharmacist, other health professionals, media, friends, or neighbours. Though some information may be accurate, other information may not. As well, accurate information may be misunderstood due to sensory or language factors. A person who legitimately believes that a medication is—or could be—harmful may not take the medication or not take it consistently.

Previous Experience or Concern

In some cases a person experiences a reaction or a side effect to a medication. The person may not tell anyone but may avoid the medication.

Complexity

Sometimes, a medication plan is too complex for a person to follow. For example, a client may be asked to take four medications. Each one is to be taken twice a day, but at different times. This requires the person to remember eight separate events each day. This can happen when a person has more than one doctor prescribing medications (for example, a family doctor and a specialist). Sometimes, the schedule can be made simpler.

Cognitive Ability

Some persons have difficulty remembering to take medication, do not think that the medication they have is the "right" medication, or feel that their medication is not appropriate. Alternately, the person may take multiple doses, forgetting that she or he has already taken the medication.

Financial Limitations

Contrary to popular belief, not all medications are covered by provincial health plans. Some medications may not be covered at all; others may be subject to a co-payment. The person may not have the resources to pay for these medications.

STOP AND REFLECT **26-2**

You are caring for your client. She is alert and cognitively aware. She uses a dossette to manage her medications. Your role is to bring her water at the appropriate time so that she may take her pills. As she is arthritic, her husband fills the dossette on Fridays. This Thursday, your client accidentally knocks the dossette off the table. There is a full week's worth of pills in the dossette. There should only be two day's worth. When you ask the client, she becomes upset and tells you that her husband filled the dossette yesterday.

You know that her husband rarely varies from his routine. What would you do?

_____

_____

You should report the event to your supervisor.

SPOTLIGHT 26-2 CPA'S A.C.T.I.O.N PLAN FOR ADDRESSING MEDICATION PROBLEMS

A Assess/observe the situation

C Contact your supervisor

T Talk to family member (if present)

I Identify how you can help

O Open the chart and document

N Note to follow up

CASE EXAMPLE 26-3

Fran is asked to remind Mr. Singh to take his medication. One of Mr. Singh's medications is to be taken with milk. Mr. Singh does not drink milk, as it has never been a part of his diet. Fran notices this and suggests that Mr. Singh discuss this with his doctor or his daughter (who goes with him to see the doctor). She also advises her supervisor that she has done this.

ADMINISTERING MEDICATIONS

Pills and Capsules

Procedure 26-1
Administering Pills and Capsules That Are to Be Swallowed

EQUIPMENT

medication

liquid for swallowing

Unless otherwise indicated, oral medications must be swallowed in order to be effective. As stated earlier, you must ensure that the liquid given to help your client swallow is appropriate for the medication.

Never open capsules or split or crush medication unless specifically told to do so by the appropriate person. Medications altered in this way may cause unintended side effects.

1. Follow the seven rights listed earlier.
2. Wash your hands.
3. Explain to the client what you are doing.
4. Assist the client to sit up if possible. Prop with pillows or raise the head of the bed if necessary.
5. Pour the correct amount of pills or capsules into the inverted cap of the prescription bottle. Check again to ensure that number and strength are correct.
6. Pour medication into the client's hand.
7. Ask client to put the pill or capsule into mouth. Ask client to place it on the top of his or her tongue. Watch to see that the client does so.
8. Offer a full glass of water, juice, or other liquid to help the client swallow the medication. Make sure liquid offered is not contraindicated.
9. Remain with the client until the medication is swallowed.
10. If the client vomits immediately after taking the medication, check the emesis for the pill. Contact the appropriate person for directions.
11. Record as per the agency's requirements.

Procedure 26-2
Administering Buccal Tablets

A **buccal tablet** is medication in a form that is dissolved in the mouth and absorbs through the mucous membrane of the mouth. Buccal tablets work best when they are placed in the pouch between the teeth and the cheek (Figure 26-2).

1. Follow the seven rights listed earlier.
2. Wash your hands.
3. Explain to the client what you are doing.
4. Assist the client to sit up if possible. Prop with pillows or raise the head of the bed if necessary.
5. Pour the correct amount of pills or capsules into the inverted cap of the prescription bottle. Check again to ensure that number and strength are correct.
6. Pour medication into the client's hand.
7. Ask client to put the pill or capsule into the pouch between the mouth and the cheek.
8. Ask client to close mouth and let tablet dissolve completely. Remind client not to swallow or chew the tablet. Do not give liquids or foods while tablet is dissolving.
9. If necessary, ask client to open mouth and pull cheek to the side so that you can ensure that the pill has dissolved.
10. Record as per the agency's requirements.

EQUIPMENT

medication

FIGURE 26-2
Placement of a buccal tablet

Procedure 26-3
Administering Sublingual Tablets

Sublingual tablets are a form of medication that is dissolved under the tongue and absorbed through the mucous membrane of the mouth. This is best done by placing the medication under the tongue (Figure 26-3).

1. Follow the seven rights listed earlier.
2. Wash your hands.
3. Explain to the client what you are doing.
4. Assist the client to sit up if possible. Prop with pillows or raise the head of the bed if necessary.

EQUIPMENT

medication

5. Pour the correct amount of pills or capsules into the inverted cap of the prescription bottle. Check again to ensure that number and strength are correct.
6. Pour medication into the client's hand.
7. Ask client to put the pill or capsule under the tongue.
8. Ask client to close mouth and let tablet dissolve completely. Remind client not to swallow or chew the tablet. Do not give liquids or foods while tablet is dissolving.
9. If necessary, ask client to open mouth and lift tongue so that you can ensure that the pill has dissolved.
10. Record as per the agency's requirements.

FIGURE 26-3
Placement of a sublingual tablet

Oral Liquid Medications

If at all possible, use a calibrated spoon, cup, or oral syringe when giving liquid medications. A calibrated dose cup may be provided with the medication. A **syringe** is a hollow tube that can be filled with a medication and then administered. You should wash the cup, spoon, or syringe after use and dry it thoroughly. It is always best to use the cup, spoon, dropper, or syringe that the pharmacist provided with the medication. If no device was provided, ask the pharmacist for one or for advice.

Measuring Oral Liquid Medications Using an Oral Syringe

It is very important to accurately measure liquid medications. A slight error in the amount measured can significantly change the dosage.

1. Follow the seven rights listed earlier.
2. Wash your hands.
3. Explain to the client what you are doing.
4. Shake the medication unless the instructions advise otherwise. If the medication tends to foam when shaken, be careful not to shake the liquid too vigorously.

Procedure 26-4
Filling a Syringe Using a Bottle Adapter

EQUIPMENT

oral syringe

bottle adapter

medication

1. Many oral syringes come with an adapter that fits into the top of the bottle. Ensure that the adapter is clean. Dampen the adapter with tap water to make it more easily fit into the mouth of the medication bottle and insert it. Ensure that the adapter fits snugly.
2. If the oral syringe has a cap, remove it. Insert the tip of the oral syringe into the upper part of the adapter, as shown in Figure 26-4.

3. Make sure that you can easily read the markings on the syringe. Turn the syringe if necessary.

4. Hold the bottle and syringe vertically with the bottle upside-down at the top, as shown in Figure 26-4.

5. Draw the syringe's plunger out. This will draw the medication into the syringe. Make sure that you keep the tip of the syringe firmly inserted in the adapter so as to prevent air from entering the syringe.

6. If air enters the syringe, depress the plunger fully and draw the liquid into the syringe again.

7. Carefully measure the amount of medication as per the support plan. It's often easier to get the exact amount if you slightly overfill the syringe then depress the plunger until only the correct amount is remaining.

8. Carefully remove the syringe from the adapter. Avoid touching the syringe's tip to avoid contamination.

FIGURE 26-4
Measuring oral liquids into a syringe

Procedure 26-5
Filling a Syringe Without a Bottle Adapter

If there is no suitable adaptor available, you will have to fill the syringe from medication poured into a clean cup. Bear in mind that medication poured has become exposed to the air, the cup, and other items that may contaminate it; thus it cannot be returned to the bottle. Do not pour more than you need to fill the syringe with the prescribed amount.

1. Pour a small amount of the medication into a clean cup or glass. Do not pour an excessive amount as you will not be able to return the excess to the medication bottle.

2. Place the syringe upright into the liquid. Do not push the syringe to the bottom of the cup as this will make it very difficult for you to draw up the liquid.

3. Draw the syringe's plunger out. This will draw the medication into the syringe. Make sure that you keep the tip of the syringe in the liquid to prevent air from entering the syringe.

4. If air enters the syringe, depress the plunger fully and draw the liquid into the syringe again.

5. Carefully measure the amount of medication as per the support plan. It's often easier to get the exact amount if you slightly overfill the syringe then depress the plunger until only the correct amount is remaining.

6. Remove the syringe from the cup. Avoid touching any surface with the syringe's tip to avoid contamination.

EQUIPMENT

syringe

clean cup or glass

medication

Procedure 26-6
Administering Liquid Medication to an Adult Using an Oral Syringe

EQUIPMENT

filled oral syringe

Some clients may be able to swallow without problem, but have difficulty taking liquid medications from a spoon or medication cup. In these situations, you may be asked to administer the medication with an oral syringe. It is very important that you gently depress the syringe's plunger so as to administer an appropriate amount of liquid into the client's mouth. Depressing the plunger too quickly may cause the client to gag or choke.

1. Ask the client to sit upright. If necessary, assist the client or raise the head of the bed.
2. Slide the oral syringe tip along the inside cheek or point toward the back of the mouth. To avoid choking, make sure that the tip of the syringe is not far from the front of the mouth.
3. Slowly depress the plunger. Allow the person to swallow the liquid normally.
4. If permissible, offer a drink.

Procedure 26-7
Administering Liquid Medication to an Infant Using an Oral Syringe

EQUIPMENT

filled oral syringe

It is often safer and easier to administer liquid medication to an infant using an oral syringe. A medication spoon may be too large for the infant's mouth or may frighten him or her. Using a syringe allows you to control the flow of the medication so that the infant does not choke.

1. Hold the infant as though you were feeding him or her a bottle. Make sure that the infant's head and neck are well supported.
2. Use your thumb to gently push down on the infant's chin to open the infant's mouth.
3. Slide the oral syringe tip along the inside lower cheek or point toward the back of the mouth (Figure 26-5). To avoid choking, make sure that the tip of the syringe is approximately 1.5–2 cm from the front of the mouth.
4. Slowly depress the plunger to flow the liquid into the infant's mouth. Allow the infant to swallow the liquid normally. You may have to pause once or twice to allow the infant to swallow.

FIGURE 26-5
Administering liquid medications to an infant using an oral syringe

Procedure 26-8
Cleaning the Syringe

As with all equipment, medication syringes must be thoroughly cleaned after each use. Improper cleaning may result in medication residue remaining in the syringe. Residue may contaminate any new dose or may affect the function of the syringe. Following this procedure will ensure the syringe is properly cleaned.

1. Pull the plunger out of the barrel of the syringe.
2. Wash and thoroughly rinse all parts.
3. Shake the barrel out to remove excess water and position it upright to drain any remaining water.
4. Dry the plunger completely.
5. Store the parts in a clean area until the next use. Do not reassemble the syringe until both barrel and plunger are completely dry.
6. Wash and thoroughly rinse the cup or adapter. Shake the adapter to remove excess water. Dry the cup. Store with the syringe.

EQUIPMENT

oral syringe

clean water

towel for drying

Procedure 26-9
Administering Oral Liquid Medication Using a Medicine Spoon or Cup

1. Follow the seven rights listed earlier.
2. Wash your hands.
3. Explain to the client what you are doing.
4. Make sure that you can easily see the measurement markings on the spoon or cup.
5. Slowly pour medication into the spoon or cup until you reach the prescribed amount.
6. Ask the client to sit upright. If necessary, assist the person or raise the head of the bed.
7. Place the rim of the spoon or cup in the client's mouth.
8. Slowly tilt the spoon or cup so that the liquid runs into the client's mouth (Figure 26-6). Pause to allow the client time to swallow if necessary.
9. Make sure that the client receives all the medication.
10. If permissible, offer liquid to drink.
11. Wash, rinse, and dry the spoon or cup.

EQUIPMENT

medicine cup or spoon

medication

FIGURE 26-6
Administering oral liquid medications using a medication spoon

Procedure 26-10
Administering Oral Liquid Medication Using a Built-In Dropper

EQUIPMENT

medication with
built-in dropper

Some medications require that you administer a specific number of drops of medication. These medications are often packaged in a bottle with a dropper built into the cap.
1. Follow the seven rights listed earlier.
2. Wash your hands.
3. Explain to the client what you are doing.
4. Open the bottle.
5. Make sure that the tip of the dropper is in the liquid. Squeeze the bulb on the dropper to expel the air in the dropper.
6. Release the bulb, allowing liquid to rise into the dropper.
7. Administer the proper number of drops onto the client's tongue.

Procedure 26-11
Administering Oral Liquid Medication Using a Calibrated Dropper

EQUIPMENT

medication

calibrated dropper

Using a calibrated dropper requires you to carefully measure the liquid. It can be difficult to attain the desired amount.
1. Follow the seven rights listed earlier.
2. Wash your hands.
3. Explain to the client what you are doing.
4. Open the bottle.
5. Make sure that the tip of the dropper is in the liquid. Squeeze the bulb on the dropper to expel the air in the dropper.
6. Release the bulb, allowing liquid to rise into the dropper.
7. Remove the dropper from the liquid when you have drawn the prescribed amount. If you have drawn too much, carefully squeeze out the excess amount.
8. Administer the medication in the same manner as described in the procedure for administering medication with an oral syringe.
9. Clean the dropper in accordance with the procedure described in Procedure 26-8 on page 571.

Photo 26-7
Calibrated dropper
Source: Jupiter Unlimited

Transdermal Patch

Transdermal patches provide a constant flow of medication to a client. These patches release medication slowly so that the amount administered is constant over the period of time that the patch is applied. The medication is absorbed through the skin. In order to make sure that the amount of medication remains constant, the patch should be applied at the same time each day.

In order for a transdermal patch to be effective, it must be applied without wrinkles and without the adhesive side having come in contact with your hands or other surfaces. The patch must also be applied to clean, dry, and unbroken skin. Procedure 25-12 will help you properly apply a transdermal patch.

SPOTLIGHT 26-3 TRANSDERMAL PATCHES

You can be exposed to the medication in a transdermal patch by touching the sticky side. Even used patches may contain enough medication to pose a risk. Always handle patches (new or used) with care.

Procedure 26-12
Applying a Transdermal Patch

1. Follow the seven rights listed earlier.
2. Wash your hands.
3. Explain to the client what you are doing.
4. Identify the area to which the patch is to be applied. Be aware that some patches must be applied to a specific area of the body.
5. Do not apply the patch to skin that is broken, scratched, or has a rash or scar tissue, as these things can affect the absorption of the medication. Avoid skin folds and areas that usually are moist because the patch may not adhere securely. Avoid hairy areas as the patch may not adhere securely or work properly. As well, removing a patch from a hairy area can be painful.
6. Rotate patch locations to avoid skin irritation.
7. Wash and dry your hands thoroughly.
8. Wash the client's skin where the patch is to be applied. Thoroughly dry the area.
9. Open the package containing one patch (Figure 26-7). Be careful not to tear the patch.
10. Remove the backing from the patch. Do not touch the sticky side.
11. Apply the patch so that there are no wrinkles. Press the patch in place and maintain pressure on the patch for ten to fifteen seconds to ensure that the patch adheres properly and is secure.
12. Dispose of the wrapper and wash your hands.

EQUIPMENT

transdermal patch

water and soap to wash skin

towel for drying

FIGURE 26-7
Applying a transdermal patch

Lotions, Creams, Gels, and Other Topical Medications

You can easily absorb these medications by applying them with your bare hands. Use gloves when applying these medications.

Procedure 26-13
Applying Medicated Creams, Ointments, Gels, and Lotions

EQUIPMENT

medication

gloves

water and soap for washing

towel

gauze or bandage if required

It's important to bear in mind that medicated creams and lotions are just like any other medication and must be handled with the same care. Application of too much or too little may not yield the desired effect and may harm the client. The following procedure will ensure that you appropriately apply these medications.

1. Follow the seven rights listed earlier.
2. Wash your hands.
3. Explain to the client what you are doing.
4. If recommended or if you are applying the medication to broken skin, wear gloves.
5. Wash the area of the client's skin where the medication is to be applied. Pat off excess water, but leave the skin moist.
6. Apply a small amount of the medication to the client's skin (Photo 26-8). Remember that a thick layer of medication is no more effective than a thin layer.
7. Spread the medication over the designated area.
8. Do not cover with gauze or a bandage unless required.
9. Cap the medication.
10. Wash your hands.

Photo 26-8
Proper application of a medicated lotion

Source: © Design Pics Inc./Alamy

Eye Drops and Ointments

Eye drops and ointments must reach the surface of the eye to be effective. We all have a tendency to blink when something is dropped onto our eye. You will need to use caution to ensure that the eye drop or ointment makes contact with the eye, without touching the eye with the dropper or tube.

Procedure 26-14
Administering Eye Drops

EQUIPMENT

eye drop medication

1. Follow the seven rights listed earlier.
2. Wash your hands.
3. Explain to the client what you are doing.
4. Ask the client to lie down or to tilt his or her head back.

5. Ask the client to look up at the ceiling.

6. Open the eye drops. Do not allow the tip of the eye dropper to touch any surface.

7. Gently pull down the lower eyelid to form a pouch between the lid and the client's eye (Figure 26-8).

8. Position the eye dropper at the side of the client's eye. Do not allow the tip of the eye dropper to touch the eye. You may find it easier to control the position of the dropper if you rest the palm of your hand on the client's forehead.

9. Squeeze the dropper slightly to administer the prescribed number of drops into the pouch.

10. Ask the client to close her or his eyes and place light pressure on the inner corners of the eye to prevent the drops from leaving the eye. Ask the client to avoid rubbing or squeezing his or her eye shut to avoid forcing the medication out of the eye.

11. Recap the bottle.

12. Wash your hands.

FIGURE 26-8
Administering eye drops

Procedure 26-15
Administering an Eye Ointment

1. Follow the seven rights listed earlier.

2. Wash your hands.

3. Explain to the client what you are doing.

4. Ask the client to lie down or to tilt his or her head back.

5. Ask the client to look up at the ceiling.

6. Open the eye ointment. Do not allow the tip of the tube to touch any surface.

7. Gently pull down the lower eyelid to form a pouch between the lid and the client's eye (Figure 26-9).

8. Squeeze the tube gently to place the prescribed amount of ointment in the pouch at the side of the client's eye. Do not allow the tip of the tube to touch the eye. You may find it easier to control the position of the tube if you rest the palm of your hand on the client's forehead.

EQUIPMENT

eye ointment

9. Ask the client to close her or his eyes and place light pressure on the inner corners of the eye to prevent the ointment from leaving the eye. Ask the client to avoid rubbing or squeezing his or her eye shut to avoid forcing the medication out of the eye.
10. Recap the tube.
11. Wash your hands.

FIGURE 26-9
Administering eye ointment

Ear Drops

Bear in mind that the correct procedure for administering ear drops to an adult differs from the procedure used for an infant. Ensure you are using the appropriate technique. Contact your supervisor or the designated contact, if you are uncertain as to the correct approach with a very young child.

Procedure 26-16
Administering Ear Drops

EQUIPMENT

ear drops

towel

1. Follow the seven rights listed earlier.
2. Wash your hands.
3. Explain to the client what you are doing.
4. Ask the client to lie down or to tilt his or her head so that the ear to be treated is facing up.
5. Shake the ear drops. Warm the bottle in your hands before opening.
6. Open the bottle and squeeze and release the dropper to draw the medication into the dropper.
7. If you are administering the ear drops to an infant or toddler, pull the ear down and back slightly to straighten the ear canal (Figure 26-10). If you are administering the drops to a child, youth, or adult, pull the ear up and back slightly to straighten the ear canal (Figure 26-11).

8. Administer the prescribed number of drops into the ear canal. Do not insert the dropper into the ear canal or allow the dropper to touch any surface.

9. Ask the client to keep the treated ear "up" for 5–10 minutes to allow the drops to be absorbed. If both of the client's ears must be treated, allow 10–15 minutes between each ear to allow the drops to be absorbed in each ear.

10. Dry excess medication from the client's ear lobe.

11. Wash your hands.

FIGURE 26-10
Administering ear drops to infants

FIGURE 26-11
Administering ear drops to children and adults

Nose Drops

Like eye drops, nose drops can be uncomfortable for many people. Carefully follow the instructions for the medication. Many nose drops can be placed on the mucous membrane in the nose, making it less uncomfortable and less likely that the client will cough or sneeze. Use the following procedure to ensure that you appropriately administer nose drops.

Procedure 26-17
Administering Nose Drops

1. Follow the seven rights listed earlier.
2. Wash your hands.
3. Explain to the client what you are doing.
4. Ask your client to gently blow his or her nose to clear the nostrils.
5. Ask the client to sit in a chair and tilt his or her head backward. If more comfortable for the client, he or she can lie on a bed with a pillow under the shoulders so that the head can tip back. A small child or infant can lie on the worker's lap with his or her head tilted back and neck supported.

EQUIPMENT

nose drops

tissues

6. Shake the nose drops. Warm the bottle in your hands before opening.
7. Open the bottle and squeeze and release the dropper to draw the medication into the dropper.
8. Administer the prescribed number of drops into each nostril (Figure 26-12). Do not allow the dropper to touch any surface.
9. Ask the client to bend forward with his or her head toward the knees. Ask the client to hold this position for five to ten seconds, then sit upright for five minutes. This helps the drops reach the desired spot.
10. Wash your hands.

FIGURE 26-12
Administering nose drops

IF PROBLEMS ARISE

When you are asked to administer medication, you should know the name and telephone number of the person to call if a problem arises. You should contact that person and your supervisor if any of the following occur:

1. The client refuses to take the medication or says that the medication is not the correct one.
2. The client appears to have taken too much medication.
3. The client has skipped a dose of medication.

Key Points

1. Medications (also called drugs or medicines) include prescription drugs, over-the-counter drugs, vitamins, herbal compounds, alcohol, and tobacco. Each has the potential to cause harm if used improperly.
2. Four factors—the province in which you work, the policy of your employer, possibly the decision of a regulated health professional who supervises your care to a particular client, and your ability to safely carry out the correct procedure—determine whether you may administer medications.
3. Medication administration is far more than the physical act of administering a pill.
4. There are four common types of assistance: reminding the client; helping the client with the physical task, such as opening the bottle; handing the client the medication at the proper time; and administering the medication.
5. Page 558 lists ten specific things you need to know when assisting the client with medications.
6. Knowing and following the Seven Rights will help to ensure that you have administered the medication properly.

7. A person may not follow prescribed medication regimes because of physical, cultural, communication, misinformation, past or current experiences, complexity of the plan, cognitive ability or financial factors.
8. Medication monitoring is essential to good client support.
9. Accurate measuring of medication is essential to proper assistance.
10. Syringes and other medication supplies must be cleaned thoroughly after each use.

Questions for Review

1. What are four factors that must be considered before a support worker may administer a medication to a client?

2. What is medication monitoring? Why is it important?

3. Are herbal medicines drugs?

4. If taken incorrectly, can over-the-counter medications be as harmful as a prescription medication?

5. Is a generic medication exactly the same as the brand-name version? Why or why not?

6. What are the four types of assistance?

7. You have been asked to administer medication to Mr. London. What ten things must you know before you can safely do this?

8. What are the seven rights of medication administration?

9. What provincial legislation (if any) limits your ability to administer medication? What is this legislation called? What branch of the government administers it?

10. What does the acronym A.C.T.I.O.N. represent?

Questions for Discussion

1. Should support workers be able to administer medications? What are the risks of this? What are the benefits?

2. How do you feel about assisting a client to take medication? What types of assistance are easier for you to provide? Which are harder to do?

3. You have been asked to give Mrs. Jaeger her medication. When you bring it to her, she says, "That's not the right pill." The medication in the bottle is identical to the pill you gave her. The name on the label of the bottle matches the name of the medication you are to give. What do you do?

4. You are assigned to assist Mr. Cadieux. Your assignment does not include assisting Mr. Cadieux with medication. However, when you open the refrigerator to get Mr. Cadieux's lunch, you find a cup with two pills in it. A note in the cup says, "Make sure Mr. Cadieux takes these pills. They are essential." What do you do? Why?

Chapter 27

Preparing for Work

Learning Objectives

Through reading this chapter, you'll be able to

1. Define employability.
2. Describe the work settings most appropriate for you.
3. Use the seven-step method to prepare a resume that includes the proper content, is well organized, and is formatted so as to be attractive and easy to read.
4. Accurately complete a standard job application.
5. Conduct an effective job search.

Chapter at a Glance

- Employability
- Work Settings
- Your Resume
- The Job Application

Terms You'll Use

Chronological Resume A resume that organizes the information in each section by date.

Employability The ability to do the tasks of a job.

Functional Resume A resume that groups skills and experiences gained from a variety of employment situations.

Fundamental Skills Skills that provide the basic foundation to get, keep, and progress in a job.

Personal Management Skills The combination of skills, attitudes, and behaviours required to get, keep, and progress in a job.

Police Record Check A check done to provide proof that a person has not been convicted of a crime that would affect that person's employability.

References People who have agreed to give information regarding your abilities to potential employers.

Teamwork Skills Skills that are needed to work with others in a job.

EMPLOYABILITY

Employability is the ability to do the tasks of a job, and it is just a part of what you need to gain employment. Employers want employees who are also adaptable, take responsibility for their actions, and communicate and work well with others. These types of skills are classified into three groups: fundamental skills, personal management skills, and teamwork skills. Table 27-1 describes these three types of skills.

As you can see, these skills are complementary, but different. Many of these skills are discussed in this text and are covered in your training. To succeed as a personal support worker, you must excel in all three types of skills.

TABLE 27-1	Employability Skills		
Fundamental Skills	**Personal Management Skills**	**Teamwork Skills**	
The skills needed as a base for further development	The personal skills, attitudes, and behaviours that drive one's potential for growth	The skills and attributes needed to contribute productively	
You will be better prepared to progress in the world of work when you can: **Communicate** - read and understand information presented in a variety of forms (e.g., words, graphs, charts, diagrams) - write and speak so others pay attention and understand - listen and ask questions to understand and appreciate the points of view of others - share information using a range of information and communications technologies (e.g., voice, e-mail, computers) - use relevant scientific, technological, and mathematical knowledge and skills to explain or clarify ideas **Manage Information** - locate, gather, and organize information using appropriate technology and information systems - access, analyze, and apply knowledge and skills from various disciplines (e.g. the arts,	You will be able to offer yourself greater possibilities for achievement when you can: **Demonstrate Positive Attitudes and Behaviours** - feel good about yourself and be confident - deal with people, problems, and situations with honesty, integrity, and personal ethics - recognize your own and other people's good efforts - take care of your personal health - show interest, initiative, and effort **Be Responsible** - set goals and priorities balancing work and personal life - plan and manage time, money, and other resources to achieve goals - assess, weigh, and manage risk - be accountable for your actions and the actions of your group - be socially responsible and contribute to your community	You will be better prepared to add value to the outcomes of a task, project, or team when you can: **Work with Others** - understand and work within the dynamics of a group - ensure that a team's purpose and objectives are clear - be flexible: respect, be open to, and supportive of the thoughts, opinions, and contributions of others in a group - recognize and respect people's diversity, individual differences, and perspectives - accept and provide feedback in a constructive and considerate manner - contribute to a team by sharing information and expertise - lead or support when appropriate, motivating a group for high performance - understand the role of conflict in a group to reach solutions - manage and resolve conflict when appropriate	

▶▶│

TABLE 27-1	Employability Skills *(continued)*	
Fundamental Skills	**Personal Management Skills**	**Teamwork Skills**
The skills needed as a base for further development	The personal skills, attitudes, and behaviours that drive one's potential for growth	The skills and attributes needed to contribute productively
languages, science, technology, mathematics, social sciences, and the humanities) **Use Numbers** ▪ decide what needs to be measured or calculated ▪ observe and record data using appropriate methods, tools, and technology ▪ make estimates and verify calculations **Think and Solve Problems** ▪ assess situations and identify problems ▪ seek different points of view and evaluate them based on facts ▪ recognize the human, interpersonal, technical, scientific, and mathematical dimensions of a problem ▪ identify the root cause of a problem ▪ be creative and innovative in exploring possible solutions ▪ readily use science, technology, and mathematics as ways to think, gain and share knowledge, solve problems, and make decisions ▪ evaluate solutions to make recommendations or decisions ▪ implement solutions ▪ check to see if a solution works, and act on opportunities for improvement	**Be Adaptable** ▪ work independently or as part of a team ▪ carry out multiple tasks or projects ▪ be innovative and resourceful: identify and suggest alternative ways to achieve goals and get the job done ▪ be open and respond constructively to change ▪ learn from your mistakes and accept feedback ▪ cope with uncertainty **Learn Continuously** ▪ be willing to continuously learn and grow ▪ assess personal strengths and areas for development ▪ set your own learning goals ▪ identify and access learning sources and opportunities ▪ plan for and achieve your learning goals **Work Safely** ▪ be aware of personal and group health and safety practices and procedures, and act in accordance with these	**Participate in Projects and Tasks** ▪ plan, design, or carry out a project or task from start to finish with well-defined objectives and outcomes ▪ work to agreed quality standards and specifications ▪ select and use appropriate tools and technology for a task or project ▪ adapt to changing requirements and information ▪ continuously monitor the success of a project or task and identify ways to improve

Source: Employability Skills 2000+. *Brochure 2000 E/F (Ottawa: The Conference Board of Canada, 2000)*

WORK SETTINGS

Where do you want to work? In Chapter 2, we discussed the various types of work settings. Depending upon where you live, there may be many types of work settings readily available to you.

What's Available? Seeking Out the Opportunities

A good first step to starting your job search is finding out what opportunities are available in your community. There are several ways to do this:

1. **Ask family and friends who work in health care or support services for their recommendations.** This often is a good method of finding out a bit about an agency as well.
2. **Check with your teacher or your school's career counsellor.** Many teachers work (or have worked) in the field. Career counsellors are usually in contact with area employers. Teachers and counsellors can be a rich source of information and advice.
3. **Contact the local home care program for information on area agencies.** Many home care agencies produce lists of agencies and facilities for clients.
4. **Visit your local library or information centre.** Libraries and centres often have information on the services available in your area.
5. **Look in the yellow pages.** Many agencies are found under the headings of "Home Health Care,""Home Health Services,""Nursing Homes,""Retirement Homes," and "Nursing Services."
6. **Check employment ads in your local newspapers.** Most agencies regularly advertise for staff.
7. **Contact your local Canada Employment Centre.** These offices often have information about area employers even if the employers have not posted jobs with the centre.
8. **Attend job fairs held in your community.** Job fairs are usually advertised in local newspapers, on the community information channel of your local cable company, or even by flyers posted in local stores. These fairs usually provide an opportunity to learn about a number of agencies in a very short period of time.

Keep in mind that any time you visit an employer, attend a job fair, or visit an agency to make enquiries about potential employers, you are making an impression. Make sure that you dress professionally and appropriately for the visit. Do not take children or friends with you. Chapter 28 discusses professional appearance and behaviour in greater detail.

What Do I Want to Know?

When you are first seeking out the opportunities in your area, there are several questions you will want to answer:

1. What kinds of work do support workers do in the agency?
2. What types of clients does the agency serve?
3. Where is the agency located? Does the agency serve clients at other centres or in their homes?
4. Are there many types of jobs that support workers do? Do support workers have the opportunity to work in more than one type of job?
5. What types of training, experience, skills, and abilities does the agency look for in a support worker?
6. What are the hours of work? Do support workers work different shifts? Weekends? Holidays?
7. Do most of the support workers work full-time or part-time?
8. Does the agency encourage support workers to take additional training? If so, what opportunities are available?

9. What kind of supervision and guidance do support workers have?
10. What is the agency's mission or philosophy?
11. What is the agency's reputation?

What If the Agency Isn't Hiring?

It's likely that your search will turn up agencies that are not hiring support workers at that time. This is fine. You still can learn about the agency and perhaps submit an application for consideration in the future.

Getting the Right Fit

Once you have gathered information about the agencies in your area, you can begin to identify those that are most promising. The questions posed in Chapter 2 will assist you in refining your search. For each agency, answer the following:

1. Does the type of work interest me? Am I excited by the job?
2. Can I perform the tasks required? Do I have all the training I'll need? If not, will the agency provide the necessary training?
3. Do I like working with people in that kind of work setting?
4. Can I get to the work site? Can I travel from client to client if the job requires it? Do I like the amount of travel required?
5. Am I comfortable with the agency or client? Will I be proud to work for them?
6. Are the wages and benefits (if any) competitive?
7. Is there an opportunity to learn additional skills and take on different responsibilities if I would like to?

Police Record Checks

Many agencies now require that employees provide a **police record check** that provides proof that the person has not been convicted of a crime that would affect the employee's ability to work as a support worker. Exactly what convictions would affect a person's ability to work as a support worker will depend upon the specific job. For example, a conviction for impaired driving may not matter in some cases, but probably would matter if the position applied for involved driving clients.

Each agency has its own policy with regard to police record checks. Generally, the agency considering you for employment will tell you where you must go to obtain the record check. In some areas, the local police department handles record checks. In other areas, the provincial police or the Royal Canadian Mounted Police (RCMP) handles these requests. Most police departments charge a fee to provide a record check. Some will reduce the fee if you are requesting the record check in order to apply for a job.

If you have a criminal record for which you have not received a pardon, any convictions will be listed on the form you receive from the police department. You must be prepared to discuss any items appearing on your record. Note that you may apply for a pardon to remove a conviction from your record. Pardons are obtained through the federal government and are usually limited to convictions that occurred many years ago. Contact your local police department for information on how to apply for a pardon.

YOUR RESUME

What Is a Resume?

A resume advertises your skills and experience to a prospective employer. Its purpose is to make the employer so interested in you that you are granted an interview.

If the resume is to be effective, it must highlight your skills and make it easy for the employer to see how you might contribute to the organization. The resume must include the information an employer will want to see, be well organized, and be formatted so as to be professional, attractive, and easy to read.

The Seven-Step Method

Developing your resume has seven steps: information gathering, focusing, organizing, summarizing, checking, formatting, and printing. Let's take a look at each of these steps.

Information Gathering

Most employers want to know the relevant skills and experience you would bring to the job. Gather information for this section by writing down your previous and current experience using the categories in this section. For now, don't worry about organizing the information too much—simply write down the details.

Education Answer these five questions:

1. Do you have a certificate or diploma in support work or a similar field?
2. What is the exact name of the certificate (e.g., Support Service Worker or Personal Support Worker)?
3. From what educational institution did you get your certificate or diploma? In what year?
4. Do you have a high-school diploma? When and where did you get this certificate?
5. Are there other relevant certificates you have attained (e.g., a certificate in palliative care or mental health support)? When and where did you get these certificates?

As you gather this information, focus on any items that may be attractive to an employer. Did you complete a field placement in a setting that gave you special skills, such as an Alzheimer day centre, an infant stimulation program, or a palliative care centre? Did you take classes from someone who is well known in the field? Did you receive any awards or honours for your work?

At first glance, you may feel that including your high-school diploma is unnecessary. It may be. Include the diploma if it was recently granted and you feel that it will demonstrate your commitment to learning and attest to your self-discipline. For example, if you returned to school as an adult and completed your diploma while working, you are demonstrating that you can set realistic goals, balance priorities, and achieve success under difficult circumstances. These are qualities that most employers desire.

Experience Experience is gained through paid employment and volunteer work. It also includes experience you have gained from work not directly related to your career.

For example, you might have gained valuable problem-solving skills through volunteer work with an organization like the Girl Guides, Block Parents, or Big Sisters. Ask yourself if the experience is something that you could use as a support worker. If the experience is relevant, jot it down.

Abilities and Skills Skills are techniques that you have developed. Abilities are often traits that you may have had all of your life. As you identified your experience, you likely began to identify abilities you have used and skills you have gained. For example, you may have been able to creatively tailor your approach to your clients' needs. Or, you may have developed problem-solving or teamwork skills. Make a list of these abilities and skills.

Interests You may want to consider including a brief description of your interests or hobbies. Sometimes, these help to give a more complete picture of you as a person. Interests and hobbies can also tell a bit about your self-discipline, commitment, and organization.

Make sure that you are specific in your description and include only two or three significant interests. For example, if you are a long-distance runner, you might say, "I am a long-distance runner who has completed fifteen races in the past three years."

Focusing

What do you offer an employer? Look at the answers you've written down during the information-gathering phase. Compare what you offer to the things you have learned employers look for in a support worker. You might want to ask your instructor or another person who knows you well to look over your answers and give you other ideas. The employability skills listed earlier in this chapter may also help you recognize attributes you have. Make a list of the information that is most relevant to potential employers.

It's important to be specific about your attributes. If you can communicate well with clients who have some type of dementia, say so. Don't use a vague phrase like "good communication skills" if you can give a really relevant example.

Organizing

You now have all the information you need to develop your resume. In the organizing phase, you'll put this information in order so that the most important information is the easiest to find.

There are two basic methods of organizing your information. The first method organizes information chronologically, starting with the most recent information. The second method organizes information by function. Each method has its particular uses. In this section, we'll discuss each in terms of what it is and when you should consider using it.

Chronological Resume In a **chronological resume**, you organize the information in each section by date. It is most appropriate when your work experience is in the same field as is the job you'd like to get, and most of your work experience has been with one or two employers over that period of time. For example, you would use a chronological resume when you have worked as a support worker for a period of time and you are applying for a similar position. As this method illustrates your work history, it's not a good choice if you have held positions with a number of employers.

Exhibit 27-1 illustrates a sample chronological resume. Refer to this resume as we discuss the various components.

A chronological resume usually begins with a section on work experience. Within this section, list the positions you have held starting with the most recent employer. If you are working in the field, you should include information about your present employment first. For each employment situation, state the position held, the employer, and the dates of employment. In a sentence or two, describe the most significant aspects of your work for that employer. Any skills you developed are usually listed with the employment, although they can be summarized in a separate section.

A section on education usually follows the section on work experience. The most recent certificate or diploma is usually listed first unless there is a specific certificate or diploma you know the employer prefers. For example, if you are applying for a support worker position, you might list a support worker certificate first even though you may have taken other certificates more recently.

After the section on education, you may choose to list skills and interests in separate sections.

Functional Resume **A functional resume** groups skills and experiences gained from a variety of employment situations. It is most appropriate when you have had a number of positions, have gaps in your work history, have had positions that vary in responsibility or skills, or have held a number of part-time positions in the field. Exhibit 27-2 illustrates a functional resume created by a person who holds three part-time positions in the field.

In this method, the skills gained through the various positions are identified at the beginning of the resume. Skills should be organized to highlight the most significant skills. (The resume in Exhibit 27-2 includes a section on the type of clients with whom the worker has experience as this is seen as important to employers.) Sources of the experience are listed after the skill set but without describing which skills came from each setting. Education and interests follow experience.

Summarizing

Summarizing includes three components: identifying data, a career objective, and a summary statement.

Identifying Information You must include some identifying data: your name, address, telephone number, as well as a statement that you are legally able to work in Canada. You should not include your social insurance number or any information about your age, race, citizenship, marital status, children, or religious affiliation. Because your age can be determined from some provincial driver's licence numbers, you should not include your licence number on your resume.

Place the identifying information at the top of the first page of the resume. Centre the information or use a bold or larger typeface to make sure your name stands out.

Career Objectives and Summary Statements Including a career objective or summary statement is optional. Many resumes include a career objective (as illustrated in Exhibits 27-1 and 27-2). Others include a summary of the candidate's significant background. The choice of including one or both is a personal one. Use the guidelines below to determine whether you should include these items.

EXHIBIT 27-1
A sample chronological resume

AUDREY O'SHEA
123 Anywhere Road · Anytown, British Columbia V7B 1J2 · 604-555-1234

Objective

To secure a full-time or part-time position providing personal support to clients who live in the community.

Employment

SOUTHWESTERN HOME HEALTH & SUPPORT	Central, B.C.
HOMEMAKER	OCTOBER 2007–PRESENT

I provide assistance with: personal care (bathing, dressing, grooming, eating, etc.) and exercise and ambulation, including follow-up on physiotherapy/occupational therapy orders as appropriate. I also provide relief for caregivers of clients with dementia.

MID-REGIONAL MS SUPPORT SERVICES	Burnaby, B.C.
ATTENDANT	JUNE 2004–OCTOBER 2007

Responsible to tailor approach and service to clients with Multiple Sclerosis whose needs often varied from day to day. Demonstrated creativity and flexibility in determining with clients what tasks were to be performed and how they were to be done.

VILLA LIVING CENTRE	North Vancouver, B.C.
HEALTH CARE AIDE	JUNE 2003–MAY 2004

Responsible to assist 15 cognitively impaired residents with routine activities of living. Developed strong communication, problem-solving, and time management skills.

Education

PERSONAL SUPPORT WORKER CERTIFICATE	November 2005	
Bytown College	*Bytown, B.C.*	

SECONDARY SCHOOL DIPLOMA	June 2003	
Bytown District School Board	*Bytown, B.C.*	

Skills & Abilities

- Manage multiple demands
- Flexible
- Work in a variety of settings
- Organized
- Responsible
- Reliable
- Strong problem-solving skills
- Thorough

I speak the following languages:

English	Gujrapi
Katcsi	Swahili

Career Objective A career objective is useful only when it indicates a specific objective that meets a unique employment need. Avoid vague objectives like "To use my skills in a community agency." Table 27-2 lists sample specific objectives.

TABLE 27-2	Examples of Specific Objectives

> **"Providing personal support to clients with dementia in a day program setting."**
>
> **"Assisting with recreation programs in a long-term care facility."**
>
> **"Working with clients receiving palliative care service at home."**

EXHIBIT 27-2
A functional resume

AUDREY O'SHEA
123 Anywhere Road · Anytown, British Columbia V7B 1J2 · 604-555-1234

Objective

To secure a full-time or part-time position providing personal support to clients who live in the community.

Skills and Abilities

- Manage multiple demands
- Flexible
- Responsible
- Work in a variety of settings
- Organized
- Calming
- Reliable
- Thorough
- Caring
- Strong problem-solving skills
- Gentle
- Professional

I have worked successfully with clients in a variety of settings:
- Palliative
- Cognitively Impaired
- Rehabilitation
- Clients with Chronic Pain
- Post-Surgical Recovery

I speak the following languages:
- English
- Gujrapi
- Katcsi

Employment

I currently work with three local agencies on an on-call basis. With each, I provide the following:
- Assistance with personal care (bathing, dressing, grooming, eating, etc.)
- Assistance with exercise and ambulation, including follow-up on physiotherapy/occupational therapy orders as appropriate.
- Assess changes in client condition and report observations to supervisor
- Caregiver relief
- Housekeeping and meal preparation

The agencies with which I currently work are:

SOUTHWESTERN HOME HEALTH & SUPPORT HOMEMAKER	Central, B.C. OCTOBER 2007–PRESENT
MID-REGIONAL MS SUPPORT SERVICES ATTENDANT	Burnaby, B.C. JUNE 2004–OCTOBER 2007
VILLA LIVING CENTRE HEALTH CARE AIDE	North Vancouver, B.C. JUNE 2003–MAY 2004

Education

PERSONAL SUPPORT WORKER CERTIFICATE *Bytown College*	NOVEMBER 2005 *Bytown, B.C.*
SECONDARY SCHOOL DIPLOMA *Bytown District School Board*	JUNE 2003 *Bytown, B.C.*

If you have more than one specific area of interest, you might consider creating a separate resume for each area. If your resume was created on a computer, it is often very easy to create two resumes from the same information.

Summary Statement Summary statements are statements that give a brief overview of your relevant background. These statements are usually placed at the beginning of the resume, just after the career objective.

Include a summary statement only if you want to highlight an aspect of your background that is truly desirable to an employer or that gives a context to your application. For example, if you have specialized in working with children with multiple needs and are applying to work in an agency serving children, you might create a summary statement that highlights your years of experience and training in that capacity.

A summary statement should not be used to highlight general skills or to highlight interests or attitudes. Table 27-3 illustrates some well-defined—and some ill-defined—summary statements.

TABLE 27-3	Summary Statements
Try This...	**Not This...**
To indicate expertise in a specific field: Over the past 10 years, I have focused my training and work in the area of dementia care. I have received three awards for my work with clients.	*Not focused on a specific need:* I am an outgoing person who is interested in clients. I enjoy working with people who need assistance.
To explain a career shift: After 15 years in accounting, I left the field to train in personal support. This change has enabled me to use my interpersonal and problem-solving skills to assist people to live independently.	*Not directly related to the profession:* I have won several awards for my artwork in local competitions.

Formatting and Printing

Formatting includes the layout and typesetting that help to make your resume look professional. Proper formatting makes it easy for the reader to find the information he or she is seeking. Printing means the way the resume is copied.

Formatting and printing make the first impression on your reader. A neat, well-formatted resume will encourage the reader to consider what you have to say. A poorly laid-out or printed resume will not be considered. Remember that the average employer spends only a few seconds looking at each resume he or she receives. If your resume doesn't catch the employer's eye, you won't be considered for the position.

Formatting Many computer programs such as WordPerfect® or Microsoft Word® have predefined layouts that you can use to create a professional-looking resume. If you have a computer, or have access to one at school, you may be able to use one of these layouts. Ask a colleague or teacher for help in using the layout. Remember to save your work on a disk so that you can easily edit the information.

If you have access to a computer but do not want to use a predefined layout, consider using a layout that you have seen and liked. You might copy a layout used by a colleague or use one found in a resume preparation handbook (usually available at your local library).

A third option is to have your resume formatted by a professional typist or resume preparer. You might be able to have this done through the career centre at your school. Typists and professional preparers charge for their services. Make sure that you know what you will receive and how much it will cost before arranging for the service. Career centres may charge a nominal fee for their service. Be aware that you are responsible for the accuracy of the information in your resume, even if you use a professional resume service to prepare it.

No matter who formats your resume, make sure to use professional and easy-to-read typefaces. Use no more than two typefaces, preferably one for the section headings and another for the information under each heading. Do not use script fonts, headline fonts, or other decorative fonts. Table 27-4 illustrates some good—and not so good—choices.

TABLE 27-4	Good—and Not So Good—Choices
Use This...	Not This...
I have worked as a support worker (Times New Roman typeface)	I have worked as a support worker (Nickelodeon typeface)
I have worked as a support worker (Arial typeface)	*I have worked as a support worker (Snell Black typeface)*

Checking Before you print your resume, take a good look at it. Make sure that it is attractive, clear, and complete. Use the following questions to examine your resume's components:

1. Are my name, address, and telephone number at the top of the first page of the resume? Are they correct? Are they in slightly larger type and easy to read?
2. Does the typeface and size make the resume look professional and easy to read?
3. Is the resume free from spelling and typographical errors? Remember that a computer spell-checker will not flag a word that is spelled correctly, even if it is not the right word. Make sure that another person reads your resume to catch these errors.
4. If you stated a career objective, is it specific enough to be useful without being so specific that you might be excluded from consideration from a position you might want? Is your objective no longer than two sentences?
5. If you stated a summary, does it reflect the events in your career that are most significant to the position for which you are applying? Is your summary no longer than two sentences?
6. Have you included all the information that would be significant to a potential employer? Have you removed any "extra" information that is not essential?
7. Does your resume use a consistent writing style from beginning to end?
8. Have you included the names and contact information of persons who have agreed to give professional, academic, and personal **references** on your behalf? Make sure that you obtain each person's permission before you include his or her name as a reference.

Printing Your resume should be printed on high-quality paper in a light colour (grey, off-white, or white) using a laser or ink-jet printer. Avoid using a dot-matrix printer or a low-quality printer that smears ink or prints poorly.

If possible, have several copies of your resume printed on a laser printer or good-quality ink-jet printer. If this is not possible, then make sure that you make copies on a high-quality photocopier. Many office supply stores now offer high-quality printing and copying at reasonable prices.

THE JOB APPLICATION

Most employers require applicants to complete a job application even if the applicant has submitted a resume. An employer may do this for several reasons: to make sure that all applicants submit information in the same format; to make sure that specific information is provided by all applicants; and even to make sure that applicants can understand and complete a simple form.

You must be prepared to complete an application. Although most employers design their own form, most forms ask for similar information. Use the sample application form in Exhibit 27-3 to make sure you have the information you need to complete a basic application form.

Remember that you must be truthful and accurate in your answers. If an answer to a question points out a shortcoming (for example, if you were fired from a recent job), answer the question honestly and attach an explanation if necessary.

EXHIBIT 27-3

Sample application form

Questions for Review

1. What is employability? Why is it important?

2. What do you need to do to prepare a resume that includes the proper content, is well organized, and is formatted so as to be attractive and easy to read?

3. What makes up an effective job search?

Questions for Discussion

1. What work settings are most appropriate for you? What makes a particular setting a good one for you? Compare your answers with those of your colleagues.

2. When you are preparing your resume, is it ever a good idea to leave out information about your work or education? Why or why not?

3. You were out of the workforce for seven years when your children were young. How might you describe this period in your resume?

Chapter 28

Presenting Yourself to an Employer

Learning Objectives

Through reading this chapter, you'll be able to

1. Explain the importance of professional appearance at all phases of your job search.
2. Describe the proper attire for visiting the employer.
3. Appropriately reply to advertisements for employment.
4. List the eight things you should do in any interview.
5. Outline the steps you should take if accepting an offer of employment.
6. Describe the steps you should take as a follow-up when you are not the successful candidate.

Chapter at a Glance

- Professional Appearance and Behaviour
- Contacting Prospective Employers
- Your Cover Letter
- The Interview
- The Offer of Employment
- When You Have Not Been Offered Employment

Terms You'll Use

Attire Clothing.

Conditional Offer of Employment An offer of employment that is conditional upon you providing certain documents before you can be hired.

Probationary Period A trial period of employment.

Professional Appearance All aspects of how you appear, including clothing, cleanliness, and the attention paid to the details of grooming.

Professional Behaviour Conducting yourself in a polite and businesslike manner.

PROFESSIONAL APPEARANCE AND BEHAVIOUR

You must take every opportunity to make a positive impression on a potential employer. Remember that even the most casual contact, such as dropping in to the agency to obtain a brochure, gives the employer an opportunity to see you. How you dress, how you act, who is with you, will all be observed. These observations form the employer's first impression of you. First impressions are lasting impressions. It is difficult for most people to change their first impression. If you look and behave in a professional manner, you will make a positive impression. If your appearance or behaviour is unprofessional, you will make a negative impression.

What Is Professional Appearance?

Professional appearance includes all aspects of how you appear: your clothing, your cleanliness, and the attention you pay to the details of your grooming. Use the following guidelines to help you attain a professional appearance. Photo 28-1 shows a professional-looking applicant.

Photo 28-1
Professional appearance
Source: *Preferred Health Care*

Clothing

1. You should dress in business-type **attire**. This means a dress, a suit, or coordinating shirt with pants or a skirt. Do not wear casual clothing such as T-shirts, tracksuits, tube tops, jeans, or shorts. Select clothing that fits properly and make sure that any undergarment (such as a slip or bra strap) does not show.
2. All clothing should be clean, without stains, and in good repair. Replace missing buttons and repair sagging hems.
3. Hosiery should be appropriate and in good repair. Stockings should be free of holes and runs. Avoid ankle socks and gym socks, as they are too casual.
4. Shoes should be polished and in good condition. Do not wear casual shoes such as running shoes or sandals.

Grooming

1. You must be clean and fresh. Shower or bathe before your interview. Wash your hands just before the interview so that they are clean.
2. Make sure that your hair is freshly washed and neat. Keep hair ornaments (barrettes, bows, clips, or headbands) to a minimum.
3. Makeup should be subtle.
4. Wear minimal jewellery. Avoid large rings, earrings, or bracelets. Remove obvious body ornaments, such as tongue studs, eyebrow studs, and nose rings.
5. Make sure that your nails are clean and neatly trimmed. If you wear nail polish, choose a neutral colour.
6. Make sure your teeth are clean and your breath is fresh. If you have eaten or smoked, chew a breath mint before the interview.

Professional Behaviour

Professional behaviour means conducting yourself in a polite and businesslike manner. Observe the following guidelines to help ensure a good impression:

1. Do not take children, family members, or friends along to the interview.
2. Arrive five to ten minutes early for any scheduled appointment. Avoid dropping in to the agency at busy times, even if you are just picking up or dropping off information.
3. Make sure that you have a clean, unwrinkled copy of your resume to leave with the prospective employer. Invest in a portfolio to protect your resumes from damage.
4. Make sure you have a pen that writes cleanly. Bring a spare in the event that the first runs dry. Make sure the ink is blue or black. Do not use red, green, violet, or fluorescent inks to fill out forms.
5. Neatly and fully complete any forms given to you to fill out. Complete the form on-site unless you are told that the form may be taken home.
6. Make your communication respectful. For example, if you have someone who is picking you up at the conclusion of the visit, politely ask the employer if you can tell that person how long you might be. Don't say something like "Will this be long? I have someone waiting for me."
7. If you carry a cell phone, turn it off during an interview.
8. Thank the employer for his or her time.

CONTACTING PROSPECTIVE EMPLOYERS

Submitting an Unsolicited Application or Resume

You need not wait until you see an advertisement to make an application or submit a resume for employment. Many agencies accept applications or resumes at any time, although others accept them only at specific times. Be sure to call the agency first to see if it is accepting applications or resumes.

When you submit an unsolicited application or resume, make sure that you include a cover letter. Your cover letter should follow the format described later in this chapter. It should indicate that you are aware that the agency is not currently hiring and that you wish to have your application on file if a position becomes available.

Responding to an Advertisement

Employers may post advertisements in local newspapers, at the local Canada Employment Centre, at schools, or even on the public service boards in supermarkets and shopping centres. Get into the habit of checking the locations where employers in your area post advertisements.

An advertisement for a support worker position will usually contain some information about the duties involved, the experience and academic requirements, as well as the procedure to follow to submit a resume or application. The information contained in the advertisement can give valuable clues as to how you should present yourself to the employer. Let's take a look at the components of a sample advertisement, using Exhibit 28-1 as an example.

EXHIBIT 28-1
Sample advertisement

Omega Support Services Association
is seeking
Support Workers (with certificate)

We have immediate openings in our outreach
and assisted-living programs for support workers
(with certificate). The successful candidates will be
enthusiastic and have experience working with clients with
a wide range of disabilities. Experience in providing
support in a community setting and in working with
clients with communication disorders is preferred.
A car is essential for the outreach position.

You may apply in person at:

12345 Bytown Road
Anytown, B.C.
on **October 15 & 16, between the hours of 1–4 p.m. only**

Please bring resume and a copy of all relevant certificates.

Employer

Who is advertising? In this case, it is Omega Support Services Association. In order to personalize your cover letter, you will want to find out the name of the person who will receive your resume. If possible, find out this information through a colleague or friend who works at the agency, not by calling the agency. The agency may receive many such calls and become a bit frustrated at the time it takes to respond to each one.

Type of Position

What positions are being offered? In this instance, both assisted living and outreach positions are available. You would have to decide whether you are interested in applying for either or both. Your interest would be reflected in your cover letter.

What Requirements Does the Agency Have?

Requirements are "must-haves." These are usually stated as "necessary for the position," "essential," or "at a minimum, the candidate must have." Make sure you distinguish the requirements from the preferred characteristics.

Omega Support Services requires four things for either position: enthusiasm, a certificate as a Support Worker, experience working with people with a wide range of disabilities, and the ability to start as soon as possible. The outreach position also requires that the candidates have a vehicle. All other characteristics are preferences.

In general, you must make sure that you possess the requirements stated before you apply. An agency may feel that you did not take the time to read its advertisement thoroughly, or that you are wasting its time if you apply without the necessary qualifications. Your cover letter should state that you have the requirements.

What Qualities Does the Agency Desire?

Many agencies will list preferred characteristics in their advertisements. Preferred characteristics are things that will cause the agency to prefer one applicant over another but that are not absolute requirements. In Exhibit 28-1, experience in community settings and experience with clients who have communication disorders are preferred characteristics.

If you have one or more of the preferred characteristics, point out this information in your cover letter.

Keep in mind that the agency may not state in its advertisement all the characteristics it prefers. This is where any prior knowledge you have about the agency can be useful. For example, you may learn from colleagues that Omega Support Services emphasizes teamwork. Even though this is not explicitly stated in the advertisement, you might refer to this in your cover letter.

How Do Candidates Apply?

Be certain to carefully follow the instructions for making applications. The agency may have arranged for extra staff members to be present to process the applications and may have made other preparations to receive applications in a specific way. If you do not follow the agency's instructions, you run the risk of irritating the people you want to hire you. In some cases, your application may not be considered if you do not submit it in accordance with the stated instructions.

Omega Support Services wants candidates to apply in person between 1 p.m. and 4 p.m. on October 15 and 16. Thus, you could visit the agency on either date. In order to allow for ample time for your application to be reviewed, you should arrive no later than 3:30 p.m.

Some agencies will ask that you fax or mail a resume. In most cases, you can drop off a resume instead. If so, you can use the visit to make a positive impression. If the agency does not want resumes submitted in any other way, respect its wishes.

YOUR COVER LETTER

When you submit a resume, you should always include a cover letter. This letter should be no longer than one page and should be typewritten. It should also meet the following criteria:

1. It is addressed to the appropriate person, by name. For example, if the person hiring support workers is Jane Harberry, the Coordinator, you should address your cover letter to "Ms. Jane Harberry." Take the time to find out the name of the person and make sure that you have the correct spelling of the person's name.
2. It highlights your skills and abilities that directly relate to the position for which you are applying.
3. It focuses on how you can contribute to the agency, not on the challenges and opportunities you expect the agency to give you.
4. It does not contain misleading information.
5. It is grammatically correct and has no spelling or typographical errors.
6. It is typed on the same kind of paper as you used for your resume.
7. It is signed in blue or black ink.

THE INTERVIEW

The interview provides you and the employer the opportunity to find out more about each other. It is also your opportunity to show how well you can contribute to the agency.

Plan Ahead

If you have planned ahead, you will have investigated the agency as a part of the job search described in Chapter 27. You will have learned about the agency, its clients, services, and philosophy. If not, you should take the time to learn about the agency before you go to the interview.

Your initial investigation probably answered many questions. It likely raised some questions about the agency. These questions may be ones to ask in the interview. Review these questions with a teacher or trusted friend before the interview.

Another aspect of planning ahead is knowing your own strengths and weaknesses. What parts of your career have been most satisfying for you? Are there types of work you do better than others? Reviewing this information in your mind will help prepare you for any questions.

Arrive on Time

Make sure that you allow plenty of time to get to the interview. If you are unfamiliar with the area, consider taking a trial trip from your home to the site. Plan to arrive at least ten minutes before the scheduled appointment time. This will allow you a few minutes to collect your thoughts before the interview begins.

Allow Plenty of Time

Allow plenty of time for the interview. If you have a friend waiting for you, make sure that the person knows that you may be an hour or more, particularly if the interview goes well.

During the Interview

Be Confident

It's normal to be a bit nervous in an interview. However, you don't want to let any nervousness get in the way of giving your best impression. In particular, you want to put forth an image of confidence. Make sure that your body language says that you are comfortable and confident of your skills and that you are interested and excited about the potential opportunity. If you have a "nervous habit," such as playing with your pen or picking at your cuticles, make sure that you do your best to control it.

Prepare for Commonly Asked Questions

Most interviewers have questions they prefer to use in an interview. If possible, find out what questions are likely to be asked (colleagues and friends who have interviewed with the same agency can be a good source of information). Prepare for these questions, but also be prepared for other questions as well. Some common questions include the following ones:

1. What interests you about working for our agency?
2. What type of client poses the greatest challenge to you and why?
3. What do you plan to do five years from now?
4. What makes you feel that you are particularly well suited to this type of work?

You may be asked "what would you do" questions. These are often case studies for which you are asked to describe the action you might take in a situation. Be aware that the agency probably has a policy that it would ask staff to follow in the situation. Consider beginning your response to questions like these with a phrase such as "As an employee, I would follow your procedure for handling this type of situation. Without knowing your procedure I would likely do the following." Then, outline what you would do. This allows you to demonstrate good problem-solving skills without appearing to go against an agency's policy.

Answer Questions Directly and Honestly

When you are asked a question, make sure that you answer the question directly and honestly. If the answer leads to a weakness, own up to it. For example, you might be asked why you left a previous position. If you were fired because you were often late, you must be forthright. If you have corrected the problem, make sure that you use the opportunity to include this information. For example, you might say something like "I was fired from that position because I was frequently late. Afterward, I made certain that I did not allow other things to interfere with my ability to get to work on time. I have not been late for work since then."

Handle the Conclusion of the Interview Professionally

You will often have the opportunity to ask questions at the end of the interview. This is an appropriate time to ask any remaining questions you have about the position. It is not an appropriate time to ask about salary or benefits.

At the conclusion of the interview, remember to thank the interviewer for his or her time. At that time, you may ask when you can expect to hear the agency's decision. Be careful to word your question carefully so that it does not sound as though you are demanding that the person contact you. Consider using this type of question: "Do you have an idea of when you'll be making your decision?" or "Would it be appropriate for me to contact you in the next week or so?"

Follow-Up

It's always a good idea to write a brief note of thanks to the interviewer. Exhibit 28-2 shows a typical thank-you note. The note shows that you appreciate the amount of time and effort that the interview process takes. It also shows that you pay attention to details and are organized in your job search. This note should be sent to the person who interviewed you no later than two days after the interview. The note should be handwritten on a blank note card. Do not send a letter or a thank-you card that has a printed verse inside.

Your note should express your appreciation for the interviewer's time. You should also include a sentence about something that impressed you about the agency or about the way the interviewer conducted the interview. Make sure that any compliment you offer is specific and genuine. For example, you might say, "The way you

EXHIBIT 28-2
A typical note

Dear Ms. Harberry,

Thank you for your time Monday. I really appreciated the opportunity to interview for the outreach support worker position in your new program. From what you told me, I'm sure that the program will make it much easier for clients to remain in their own homes.

Thank you again for your time.

Sarah Jones

asked questions really put me at ease," or "I was impressed with the way you have involved clients in the development of the assisted-living project." It's usually a good idea to write out a rough draft of your note on plain paper first. Make any changes before you write the final version on the card. Make sure that you sign your name on the card.

THE OFFER OF EMPLOYMENT

When Will I Hear?

Although it's possible that you will be offered employment at the conclusion of the interview, an offer is most likely to come after the agency has held all the interviews scheduled for a particular period of time. Don't be disappointed if your interview does not conclude with an immediate job offer.

Conditional Offer of Employment

If you are offered a job, it is likely to be a conditional offer of employment. This means that you must provide certain documents before you can be hired. The most common conditions are: a medical report that certifies that you are free from infectious diseases and able to perform the duties of the position; and a criminal record check or a vulnerable sector screening that shows no offences unacceptable to the employer. You will usually have to supply the required information before you can begin to work for the agency.

Probationary Periods

Employers usually make an initial offer of employment on a trial basis. This situation is called a probationary period. Most provinces have legislation that governs this probationary period, but it is usually a few months long. This gives both you and the agency the opportunity to see how well your employment works out. Usually, if the probationary period is successful, you become a regular employee.

Your Responsibilities

It is particularly important to submit all required documents as soon as possible so that you can begin work. If your agency requires that a particular form be completed, obtain the form and get it to the proper person as soon as you can.

You will likely have to complete tax forms and other payroll documents. Have all the information that is required when you complete the form and make sure that any information you write down is correct and legible.

WHEN YOU HAVE NOT
BEEN OFFERED EMPLOYMENT

Not every interview will result in an offer of employment. This may be for several reasons: the agency had more qualified applicants than it could hire; your skills were not exactly what the agency was seeking; or you were simply not the strongest candidate.

You should follow up with the agency to see if you can learn why you were not the appropriate candidate and what you can do to improve your chances for employment. Most agencies will share their impressions with you, provided that you let them know that you are seeking for ways to improve your interview skills and nothing more.

If you are able to discuss your performance with the interviewer, keep in mind that you are there to learn, not to debate the interviewer's opinion. Listen carefully to what the person has to say. Focus on how you can improve your skills. Take notes if possible, and ask questions so that you fully understand what the interviewer is saying. At the conclusion, thank the interviewer for his or her time. Be sure to send a written thank-you note as soon as possible after the session.

When you return home, review the notes that you have made. Make the changes that you need to make. If the interviewer made suggestions as to how you may better answer interview questions, practise these suggestions with a friend.

Questions for Review

1. Describe how you would dress to give a professional appearance.

2. What are eight ways you can demonstrate professional behaviour when contacting an employer?

3. What five types of information must you find in an advertisement?

4. Why should you send a cover letter with any resume or application?

Questions for Discussion

1. You are being interviewed for a job in a new long-term care facility. The clients will all be over 90 and many will have a cognitive impairment. How would you answer the following questions?
   a. What do you see yourself doing two years from now?
   b. What interests you most about this position?
   c. Working with clients with cognitive impairment poses real challenges to support staff. How have your training and experience prepared you for this role?

2. Generate a list of interview questions you feel an employer is likely to ask. Share your questions with your colleagues. Then use these questions to help each other practise responding.

3. You are in an interview. The employer asks you why you left a position you held two years ago. You were not the right person for that position and were let go before your probationary period was over. How do you respond to the employer's question?

Canadian Charter of Rights and Freedoms

Schedule B

Constitution Act, 1982 (79)

Enacted as Schedule B to the Canada Act 1982 (U.K.) 1982, c. 11,
which came into force on April 17, 1982

PART I

Canadian Charter of Rights and Freedoms

Whereas Canada is founded upon principles that recognize the supremacy of God and the rule of law:

Guarantee of Rights and Freedoms

1. The Canadian Charter of Rights and Freedoms guarantees the rights and freedoms set out in it subject only to such reasonable limits prescribed by law as can be demonstrably justified in a free and democratic society.

Rights and freedoms in Canada

Fundamental Freedoms

2. Everyone has the following fundamental freedoms:
   a) freedom of conscience and religion;
   b) freedom of thought, belief, opinion and expression, including freedom of the press and other media of communication;
   c) freedom of peaceful assembly; and
   d) freedom of association.

Fundamental freedoms

Democratic Rights

3. Every citizen of Canada has the right to vote in an election of members of the House of Commons or of a legislative assembly and to be qualified for membership therein.

Democratic rights of citizens

4. (1) No House of Commons and no legislative assembly shall continue for longer than five years from the date fixed for the return of the writs of a general election of its members.

   (2) In time of real or apprehended war, invasion or insurrection, a House of Commons may be continued by Parliament and a legislative assembly may be

Maximum duration of legislative bodies

Continuation in special circumstances	continued by the legislature beyond five years if such continuation is not opposed by the votes of more than one-third of the members of the House of Commons or the legislative assembly, as the case may be.
Annual sitting of legislative bodies	5. There shall be a sitting of Parliament and of legislative each legislature at least once every twelve months.

Mobility Rights

Mobility of citizens	6. (1) Every citizen of Canada has the right to enter, remain in and leave Canada.
	(2) Every citizen of Canada and every person who has the status of a permanent resident of Canada has the right
Rights to move and gain livelihood	a) to move to and take up residence in any province; and
	b) to pursue the gaining of a livelihood in any province.
	(3) The rights specified in subsection (2) are subject to
Limitation	a) any laws or practices of general application in force in a province other than those that discriminate among persons primarily on the basis of province of present or previous residence; and
	b) any laws providing for reasonable residency requirements as a qualification for the receipt of publicly provided social services.
Affirmative action programs	(4) Subsections (2) and (3) do not preclude any law, program or activity that has as its object the amelioration in a province of conditions of individuals in that province who are socially or economically disadvantaged if the rate of employment in that province is below the rate of employment in Canada.

Legal Rights

Life, liberty and security of person	7. Everyone has the right to life, liberty and security of the person and the right not to be deprived thereof except in accordance with the principles of fundamental justice.
Search or seizure	8. Everyone has the right to be secure against unreasonable search or seizure.
Detention or imprisonment	9. Everyone has the right not to be arbitrarily detained or imprisoned.
Arrest or detention	10. Everyone has the right on arrest or detention
	a) to be informed promptly of the reasons therefor;
	b) to retain and instruct counsel without delay and to be informed of that right; and
	c) to have the validity of the detention determined by way of *habeas corpus* and to be released if the detention is not lawful.
Proceedings in criminal and penal matters	11. Any person charged with an offence has the right
	a) to be informed without unreasonable delay of the specific offence;
	b) to be tried within a reasonable time;
	c) not to be compelled to be a witness in proceedings against that person in respect of the offence;

d) to be presumed innocent until proven guilty according to law in a fair and public hearing by an independent and impartial tribunal;

e) not to be denied reasonable bail without just cause;

f) except in the case of an offence under military law tried before a military tribunal, to the benefit of trial by jury where the maximum punishment for the offence is imprisonment for five years or a more severe punishment;

g) not to be found guilty on account of any act or omission unless, at the time of the act or omission, it constituted an offence under Canadian or international law or was criminal according to the general principles of law recognized by the community of nations;

h) if finally acquitted of the offence, not to be tried for it again and, if finally found guilty and punished for the offence, not to be tried or punished for it again; and

i) if found guilty of the offence and if the punishment for the offence has been varied between the time of commission and the time of sentencing, to the benefit of the lesser punishment.

12. Everyone has the right not to be subjected to any cruel and unusual treatment or punishment.

Treatment or punishment

13. A witness who testifies in any proceedings has the right not to have any incriminating evidence so given used to incriminate that witness in any other proceedings, except in a prosecution for perjury or for the giving of contradictory evidence.

Self-crimination

14. A party or witness in any proceedings who does not understand or speak the language in which the proceedings are conducted or who is deaf has the right to the assistance of an interpreter.

Interpreter

Equality Rights

15. (1) Every individual is equal before and under the law and has the right to the equal protection and equal benefit of the law without discrimination and, in particular, without discrimination based on race, national or ethnic origin, colour, religion, sex, age or mental or physical disability.

Equality before and under law and equal protection and benefit of law

(2) Subsection (1) does not preclude any law, program or activity that has as its object the amelioration of conditions of disadvantaged individuals or groups including those that are disadvantaged because of race, national or ethnic origin, colour, religion, sex, age or mental or physical disability.

Affirmative action programs

Official Languages of Canada

16. (1) English and French are the official languages of Canada and have equality of status and equal rights and privileges as to their use in all institutions of the Parliament and government of Canada.

Official languages of Canada

(2) English and French are the official languages of New Brunswick and have equality of status and equal rights and privileges as to their use in all institutions of the legislature and government of New Brunswick.

Official languages of New Brunswick

Advancement of status
and use

(3) Nothing in this Charter limits the authority of Parliament or a legislature to advance the equality of status or use of English and French.

English and French
linguistic communities
in New Brunswick

16.1 (1) The English linguistic community and the French linguistic community in New Brunswick have equality of status and equal rights and privileges, including the right to distinct educational institutions and such distinct cultural institutions as are necessary for the preservation and promotion of those communities.

Role of the legislature
and government of
New Brunswick

(2) The role of the legislature and government of New Brunswick to preserve and promote the status, rights and privileges referred to in subsection (1) is affirmed.

Proceedings of Parliament

17. (1) Everyone has the right to use English or French in any debates and other proceedings of Parliament.

Proceedings of the New
Brunswick legislature

(2) Everyone has the right to use English or French in any debates and other proceedings of the legislature of New Brunswick.

Parliamentary statutes
and records

18. (1) The statutes, records and journals of Parliament shall be printed and published in English and French and both language versions are equally authoritative.

New Brunswick statutes
and records

(2) The statutes, records and journals of the legislature of New Brunswick shall be printed and published in English and French and both language versions are equally authoritative.

Proceedings in courts
established by Parliament

19. (1) Either English or French may be used by any person in, or in any pleading in or process issuing from, any court established by Parliament.

Proceedings in New
Brunswick courts

(2) Either English or French may be used by any person in, or in any pleading in or process issuing from, any court of New Brunswick.

Communications by public
with federal institutions

20. (1) Any member of the public in Canada has the right to communicate with, and to receive available services from, any head or central office of an institution of the Parliament or government of Canada in English or French, and has the same right with respect to any other office of any such institution where
   a) there is a significant demand for communications with and services from that office in such language; or
   b) due to the nature of the office, it is reasonable that communications with and services from that office be available in both English and French.

Communications by public
with New Brunswick
institutions

(2) Any member of the public in New Brunswick has the right to communicate with, and to receive available services from, any office of an institution of the legislature or government of New Brunswick in English or French.

Continuation of existing
constitutional provisions

21. Nothing in sections 16 to 20 abrogates or derogates from any right, privilege or obligation with respect to the English and French languages, or either of them, that exists or is continued by virtue of any other provision of the Constitution of Canada.

Rights and privileges
preserved

22. Nothing in sections 16 to 20 abrogates or derogates from any legal or customary right or privilege acquired or enjoyed either before or after the coming into force of this Charter with respect to any language that is not English or French.

Minority Language Educational Rights

23. (1) Citizens of Canada

    a) whose first language learned and still understood is that of the English or French linguistic minority population of the province in which they reside, or

    b) who have received their primary school instruction in Canada in English or French and reside in a province where the language in which they received that instruction is the language of the English or French linguistic minority population of the province, have the right to have their children receive primary and secondary school instruction in that language in that province.

(2) Citizens of Canada of whom any child has received or is receiving primary or secondary school instruction in English or French in Canada, have the right to have all their children receive primary and secondary school instruction in the same language.

(3) The right of citizens of Canada under subsections (1) and (2) to have their children receive primary and secondary school instruction in the language of the English or French linguistic minority population of a province

    a) applies wherever in the province the number of children of citizens who have such a right is sufficient to warrant the provision to them out of public funds of minority language instruction; and

    b) includes, where the number of those children so warrants, the right to have them receive that instruction in minority language educational facilities provided out of public funds.

Language of instruction

Continuity of language instruction

Application where numbers warrant

Enforcement

24. (1) Anyone whose rights or freedoms, as guaranteed by this Charter, have been infringed or denied may apply to a court of competent jurisdiction to obtain such remedy as the court considers appropriate and just in the circumstances.

(2) Where, in proceedings under subsection (1), a court concludes that evidence was obtained in a manner that infringed or denied any rights or freedoms guaranteed by this Charter, the evidence shall be excluded if it is established that, having regard to all the circumstances, the admission of it in the proceedings would bring the administration of justice into disrepute.

Enforcement of guaranteed rights and freedoms

Exclusion of evidence bringing administration of justice into disrepute

General

25. The guarantee in this Charter of certain rights and freedoms shall not be construed so as to abrogate or derogate from any aboriginal, treaty or other rights or freedoms that pertain to the aboriginal peoples of Canada including

    a) any rights or freedoms that have been recognized by the Royal Proclamation of October 7, 1763; and

    b) any rights or freedoms that now exist by way of land claims agreements or may be so acquired.

Aboriginal rights and freedoms not affected by Charter

26. The guarantee in this Charter of certain rights and freedoms shall not be construed as denying the existence of any other rights or freedoms that exist in Canada.

Other rights and freedoms not affected by Charter

Multicultural heritage

27. This Charter shall be interpreted in a manner consistent with the preservation and enhancement of the multicultural heritage of Canadians.

Rights guaranteed equally to both sexes

28. Notwithstanding anything in this Charter, the rights and freedoms referred to in it are guaranteed equally to male and female persons.

Rights respecting certain schools preserved

29. Nothing in this Charter abrogates or derogates from any rights or privileges guaranteed by or under the Constitution of Canada in respect of denominational, separate or dissentient schools.(93)

Application to territories and territorial authorities

30. A reference in this Charter to a Province or to the legislative assembly or legislature of a province shall be deemed to include a reference to the Yukon Territory and the Northwest Territories, or to the appropriate legislative authority thereof, as the case may be.

Legislative powers not extended

31. Nothing in this Charter extends the legislative powers of any body or authority.

Application of Charter

Application of Charter

32. (1) This Charter applies
   a) to the Parliament and government of Canada in respect of all matters within the authority of Parliament including all matters relating to the Yukon Territory and Northwest Territories; and
   b) to the legislature and government of each province in respect of all matters within the authority of the legislature of each province.

Exception

(2) Notwithstanding subsection (1), section 15 shall not have effect until three years after this section comes into force.

Exception where express declaration

33. (1) Parliament or the legislature of a province may expressly declare in an Act of Parliament or of the legislature, as the case may be, that the Act or a provision thereof shall operate notwithstanding a provision included in section 2 or sections 7 to 15 of this Charter.

Operation of exception

(2) An Act or a provision of an Act in respect of which a declaration made under this section is in effect shall have such operation as it would have but for the provision of this Charter referred to in the declaration.

Five year limitation

(3) A declaration made under subsection (1) shall cease to have effect five years after it comes into force or on such earlier date as may be specified in the declaration.

Re-enactment

(4) Parliament or the legislature of a province may re-enact a declaration made under subsection (1).

Five year limitation

(5) Subsection (3) applies in respect of a re-enactment made under subsection (4).

Citation

Citation

34. This Part may be cited as the *Canadian Charter of Rights and Freedoms.*

National and Provincial Long-Term Care Associations

All provinces have long-term care services. However, the exact services each province provides are different. The following list provides information on selected provincial and national associations. It is current as of September 2007. Please note that this is not an exhaustive list. There may be other associations or organizations in your area.

International

World Health Organization
http://www.who.int/

National

Canadian Healthcare Association
17 York Street
Ottawa, Ontario K1N 9J6
tel: (613) 241-8005
fax: (613) 241-5055
http://www.cha.ca

Canadian Mental Health Association
180 Dundas Street West, Suite 2301
Toronto ON M5G 1Z8
tel: (416) 484-7750
fax: (416) 484-4617
http://www.cmha.ca

Public Health Agency of Canada
(federal government)
http://www.phac-aspc.gc.ca/

The Vanier Institute of the Family
94 Centrepointe Drive
Ottawa, Ontario K2G 6B1
tel: (613) 228-8500
fax: (613) 228-8007
http://www.vifamily.ca/

Alberta

Alberta Continuing Care Association
509 5241 Calgary Trail
Edmonton, Alberta T6H 5G8
tel: (780) 435-0699
fax: (780) 436-9785
http://www.longtermcare.ab.ca

Alberta Health & Wellness
http://www.health.gov.ab.ca/default.htm

Health Sciences Association of Alberta
http://www.hsaa.ca/
Edmonton
10212 - 112 Street
Edmonton, Alberta T5K 1M4
tel: (780) 488-0168
toll-free: 1-800-252-7904
fax: (780) 488-0534
Calgary
Suite #204 - 200 Country Hills Landing NW
Calgary, Alberta T3K 5P3
tel: (403) 250-8999
toll-free: 1-800-252-7904
fax: (403) 250-8576
Lethbridge
#404, 515 - 7 Street South
Lethbridge, Alberta T1J 2G8
tel: (403) 328-8005
toll-free: 1-866-328-8005
fax: (403) 328-8025

HBA Services
(Assumed role of Provincial Health Authorities
of Alberta)
900, 9925-109 Street
Edmonton AB T5K 2J8
Phone: (780) 426-8500
Fax: (780) 424-4309
http://www.hbas.ca

British Columbia

British Columbia Care Providers Association
#301 -1338 West Broadway
Vancouver, BC V6H 1H2
tel: (604) 736-4233
fax: (604) 736-4266
http://www.bccare.ca

British Columbia Paraplegic Association
780 S.W. Marine Drive
Vancouver, B.C. V6P 5Y7
tel: (604) 324-3611
toll-free: 1-877-324-3611
fax: (604) 326-1229
http://www.bcpara.org/default.aspx

Public Health Association of BC
#219 - 2187 Oak Bay Ave
Victoria BC V8R 1G1
tel: (250) 595-8422
fax: (250) 595-8622
http://www.phabc.org

New Brunswick

New Brunswick Home Support Association
P.O. Box 21004, (By Pass Postal Outlet)
1715 Woodstock Road,
Fredericton, New Brunswick E3B 7A3
http://www.sjfn.nb.ca/community_hall/N/
newxxxxx.html

**The New Brunswick Association
of Nursing Homes Inc.**
1113 Regent Street, Suite 302
Fredericton, NB E3B 3Z2
tel: (506) 460-6262
fax: (506) 460-6253
http://www.nbanh.com

**Family and Community Services Department,
Province of New Brunswick**
Sartain MacDonald Building
551 King Street
Fredericton, New Brunswick E3B 1E7
tel: (506) 453-2001
fax: (506) 453-7478
http://www.gnb.ca/0017/index-e.asp

Newfoundland and Labrador

**Newfoundland and Labrador Health Boards
Association**
2nd Floor Beothuck Building
20 Crosbie Place
St. John's, NL A1B 3Y8
tel: (709) 364-7701
fax: (709) 364-6460
http://www.nlhba.nl.ca/

Nova Scotia

**Continuing Care Association of Nova Scotia
(CCANS)**
tel: (902) 956-0090
http://www.nsnet.org/ccans/index.html
Home Support Nova Scotia Association
Armdale Professional Building
2625 Joseph Howe Drive, Suite 35
Halifax, Nova Scotia B3L 4G4
tel: (902) 479-0989
fax: (902) 479-0990

**Nova Scotia Association of Health Organizations
(NSAHO)**
2 Dartmouth Road,
Bedford, Nova Scotia B4A 2K7
tel: (902) 832-8500
fax: (902) 832-8505
http://www.nsaho.ns.ca

Ontario

Ontario Home Care Association
19 Melrose Avenue South
Hamilton, Ontario L8M 2Y4
tel: (905) 543-9474
fax: (905) 545-1568
http://www.homecareontario.ca/

Ontario Association of Non-Profit Homes and Services for Seniors
7050 Weston Road, Suite 700
Woodbridge, Ontario L4L 8G7
tel: (905) 851-8821
fax: (905) 851-0744
http://www.oanhss.org

Ontario Community Support Association
104–970 Lawrence Avenue West
Toronto, Ontario M6A 3B6
tel.: (416) 256-3010
toll-free: 1-800-267-6272
fax: (416) 256-3021
http://www.ocsa.on.ca

Ontario Retirement Communities Association
2155 Leanne Blvd., Suite 218
Mississauga Ontario L5K 2K8
tel: (905) 403-0500
toll-free: 1-800-361-7254
fax: (905) 403-0502
http://www.orca-homes.com

Ontario Long-Term Care Association
345 Renfrew Drive, 3rd Floor
Markham, Ontario L3R 9S9
tel: (905) 470-8995
fax: (905) 470-9595
http://www.oltca.com/

Personal Support Network of Ontario
104–970 Lawrence Avenue West
Toronto, Ontario M6A 3B6
tel.: (416) 256-3010
toll-free: 1-800-267-6272
fax: (416) 256-3021
http://www.personalsupportontario.ca/

Prince Edward Island

PEI Council of the Disabled Inc.
25 University Ave., Suite 300
Charlottetown, Prince Edward Island C1A 7N7
tel: (902) 892-9149
toll-free: 1-888-473-4263
fax: (902) 566-1919
http://www.peicod.pe.ca/

Community Hospitals and Continuing Care, Province of Prince Edward Island
http://www.gov.pe.ca/health/chacc-info/index.php3

Health Association of PEI
10 Pownal Street
Charlottetown, Prince Edward Island C1A 3V6
tel: (902) 368-3901
fax: (902) 368-3231
http://www.cha.ca/members.htm#Health_Association_of_PEI_(HAPEI)_

Quebec

Santé et Services Sociaux Quebec
Quebec City area: (418) 644-4545
Montreal area: (514) 644-4545
Elsewhere in Quebec: 1 877 644-4545 (toll-free)
http://www.msss.gouv.qc.ca/en/index.php

Saskatchewan

Saskatchewan Association of Health Organizations
600-2002 Victoria Ave.
Regina, Saskatchewan S4P 0R7
tel: (306) 347-5500
fax: (306) 525-1960
http://www.saho.org

Glossary

Abdomen The portion of the body between the pelvis and the diaphragm.

Abduction moving an arm or leg away from the centre of the body.

Abuse Harm to a victim caused by anyone upon whom the victim relies for basic needs or support.

Accountability Being personally responsible for your actions.

Acquired Brain Injury Brain injury that occurs as the result of trauma, anoxia, hemorrhage, seizure, or toxins.

Acquired Immune Deficiency Syndrome A condition caused by HIV in which the person experiences opportunistic diseases.

Active Range of Motion Exercise Movement completed by the client.

Acute Care The type of care provided in hospitals. Clients in an acute care setting are usually called patients.

Acute Care Facility A setting in which a person receives treatment for a specific medical condition on a short-term basis. This is another term for a hospital.

Adaptive Communication A form of communicating in which a group of techniques is used to adapt communication to the specific needs of the sender or receiver.

Adolescence The period from 12–19 years of age.

Adduction Moving an arm or leg toward the centre of the body.

Age-Related Changes The changes that are part of the aging process that happen to everyone if they live long enough.

Alignment The positioning of the body along a straight line.

Alimentary Canal The structure that links the organs of the digestive system. It is also called the gastrointestinal tract.

Anatomy The study of the body's structure.

Antibacterial An agent that destroys bacteria and/or prevents bacterial growth.

Antibiotics Medications that treat bacterial infections.

Anticipatory Grief The sense of loss, grieving, and preparing to move on that can occur before an expected loss happens.

Anxiety Disorders A group of conditions in which anxiety becomes extremely disabling over a long period of time.

Aphasia The complete or partial loss of language skills because of an injury to the brain.

Appearance Observations about body language, dress, and cleanliness.

Apraxia A condition that results from an injury to the brain, making voluntary, physical control of purposeful movement difficult.

Arthritis A condition that causes pain, stiffness, and sometimes swelling in or around joints. It can also affect other tissues.

Assertiveness A technique that helps you respect others' views, concerns, and needs while not compromising your own.

Assessment The phase of support planning that determines the type of support needed.

Assisted Living A setting in which clients live in their own apartments or townhouses but receive services from an agency in the building. Assisted living is also called supportive housing or assisted housing.

Attendant A person who assists a client with physical disabilities, who directs his or her own care.

Attire Clothing.

Augmentative Communication A form of communicating in which physical aids are used in communication.

Autism Spectrum Disorder A group of disorders that affect verbal and non-verbal communication and social interaction caused by abnormalities in brain structure or function.

Autonomy Each person's right to have his or her decisions respected.

Bacteria Microscopic organisms that we commonly call germs.

Barriers Things that prevent the message from getting across when communicating, such as language or hearing impairment.

Base of Support That part of the body that is in contact with the supporting surface—the weight-bearing surface most often defined by the position of your feet.

Behaviour Observations about actions, awareness and interest in surroundings, and awareness and interest in others.

Beneficence The obligation to prevent or remove what is bad and to promote what is good.

Biodegradable A material that is easily broken down into chemicals that do not harm the environment.

Bipolar Disorder A condition in which a person has alternating periods of hyperactivity and depression; also called manic depression.

Blister Pack A card containing single doses of one or more medications prescribed for a person.

Blood Assists in nutrition and elimination, regulation, protection, and oxygenation of the body.

Blood Pressure The pressure of the blood within the arteries.

Body Language Communication through posture, facial expressions, and movements. This is often called nonverbal communication.

Bones Hard, rigid, living structures that provide support for the body.

Buccal Tablet A dose of medication that is dissolved in the mouth and absorbs through the mucous membrane of the mouth.

Canada's Food Guide A guide that is based on nutritional needs and provides an easy way to ensure that people obtain the nutrients required to build and maintain a healthy body. *Canada's Food Guide* was revised in 2007.

Cancer A disease in which cells grow abnormally and out of control.

Carbohydrates Substances formed of starches and sugars that provide energy.

Care Plan A written document that outlines the support a client is to receive. This document often describes client needs and support goals, and includes names and contact information for family members and other services involved in the client's support. There are many forms of care plans. These plans are also called support plans or service plans.

Caregiver A person who assists the client. Caregivers can include people who are not paid (e.g., family, friends, neighbours, and volunteers) as well as those who are paid (e.g., support workers or companions).

Cell The basic element of the human body and all living things.

Centre of Gravity The point where mass is equally distributed.

Cerebral Palsy A condition that results from an anomaly or injury to the brain as it develops.

Chain of Infection The process of transmission of an infection.

Chronic Care The type of care provided to people whose condition is stable, but who need more professional care than residents of long-term care facilities. Some provinces have separate buildings for chronic care facilities; others provide chronic care services in acute care centres.

Chronic Obstructive Pulmonary Disease A group of irreversible lung diseases.

Chronological Resume A resume that organizes the information in each section by date.

Circumcision The surgical removal of the foreskin of the penis.

Clarifying Describing things clearly so that others understand or asking questions so that you understand.

Clean Technique A method of destroying many pathogens to prevent transmission of infection; also called medical asepsis.

Cleft Lip A congenital fissure or opening in the upper lip.

Cleft Palate A congenital fissure in the roof of the mouth, resulting from incomplete fusion of the palate during embryonic development.

Client A person who uses community support services. Throughout this text, we will use the term client to refer to clients, residents, and consumers.

Client Teaching The instruction given to a client by a support worker.

Club Foot A congenital condition that may result in the following: an infant's foot (especially the heel) being smaller than normal, pointing downward, the front of the foot rotating toward the other foot, or the entire foot turning in. In extreme cases, the bottom of the foot can point up.

Code of Conduct A statement that is intended to guide support worker practice. It is often made up of ethical principles, support worker qualities, and skills. It is sometimes called a code of ethics.

Cognition The ability to process information; it includes six cognitive processes.

Cognitive Impairment A situation that disrupts the way the brain works to think, use language, remember, and coordinate movements.

Cognitive Processes The six factors that contribute to cognition: perceiving, recognizing, interpreting, and organizing information; judging; and reasoning.

Communication The ability to share your ideas, explore others' ideas, and resolve conflicts. The aim of communication is to understand and to be understood. In reporting, this means observations about messages, including what is said and how it is said.

Community A setting in which a person lives in her or his own home (house or apartment) without support services located in the same building.

Conditional Offer of Employment An offer of employment that is conditional upon you providing certain documents before you can be hired.

Confidentiality The obligation to keep the client's personal information private.

Congenital Hip Dysplasia A condition resulting in partial or total hip dislocation.

Connective Tissue The tissue that forms bones, tendons, cartilage and other fibrous tissues.

Consumer In this book, we use the term to describe a person with temporary or permanent physical disability who uses support services.

Content Information communicated through words.

Continence The ability to control bowel or bladder function.

Continuing Care The type of care provided on a long-term basis. Continuing care can refer to long-term services provided in facilities or for people who live in their own homes.

Continuum A range.

Contracture A tightening of muscles, tendons, ligaments or skin that prevents normal movement.

Crisis Plan A document that includes information to help address any worsening symptoms to avoid further deterioration and list the client's wishes for support or care if the client becomes unable to express these wishes because of a mental health crisis.

Cycle of Abuse A term used to describe the three phases of abuse: abuse, remorse, and anger escalation.

Day Program Programs that provide clients an opportunity to take part in activities and be with others in a secure setting. Some day programs offer rehabilitation services to help clients recover from illness or injury. Other programs are geared toward clients with specific conditions, such as clients who have dementia or who have had a stroke.

Decubitus Ulcers Skin breakdown caused when tissue is trapped between a hard surface and a bony prominence. Often occur when clients are not repositioned frequently; also called pressure sores.

Delirium A reversible cognitive impairment often related to extremely high fever, medications, or infections.

Dementia A term used to describe a set of symptoms that occur in some types of cognitive impairment.

Development The progression from simple to more complex communication, language, thinking, movements and behaviours.

Depression A range of conditions from a feeling of sadness to a clinical syndrome.

Developmental achievements The expected physical, emotional, or psychological and social skills at a particular age, stage or situation.

Developmental delays When physical skills and behaviours expected at a particular point in an individual's life are not present.

Diabetes A disease resulting from the pancreas's inability to produce enough insulin or to properly use the insulin that is produced.

Disability A limitation to a person's functioning, caused by an impairment, that affects things the person needs or wants to do.

Disinfection The process of destroying pathogens.

Distress Stress that prevents us from functioning in the way we would like.

Documentation Written reports such as notes, reports, and checklists.

Do-Not-Resuscitate Orders A document that states a person is not to receive life-sustaining measures.

Dossette A container that holds individual doses of medication.

Down Syndrome A condition caused by an unusual arrangement of chromosomes, most often due to the presence of an additional copy of chromosome 21 in each cell.

Drug An agent that alters the body's mechanisms.

Dysarthria A condition that results from a weakness or lack of coordination in some of the muscles involved in speaking.

Early-Onset Dementia Dementia that occurs in younger people.

Embolus A mass, such as an air bubble, a blood clot or clump, or a foreign body that travels through the bloodstream and lodges in a way that blocks a blood vessel.

Empathy The ability to sense what others are feeling while respecting that you will never fully understand their emotions.

Employability The ability to do the tasks of a job.

Engorgement A painful overfilling of the breasts.

Epithelial Tissue The tissue that covers the internal and external body tissues.

Ethics The principles that guide how people behave.

Ethnicity A person's ethnic origin.

Evaluation The phase of support planning that reviews the client's situation, needs, and preferences.

Extension Straightening the joint.

Facility A setting in which a person lives that has shared dining and recreational areas. In facilities, the person receives support from services housed in the same building. Throughout this text, the term facility will refer to long-term care facilities, retirement homes, and rest homes.

Failure to Thrive A condition that occurs when abuse causes a child to fail to grow and develop.

Fat The substance that allows fat-soluble vitamins to be used by the body. Fat forms adipose tissue in the body and serves as an energy reserve.

Feelings Emotions communicated through words and body language.

Fetal Alcohol Effect (FAE) A disorder that can occur when a woman drinks alcohol during pregnancy; milder than FAS.

Fetal Alcohol Syndrome (FAS) A disorder that can occur when a woman drinks alcohol during pregnancy; more serious than FAE.

Filters Things that affect how we communicate, including body language, mood, and stress.

Fine motor skills The delicate movements of the human body that require small muscles and coordination.

Fire Hazards Things in the environment that pose a risk of fire or could make a fire spread.

Flexibility The ability to adapt to changes in a relationship, setting, or situation.

Flexion Bending the joint.

Fragile X Syndrome A genetic disorder caused by a weakness or break in a portion of a child's X chromosome.

Functional Change The way in which a particular condition affects a client.

Functional Resume A resume that groups skills and experiences gained from a variety of employment situations.

Fundamental Skills Skills that provide the basic foundation to get, keep, and progress in a job.

Fungi A microscopic plant that lacks chlorophyll and must rely on a host to survive.

Goal Setting The phase of support planning in which client goals are identified, along with the methods that will be used to attain the goals.

Generic Name The name of the active ingredient in a medication.

Good Body Mechanics Using your body in a safe and efficient manner to avoid injury and/or repetitive strain.

Grief Work Tasks associated with moving through the phases of grieving.

Gross motor skills The movements of the body that primarily involve the body's large muscles.

Group Home A home in which a small number of people live—in most cases, no more than eight people. The group home has round-the-clock staff members, and it is usually located in a residential neighbourhood.

Growth A measurable increase.

Habilitation A process by which a person chooses to gain or regain function, or to adapt to a change in function in order to attain self-fulfillment.

Handicap Commonly used to refer to a disability or activity limitation; not as widely used as it once was.

Health "A state of complete physical, social, and mental well-being, not merely the absence of disease or infirmity" (WHO, 1998).

Health Condition Something that causes a change in a person's health status.

Hemiplegia Partial or total paralysis of one side of the body.

Herbal Medications Substances that contain naturally occurring chemicals.

Heredity The traits and attributes a person inherits from his or her parents.

Heterotopic Ossification Abnormal bone growth in joints after a brain injury.

Holistic Approach A way of seeing all aspects of a person instead of just one.

Home Care Services provided to clients in their own homes through a provincially funded program. Different provinces include different services, although most include personal support as well as nursing, physiotherapy, and occupational therapy services.

Home Management The process of taking care of the client's home.

Hospice A form of support and care for people who are terminally ill.

Human Immunodeficiency Virus The virus that causes AIDS.

Huntington's Disease An inherited neurological disease characterized by progressive physical and cognitive decline.

Hydrocephalus A condition related to an increase of intracranial fluid in the brain that causes increased head size and pressure in the brain.

Illness An acute or short-term condition of poor health.

Impairment A change in a person's functioning that differs from that expected of others of the same age or sex.

Implementation The phase of support planning in which the methods identified in the goal-setting phase are put into practice.

Incontinence The lack of ability to control bowel or bladder function.

Independence The ability to do things for oneself.

Infantilize The treatment of an adult like a child.

Infectious Agent Microorganism capable of causing disease. These are also called pathogens.

Integumentary System The system that includes the skin, nails, oil and sweat glands, and hair.

Interdependence The reliance we all have on others to help us do things.

Irreversible Not curable or capable of being restored to a previous state.

Isolation Precautions Techniques used to prevent transmission of serious or highly contagious diseases.

Jaundice A condition that causes yellowing of the skin.

Joints The points where two or more bones meet and may move.

Lateral Lying on your side; also refers to body parts away from the midline.

Laundry Symbols Symbols that indicate the type of care a garment should receive.

Learning Changes in behaviour that result from new information.

Life Satisfaction Being content with our lives.

Life Span Perspective The development of a person that occurs from birth to death.

Life-Threatening Illness An illness that is likely to cause death.

Line of Gravity The imaginary line in the middle of your body mass where each side is equally balanced.

Living Will A document that gives specific instructions as to the care and treatment a person wants; also called an advance directive.

Long-Term Care Facility A setting in which a person lives and receives assistance with routine activities of living as well as some nursing care.

Matrix The substance found between the cells in connective tissue.

Maturation The sequence of growth and development.

Means of Transmission The method of transfer of a causative agent from a reservoir to a susceptible host.

Medical Asepsis The destruction of many pathogens to prevent transmission of infection; also called clean technique.

Mental Health The ability to deal with the conditions of life effectively.

Mental Health Conditions Conditions that affect a person's self-concept, behaviour, thoughts, or feelings to such an extent that they interfere with the person's ability to deal with situations effectively.

Mental Health Facility A facility designed to provide service to people with mental health concerns. Many such facilities provide both short-term and long-term services. Some mental health facilities are located in acute care settings, whereas others are completely separate. Increasingly, mental health services are provided to clients who live in their own homes.

Microorganisms Organisms that cannot be seen without a microscope, including bacteria, viruses, protozoa, and fungi.

Milestone The time at which particular events, skills, or behaviours are generally expected to occur.

Minerals Inorganic materials that the body requires.

Mobility Aids Aids that are designed to improve a person's stability by expanding his or her base of support.

Motor Skills The coordinated movements of the human body that require either large or small muscles.

Multidisciplinary Teams A support team made up of members from different professions or backgrounds.

Multiple Births The birth of more than one baby during one pregnancy.

Multiple Loss The loss of more than one thing at a time.

Multiple Sclerosis A central nervous system disease caused by the inflammation and scarring of the myelin sheath that protects nerve fibres.

Muscle Tissue The tissue that can contract and relax; may be smooth, striated, or cardiac.

Muscles Part of the musculoskeletal system that helps to maintain posture, causes movement, and produces and helps to maintain body heat.

Muscular Dystrophy A condition that causes muscle tissue to degenerate and be replaced by fatty and connective tissue.

Mutuality The ability to see how both people in a relationship benefit from it.

Narcotics Medications that dull the senses to provide pain relief and may be addictive.

Need Something we must meet in order to survive or feel satisfied with our lives.

Neglect The intentional or unintentional failure to provide the essentials of life.

Negotiating The give-and-take used in problem solving.

Nerve Tissue The tissue made of nerve cells, or neurons, that transmits electrical signals from the central nervous system to various parts of the body.

Nonmalificence The obligation to do no harm to another person.

Nosocomial Infections Infections acquired after admission to a facility.

Nutrients Vitamins, minerals, proteins, fats, carbohydrates, and water that your body needs to be healthy.

Omnipotent The state of being above all harm.